PROTEIN PHOSPHORYLATION IN HUMAN HEALTH

Edited by **Cai Huang**

Protein Phosphorylation in Human Health
http://dx.doi.org/10.5772/2944
Edited by Cai Huang

Contributors

Elena Tchevkina, Andrey Komelkov, Andrei V. Budanov, Björn Stork, Sebastian Alers, Antje S. Löffler, Sebastian Wesselborg, Jing Pu, Pingsheng Liu, Olga Calvo, Alicia García, Martin Lützelberger, Norbert F. Käufer, Katrin Deinhardt, Freddy Jeanneteau, Andres Joaquin Lopez-Contreras, Oscar Fernandez-Capetillo, Dmytro Pavlov, John G. Mielke, Nina Kurrle, Bincy John, Melanie Meister, Ritva Tikkanen, Masataka Oda, Masahiro Nagahama, Keiko Kobayashi, Jun Sakurai, Yamuna D. Gandaharen, Rachel S. Welt, David Kostyal, Sydney Welt, Roberta Fraschini, Erica Raspelli, Corinne Cassani, C. Frazer, P.G. Young, Shuishu Wang

Published by InTech

Janeza Trdine 9, 51000 Rijeka, Croatia

Copyright © 2012 InTech

Notice

Publishing Process Manager Vedran Greblo
Technical Editor InTech Prepress, Novi Sad
Cover InTech Design team

Additional hard copies can be obtained from orders@intechopen.com

Protein Phosphorylation in Human Health, Edited by Cai Huang
p. cm.
ISBN 978-953-51-0737-8

For EU product safety concerns:
IN TECH d.o.o., Prolaz Marije Krucifikse Kozulić 3, 51000 Rijeka, Croatia,
info@intechopen.com or visit our website at intechopen.com.

Meet the editor

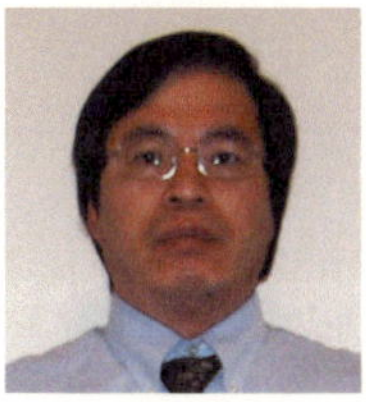

Dr Cai Huang, Ph.D., is an Assistant Professor in the Markey Cancer Center and Department of Molecular and Biomedical Pharmacology, University of Kentucky, USA. His laboratory engages in elucidating the molecular mechanism of cancer cell migration and metastasis. He characterized multiple phosphorylation pathways and identified their role in cell migration. Currently his research is focusing on the role of protein kinases and E3 ubiquitin ligases in focal adhesion dynamics, cell migration and metastasis in cancer cells. Dr Huang earned Ph.D. in Cell Biology at the University of North Carolina at Chapel Hill, USA. After graduating, he did his Postdoctoral training at the University of California-San Diego, USA. He joined the University of Kentucky as an assistant professor in 2010.

Contents

Preface

Protein phosphorylation is a reversible posttranslational modification catalyzed by protein kinases and reversely by protein phosphatases. There are about 500 protein kinases and 25-30 phosphatases in human genome. Each kinase and phosphatase targets multiple substrates. Thus, protein phosphorylation is a most versatile signaling regulatory mechanism and constitutes a most complicated signaling network in living organisms. In fact, protein phosphorylation governs all aspects of physiological and pathological processes in human health. During last decades, more than 180,000 scientific papers on protein phosphorylation have been published. To handle and digest so much knowledge and information is a big challenge to our students, college teachers and investigators. Therefore, we invited expert scientists to write 15 chapters on specific fields of protein phosphorylation where their expertise lies. We also asked our authors to relate their protein phosphorylation pathways to human health. We hope that this book could be a good hand for our students, teachers and investigators who want to extend their knowledge on the role of protein phosphorylation in human health. Please also keep in mind that no any single book can cover all aspects of protein phosphorylation pathways.

The chapters have been organized into 5 different sections, based on the similarity of protein phosphorylation pathways. The first section has 4 chapters summarizing on the role of Akt, mTOR and AMPK in cancer and metabolic disorders. The section focuses on the structure, function and regulation of mTOR1 and mTOR2 and their role in cancer, neurodegeneration, and diabetes, the role of Sestrins, a family of stress-responsive genes in regulating AMPK-mTOR pathway and their role in cardiovascular diseases, muscle- and neuro- degeneration, diabetes and cancer, the signaling pathways that regulate autophagy, including Akt, AMPK and mTOR, and the role of Akt/AMPK and PI3K/Erk pathways in fatty acids-stimulated glucose uptake. The second section has 4 chapters reviewing the role of protein phosphorylation in transcription, pre-mRNA splicing and DNA damage. The section emphasizes the regulation of RNA polymerase II sequentially by protein kinases and phosphatases in gene expression and therapeutically potentials, the genetic interactions, biochemical properties, and substrate specificity of Prp4 kinase and its role in pre-mRNA splicing, the regulation of Trk/Erk/CREB pathway by BDNF and the role in neuronal growth, synaptic plasticity and cell survival, and the signaling pathways in regulating DNA damage. The third section has 4 chapters covering the role of protein tyrosine kinases in receptor signaling and human diseases. This section accentuates the tyrosine phosphorylation of NMDA receptor by Src family kinases and its role in cerebral ischaemia, the role of flotillins in regulating receptor tyrosine kinase and in cancer, Alzheimer's Disease and diabetes, the role of TrkA/PKCθ/Erk pathway in alpha-toxin-mediated inflammation, and distinct regulation of HER2 tyrosine/threonine phosphorylation by trastuzumab (anti-HER2 monoclonal antibody) and lapatinib (small molecule HER2/1 tyrosine kinase inhibitor). The fourth section has 2 chapters: one summarizes the regulation of cdc25 phosphatase by phosphorylation during cell-cycle and DNA damage, and another illustrates the role of protein phosphorylation in cell cycle regulation using Swe1, Kin4, Cyk3, Hof1 and Chs2 as examples. The fifth section has only 1 chapter describing the role of histidine kinases in the bacterium two-component system.

The study on protein phosphorylation is one of most exciting fields in biomedical research. This book provides detailed and comprehensive review on 5 different areas of protein phosphorylation signaling pathways and their roles in human health. This book is our attempt to bridge the basic phosphorylation pathways with human health and diseases. We hope that this book will be of help to students, teachers and researchers who need to deepen their knowledge in these specific areas and promote progress in multi-disciplines of biomedical science.

Cai Huang, Ph.D.
Markey Cancer Center and Department of Molecular & Biomedical Pharmacology,
University of Kentucky,
USA

Section 1

Akt, mTOR and AMPK in Cancer and Metabolic Disorders

Chapter 1

Protein Phosphorylation as a Key Mechanism of mTORC1/2 Signaling Pathways

Elena Tchevkina and Andrey Komelkov

Additional information is available at the end of the chapter

http://dx.doi.org/10.5772/48274

1. Introduction

The mammalian target of rapamycin (mTOR) has attracted growing attention during the past decade due to the increase realization of it's extraordinarily significance in cellular life-sustaining activity on the one hand, and because of its crucial role in a variety of diseases, (including cancer, hamartoma syndromes, cardiac hypertrophy, diabetes and obesity) on the other. mTOR is an atypical serine/threonine protein kinase, belonging to the phosphatidylinositol kinase-related kinase (PIKK) family. Cumulative evidence indicates that mTOR acts as a 'master switch' of cellular energy-intensive anabolic processes and energy-producing catabolic activities. It coordinates the rate of cell growth, proliferation and survival in response to extracellular mitogen, energy, nutrient and stress signals [1, 2]. mTOR functions within two distinct multiprotein complexes, mTORC1 and mTORC2, responsible for the different physiological functions. Thus, mTORC1 is considered mostly involved in the regulation of the translation initiation machinery influencing cell growth, proliferation, and survival, while mTORC2 participates in actin cytoskeleton rearrangements and cell survival. mTORC1 and mTORC2 were initially identified in yeast on the basis of their differential sensitivity to the inhibitory effects of rapamycin, mTORC1 being originally considered as rapamycin-sensitive and mTORC2 as rapamycin-insensitive [3-5].

The history of TOR began in the early 1970s when a bacterial strain, *Streptomyces hygroscopicus*, was first isolated from Rapa Nui island during a discovery program for anti-microbial agents. These bacteria secrete a potent anti-fungal macrolide that was named rapamycin after the location of its discovery [6-9]. Later rapamycin was proven to have anti-proliferative and immunosuppressive properties. In the beginning of 1990s, two rapamycin target genes titled TOR1 (the target of rapamycin 1) and TOR2 were discovered through the yeast genetic screens for mutations that counteract the growth inhibitory properties of rapamycin [10, 11]. Further studies revealed that rapamycin forms the complex with its intracellular receptor, FK506-binding protein 12 kDa (FKBP12), This complex binds a region in the C-terminus of TOR kinase named FRB (FKB12-rapamycin binding) domain, what leads to the inhibition of TOR functions [12-14].

At present, it becomes clear that mTORC1 and mTORC2 activities are mediated through diverse signaling pathways depending on the type of extracellular signal. Thus, signaling from growth factors is mediated predominantly through PI3K-Akt-TSC1/2 pathway and upregulates mTORC1 to stimulate translation initiation, while energy or nutrient depletion and stresses suppress mTORC1 via LKB1–AMPK cascade to trigger off the process of autophagy. In contrast, mTORC2 is insensitive to nutrients or energy conditions. mTORC2 phosphorylates Akt and some other protein kinases regulating actin cytoskeleton and cell survival in response to growth factors and hormones. The physiological functions of mTOR continue to expand. It should be stressed, that the signaling throughout the complicated mTOR network, including branched pathways and feedback loops, is regulated predominantly by phosphorylation and includes myriads of phosphorylation events. Moreover, the complexity of mTOR regulation is amplified by the crosstalk with other signaling pathways, such as MAP kinase- or TNFα-dependent cascades, which activity is also determined by vast number of phosphorylations. The complication of mTOR signaling additionally increases due to the hierarchical character of multiple site-specific phosphorylations of the main mTOR targets. Up to date there are no full clarity, concerning which kinase is responsible for each site phosphorylation as well as functional role and precise mechanisms of each phosphorylation event. The better understanding of underlying molecular mechanisms is now especially essential since inhibitors of mTOR signaling are widely used as drugs in the therapy of cancer and neurodegenerative diseases.

2. mTOR kinase structural organization

Although mTOR has limited sequence similarities in eukaryotes, it demonstrates a high level of conservation in its key cellular functions. mTOR, also known as FRAP (FKBP12-rapamycin-associated protein), RAFT1 (rapamycin and FKBP12 target), RAPT 1 (rapamycin target 1), or SEP (sirolimus effector protein), is a large 289 kDa atypical serine/threonine (S/T) kinase [15-18] and is considered a member of the phosphatidylinositol 3-kinase (PI3K)-kinase-related kinase (PIKK) superfamily since its C-terminus shares strong homology to the catalytic domain of PI3K [19, 20]. mTOR and yeast TOR proteins share > 65% identity in carboxy-terminal catalytic domains and about 40% identity in overall sequence [21]. At the amino-acid level, human, mouse and rat TOR proteins share a 95% identity [22, 23]. The knockout of mTOR in mice is embryonic lethal, indicating its physiological importance [24, 25].

Structurally, mTOR contains 2549 amino acids and the region of first 1200 N-terminal amino acids contains up to 20 tandem repeated **HEAT** (a protein-protein interaction structure of two tandem anti-parallel α-helices found in **H**untingtin, **E**longation factor 3 (EF3), PR65/**A** subunit of protein phosphatase 2A (PP2A), and **T**OR) motifs [26]. Tandem HEAT repeats are present in many proteins and may form an extended superhelical structure responsible for protein-protein interactions. HEAT repeats region is followed by a **FAT** (**F**RAP, **A**TM, and

TRRAP (PIKK family members)) domain and **FRB** (**F**KPB12-**r**apamycin **b**inding domain), which serves as a docking site for the rapamycin -FKBP12 complex formation. Downstream lies a catalytic kinase domain and a **FATC (FAT C**arboxyterminal) domain, located at the C-terminus of the protein (**Figure 1A).** The FAT and FATC domains are always found in combination, so it has been hypothesized that the interactions between FAT and FATC might contribute to the catalytic kinase activity of mTOR via unknown mechanisms [26, 27].

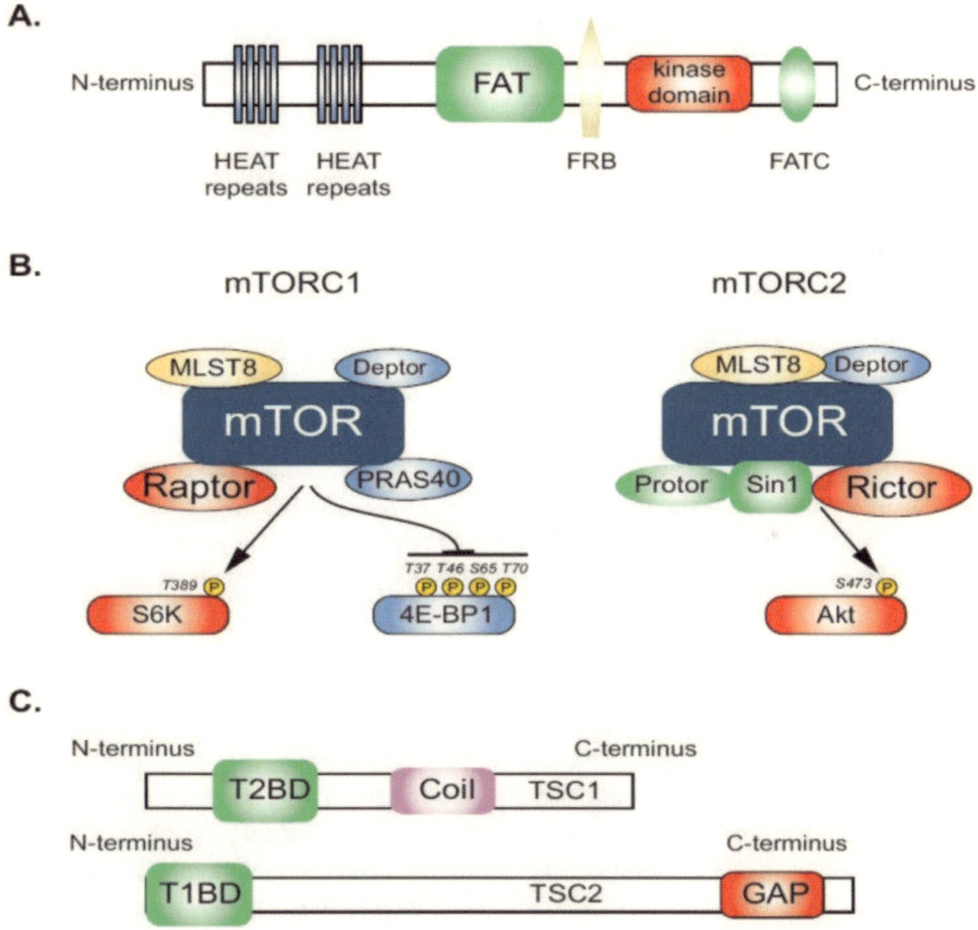

Figure 1. A. The domain structure of mTOR. mTOR contains tandem HEAT repeats, central FAT domain, FRB domain, a catalytic kinase domain and the FATC domain. Rapamycin associates with its intracellular receptor, FKBP12, and the resulting complex interacts with the FRB domain of mTOR. Binding of rapamycin–FKBP12 to the FRB domain disrupts the association of mTOR with the mTORC1 specific component Raptor and thus uncouples mTORC1 from its substrates, thereby blocking mTORC1 signaling. **B.** Composition of mTORC1 and mTORC2. mTORC1 consists of mTOR, Raptor, PRAS40, mLST8 and Deptor. mLST8 binds to the mTOR kinase domain in both complexes, where it seems to be crucial for their assembly. Deptor acts as an inhibitor of both complexes. Other protein partners differ between the two complexes. mTORC2 contains Rictor, mSIN1, and Protor1. **C.** Schematic of the TSC1 and TSC2 proteins. The functional domains (including GAP) on TSC1 and TSC2 are represented schematically. T2BD/T1BD — TSC2 and TSC1 binding domains respectively.

Up to date quite a few phosphorylation sites in mTOR have been reported, namely T2446, S2448, S2481 and S1261 and this list will be probably appended. S2481 is considered to be a site of autophosphorylation [28]. S2481 is the only site the phosphorylation of which is well established for regulating mTOR intrinsic activity [29, 30]; the significance of other phosphorylation sites for mTOR activity are not entirely clear. Recently, S1261 has been reported as a novel mTOR phosphorylation site in mammalian cells and the first evidences of this phosphorylation in regulating mTORC1 autokinase activity has been provided [31]. Although phosphorylation at T2446/S2448 was shown to be PI3K/Akt-dependent, mTORC1 downstream kinase S6K has been also reported to phosphorylate these two sites [32]. The significance of this potential feedback loop is unknown, as it is not yet clear whether and how these phosphorylations influence mTOR activity

Binding of rapamycin–FKBP12 to the FRB domain of mTOR disrupts the association of mTOR with mTORC1-specific component Raptor and thus divide mTORC1 from its targets, blocking mTORC1 signaling. However, whether rapamycin directly inhibits mTOR's intrinsic kinase activity is still not entirely clear [3, 33, 34].

The TOR complexes mTORC1 and mTORC2

The mammalian mTORC1 and mTORC2 complexes perform non-overlapping functions within the cell. Thus, the best-known function of TORC1 signaling is the promotion of translation. Other mTORC1 functions include autophagy inhibition, promotion of the ribosome biogenesis and of the tRNA production. The main known mTORC2 activity is the phosphorylation and activation of AKT and of the related kinases — serum/glucocorticoid regulated kinase (SGK) and protein kinase C (PKC) [35]. It is also involved in cytoskeletal organization. Although both mTOR complexes exist predominantly in the cytoplasm, some data indicate that they could function in different compartments. Thus, upon nutrients and energy availability mTORC1 is recruited to lysosomes where it could be fully activated [36] and where it functions to suppress autophagy. Unlike mTORC1, mTORC2 according to the most recent data localizes predominantly in ER compartment where it could directly associate with ribosomes [37, 38]. Additionally, some data evidence that mTOR may actually be a cytoplasmic-nuclear shuttling protein. The nuclear shuttling could facilitate the phosphorylation of mTORC1 substrates under the mitogenic stimulation [39]. The unique compositions of mTORC1 and mTORC2 determine the selectivity of their binding partners. Up to date we know more about mTORC1 rather then mTORC2 probably due to the lack of available and wide-spreaded inhibitors of mTORC2 activity.

TORC1 composition. Within the mammalian cells, TORC1 functions as a homodimer. Each monomer consists of mTOR, **r**egulatory **a**ssociated **p**rotein of m**TOR** (Raptor), **p**roline-rich **A**KT **s**ubstrate **40** kDa (PRAS40), **DEP** domain **TOR**-binding protein (Deptor) and **m**ammalian **l**_ethal_ with **S**ec-13 protein **8** (mLST8, also known as GbL) [40, 41]**(Figure 1B).**

Raptor is a 150 kDa presumably non-enzymatic subunit of mTORC1 that is essential for the kinase mTORC1 activity *in vitro* and *in vivo* in response to insulin, nutrient and energy level. [42, 43]. It includes a highly conserved N-terminal region followed by 3 HEAT repeats and 7

WD40 (about **40** amino acids with conserved **W** and **D** forming four anti-parallel beta strands) repeats. The Raptor-mTOR interaction is very dynamic, and is thought to require the HEAT repeats of mTOR. It is established that Raptor is indispensable for mTOR to phosphorylate its main effectors p70S6 kinase (S6K1) and **e**ukaryotic **i**nitiation **f**actor **4E** (eIF4E) **b**inding **p**rotein 1 (4E-BP1), but whether Raptor positively or negatively regulates mTOR itself remains controversial [43]. Raptor is essential for mTORC1 complex formation and for the dimerization of TORC1 complexes as it provides direct interaction between TOR proteins from each monomer. Thus it can be considered to be a scaffolding protein that recruits substrates for mTOR thereby demonstrating a stimulating effect on mTOR activity [43]. Alternatively, other study has demonstrated that Raptor negatively regulates mTOR being tightly bound to the kinase [42]. There are also a hypothesis according to which at least two types of interaction exist between Raptor and mTOR depending on nutrients availability. One mTOR-Raptor complex that forms in the absence of nutrients is stable and leads to a repression of the mTOR catalytic activity. In contrast, the other complex that forms under nutrients-rich conditions is unstable, but it is important for *in vivo* mTOR function [42] (reviewed in [44]). Recent studies suggested that the phosphorylation status of Raptor could influence mTORC1 activity [45]. Phosphorylation on S722/792 is mediated by AMPK (AMP-activated protein kinase) and is required for the inhibition of mTORC1 activity induced by energy stress [45], whereas phosphorylation of Raptor on S719/721/722 is mediated by the p90 ribosomal S6 kinases (RSKs) and contributes to the activation of mTORC1 by mitogen stimulation [45, 46]. Most recently, S863 in Raptor was identified as mTOR-mediated phosphorylation site responsible for the insulin-dependent activation of mTORC1 [47].

PRAS40, another subunit of mTORC1, has been defined as a direct negative regulator of mTORC1 function [48]. Initially, PRAS40 was identified as a novel substrate of Akt being directly phosphorylated at T246 near its C-terminus [49]. This phosphorylation releases inhibition of mTORC1 by PRAS40. Subsequent studies showed that PRAS40 associates with mTORC1 via Raptor and inhibits mTORC1 activity [48]. A putative TOR signaling motif, FVMDE, has been identified in PRAS40 and shown to be required for interaction with Raptor. Upon binding to Raptor, PRAS40 is phosphorylated on S183 by mTORC1 both *in vivo* and *in vitro* [50] Thus, PRAS40 has been implicated as a physiological substrate of mTORC1. Most recently, two novel sites in PRAS40 phosphorylated by mTORC1, S212 and S221, have been identified [51]. Rapamycin treatment reduced the phosphorylation of S183 and S221 but not S212, indicating that besides mTORC1, other kinases may also regulate the phosphorylation of S212 *in vivo* [51].

mLST8 has been identified after Raptor as a stable component of both mTOR complexes [52]. It consists almost entirely of seven "sticky" WD40 repeats, and has been initially shown to bind to the kinase domain of mTOR, leading to the hypothesis that mLST8 positively regulates mTOR kinase activity. It was proposed that mLST8 is essential for a nutrient- and rapamycin-sensitive interaction between Raptor and mTOR [52]. However, there is no substantial evidence to support this idea. It has been speculated, that mLST8 may participate in the amino acids mediated activation of TORC1 being insignificant for other mechanisms of TORC1 activation [52]. Alternatively, recent studies demonstrated functional importance of mLST8 for the Rictor-mTOR interaction, evidencing that mLST8 is involved in mTORC2 rather than in mTORC1 activity.

Deptor binds to mTOR at the FAT domain thus originally proposed to be a part of TORC1. Recently it has been identified as mTOR inhibitor that acts on both TORC1 and TORC2. The upstream regulators of Deptor still remain unknown [41].

mTORC2 composition and distinctions from mTORC1

In 2004, mTORC2, containing mTOR, mLST8 and Rictor was identified [3, 4]. Since mTORC2 complex was discovered later than mTORC1, its functions and regulatory mechanisms are less understood [3]. TORC2 and TORC1 contain common subunits, as is mTOR itself, mLST8 and Deptor, but instead of Raptor, mTORC2 includes two different subunits, Rictor (**r**apamycin-**i**nsensitive **c**ompanion of m**TOR)** and mSin1 (**m**ammalian **s**tress-activated protein kinase (SAPK)-**in**teracting protein **1**) [3, 4, 53]. In addition, Protor (**pro**tein **o**bserved with Rictor) was also considered a component of mTORC2 (**Figure 1B**) [54, 55]. mTORC2 was originally thought to be rapamycin-insensitive [3], however, further studies demonstrated that prolonged rapamycin treatment inhibits the assembly of mTORC2 as well as its activity towards Akt phosphorylation in certain cell lines [56].

Rictor is the first identified TORC2 specific component [3, 4]. It represents a large protein with a predicted molecular weight of about 200 kDa. Although Rictor contains no apparent catalytic domain motifs [4], knockdown of Rictor results in the loss of actin polymerization and cell spreading, the main known mTORC2 functions [4]. It was shown that the Rictor-mTOR complex does not affect the mTORC1 effectors S6K1 and 4E-BP1, but influence the activities of several proteins known as mTORC2 downstream targets, including phosphorylation of Akt, PKC and the focal adhesion proteins.

mSin1 was recently identified as a novel component of mTORC2, which is important for both the complex assembly and function [57-59]. *Sin1* is conserved among all eukaryotic species especially in the middle part of the sequence [60]. A Ras-binding domain and a C-terminal PH domain have been identified recently [61]. The several experimental techniques showed the importance of Sin1 for mTORC2 function [62]. The interaction *in vivo* between Sin1 and Rictor is more stable than their interactions with mTOR probably due to the ability of Sin1 and Rictor to stabilize each other [59]. Thus knockdown of Sin1 decreases the interaction between mTOR and Rictor, suggesting that Sin1 is important for mTORC2 assembly. Knockdown of Sin1 by RNAi in *Drosophila and* mammals crucially diminishes the Akt phosphorylation on S473 *in vitro*. The same effect was observed in Sin1−/− cells [58].

Protor-1 and Protor-2 (also known as Proline rich protein 5 (PRR5) [54, 55] and PRR5-like (PRR5L) [63] are two newly identified mTORC2 interactors which have been identified as Rictor-binding or SIN1 binding proteins [54]. Up to date their functions remain unclear. It is currently accepted that they are dispensable for mTORC2 assembly as well as for its catalytic activity [54], although Protor stability is dependent on the production of other TORC2 components. It is possible that Rictor and Sin1 act as scaffold proteins for various complexes involving different kinases.

mLST8 and Deptor, as was mentioned above, are the components of both mTORC1 and mTORC2 complexes.

3. Upstream regulation of mTOR signaling

3.1. PI3K-AKT-TSC1/2 -"Classical" pathway of mTOR regulation

Although this pathway is still considered to be the main way exerting multi-faceted control over mTORC1 activity which sense insulin and growth factors signals to regulate cell growth, at present it becomes clear that at least some of its components also function to mediate responses on other stimulus, such as energy, stress or nutrients which are provided by discrepant signaling pathways, described below.

3.1.1. TSC1/TSC2 complex and Rheb protein

The TSC1/TSC2 complex (tuberous sclerosis complex 1/2, TSC1/2) has been established as the major upstream inhibitory regulator of mTORC1 [64, 65]. This complex mediates signals from a large number of distinct signaling pathways to modulate mTORC1 activity predominantly via different phosphorylations of TSC2. Functioning as a molecular switch, TSC1/2 suppresses mTOR's activity to restrict cell growth during the stress, and releases its inhibition under the favorable conditions. The *TSC1* and *TSC2* genes were identified in 1997 and 1993 respectively as the tumor-suppressor genes mutated in the tumor syndrome TSC 1(tuberous sclerosis complex) [66-68]. TSC is a multisystem disorder characterized by the development of numerous benign tumors (e.g. hamartomas) most commonly detected at the brain, kidneys, skin, heart and lungs. Genetic studies of *TSC1* and *TSC2* in humans, mice, *Drosophila* and yeast strongly suggest that these proteins act mainly as a complex. The 140 kDa TSC1 (also known as hamartin) and 200 kDa TSC2 (also known as tuberin) proteins share no homology with each other and very little with other proteins **(Figure 1C)** TSC1 and TSC2 associate through certain regions [69] giving a heterodimeric complex. The only known functional domain throughout these two proteins is a region of homology at the C-terminus of TSC2 to the GAP domain of small G-protein Rap1. Searches for a GTPase target regulated by the TSC2 GAP (GTPase-activating protein) domain revealed the small G-protein Rheb. Mammalian TSC2 was shown to accelerate the rate of GTP hydrolysis of Rheb, converting Rheb from the active GTP-bound to the inactive GDP-bound state [69, 70]. This evidences that Rheb is a direct target of TSC2 GAP activity, and TSC2 suppress Rheb function. While the GAP activity of TSC2 is necessary for the complex functionality, TSC1 is required to stabilize TSC2 and prevent its ubiquitin-mediated degradation [71, 72]. Under growth conditions, the TSC1/2 complex is inactive, thereby allowing Rheb-GTP to activate TORC1.

Rheb is a member of the Ras superfamily that appears to be conserved in all eukaryotes and, despite the term 'brain' in its name, is in fact ubiquitously expressed in mammals. Whether a GEF protein (guanine-nucleotide exchange factor responsible for reverse process, i.e. change GDP-bound to GTP-bound state) for Rheb exists remains unknown. Several evidences demonstrate that Rheb positively regulates mTORC1. In particular, Rheb overexpression stimulates S6K1 and 4EBP1 phosphorylation, which are indicators of mTORC1 activity. This effect can be reversed by mTOR inactivation or by rapamycin treatment, suggesting that Rheb primarily functions through TORC1 [59]. Although genetic and biochemical studies strongly suggest that GTP-bound Rheb potently activates mTORC1, the molecular mechanism is still unclear. Overexpressed Rheb was shown to bind to mTOR [73, 74]. Associations between endogenous Rheb and mTORC1 components have not been reported. In general, Ras-related small G-proteins bind to their downstream effectors mostly in the GTP-bound state. Surprisingly, Rheb has been found to bind stronger to mTOR in its GDP-bound or nucleotide-free states [74]. At the same time it has been shown that GTP-bound Rheb rather than the GDP-bound stimulates mTOR kinase activity *in vitro* [74]. Although the mechanism by which Rheb-GTP activates mTORC1 has not been fully understood, it needs Rheb farnesylation and can be blocked by farnesyl transferase (FT) inhibitors. Recently, it was found that Rheb can directly interact with the FKBP12 homologue FKBP38 (named also FKBP8), and this binding seems to be tighter with Rheb-GTP [75]. That study suggests that Rheb-GTP binds to FKBP38 and triggers its release from mTORC1, stimulating mTORC1 activity **(Figure 2).** In support of this model, an independent study carried out that decreasing FKBP38 expression with antisense oligonucleotides blocked the growth inhibitory effects of TSC1–TSC2 overexpression [76]. Although more studies are needed, these findings suggest that FKBP38 might be a Rheb effector that regulates mTORC1 and, perhaps, unknown targets downstream of the TSC1/TSC2 complex and Rheb.

3.1.2. The PI3K-AKT pathway joins TSC-mTORC1 regulation

The responsiveness of mTORC1 signaling to growth factors and insulin is provided through activation of PI3K (phosphatidylinositol-3-kinase) and Akt kinase, but the precise mechanism is still not clear. Through PI3K signaling, Akt also termed PKB (serine/threonine protein kinase B) is activated by most growth factors to phosphorylate several downstream substrates [77].

PI3K is a heterodimeric protein containing an 85-kDa regulatory and a 110-kDa catalytic subunits (*PIK3CA*) [78, 79]. PI3K acts to phosphorylate a number of membrane phospholipids to form the lipid second messengers phosphatidylinositol 3,4-bisphosphate (PtdIns(3,4)P2 or PIP2) and phosphatidylinositol 3,4,5-trisphosphate (PtdIns(3,4,5)P3 or PIP3). In response to the upstream inputs, PI3K at the cell membrane is activated through the association of a ligand with its receptor, stimulating p85 to bind phosphorylated tyrosine residues of Src-homology 2 (SH2) domain on the receptor. This association promotes the p110 catalytic subunit to transfer phosphate groups to the membrane phospholipids [78, 80]. Consequently these lipids, particularly PtdIns(3,4,5)P3, attract several kinases to the plasmalemma initiating the signaling cascade [78, 80]. PIP3 accumulation is antagonized by the well-known tumor suppressor, lipid phosphatase PTEN (**p**hosphatase and **te**nsin homolog deleted on chromosome 10), which converts PIP3 to PIP2. One important function of PIP3 is to recruit Akt as well as PDK1 (or PDPK1, 3-phosphoinositide-dependent protein kinase-1) [81] via their PH (**p**leckstrin **h**omology) domains to the plasma membrane (**Figure 2).**

Akt, known as one of the major survival kinases, belongs to the AGC (PKA/PKG/PKC) protein kinase family and is involved in regulating a vast number of cellular processes, including transcription, proliferation, migration, growth, apoptosis and various metabolic processes [3, 82]. Being translocated to the plasma membrane, Akt undergoes partial activation through the phosphorylation of T308 residue within the activation loop by PDK1 and following full activation through the additional phosphorylation at the hydrophobic motif site S473 by PDK2 [83]. After activation Akt quits the cell membrane to phosphorylate intracellular substrates. Particularly, Akt can translocate to the nucleus [80] where it influences the activity of transcriptional factors, including CREB *(cAMP response element-binding)*, E2F (eukaryotic transcription factor 2), NF-κB (nuclear factor kappa from B cells) through Iκ-K (inhibitor kappa B protein kinase), the forkhead transcription factors, in particular, FOXO1 and FOXO3 and murine double minute 2 (MDM2) which regulates p53 activity [84, 85]. In addition, Akt is able to target some other molecules to influence cell survival including GSK-3β (glycogen-synthase kinase-3β), which regulates β-catenin protein stability, and BAD (the pro-apoptotic molecule Bcl-2-associated death promoter).

Akt was the first kinase demonstrated to phosphorylate directly the TSC1/TSC2 complex in response to growth factors. Human TSC2 contains five predicted Akt sites (S939, S981, S1130, S1132 and T1462 on full-length human TSC2), all of which have been suggested to be subjects of phosphorylation by Akt (**Figure 2**). Importantly, the two sites were shown definitively to be targeted by Akt in mammalian cells, S939 and T1462 [86]. There is also evidence that either S1130 or S1132 is phosphorylated by Akt *in vivo* [87]. Finally, Akt can phosphorylate a peptide corresponding to the sequence surrounding S981 *in vitro* [88]. This residue has been identified as an *in vivo* phosphorylation site on TSC2 by tandem-MS analyses [89]. However, whether Akt phosphorylates S981 on full-length TSC2 within cells has not been conclusively demonstrated.

The majority of studies postulated that activated AKT promotes TORC1 signaling by phosphorylating multiple sites on TSC2, thereby relieving inhibition of Rheb and activating TORC1 [86, 87, 90, 91]. The data obtained using phosphorylation-site mutants of TSC2 demonstrate that Akt mediated phosphorylation of these sites inhibits the function of the TSC1–TSC2 complex in cells, however the molecular mechanism of this inhibition has been the subject of much debate (reviewed in [92]). One proposed mechanism involves disruption of the TSC1–TSC2 complex. However, this does not occur rapidly and, although it might contribute to the long-term effects of Akt on mTORC1 signaling, it cannot explain the immediate effects of Akt activation on mTORC1, which are blocked by Akt phosphorylation-site mutants of TSC2. Another proposed mechanism is based on the possibility that phosphorylation of TSC2 alters its subcellular localization, such that it can no longer act as a GAP for Rheb. One study supporting this mechanism found that growth factor stimulation led to increase of the TSC2 levels within the cytosolic fraction [93]. This effect was PI3K-dependent, stimulated by activated Akt and required both S939 and S981 on TSC2. In that study, both TSC1 and Rheb were found exclusively in the membrane fraction, and unlike TSC2, did not show an increase in the cytosolic fraction following growth-factor stimulation. From these findings it was concluded that Akt-mediated phosphorylation of

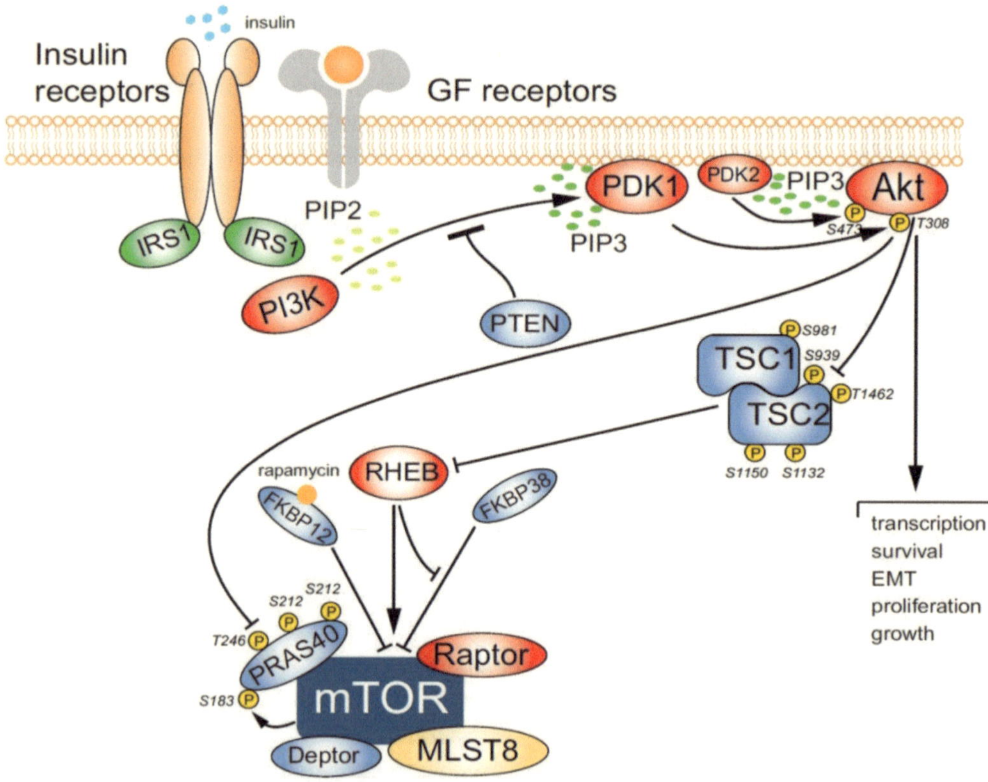

Figure 2. Growth factors and insulin regulation of mTORC signaling. mTORC1 activity is modulated by a number of positive (shown in red) and negative (shown in blue) regulators. Growth factors activate mTORC1 indirectly by suppressing the function of its negative regulator TSC1/TSC2 complex. TSC2 contains a GAP domain that converts Rheb to its inactive, GDP-bound form. PI3K-AKT dependent phosphorylation inhibits the TSC1/2 complex, thereby relieving the TSC1/2-mediated repression of Rheb and allowing activation of TORC1. AKT also activates mTORC1 through negative phosphorylation of mTORC1 suppressor, PRAS40. FKBP38 appears to associate through the FRB domain of mTOR and trigger its release from mTORC1, thereby stimulating mTORC1 activation.

TSC2 on S939 or S981 inhibits the TSC1/TSC2 complex by triggering release of TSC2 from TSC1 at an intracellular membrane also occupied by Rheb. This model points on the significant and rapid dissociation of TSC2 from TSC1 upon phosphorylation – something that has not been detected in the majority of studies to date. Recent studies have suggested that AKT mediated phosphorylation of TSC2 at S939 and S981 creates a binding site for a cytosolic anchor protein, 14-3-3 (tyrosine 3-monooxygenase/tryptophan 5-monooxygenase activation protein, theta polypeptide also known as YWHAQ, 1C5; HS1), a mechanism of regulation shared by several other Akt substrates [77]. Examining interactions between endogenous 14-3-3 proteins and TSC2, another study found that S939 and T1462 were both required for 14-3-3 binding to TSC2 downstream of PI3K signaling. It seems likely that 14-3-3 binding to TSC2 (provided by some combination of phosphorylated S939, S981 and T1462) contributes to Akt-mediated inhibition of TSC2. Binding of 14-3-3 to TSC2 can disrupt binding TSC2 to TSC1 and RHEB, which are associated with endomembranes [93]. However, in 14-3-3 pull-down experiments, both TSC1 and TSC2 were found to bind, and 14-3-3 did not affect the association between TSC1 and TSC2 [94, 95]. It also remains unclear whether TSC2 binding to14-3-3 hindered its GAP activity towards Rheb. Importantly, TSC2 is not an essential target of AKT during normal *D. melanogaster* development [96], suggesting the presence of possible additional targets for the AKT mediated regulation of mTORC1.

Growth factors control mTORC1 independently of the TSC complex

As was mentioned above, the PRAS40 binds Raptor and thereby inactivates mTORC1 [48, 50, 57, 63]. In response to growth factors, Akt phosphorylates PRAS40 at T246. This phosphorylation leads to the dissociation of PRAS40 from mTORC1 resulting in a reduced ability of PRAS40 to inhibit TORC1 [48, 49, 57]. This was proposed to be mediated through 14-3-3 binding of the phosphorylated PRAS40 [57]. Thus, bypassing TSC2, AKT phosphorylates PRAS40 and prevents its ability to suppress mTORC1 downstream effectors. The inhibition of PRAS40 by AKT is conserved; in *Drosophila*, the PRAS40 ortholog Lobe regulates TORC1 signaling [97]. PRAS40 is in turn a substrate of mTORC1, and mTORC1 mediated phosphorylation of PRAS40 S183, [50, 63] has been proposed to negatively regulate mTORC1 signaling by competing with 4EBP1 and S6K for interaction with Raptor. PRAS40 is a direct inhibitor of mTORC1 and antagonizes the activation of the mTORC1 by Rheb•GTP. However, constitutive mTORC1 signaling in TSC2 null mouse embryonic fibroblasts, in which AKT signaling is largely inhibited owing to a negative feedback mechanism (see below), indicates that hyperactive Rheb can overcome PRAS40 mediated inhibition of mTORC1 [48]. Thus, the AKT pathway might stimulate mTORC1 through two interconnected mechanisms: by activating Rheb and/or by inhibiting PRAS40.

3.2. mTORC1 activation by nutrients

3.2.1. hVps34 PI-3-P kinase and Rag GTPases

It has long been known that mTORC1 signaling is strongly inhibited in cells under the conditions of nutrient deficiency and that the re-addition of amino acids to starved cells can strongly stimulate mTORC1 activity [22, 98]. However, the mechanisms by which amino acids convey signals to mTORC1 remain largely unknown. Earlier studies demonstrated that silencing expression of TSC1/2 confers resistance to amino acid deprivation, indicating that TSC1/2 is involved in the regulation of mTOR function by amino acids [90]. It has been suggested that branched-chain amino acids, (such as leucine), activate mTORC1 by inhibiting TSC1/TSC2 or stimulating Rheb [62]. Consequently, inhibition of Rheb binding to mTOR is critical for the inhibitory effect of amino acid withdrawal on mTOR signaling [99]. However, other studies do not support this idea. Thus, in TSC-null cells (that lack either TSC1 or TSC2), the mTORC1 activity remains sensitive to amino acid deprivation, suggesting that other than TSC2, additional mechanisms may also be involved in the regulation of mTOR by amino acids [100]. Although Rheb is required for the amino acid stimulation of mTORC1, starving of amino acids has no effect on GTP loading [99-102].

Therefore, while there is a requirement for GTP-bound Rheb to induct of mTORC1 by amino acids, amino acids probably do not affect Rheb activity – indicating that regulation of Rheb does not stimulate mTORC1 in response to amino acids.

Recently, Ste20-related kinase MAP4K3 (mitogen activated protein kinase kinase kinase kinase 3) and the class III PI3K hVps34 (human vacuolar protein sorting 34) were proposed to be activated by amino acid and be involved in the transduction of signals from amino acids to mTORC1 [103-107]. While the mechanism by which MAP4K3 regulates mTORC1 remains unknown, a mechanism for hVPS34 was recently proposed (**Figure 3**). According to this proposed mechanism, amino acids induce an extracellular calcium influx that activates calmodulin, which in turn binds and activates hVps34 [108]. hVps34 then generates PI-3-phosphate (PI-3-P) instead of the PI-3,4,5-tris-phosphate generated by type I PI3Ks [109], that somehow activates mTORC1. The mechanism also involves the formation of a calmodulin-hVps34-mTORC1 supercomplex. However, the regulation of mTORC1 by hVps34 is thought to be specific to mammalian cells because in flies Vps34 does not regulate TORC1 [106]. This is unexpected because regulation of TORC1 by amino acids is known as very conserved. Furthermore, in certain mammalian cells, amino acids appear to inhibit rather than activate mVps34 [110]. However, additional studies are needed to clarify the roles of these proteins in TORC1 activation.

Most recent studies identified Rag GTPases as activators of mTORC1 by sensing amino acid signals [111, 112]. Rag-mediated activation of TORC1 still requires Rheb, indicating that, during amino acid signaling, Rag complexes act upstream of Rheb. Rag family members (Rag A-D) belong to the Ras superfamily of GTPases. They are unique in their ability to dimerize through long C-terminal extensions. In the presence of amino acids, the dimeric Rag complex, which consists of a Rag A/B monomer and a Rag C/D monomer, binds Raptor and transport mTORC1 to lysosomes, the same intracellular compartment that contains Rheb [36, 111, 112]. Rag complexes are recruited to the lysosomal membrane by the trimeric Ragulator complex [36], which contains the proteins MP1 (MEK partner 1), p14 and p18. The GTP-loading of Rag A/B appears to be regulated by amino acids, and binding to TORC1 is observed most robustly under nutrient-rich conditions – when Rag A/B is in the GTP-bound state and Rag C/D is in the GDP-bound state [111, 112]. This model answers the question why mTORC1 activity cannot be stimulated by growth factors in the absence of amino acids. It also explains why Rag GTPases are not able to activate mTORC1 activity *in vitro* [111]. mTORC1 can be fully activated only under the conditions of amino acids availability, Rab-dependent mTORC1 translocation to a Rheb-containing compartment, and Rheb activated by growth factors. However, there are many key aspects that remain to be discovered, such as how branched amino acids are detected by Rag GTPases and the identification of the Rag guanine exchange factor (GEF).

3.2.2. PLD joins to amino acids dependent mTORC1 regulation

Several data evidence that phosphatidic acid (PA) is essential for mTORC1 activation. The main mechanism for generating PA is the hydrolysis of phosphatidylcholine (PC) by phospholipase D (PLD). In mammals PLD exists as two isoforms (PLD1 and PLD2) possessing different mechanisms of regulation and subcellular distribution [113]. PLD1 is predominantly localized under steady-state conditions at the Golgi complex, endosomes, lysosomes and secretory granules, and is regulated by two major signaling categories: growth factors/mitogens like EGF, PDGF, insulin and serum that implicate tyrosine kinases, and the small GTPase proteins from Arf, Ral and Rho families. PLD2 is largely associated with lipid rafts on the membrane surface. [113]. Both PLD1 and PLD2 have a strong requirement for PIP2 as a co-factor [113]. It has been shown that PLD1 activation stimulates PLD2 by increasing levels of PIP2 (product of PA metabolic modifications) [114]. This makes more clear the involvement of both PLD1 and PLD2 in the mTORC1 activation. The generation of PA by PLD can be suppressed by primary alcohols (such as 1-butanol) through the transphosphatidylation reaction whereby inert phosphatidyl-alcohol is generated instead of PA. This reaction has been widely used to examine PLD significance, and several studies have demonstrated that the activation of mTOR was sensitive to primary alcohols. Thus, 1-butanol was able to block almost completely the serum-stimulated phosphorylation of mTOR downstream targets, S6K1 and 4E-BP1 [115]. From these findings, it can be asserted that PLD production of PA plays an essential role in the mTOR signaling pathway). In skeletal muscle, PA stimulated S6 kinase phosphorylation, and 1-butanol suppressed S6 kinase phosphorylation [116]. Nutrient-dependent multimerization of mTOR was also suppressed by 1-butanol [117]. Therefore, primary alcohols-dependent suppression of PLD activity has been shown to suppress mTORC1 signaling in several cell models [114].

Several laboratories have shown that mTORC1 is activated in response to exogenously supplied PA. For example, exogenously provided PA stimulated the activation of S6 kinase and phosphorylation of 4E-BP1 in cancer HEK293 cells. The effect of PA was sensitive to rapamycin [115, 118] and was dependent on the presence of amino acids [115]. Coexpression of TSC1/2 was shown to inhibit PA-dependent stimulation of S6K. This indicates that PA-induced S6K activity is mediated through TSC1/2-mTOR signaling. PA was also shown to activate mTOR in macrophages in an Akt-dependent manner [119].

In addition, several studies have explored the influence of PLD1 and PLD2 expression on mTORC1 activation. Particularly it was reported that PLD2 overexpression increases S6K phosphorylation in MCF7 cells [120]. Overexpression of PLD1 also stimulated S6K phosphorylation in rat fibroblasts [121]. siRNA-mediated knockdown of PLD1 blocked S6K phosphorylation in B16 melanoma cells, and suppression of either PLD1 or mTOR led to melanoma cells differentiation [122].

At the same time, up to date the precise mechanism of PA-dependent stimulation of mTOR signaling remains unclear. One possibility is that PA binds to mTOR at the FRB domain, the region where the rapamycin-FKBP12 molecule binds mTOR as well. This binding was specific for PA as other phospholipids were unable to bind the FRB with such specificity. It was hypothesized that the competition between the rapamycin-FKBP12 complex and PA for the FRB site may be one of the regulating factors in mTOR activation [115]. According to the

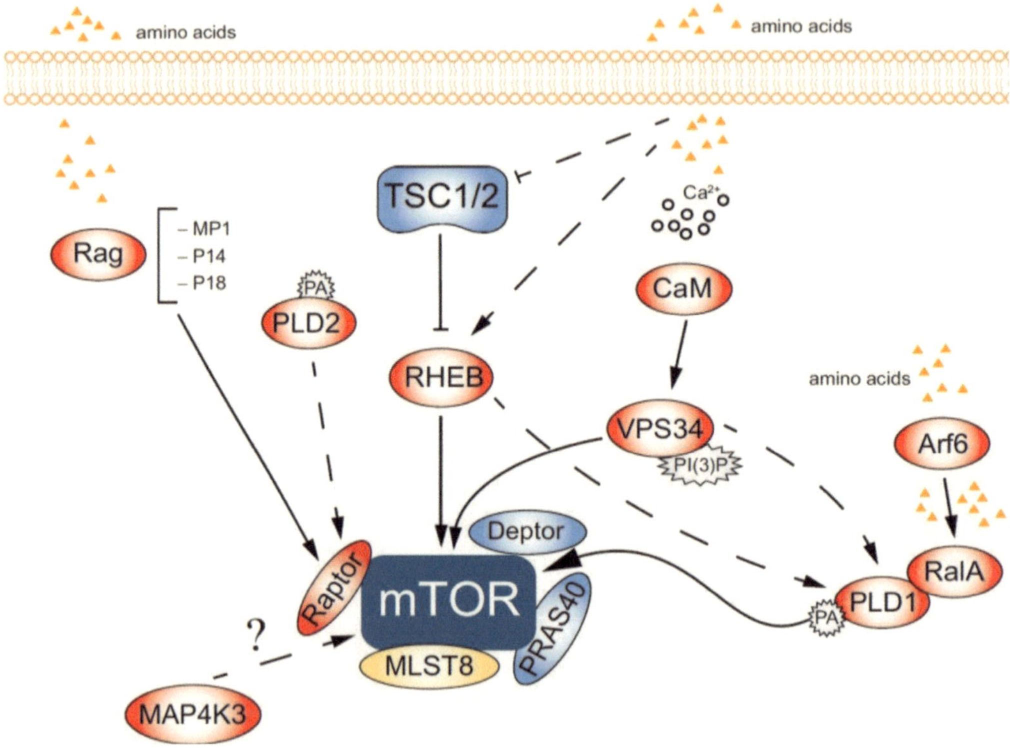

Figure 3. Nutrients regulation of mTORC signaling. mTORC1 could be activated by amino acids through few proposed molecular mechanisms. In the response to amino acid sufficiency Rag complex is recruited to the lysosomal membrane by the trimeric Ragulator complex which consists of MP1, p14 and p18 thereby allowing Rheb to activate mTORC1. Amino acids also induce an extracellular calcium influx that activates calmodulin, which in turn binds and activates hVps34 that generates PI-3-P, what leads somehow to the mTORC1 activation. One model puts PLD downstream of hVps34 suggesting hVps34(PI-3-P)-PLD-mTORC1 pathway mediating response to amino acids. According to this model nutrient activation of PLD requires interaction with small G proteins RalA and Arf6. In addition, several studies evidence that PLD probably via generation of PA contributes to the mTORC1 activation in response to the nutrient stimulation. Particularly, PA could compete with rapamycin-FKBP12 complex for the mTOR FRB domain binding or reduce the pH around mTOR. PLD2 has also been reported to form a functional complex with mTOR and Raptor through a TOS (TOR signaling) motif. It has also been proposed that branched-chain amino acids could activate mTORC1 by inhibiting TSC1/TSC2 or stimulating Rheb.

other hypothesis the pH locally around mTOR is reduced by PA-generated PLD, which eventually promotes its kinase activity, or allows for interaction with yet unknown promoter substrates [114]. It was shown that PLD1 is an effector of the small GTPase Rheb (see above) within the mTORC1 signaling pathway [123, 124] **(Figure 3)**. It was also reported that PLD2 forms a functional complex with Raptor and mTOR via a TOS (TOR signaling) motif in PLD2, and this interaction was essential for mitogen stimulation of mTORC1 [125]. More recently, dominant negative mutants of both PLD1 and PLD2 were able to suppress the activation of mTORC1 [126]. Therefore, besides PA ability to activate mTORC1, there are several data indicating requirement of PLD itself for the activation of mTORC1. Very recent study provided additional evidence that nutrient stimulation of mTORC1 is dependent on PLD activity which in turn is activated by small GTPases RalA and Arf6 [127]. According to this study, amino acids dependent activation of PLD is mediated trough generated by Vps34 PI-3-phosphate [127], that could interact with PX domains of PLD1 and PLD2 which are known to be critical for PLD activity [128]. This activation also requires PLD interaction with both RalA and Arf6. Interestingly, these small GTPases have been earlier shown to be implicated in both responding to nutrients and the stimulation of PLD activity. RalA is constitutively associated with PLD1, but does not activate PLD1 by itself. RalA contributes to the activation of PLD1 by recruiting ARF6, which does activate PLD1 activity, into RalA/ARF6/PLD1 complex. While it is still not clear how the presence of nutrients activates RalA and ARF6, the data provided in this study indicate that PLD is a key target of RalA and ARF6 for the stimulation of mTORC1. In concordance with these findings data from our lab evidence that expression of constitutively active Arf6 stimulates PLD activity which leads to the mTORC1 dependent phosphorylation of downstream targets 4E-BP1, S6K1 kinase and its effector ribosomal protein **S6** (rpS6). We also show that mTORC1 signaling stimulation contributes to the Arf6 promitogenic activity [129].

3.3. Control of mTOR signaling in response to energy stress

AMPK (the AMP-activated protein kinase, also known as PRKAB1) is activated under the low level of intracellular ATP and found in all eukaryotes. It was initially identified as a serine/threonine kinase that negatively regulates several key enzymes of the lipid anabolism [130]. At present, AMPK is considered to be the major energy-sensing kinase that activates a whole variety of catabolic processes in multicellular organisms such as glucose uptake and metabolism, while simultaneously inhibiting several anabolic pathways, such as lipid, protein, and carbohydrate biosynthesis (reviewed in [130]). AMPK is upregulated under energy stress conditions in response to nutrient deprivation or hypoxia when intracellular ATP level decreases and AMP increases [131]. In response, AMPK turns on ATP generating pathways while inhibiting ATP consuming functions of the cell [131]. AMPK functions as heterotrimeric kinase complex, which consists of a catalytic (α) subunit and two regulatory (β and γ) subunits. Upon energy stress, AMP directly binds to tandem repeats of crystathionine-β-synthase (CBS) domains in the AMPK γ subunit [132]. Since the ratio of AMP to ATP represents the most accurate way to precisely measure the intracellular energy level, both AMP and ATP are able to oppositely regulate the activity of AMPK. While AMP binding to the γ–subunit allosterically enhances AMPK kinase activity and prevents the dephosphorylation of T172 [133], ATP is known to counteract the activating properties of AMP [130]. Although ADP does not allosterically activate AMPK, it also binds to AMPK and enhances phosphorylation at T172 [134, 135]. The phosphorylation of the activation loop T172 is absolutely necessary for AMPK activation. At present, several AMPK-phosphorylating kinases have been identified. In addition to the ubiquitously expressed and constitutively active kinase LKB1, Ca^{2+}-activated Ca^{2+}/calmodulin-dependent kinase kinase β

(CaMKKβ) [136] and transforming growth factor β-activated kinase-1 (TAK1) are both known as AMPK activators. Genetic and biochemical studies in worms, flies, and mice have identified the serine/threonine liver kinase B1 (LKB1) as major kinase phosphorylating the AMPK activation loop at T172 residue, under conditions of energy stress [130]. Within the TOR signaling pathway, LKB1 dependent activation of AMPK inhibit mTORC1 activity by two ways **(Figure 4).** Firstly, AMPK directly phosphorylates the TSC2 on S1387 and T1227 [2, 64, 70, 87, 137, 138]. AMPK phosphorylation of TSC2 has also been reported to act as a primer for the phosphorylation and enhancement of TSC2 function by glycogen synthase 3β (GSK3β). GSK3β dependent phosphorylation of TSC2 on S1341 and S1337 stimulates its GAP activity towards Rheb, leading to the inhibition of mTORC1 [138]. It is possible that GSK3β cooperates with AMPK to fully activate the GAP activity of TSC2. The second, TSC2 independent mechanism by which AMPK can signal to mTORC1, [45] is a direct phosphorylation of Raptor at two highly conserved residues – S722 and S792. These phosphorylation events induce Raptor direct binding to 14-3-3 protein, which leads to a suppression of mTORC1 kinase downstream activity [45]. Therefore, mTORC1 itself serves as an AMPK substrate for inhibiting phosphorylation.

3.4. mTOR signaling regulating by hypoxia

mTOR signaling pathway is strictly regulated by hypoxia [139, 140], since the sufficiency of oxygen is also essential for cellular metabolism. Hypoxia inhibits mTORC1 signaling via multiple signal pathways, two of them being mediated through activation of the TSC1/TSC2 complex **(Figure 4**). First, activation of AMPK by hypoxia can enhance TSC complex function. Particularly, it was shown, that brief hypoxia exposure prevents insulin-mediated stimulation of mTORC1 and phosphorylation of its targets p70S6K and 4E-BP1 [139]. Under these conditions mTOR suppression is mediated through a HIF1α (hypoxia-inducible factor 1α)-independent pathway involving AMPK-dependent activation of TSC1/TSC2 [2, 87, 141]. Second way includes the upregulation of TSC1/TSC2 through transcriptional regulation of stress-induced protein REDD1 (Regulated in Development and DNA damage responses, also known as DDIT4 or RTP801) [142, 143]. This response is mediated in part through a mechanism that involves HIF1α, a transcription factor that is stabilized under hypoxic conditions and drives the expression of several genes, including *REDD1.* Induction of REDD1 can activate the TSC1/2 complex by competing with TSC2 for 14-3-3 proteins binding [142, 144]. Thus, increased REDD1 levels that occur following exposure to hypoxia prevent the inhibitory binding of 14-3-3 to TSC2 [144], which eventually leads to the inhibition of mTORC1 signaling. Therefore inhibitory effect of REDD1 on mTOR signaling seemed to be dependent on the presence of the TSC1/2 complex, but independent on the LKB1-AMPK signaling [142, 145, 146]. However, most recent studies proposed that hypoxia and the LKB1-AMPK signaling are highly interrelated at least in some type of cells [140]. In response to prolonged hypoxia, REDD1 expression was enhanced by AMPK activation, leading to the inhibition of mTOR pathway. Indeed, it was demonstrated that prolonged hypoxia induced ATP depletion and eventually activate AMPK [140]. Taken together, under hypoxic stress, the inhibition of mTOR activity by REDD1 activation may be mediated either through AMPK-independent or -dependent mechanisms.

Hypoxia may also downregulate mTORC1 through proteins that hinder the the Rheb–mTOR interaction. The PMl (promyelocytic leukaemia tumour suppressor) has been found to bind mTOR during hypoxia and inactivate it via sequestration in nuclear bodies [147]. Likewise, the hypoxia-inducible proapoptotic protein BNIP3 (BCl2/adenovirus E1B 19 kDa protein-interacting protein 3) was found to regulate mTOR by direct association with Rheb [148]. (Reviewed in [149]).

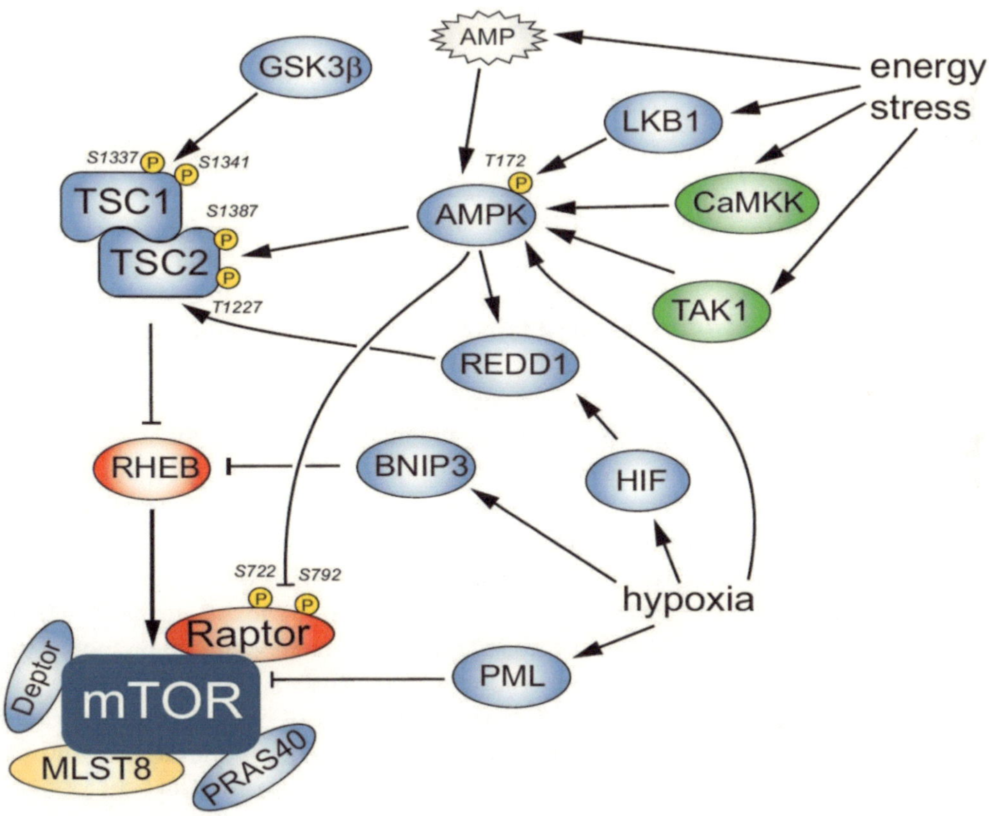

Figure 4. mTORC1 regulation in response to energy deprivation and hypoxia. Low cellular energy levels (conveyed by AMP) and hypoxia activate AMPK, which represses mTORC1 both through direct negative phosphorylation of TSC2 and through Raptor inhibition. LKB1, CaMKK and TAK1 are known as AMPK activators. AMPK- and GSK3β-mediated phosphorylation of the TSC1/2 complex positively regulates the GAP activity of TSC2 towards Rheb, abrogating its stimulative activity towards mTORC1. Under hypoxic stress, the inhibition of mTOR activity could be mediated by REDD1 either through AMPK-independent or -dependent mechanisms. Hypoxia-inducible proapoptotic protein BNIP3 is reported to regulate mTOR by direct binding to Rheb, while PML can binds mTOR and inactivate it through sequestration in nuclear bodies.

4. Signaling downstream of mTOR

4.1. TORC1 regulates translation machinery

The protein synthesis stimulation and the inhibition of autophagy are two mostly known biological outputs controlled by this pathway under the favorable conditions, such as nutrient and oxygen availability. By sensing the presence of growth factors and the sufficiency of nutrients, activated mTORC1 mediates the signals to various components of the translation initiation machinery through direct or indirect phosphorylation events [22]. Several data also evidence that mTOR regulates the synthesis of many classes of lipids (such as phosphatidylcholine, phosphatidylglycerol, and sphingolipids, unsaturated and saturated fatty acids) that are required for membrane biosynthesis and energy storage (For the detailed review see [150]. Since the best characterized effectors of mTOR signaling are proteins controlling the translational initiation machinery it is important to understand how mTORC1 signal transduction pathways contribute to protein synthesis regulation (reviewed in [151]).

The earliest identified and best-studied mTORC1 targets are S6K kinases (p70 ribosomal protein S6 kinase 1 and 2) and 4EBP1 (eIF4E binding protein 1); both proteins involved in the translation initiation process [152] **(Figure 5A**). Protein synthesis is one of the most energy consuming processes within the cell and translation rates are strictly regulated mostly through modification of the eukaryotic initiation factors (eIFs). In eukaryotes, several mRNAs are translated in a cap-dependent manner. The cap structure, m7GpppN (where N is any nucleotide), is present at the 5′ terminus of the majority cellular eukaryotic mRNAs (except those in organelles) [153]. The cap structure is bound by the eIF4F (eukaryotic initiation factor 4F) complex, which contains three initiation factors — the mRNA 5′ cap-binding protein eIF4E, an ATP-dependent RNA helicase eIF4A and a large scaffolding protein eIF4G, which provides docking sites for the other proteins. Briefly, to assemble the eIF4F complex, eIF4E binds the 5′ cap and recruits eIF4G and eIF4A. eIF4A along with eIF4B acts to unwind the mRNA 5′ secondary structure to facilitate ribosome binding [153]. It is especially essential, since stable secondary structures are often found in the 5′ UTR of specific mRNA species, many of which encode proteins that are involved in promoting cell growth and proliferation, and significantly suppress their translation efficiency [154]. As the translation preinitiation complex is recruited near the 5′ end of mRNA, this requires the structured UTR to be 'linearized' — not only for the initial binding of the 40S ribosome but also for subsequent searching for the downstream initiation codon. Although eIF4A alone exhibits low levels of RNA helicase activity the last one is substantially stimulated by its regulatory cofactor, eIF4B. Thus, eIF4B enhances the affinity of eIF4A binding to ATP, which, in turn, increases the processivity of the eIF4A helicase function [155]. eIF4G recruits the small ribosomal subunit to the mRNA (and the poly(A)-binding protein, PABP) through the ribosome associated large multisubunit factor eIF3. As a result the assembly of the 48S translation preinitiation complex takes place, allowing for the ribosome scanning and translation initiation [22, 26]. The translation initiation factors and cofactors that are regulated by mTORC1 signaling include eIF4G, eIF3, eIF4B, eIF4E and 4EBP1, of which 4EBP1 is considered to be the most well-known mTORC1 direct effector protein.

eIF4G serving as a modular scaffold for the translation preinitiation complex formation, is phosphorylated in response to growth factor stimuli at multiple sites, some of which are dependent on mTORC1. These sites are clustered in a hinge region of eIF4G that joins two structural domains, and it has thus been predicted that the modification might induce conformational changes in the protein that affect its activity [22]. Nevertheless, the precise molecular mechanism by which eIF4G phosphorylation regulates its function remains to be determined. Regulation of the mRNA cap binding protein eIF4E is mediated mainly in two ways, firstly, through phosphorylation at S209 in its C-terminus by MAP kinase signaling integration kinases 1 and 2 (Mnk1/2) [156] and, secondly, through the sequestration by small, heat stable phosphoproteins termed 4E-binding proteins, 4E-BPs [153] belonging to the 4E-BPs translation repressors family. One of these proteins, 4E-BP1 is a direct mTORC1 phosphorylation target. In quiescent cells, hypophosphorylated 4EBP1 binds tightly to eIF4E. As 4EBP1 and eIF4G share the same eIF4E-binding motif 4EBP1 competes with eIF4G for an overlapping binding site on eIF4E, and prevents eIF4G from interacting with eIF4E. On mTORC1 activation, hyperphosphorylated 4EBP1 dissociates from eIF4E, allowing for the recruitment of eIF4G and eIF4A to the 5′ end of an mRNA. Thus, the effects of 4E-BP1 on protein translation are not limited to switching 'off ' or 'on' protein synthesis; they can also alter the range of nascent proteins by mediating a switch between cap-dependent and cap-independent translation. Indeed, during specific stress conditions, such as nutrient depletion, hypoxia or metabolic stress, the cell can reduce the activity of mTORC1, resulting in the cessation of cap-dependent translation and the concomitant promotion of cap-independent translation of essential pro-survival factors. Rapamycin inhibits mTORC1-dependent 4E-BP1 phosphorylation, stimulating the interaction between eIF4E and 4E-BP1, what leads to cap-dependent translation inhibition [157].

Control of the 4E-BPs by mTOR

Upon the stimulation (by growth factors, mitogens and hormones), human 4E-BP1 is phosporylated at 7 sites, 4 of which are involved in mTOR signaling [157, 158]. These are T37, T46 and T70, and S65. The 4E-BP1 phosphorylation is proceeded in a hierarchical manner (first T37 and T46, then T70 and last S65) [157]. S65 and T70 are located near the eIF4E-binding site. Often phosphorylation of these residues is stimulated by insulin in a rapamycin-sensitive manner. Some data evidence that phosphorylation of S65 is required for release of eIF4E from 4E-BP1, however the role of phosphorylation of this site is unclear [159]. Molecular dynamics findings [160] and earlier biophysical data suggest that phosphorylation of S65 and T70 is insufficient to bring about release from eIF4E. Phosphorylation of both S65 and T70 depends upon the prior phosphorylation of the N-terminal threonines, and modification of T46 is considered to be essential for phosphorylation of T37 [157, 161]. The phosphorylation of T70 and S65 in human 4E-BP1 depends upon a further site, S101 [162]. The phosphorylation of the N-terminal threonin residues in 4E-BP1 depends upon a certain sequence in the N-terminus, which includes the Arg-Ala-Ile-Pro ('RAIP' motif) [91, 163]. This phosphorylation is not significantly influenced by TOS motif inactivation and according to some data is rather insensitive to rapamycin [158]. This suggests that it could be mediated independently of mTORC1. However, several data evidence that phosphorylation is mediated by mTORC1: (i) it is inhibited by starvation of cells for amino acids; (ii) it is activated by Rheb; (iii) it is suppressed by TSC1/2; (iv) it is sensitive to inhibitors of the kinase activity of mTOR and (v) it is decreased in cells in which mTOR levels have been knocked down [158]. Therefore, further study of this process needs to clarify the molecular mechanisms of mTOR downstream signaling.

Control of the S6Ks by mTOR

Another important target of mTORC1 is the S6 kinases family, including S6K1 and S6K2. Ribosomal protein S6 (rpS6) is highly phosphorylated protein containing at least five phosporylating sites in its C-terminus. There are two main classes of protein kinases which are responsible for rpS6 phosphorylation *in vitro*, namely the p70 S6 kinases (S6Ks) and the p90 ribosomal protein S6 kinases, also known as RSKs [164, 165], (reviewed in [151]). The observed sensitivity of rpS6 to rapamycin lead to the speculation that S6K are responsible for rpS6 phosphorylation as their activation is mediated by mTOR. Unlike S6Ks, the RSKs are not influenced by rapamycin since they are known to be activated through the classical MAP kinase (ERK) pathway (see below). There are two similar S6 kinase proteins, S6K1 and S6K2, in mammals [166], which show 70% of amino acid homology. Each p70S6K gene encodes two distinct proteins due to alternative splicing of the mRNAs. Several data confirm that activation of both the S6K1 and S6K2 are regulated by mTORC1 [118, 167, 168]. S6K1, which was discovered earlier than S6K2, is ubiquitously expressed and appears to be more critical for the control of cell growth. S6K1 can be activated by a wide variety of extracellular signals and is known as the major rpS6 kinase in mammalian cells and key player in the control of cell growth (cell size) and proliferation [169, 170].

Earlier it was thought that activated S6K1 regulates translation of a class of mRNA transcripts that bear a 5′-terminal oligopolypyrimidine (5′-TOP). Particularly, it was shown that S6K1 phosphorylates eIF4B on S422, which is located in the RNA binding region that is necessary for promoting the helicase activity of eIF4A [171]. Few data indicate that eIF4B phosphorylation by S6K1 is both sufficient and necessary for its recruitment to the translation preinitiation complex [172]. However, there are also some data that disprove this model. In S6K1/2−/− cells, 5′-TOP mRNA translation is intact and still rapamycin-sensitive [173]. These results are in concordance with earlier data showing that mitogenic-stimulated or amino acid dependent 5′-TOP mRNAs translation is dependent on PI3K mediated signaling, and does not require S6K1 activity and ribosomal protein S6 phosphorylation [174, 175]. Instead, a role for the S6 kinases in controlling the cell size has been suggested as deletion of S6K leads to animal size decrease [173]. Studies performed on 'knock-in' mice in which all sites phosphorylated by the S6 kinases were mutated also indicated a role for S6 phosphorylation in cell growth [176]. These knock-in cells still demonstrated faster rates of protein synthesis at the same time being decreased in size. This could be explained by elevated access of the S6K to other substrates involved in translation, such as eIF4B and eEF2 kinase (see below) [151].

Another pool of data connecting S6K1 activity and translation initiation occurs from the study of potential tumor suppressor, Programmed cell death 4 (PDCD4) protein **(Figure**

5A). PDCD4 binds to eIF4A and is thought to inhibit its helicase activity [177]. PDCD4 is also thought to prevent eIF4A from incorporating into the eIF4F complex by competing with eIF4G for eIF4A binding [178]. S6K1 phosphorylates PDCD4 on S67 in response to growth factor stimulation resulting in its subsequent degradation through the ubiquitin ligase βTrCP101. Therefore, S6K1-dependent phosphorylation of PDCD4 prevents the inhibitory effect of PDCD4 towards eIF4A helicase function within the eIF4F complex.

Recent data give new evidence on interconnection of the mTOR/S6K1 pathway and translation preinitiation complex assembly [172, 179]. Under the poor growth conditions, S6K1 but not mTORC1 binds with multisubunit initiation factor eIF3 that was identified as a dynamic scaffold for mTORC1 and S6K1 binding [172] **(Figure 5B).** Upon growth factors or nutrients availability, the mTORC1 is recruited to eIF3 and phosphorylates S6K1. Based on polysome analysis and cap-binding assays, it is thought that the mTORC1–eIF3 complex associates with the mRNA 5′ cap, bringing mTORC1 into proximity with 4EBP1. Phosphorylation of S6K1 at T389 leads to its dissociation from eIF3. T389-phosphorylated S6K1 binds to PDK1 **(Figure 5A**), which phosphorylates S6K1 at T229. The fully activated S6K1 is able to phosphorylate eIF4B and S6. Phosphorylation of eIF4B by S6K1 at S422 promotes its association with eIF3 [172, 180]. The interaction of mTOR with eIF3 also strengthens the association between eIF4G and eIF3 [181]. Described interactions cooperate to enhance the assembly of translation initiation complex and facilitate cap-dependent translation.

The S6 kinases are activated by phosphorylation at multiple sites. Several of them lie within the C-terminus, while two others lay immediately C-terminal to the catalytic domain. One of these, T389 in the shorter form of S6K1, which is located at a hydrophobic motif carboxyterminal to the kinase domain, is directly phosphorylated by mTOR as part of the mTORC1 complex [182, 183]. Phosphorylation here is required for the consequent phosphorylation of S6K1 by PDK1 at a T229 in the activation loop of the catalytic domain. Phosphorylation at T229 allows full activation of S6K1. S6K2 is likely regulated in a similar manner. Both S6K1 and 2 contain a TOS motif within their N-terminus region, which interacts with Raptor, promoting phosphorylation of S6Ks by mTORC1 [184]. The phosphorylation within the C-terminal region seems to open access to the sites T389/T229, phosphorylation of which provides the complete activation. It is not known exactly which kinase is responsible for C-terminal phosphorylation sites. Nevertheless mTOR also indirectly contributes to the phosphorylation of the C-terminal sites. A motif RSPRR exists in this region probably plays a significant role in the inhibitory effect of the C-terminal region. It has been speculated that a negative S6K1 regulator binds S6K via this motif and that mTOR could broke this binding [184]. The C-terminal region of S6K1 also determines whether S6K1 can be phosphorylated by mTORC2. Mutant S6K1 with deletion of this region is a substrate for mTORC2 [185]. Some data indicate that for S6K1 activation, mTOR can directly phosphorylate S371 *in vitro*, and this event modulates T389 phosphorylation by mTOR [186, 187].

In addition to the discussed above mTORC1 targets, S6Ks and 4E-BP1, both of which modulate translation initiation, mTOR signaling also regulates the translation elongation process through the phosphorylation of eukaryotic elongation factor 2 (eEF2). eEF2 is a GTP binding protein that mediates the translocation step of elongation [188]. eEF2 is phosphorylated at T56 within the GTP-binding domain and this phosphorylation impedes its ability to bind the ribosome, thus inhibiting its function [188, 189]. Insulin and other stimuli induce the dephosphorylation of eEF2, and this effect is blocked by rapamycin, indicating that this effect is also mediated through mTOR [190]. The eEF2 phosphorylation function is attributed to a highly specific enzyme called eEF2 kinase (eEF2K) [190]. Phosphorylation of eEF2 at T56 by eEF2 kinase impedes the eEF2 binding of to the ribosome and the translocation step of the elongation [188]. The calcium/calmodulin-dependent protein kinase eEF2K is an atypical enzyme since the sequence of its catalytic domain differs substantially from that of other protein kinases, and it is not a member, e.g., of the main Ser-Thr-Tyr kinase superfamily [191]. The C-terminal half of the eEF2K polypeptide contains several sites of phosphorylation including the binding site for the substrate eEF2 at the C-terminus [192]. mTOR negatively regulates eEF2 kinase and consequently activates eEF2. mTOR is considered being able to phosphorylate 3 sites, as was determined by their rapamycin- and/or amino-acid starvation sensitivities [188, 193]. S366 in the C terminus of the catalytic domain has been identified as the site being phosphorylated by S6K and by p90RSK [190]. The phosphorylation at S359 has been shown to be also regulated in a rapamycin-sensitive manner in response to insulin-like growth factor 1 (IGF1) and inactivates eEF2K [194], but the kinase responsible for this phosphorylation remains to be determined. Recently, a novel phosphorylation site located immediately adjacent to the CaM-binding site in eEF2K that is regulated markedly in response to insulin in an mTOR dependent manner has been identified. This site (S78) is not known to be phosphorylated by any known protein kinase in the mTOR pathway. Phosphorylation at this third site also causes the inactivation of eEF2 kinase, in this case by inhibiting the binding of CaM, which binds immediately C-terminal to S78 [193]. eEF2K is thought to be a target of signaling from mTOR independently of other known targets of this pathway, which implies the existence of a novel (probably mTOR-controlled) protein kinase that could acts upon S78 in eEF2K. These data provide a molecular mechanism by which mTOR could regulate peptide chain elongation.

Since the protein synthesis depends on the amount of ribosomes and transfer RNAs (tRNAs) it is important to know that mTOR signaling also contributes to the regulation of tRNA production, promotion of rRNA synthesis and ribosome biogenesis. Thus mTOR signaling tightly regulates transcription of ribosomal RNAs (rRNAs) and tRNAs by RNA polymerases I and III [195]. mTOR can associate with general transcription factor III C (TFIIIC) and relieve its inhibitor Maf1, leading to increased tRNA production. mTORC1 activity also promotes association between transcription initiation factor 1A (TIF-1A) and polymerase I (PolI), thereby promoting rRNA synthesis [35]. The activity of several other transcription factors, such as signal transducer and activator of transcription-1 and -3 (Stat-1 and Stat-3) is also suggested to be regulated by mTORC1-mediated phosphorylation in a rapamycin-sensitive manner [196].

4.2. TORC1-mediated repression of autophagy

Autophagy is a lysosomal-dependent cellular degradation process that generates nutrients and energy to maintain essential cellular activities upon nutrient starvation. A term

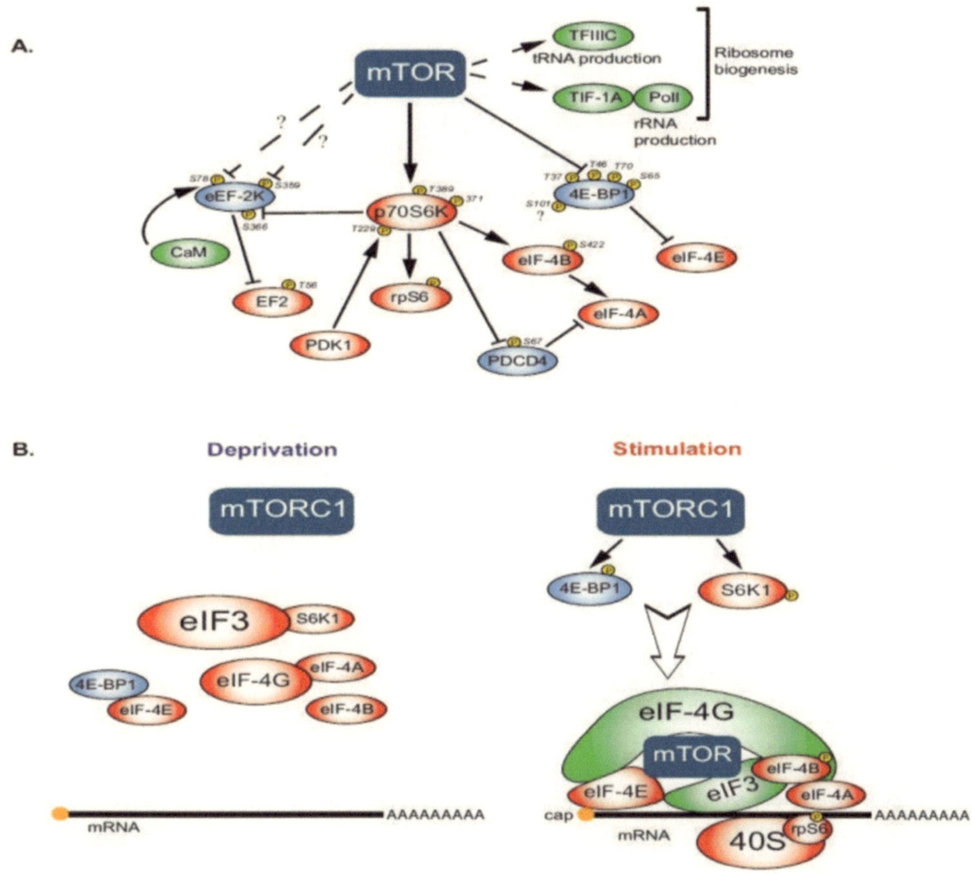

Figure 5. mTORC1 downstream signaling and translation regulation.
A. mTOR phosphorylates two major targets: 4E-BP1 and S6Ks. Hypophosphorylated 4E-BP1 binds tightly to eIF-4E, thereby preventing its interaction with eIF-4G and thus inhibiting translation. Phosphorylated 4E-BP1 is released from eIF-4E resulting in the recruitment of eIF-4G to the 5´-cap, and thereby allowing translation initiation to proceed. Phosphorylation of p70S6K stimulates its activity towards several substrates, including 40S ribosomal protein S6, translation initiation factor eIF-4B, elongation factor kinase eEF2K, and PDCD4 protein. Following S6K-mediated phosphorylation, eIF-4B is recruited to the translation pre-initiation complex and enhances the RNA helicase activity of eIF-4A. S6K1dependent phosphorylation of PDCD4 prevents its inhibitory effect towards eIF-4A helicase. mTORC1 also contributes to the translation elongation through the regulation of eEF2. mTOR negatively regulates eEF2 kinase (either directly or via p70S6K activation) and thereby activates eEF2. mTOR signaling also contributes to the regulation of tRNA production, promotion of rRNA synthesis and ribosome biogenesis activating TFIIIC and promoting the association between transcription initiation factor 1A and polymerase I respectively.
B. In the absence of extracellular stimuli, S6K1 is associated with eIF3 while 4E-BP1 binding to eIF-4E prevents its interaction with eIF-4G and thus inhibiting translation. In response to extracellular stimuli, such as growth factors or nutrients, the mTOR complex is recruited to eIF3 to phosphorylate S6K1 and 4E-BP1. Phosphorylation and activation of S6K1 leads to its dissociation from eIF3. Activated S6K1 then phosphorylates eIF4B and S6. Phosphorylation of eIF-4B 2 promotes its association with eIF3. mTOR also stimulates the association between eIF3 and eIF-4G.

autophagy appeared from Greek "auto" (self) and "phagy" (to eat), refers to an evolutionarily conserved, multi-step lysosomal degradation process in which a cell degrades long-lived proteins and damaged organelles. Three forms of autophagy have been identified, namely macroautophagy, microautophagy and chaperone-mediated autophagy that differ with respect to their modes of delivery to lysosome and physiological functions [197]. Macroautophagy (hereafter autophagy) is the major regulated catabolic mechanism that involves the delivery of cytosolic cargo sequestered inside specific intracellular double-membrane vesicles, called autophagosomes to the lysosomal compartment and subsequent fusion with lysosomes to form single-membrane-bound autophagolysosomes, in which the sequestered material is degraded by acidic lysosomal hydrolases. On one hand, autophagy is crucial for cell survival under extreme conditions through degradation of intracellular macromolecules, which provides the energy required for minimal cell functioning when nutrients are deprived or scarce. Also, autophagy-mediated elimination of altered cytosolic constituents, such as aggregated proteins or damaged organelles, preserves cells from further damages, indicating that autophagy plays a protective role in early stages of cancer [198]. On the other hand, autophagy plays a death-promoting role as type II programmed cell death (type II PCD), compared to apoptosis (type I PCD), as a bona fide tumor suppressor mechanism in cancer [199].

The ability of mTORC1 to regulate autophagy is as highly conserved as well as the process of autophagy itself. AMPK has been indicated as a main upstream regulator of mTORC1 mediated autophagy inhibition.

The mechanism by which TORC1 negatively regulates the autophagic machinery has first been described in yeast. Genetic screenings for autophagy defective mutants led to the identification of more than 30 essential autophagy-related genes (Atg).These proteins can be classified into several groups depending on their function and interdependency. Most upstream is a protein complex that comprises the serine/threonine kinase Atg1, as well as two accessory proteins Atg13 and Atg17. In mammals, two homologs of Atg1, uncoordinated 51-like kinase 1 (ULK1) and ULK2 have been identified. Accumulating evidence suggests that ULK1 is a key regulator of autophagy initiation. ULK1 is directly phosphorylated by TORC1 [200-202]. Recently, it has also been shown that mTORC1-mediated phosphorylation of ULK1 impairs its activation by AMPK and results in an overall decrease in autophagy [203]. ULK1 and ULK2 are found in a stable complex with mammalian autophagy-related protein 13 (mAtg13), the scaffold protein FAK-family interacting protein of 200 kDa (FIP200) [204] [201] and Atg101, an additional binding partner of Atg13 that has no ortholog in yeast [205]. In contrast to yeast, the composition of this complex does not change with the nutrient status. Several data evidence that the phosphorylation status within the Ulk1/2-Atg13-FIP200 complex dramatically changes with the nutrient availability. Under rich growth conditions, mTORC1 associates with the Ulk1/2-Atg13-FIP200 complex, via direct interaction between Raptor and Ulk1/2 (37). The active mTOR phosphorylates Atg13 and Ulk1/2 [201], thereby downregulating Ulk1/2 kinase activity and suppressing autophagy **(Figure 6)**. In response to starvation, the mTORC1-dependent phosphorylation sites in Ulk1/2 are rapidly dephosphorylated by yet unknown phosphatases, what stimulates Ulk1/2 autophosphorylation and phosphorylation of both

Atg13 and FIP200. Several serine and threonine residues in human Ulk1 whose phosphorylation was decreased after starvation have been recently identified from which S638 and S758 have been proposed to be most probable mTORC1 negative phosphorylation sites [203, 206]. Ulk1/2 autophosphorylation and following FIP200 and Atg13 phosphorylation in turn leads to translocation of the entire complex to the pre-autophagosomal membrane and to autophagy induction [200, 201, 205]. However, the functional relevance of Ulk1/2-mediated phosphorylation of Atg13 and FIP200 for this recruitment and the relevant phosphorylation sites has not been verified yet. Interestingly, another Ulk1-dependent phosphorylation site in human Atg13 (S318) has been identified recently [207]. The authors of that study could show that the Hsp90-Cdc37 chaperone complex selectively stabilizes and activates Ulk1.

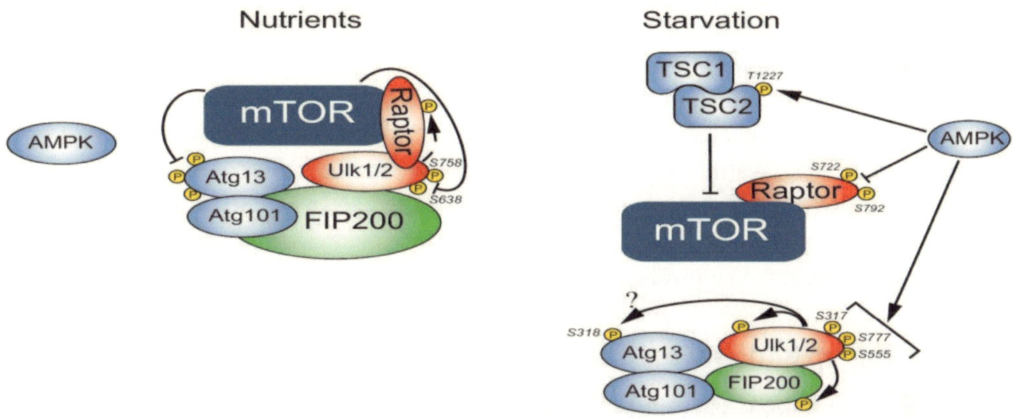

Figure 6. mTORC1 downstream signaling and autophagy regulation. Ulk1 and Ulk2 form a stable complex with Atg13, FIP200 and Atg101. Under fed conditions mTORC1 phosphorylates Ulk1/2 and Atg13, thereby inhibiting the Ulk1/2 kinase activity and complex stability. In response to starvation, the mTORC1-dependent phosphorylation sites in Ulk1/2 are rapidly dephosphorylated, and Ulk1/2 autophosphorylates and phosphorylates Atg13 and FIP200 resulting in translocation of the entire complex to the pre-autophagosomal membrane and autophagy induction. Alternatively, Ulk1/2 is phosphorylated by AMPK and thereby activated. In addition, AMPK indirectly leads to the induction of autophagy by inhibiting mTORC1 through phosphorylation of Raptor or TSC2.

In yeast, autophagosomes originate from a single preautophagosomal structure. Although an equivalent structure seems to be absent from mammalian cells, a special subdomain in the endoplasmic reticulum (ER) termed the "omegasome" has been suggested as a putative origin of autophagosomes. This structure is enriched in PI(3)P, a product of the phosphatidylinositol 3-kinase (PI3K). A hierarchical analysis of the mammalian Atg proteins could recently confirm the recruitment of Ulk1 proximal to these omegasomes [208]. The translocation of Ulk1, presumably in a complex with Atg13 and FIP200, is the initial step of autophagosome biogenesis and is completely abrogated in *FIP200–/–* cells [208]. The subsequent recruitment of the PI3K depends on Ulk1 and its kinase activity [208]. Recently, two groups found evidence for the mechanism by which Ulk1 and Ulk2 in turn negatively regulate mTORC1 signaling. Particularly, the phosphorylation of Raptor at numerous sites was strongly enhanced after overexpression of Ulk1. Interestingly, one of these residues (T792) is the abovementioned effector site through which AMPK negatively regulates mTORC1 activity [45]. The multiple Ulk1-dependent phosphorylation of Raptor either results in direct inhibition of mTORC1 kinase activity [209], or interferes with Raptor-substrate interaction [210], thus finally leads to reduced phosphorylation of mTORC1 downstream targets.

Apart from mTOR, Ulk1/2 is phosphorylated (probably on S317 and S777 or S555 according to different studies) by AMPK under glucose starvation and thereby activated [112, 203, 211, 212]. Under nutrient sufficiency phosphorylation of ULK1 S758 by active mTORC1 disrupts ULK1 interaction with, and hence activation by, AMPK [203]. Although the data concerning the role of ULK1/2 certain sites phosphorylation is rather discrepant it is clear that in mammals, phosphorylation of ULK1 by AMPK is strongly required for ULK function in the response to nutrient deprivation. Therefore, AMPK could control ULK1 via a two-pronged mechanism, ensuring activation only under the appropriate cellular conditions – firstly, by direct phosphorylation and secondly, by suppression of mTORC1-mediated ULK1 inhibition [212]. Several studies demonstrated that Ulk1 in addition directly interferes with mTORC1 downstream signaling and negatively regulates S6K1 activity, both in *Drosophila* and mammalian cells [213]. Taken together these data evidence that mTOR subnetwork occupy the key position in autophagic pathways.

5. Signaling up and downstream of mTORC2

In contrast to mTORC1, very little is known about the upstream regulation of TORC2. Rapamycin–FKBP12 complex does not bind directly to mTORC2, but long-term rapamycin treatment disrupts mTORC2 assembly in ~20% of cancer cell lines through an unknown mechanism [56]. It remains to be determined why rapamycin-mediated inhibition of mTORC2 assembly only occurs in certain cell types. One hypothesis suggests that some mTORC2 subunits could prevent the binding of rapamycin/FKBP12 complex to the mTOR FRB domain by the competing mechanism (reviewed in [62]). However, there are no enough data to support this model.

It seems that mTORC2 is activated in response to growth factors but is insensitive to nutrients and energetic stress, [214]. Thus, like TORC1, TORC2 can be stimulated by growth factors through PI3K [3]. Consequently, treatment with PI3K inhibitors can inhibit TORC2-mediated target phosphorylation [85]. Thus it was suggested that mTORC2 lies downstream of PI3K signaling [85]. Rheb which is known as a key upstream activator of mTORC1 showed negative and indirect effect on the regulation of mTORC2 both in *Drosophila* and mammalian cells [59]. Some data pointed on TSC1-TSC2 function in mTORC2 regulation [92]. Moreover, the TSC1/TSC2 complex was found to physically associate with mTORC2, but not with mTORC1. The molecular mechanism through which the TSC1/TSC2 complex promotes mTORC2 activation is unclear. It is also currently unknown whether some pathways that regulate TSC1/TSC2 ability to inhibit mTORC1, also influence on mTORC2 activation.

The best-characterized target of mTORC2 is AKT, which is phosphorylated at S473 upon TORC2 activation [53, 58, 85]. Numerous studies attempted to identify the crucial kinase(s) (often referred to as PDK2) responsible for the phosphorylation of S473 in Akt. Several enzymes are in the candidate list, including PDK1, integrin-linked kinase (ILK), Akt itself, DNA-dependent protein kinase catalytic subunit (DNA-PKcs) and mTORC2 [215]. Since mTORC2 complex fulfills the role of the Akt S473 kinase, mTORC2 has been identified as the PDK2 [85]. Akt is a member of the AGC kinase family (see above), which also includes S6Ks, serum glucocorticoid-induced protein kinase (SGKs), RSKs, and PKCs [62, 216]. mTORC2 has been shown to phosphorylate AKT, SGK and PKCα [85]. mTORC2 seems to regulate Akt by phosphorylation of its two different sites. The mTORC2-mediated Akt hydrophobic motif phosphorylation on the regulatory S473 site is dependent on growth factor signaling, whereas a basal activity of mTORC2 maintains the constitutive phosphorylation of Akt on T450 site in its turn motif [217]. This difference indicates that phosphorylation of the T450 and S473 sites on Akt by mTORC2 are separate events and might take place at different locations. It has been proposed that translocation of Akt to the plasma membrane coupled with its phosphorylation on T308 and S473 is a critical step in activation of Akt by growth factor signaling [217]. Phosphorylation of AKT on S473 enhances the activation phosphorylation motif at T308, which is absolutely required for AKT activity.

The major functions of mTORC2 include the regulation of cytoskeletal organization and the promotion of cell survival. If the last one is mediated apparently through AKT activation, the mechanisms, which realize mTORC2 function in cytoskeletal reorganization, are not obvious. Paxillin, which functions as a docking protein, localizing to the focal adhesions of adherent cells [218] has been shown to be highly phosphorylated at Tyr118. Knockdown of mTORC2 inhibited the phosphorylation of paxillin [3]. Rho, Rac and Cdc42, three best-characterized members of the Rho family of small GTPases, were demonstrated to be involved in actin cytoskeleton assembly and disassembly [219]. It was reported that mTORC2 may function as upstream regulator of Rho GTPases to regulate the actin cytoskeleton [3].

Interestingly, the TORC2-mediated activation of AKT places TORC2 upstream of TORC1 in the TOR signaling cascade. A most recent publication has highlighted a role for ribosomes in the activation of TORC2 [38]. The authors have found that active mTORC2 was physically associated with the ribosome, and insulin-stimulated PI3K signaling promoted mTORC2-ribosome binding. Interaction of mTORC2 with NIP7 (nuclear import 7, a protein responsible for ribosome biogenesis and rRNA maturation) was shown to be required for full activation of mTORC2 by insulin. Noteworthy, inhibition of protein translation had no effect on mTORC2 activation, supporting the notion that mTORC2 is activated by the ribosome, but not translation. Ribosome associated mTORC2 displays kinase activity toward AKT *in vitro*. Inhibition of PI3K activity blocks the interaction between the ribosome and mTORC2, as well as inhibits mTORC2 activation in response to insulin, confirming that NIP7-ribosome assembly activates mTORC2 downstream from PI3K. It appears that the mTORC2 components, Rictor and/or Sin1, which are not found in mTORC1, interact with the 60S subunit of ribosome. Interestingly, another study [220] has also recently reported the association of mTORC2 with the ribosome and proposed that the ribosomal association is important for the cotranslational phosphorylation of the AKT turn motif. These findings are coherent with very recent data that point on endoplasmic reticulum (ER), the cellular organelle highly enriched with ribosomes, as a major compartment of mTORC2 localization. Moreover, the signaling from growth factor does not change the ER localization of mTORC2 as well as its translocation to the plasma membrane. Besides it was suggested that the mTORC2-dependent phosphorylation of Akt on S473 occurs on the surface of ER [37]. These observations raise many interesting questions regarding the regulation of TORC2 and its ribosomal interactions, but it also indicates that additional levels of interplay between TORC2 and TORC1 may exist, as both complexes are linked to the process of ribosome biogenesis.

6. Crosstalk of mTORC1/2 and major cytokine signaling pathways

6.1. mTORC1/2 and Ras-MAP kinases pathways

Ras-Erk-RSKs

In addition to the PI3K–Akt pathway, activation of Ras-MAPK signaling can also stimulate mTORC1 activity. The Ras–mitogen-activated protein kinase (MAPK) pathway is a key signaling pathway that is involved in the regulation of normal cell proliferation, survival, growth and differentiation. This pathway includes the whole number of kinases, being regulated through phosphorylation in consecutive order. The Ras–MAPK signaling network has been the subject of intense research because mutations in (or overexpression of) many of the signaling components from this pathway are a hallmark of several human cancers and other human diseases [221]. The Ras–ERK (extracellular signal-regulated kinase-1 and -2) pathway has an established role in regulating transcription [222], but a connection between this pathway and translational regulation is less clear. Over the past few years, mitogen activated Ras–ERK pathway has been shown to trigger the activation of mTORC1 signaling. This is mediated by ERK and RSK dependent phosphorylations of TORC1 pathway components.

p90RSKs (also known as MAPKAP kinase 1 (mitogen-activated protein kinase-activated protein) kinase-1) are a family of Ser/Thr kinases that lies downstream of the Ras–MAPK cascade and has overlapping substrate specificity with Akt. The RSK isoforms are directly activated by ERK1/2 in response to growth factors, many polypeptide hormones, neurotransmitters, chemokines and other stimuli. RSKs phosphorylate several cytosolic and nuclear targets and they are involved in the regulation of different cellular processes, including cell survival, cell proliferation, cell growth and motility. Following the stimulation of cells with growth factors, RSKs are phosphorylated at multiple Ser and Thr residues by several kinases; these phosphorylation events are directly or indirectly initiated by the activation of the ERK/MAPK cascade [223]. Six different phosphorylation sites have been mapped in RSK1/2 (and are conserved in RSK3/4), of which four have been shown to be important for their activity

(S221, S363, S380 and T573 in human RSK1). Following mitogen stimulation, ERK1/2 phosphorylates T573 at the C-terminal domain (CTKD) activation loop of RSK, resulting in CTKD activation. ERK1/2 might also phosphorylate S363 (the turn motif) and T359 (unknown function) in the RSK linker region. The activated CTKD of RSK then autophosphorylates S380 in the hydrophobic motif, creating a docking site for PDK1. After binding, PDK1 phosphorylates the NTKD activation loop S221, leading to the complete activation of the protein and following phosphorylation of the substrates by the NTKD. The NTKD also phosphorylates S749 in the CTKD domain of RSK, differentially modulating the interaction of RSK isoforms with ERK1/2 and thereby completing a sequence of coordinated phosphorylation events and protein–protein interactions that culminate in RSK activation and downstream signaling throughout the cell [224]. Other factors that have been shown to be involved in the activation of RSK include the p38 MAPK, the ERK5 MAPK and fibroblast growth factor receptor-3 (FGFR3). RSK was found to phosphorylate TSC2 at the C-terminus S1798 [225] and, to a lesser extent, the two conserved Akt sites (S939 and T1462) and inactivates its suppressor function, thereby promoting mTOR signaling and translation (**Figure 7**). RSK mediated phosphorylation of TSC2 is additive to AKT mediated inhibitory modifications of TSC2, but how these phosphorylation events lead to TSC2 inhibition remains unclear.

Erk1/2 kinase itself also impacts the mTORC1 regulation. Thus, a number of additional sites on TSC2 were found to be weakly induced by PMA [89], including an ERK consensus site S664. This site, and a second site on TSC2, S540, was independently found to be directly phosphorylated by ERK and to contribute to ERK-mediated activation of mTORC1 signaling [226]. Strikingly, phosphorylation of S540 and/or S664 by ERK was found to disrupt the association between TSC1 and TSC2. This effect was also detected following phosphorylation of the TSC1/TSC2 complex *in vitro,* suggesting that it is direct and does not require other proteins.

In addition, it was recently shown that RSK also directly impacts the mTORC1 complex phosphorylating Raptor, and thereby promotes mTORC1 kinase activity [46]. RSK phosphorylates at least two evolutionarily conserved Raptor serine residues that lie within a region with no homology to known functional domains. Whereas S721 lies within a classical RSK consensus sequence (RXRXXpS/T), S719 is located within a minimal phosphoacceptor sequence (RXXpS) that was found to be sufficient in other RSK substrates, such as DAPK, c-Fos, and CREB. Although the underlying molecular mechanism of this was not fully defined, this study provided new insights into Ras–ERK signals to mTORC1. As tumor promoting phorbol esters and some growth factors activate mTORC1 signaling independently of AKT, phosphorylation of Raptor by RSK might provide a mechanism to overcome the inhibitory effects of PRAS40 inhibitory phosphorylation of TSC2 at S664 and S1798, respectively [89, 226, 227]. Collectively, these data suggest that ERK signaling activates mTORC1 through multisite phosphorylation events by both ERK and its downstream target RSK.

Erk1/2-RSK pathway also contributes to the mTORC1 downstream signaling, this includes RSK dependent *in vivo* and *in vitro* phosphorylation of eukaryotic translation initiation factor-4B (eIF4B) and rpS6 [180]. Although early studies indicated S6K1 and S6K2 as the major rpS6 kinases in somatic cells [228, 229], the role of RSK in regulating site-specific rpS6 phosphorylation and translation in somatic cells has been recently readdressed [230]. Particularly, *in vitro* and *in vivo* evidence suggests that S6Ks phosphorylate every site in rpS6, while RSK predominantly phosphorylates S235 and S236 [230]. Studies from *S6k1*/*S6k2*-knockout mice showed that there was minimal phosphorylation of rpS6 at S240/244, but there was persistent phosphorylation at S235/236 [173]. In accordance with this finding, RSK1 and RSK2 were shown to phosphorylate rpS6 on S235/236 in response to Ras–MAPK-pathway activation, using an mTOR-independent pathway [230]. The RSK mediated S235/236 phosphorylation correlated with formation of the translation pre-initiation complex and increased cap-dependent translation, pointing that RSK provides an additional mitogen- and oncogene-regulated input that links the ERK pathway to the regulation of translation initiation [230]. Translation initiation factor-4B is also phosphorylated by RSK and S6K on S422 [171, 180]. Therefore, phosphorylation and regulation of eIF4B function by RSK and S6K exemplifies the convergence of two major signaling pathways that are involved in translational control. Together, these findings suggest that the mitogen-activated Ras–ERK–RSK signaling module, in parallel with the PI3K–AKT pathway, contains several inputs to stimulate mTORC1 signaling.

6.2. mTORC1 and TNFα-IKKβ-TSC1 pathway

Although the activation of mTORC1 downstream of most cytokines including insulin and growth factors is likely to occur through the Akt and ERK signaling mechanisms described above, accumulating evidence suggests that other cytokines, such as tumor necrosis factor α (TNFα), can also induce mTORC1 activity. TNFα is a proinflammatory cytokine that is involved in many human diseases, including cancer [231, 232]. Early studies implicated the TNFα pathway in mTORC1 activation [233]. Recently, it has been shown that IKKβ (inhibitor of nuclear factor κB (NFκB) kinaseβ; also known as IKBKB), a major downstream kinase in the TNFα signaling pathway, can associate with and phosphorylates TSC1 at S487 and S511, resulting in the inhibition of TSC1–TSC2 and, therefore, the activation of mTORC1 [234]. *Tsc1–/–* mouse embryo fibroblasts expressing TSC1 mutants lacking these sites lose their responsiveness to TNFα for activation of mTORC1, whereas phosphomimetic mutation lead to a basal increase in mTORC1 signaling. Authors proposed a mechanism involving rapid dissociation of the complex and increased degradation of TSC1. However, the results suggest minimal effects on the stability of the TSC1–TSC2 complex, and the precise mechanism of acute complex inhibition by phosphorylation of these sites is not known. In certain human cancers, TNFα promotes vascular endothelial growth factor (vEGF) expression and angiogenesis through activated mTORC1 signaling as a result of IKKβ mediated suppression of TSC1 [234]. This has provided a plausible mechanism that could link inflammation to cancer pathogenesis. Moreover, TNFα also signals to AKT [231]. Activated AKT in turn induces IKKα (also known as CHUK), [232]. It has been shown that IKKα associates with mTORC1 in an AKT dependent manner [235]. Importantly, IKKα is required for efficient induction of mTORC1 activity by AKT in certain cancer cells [235, 236].

It remains unclear, however, how the association of IKKα with mTORC1 can result in the activation of mTORC1.

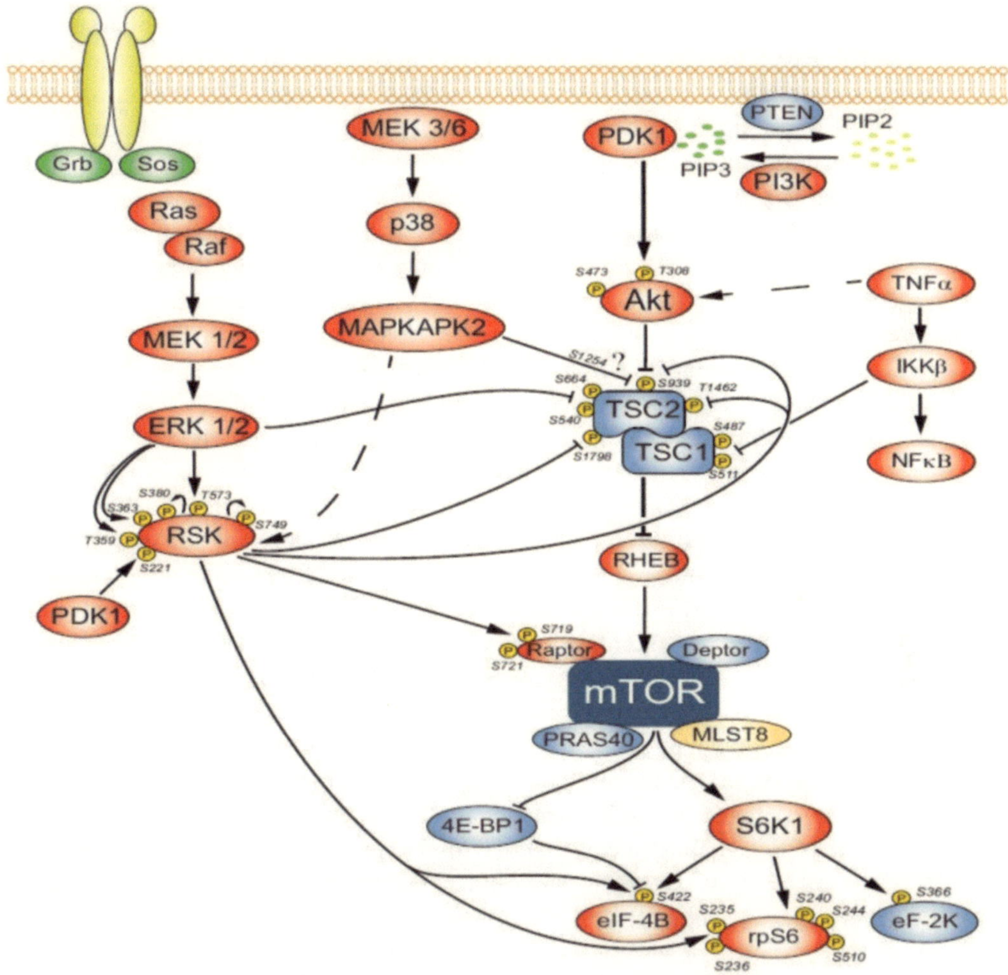

Figure 7. mTORC1 crosstalk with the major cytokine signaling pathways. MAPK pathway impinges on the mTORC1 signaling in a few ways. RSK phosphorylates TSC2 at the C-terminus and, to a lesser extent, the two conserved Akt sites thus inactivating its suppressive effect on mTORC1. RSK also directly impacts the mTORC1 complex by phosphorylation of Raptor and thereby upregulates mTORC1 kinase activity. Besides, RSK phosphorylates the rpS6 and eIF-4B to promote cap-dependent translation in response to Ras - MAPK-pathway activation. ERK1/2 kinase contributes to the activation of mTORC1 signaling through direct phosphorylation of TSC2 and probably through the disruption of the association between TSC1 and TSC2. Stress activated signaling pathway might also influence mTORC1 signaling through TSC2 phosphorylation by p38-activated MAPKAPK2 kinase. IKK β, a major downstream kinase in the TNF α signaling pathway, can associate with and phosphorylate TSC1 leading to the inhibition of TSC1/TSC2 and, therefore, the activation of mTORC1.

7. Conclusion

Maintenance of cellular energy homeostasis and life-sustaining activity requires their appropriately adaptation to the continually varying surrounding environment. This adaptation is provided by the differential expression of genes that is strictly controlled at the levels of transcription and translation. To provide the rapid response to the environmental cues cells switch vast number of intracellular signaling cascades that define the activity of key proteins responsible for transcription and translation regulation. This implies operative and directed changes in the activities of proteins mediating the signal transduction. Phosphorylation represents one of the most important intracellular regulatory molecular mechanisms since it provides the rapid and reversible activation or downregulation of protein activities. Not surprisingly, mTOR signaling network, which integrates and promotes the prompt respond to environmental changes is mainly regulated through this type of posttranslational modification. mTOR is known as a "switch master" that converts vast array of nutrient-, cytokine-, energy- and stress-sensitive signals into the alterations of cellular metabolism including protein and lipid biosynthesis and autophagy. Indeed such resources consuming processes as growth and proliferation could occur only under the conditions of nutrient and energy sufficiency. When energy or amino acids become limiting, cell growth needs to be restricted and protein production needs to be downregulated so that cells can use their limited resources to survive. mTORC1 contributes to overall cap-dependent translation including initiation and elongation steps by several different pathways. Significantly, all of these pathways use phosphorylation as common molecular mechanism of regulation. Most of the proteins from mTOR-dependent pathways (for instance TSC2, Akt, S6K, etc.) contain multiple phosphorylating sites, which mediate stimulating or negative effect on their activity. Some of mTOR partners are characterized by the hierarchical mode of phosphorylation (rpS6, Akt as the examples), whereby each previous phosphorylation opens the opportunity for the subsequent ones. Interestingly, one certain site could serve as phosphorylation target for more than one kinase, therefore implementing the competitive mechanism of regulation (for instance, eIF4B S422). The complexity of mTOR signaling increases due to the presence of positive or negative feedback loops as well as crosstalk with other pathways. The number of reported phosphorylation sites throughout mTOR pathways constantly increases although the precise molecular meaning of several already discovered phosphorylation events remains unclear. This is also true to some molecular mechanisms of mTORC1 and especially mTORC2 functioning. About mTORC1 signaling, a number of issues remain unresolved. For example, aside from S6K, 4EBP1 and ULK1, the downstream direct targets that mediate the cellular effects of TORC1 signaling are largely unaccounted for. In addition, how the specificity of TORC1 signaling is achieved and how multiple signals are integrated is not known. Concerning TORC2, the upstream regulators are poorly defined. This knowledge seems to be of great significance since mTOR is considered a central node of intracellular signaling network and deregulation of its activity strongly contributes to the wide spectrum of human diseases. Further studies will give us a better understanding of the whole picture of mTORC1/mTORC2 functioning that could be applied to the development of new approaches to the treatment of mTOR-associated diseases.

Author details

Elena Tchevkina
Corresponding Author
Oncogenes Regulation Department, N.N. Blokhin Russian Cancer Research Center, Moscow, Russia

Andrey Komelkov
Oncogenes Regulation Department, N.N. Blokhin Russian Cancer Research Center, Moscow, Russia

8. References

[1] Dennis PB, Jaeschke A, Saitoh M, Fowler B, Kozma SC, et al. (2001) Mammalian TOR: a homeostatic ATP sensor. Science.294(5544):1102-5. Epub 2001/11/03.
[2] Inoki K, Zhu T, Guan KL. (2003) TSC2 mediates cellular energy response to control cell growth and survival. Cell.115(5):577-90. Epub 2003/12/04.
[3] Jacinto E, Loewith R, Schmidt A, Lin S, Ruegg MA, et al. (2004) Mammalian TOR complex 2 controls the actin cytoskeleton and is rapamycin insensitive. Nature cell biology.6(11):1122-8. Epub 2004/10/07.
[4] Sarbassov DD, Ali SM, Kim DH, Guertin DA, Latek RR, et al. (2004) Rictor, a novel binding partner of mTOR, defines a rapamycin-insensitive and raptor-independent pathway that regulates the cytoskeleton. Current biology: CB.14(14):1296-302. Epub 2004/07/23.
[5] Loewith R, Jacinto E, Wullschleger S, Lorberg A, Crespo JL, et al. (2002) Two TOR complexes, only one of which is rapamycin sensitive, have distinct roles in cell growth control. Molecular cell.10(3):457-68. Epub 2002/11/01.
[6] Vezina C, Kudelski A, Sehgal SN. (1975) Rapamycin (AY-22,989), a new antifungal antibiotic. I. Taxonomy of the producing streptomycete and isolation of the active principle. The Journal of antibiotics.28(10):721-6. Epub 1975/10/01.
[7] Eng CP, Sehgal SN, Vezina C. (1984) Activity of rapamycin (AY-22,989) against transplanted tumors. The Journal of antibiotics.37(10):1231-7. Epub 1984/10/01.
[8] Douros J, Suffness M. (1981) New antitumor substances of natural origin. Cancer treatment reviews.8(1):63-87. Epub 1981/03/01.
[9] Sehgal SN, Baker H, Vezina C. (1975) Rapamycin (AY-22,989), a new antifungal antibiotic. II. Fermentation, isolation and characterization. The Journal of antibiotics.28(10):727-32. Epub 1975/10/01.
[10] Cafferkey R, Young PR, McLaughlin MM, Bergsma DJ, Koltin Y, et al. (1993) Dominant missense mutations in a novel yeast protein related to mammalian phosphatidylinositol 3-kinase and VPS34 abrogate rapamycin cytotoxicity. Mol Cell Biol.13(10):6012-23. Epub 1993/10/01.
[11] Heitman J, Movva NR, Hall MN. (1991) Targets for cell cycle arrest by the immunosuppressant rapamycin in yeast. Science.253(5022):905-9. Epub 1991/08/23.
[12] Chen J, Zheng XF, Brown EJ, Schreiber SL. (1995) Identification of an 11-kDa FKBP12-rapamycin-binding domain within the 289-kDa FKBP12-rapamycin-associated protein and characterization of a critical serine residue. Proceedings of the National Academy of Sciences of the United States of America.92(11):4947-51. Epub 1995/05/23.

[13] Choi J, Chen J, Schreiber SL, Clardy J. (1996) Structure of the FKBP12-rapamycin complex interacting with the binding domain of human FRAP. Science.273(5272):239-42. Epub 1996/07/12.

[14] Sabers CJ, Martin MM, Brunn GJ, Williams JM, Dumont FJ, et al. (1995) Isolation of a protein target of the FKBP12-rapamycin complex in mammalian cells. The Journal of biological chemistry.270(2):815-22. Epub 1995/01/13.

[15] Brown EJ, Albers MW, Shin TB, Ichikawa K, Keith CT, et al. (1994) A mammalian protein targeted by G1-arresting rapamycin-receptor complex. Nature.369(6483):756-8. Epub 1994/06/30.

[16] Chiu MI, Katz H, Berlin V. (1994) RAPT1, a mammalian homolog of yeast Tor, interacts with the FKBP12/rapamycin complex. Proceedings of the National Academy of Sciences of the United States of America.91(26):12574-8. Epub 1994/12/20.

[17] Sabatini DM, Erdjument-Bromage H, Lui M, Tempst P, Snyder SH. (1994) RAFT1: a mammalian protein that binds to FKBP12 in a rapamycin-dependent fashion and is homologous to yeast TORs. Cell.78(1):35-43. Epub 1994/07/15.

[18] Chen Y, Chen H, Rhoad AE, Warner L, Caggiano TJ, et al. (1994) A putative sirolimus (rapamycin) effector protein. Biochemical and biophysical research communications.203(1):1-7. Epub 1994/08/30.

[19] Keith CT, Schreiber SL. (1995) PIK-related kinases: DNA repair, recombination, and cell cycle checkpoints. Science.270(5233):50-1. Epub 1995/10/06.

[20] Kunz J, Henriquez R, Schneider U, Deuter-Reinhard M, Movva NR, et al. (1993) Target of rapamycin in yeast, TOR2, is an essential phosphatidylinositol kinase homolog required for G1 progression. Cell.73(3):585-96. Epub 1993/05/07.

[21] Wiederrecht GJ, Sabers CJ, Brunn GJ, Martin MM, Dumont FJ, et al. (1995) Mechanism of action of rapamycin: new insights into the regulation of G1-phase progression in eukaryotic cells. Progress in cell cycle research.1:53-71. Epub 1995/01/01.

[22] Hay N, Sonenberg N. (2004) Upstream and downstream of mTOR. Genes & development.18(16):1926-45. Epub 2004/08/18.

[23] Janus A, Robak T, Smolewski P. (2005) The mammalian target of the rapamycin (mTOR) kinase pathway: its role in tumourigenesis and targeted antitumour therapy. Cellular & molecular biology letters.10(3):479-98. Epub 2005/10/12.

[24] Gangloff YG, Mueller M, Dann SG, Svoboda P, Sticker M, et al. (2004) Disruption of the mouse mTOR gene leads to early postimplantation lethality and prohibits embryonic stem cell development. Mol Cell Biol.24(21):9508-16. Epub 2004/10/16.

[25] Murakami M, Ichisaka T, Maeda M, Oshiro N, Hara K, et al. (2004) mTOR is essential for growth and proliferation in early mouse embryos and embryonic stem cells. Mol Cell Biol.24(15):6710-8. Epub 2004/07/16.

[26] Gingras AC, Raught B, Sonenberg N. (2001) Regulation of translation initiation by FRAP/mTOR. Genes & development.15(7):807-26. Epub 2001/04/12.

[27] Perry J, Kleckner N. (2003) The ATRs, ATMs, and TORs are giant HEAT repeat proteins. Cell.112(2):151-5. Epub 2003/01/30.

[28] Foster KG, Fingar DC. (2010) Mammalian target of rapamycin (mTOR): conducting the cellular signaling symphony. The Journal of biological chemistry.285(19):14071-7. Epub 2010/03/17.

[29] Soliman GA, Acosta-Jaquez HA, Dunlop EA, Ekim B, Maj NE, et al. (2010) mTOR Ser-2481 autophosphorylation monitors mTORC-specific catalytic activity and clarifies rapamycin mechanism of action. The Journal of biological chemistry.285(11):7866-79. Epub 2009/12/22.
[30] Caron E, Ghosh S, Matsuoka Y, Ashton-Beaucage D, Therrien M, et al. (2010) A comprehensive map of the mTOR signaling network. Molecular systems biology.6:453. Epub 2010/12/24.
[31] Acosta-Jaquez HA, Keller JA, Foster KG, Ekim B, Soliman GA, et al. (2009) Site-specific mTOR phosphorylation promotes mTORC1-mediated signaling and cell growth. Mol Cell Biol.29(15):4308-24. Epub 2009/06/03.
[32] Chiang GG, Abraham RT. (2005) Phosphorylation of mammalian target of rapamycin (mTOR) at Ser-2448 is mediated by p70S6 kinase. The Journal of biological chemistry.280(27):25485-90. Epub 2005/05/19.
[33] Peterson RT, Beal PA, Comb MJ, Schreiber SL. (2000) FKBP12-rapamycin-associated protein (FRAP) autophosphorylates at serine 2481 under translationally repressive conditions. The Journal of biological chemistry.275(10):7416-23. Epub 2000/03/04.
[34] Edinger AL, Linardic CM, Chiang GG, Thompson CB, Abraham RT. (2003) Differential effects of rapamycin on mammalian target of rapamycin signaling functions in mammalian cells. Cancer research.63(23):8451-60. Epub 2003/12/18.
[35] Russell RC, Fang C, Guan KL. (2011) An emerging role for TOR signaling in mammalian tissue and stem cell physiology. Development.138(16):3343-56. Epub 2011/07/28.
[36] Sancak Y, Bar-Peled L, Zoncu R, Markhard AL, Nada S, et al. (2010) Ragulator-Rag complex targets mTORC1 to the lysosomal surface and is necessary for its activation by amino acids. Cell.141(2):290-303. Epub 2010/04/13.
[37] Boulbes DR, Shaiken T, Sarbassov dos D. (2011) Endoplasmic reticulum is a main localization site of mTORC2. Biochemical and biophysical research communications.413(1):46-52. Epub 2011/08/27.
[38] Zinzalla V, Stracka D, Oppliger W, Hall MN. (2011) Activation of mTORC2 by association with the ribosome. Cell.144(5):757-68. Epub 2011/03/08.
[39] Kim JE, Chen J. (2000) Cytoplasmic-nuclear shuttling of FKBP12-rapamycin-associated protein is involved in rapamycin-sensitive signaling and translation initiation. Proceedings of the National Academy of Sciences of the United States of America.97(26):14340-5. Epub 2000/12/13.
[40] Yip CK, Murata K, Walz T, Sabatini DM, Kang SA. (2010) Structure of the human mTOR complex I and its implications for rapamycin inhibition. Molecular cell.38(5):768-74. Epub 2010/06/15.
[41] Peterson TR, Laplante M, Thoreen CC, Sancak Y, Kang SA, et al. (2009) DEPTOR is an mTOR inhibitor frequently overexpressed in multiple myeloma cells and required for their survival. Cell.137(5):873-86. Epub 2009/05/19.
[42] Kim DH, Sarbassov DD, Ali SM, King JE, Latek RR, et al. (2002) mTOR interacts with raptor to form a nutrient-sensitive complex that signals to the cell growth machinery. Cell.110(2):163-75. Epub 2002/08/02.
[43] Hara K, Maruki Y, Long X, Yoshino K, Oshiro N, et al. (2002) Raptor, a binding partner of target of rapamycin (TOR), mediates TOR action. Cell.110(2):177-89. Epub 2002/08/02.

[44] Zhou H, Huang S. (2010) The complexes of mammalian target of rapamycin. Current protein & peptide science.11(6):409-24. Epub 2010/05/25.

[45] Gwinn DM, Shackelford DB, Egan DF, Mihaylova MM, Mery A, et al. (2008) AMPK phosphorylation of raptor mediates a metabolic checkpoint. Molecular cell.30(2):214-26. Epub 2008/04/29.

[46] Carriere A, Cargnello M, Julien LA, Gao H, Bonneil E, et al. (2008) Oncogenic MAPK signaling stimulates mTORC1 activity by promoting RSK-mediated raptor phosphorylation. Current biology : CB.18(17):1269-77. Epub 2008/08/30.

[47] Wang L, Lawrence JC, Jr., Sturgill TW, Harris TE. (2009) Mammalian target of rapamycin complex 1 (mTORC1) activity is associated with phosphorylation of raptor by mTOR. The Journal of biological chemistry.284(22):14693-7. Epub 2009/04/07.

[48] Sancak Y, Thoreen CC, Peterson TR, Lindquist RA, Kang SA, et al. (2007) PRAS40 is an insulin-regulated inhibitor of the mTORC1 protein kinase. Molecular cell.25(6):903-15. Epub 2007/03/28.

[49] Kovacina KS, Park GY, Bae SS, Guzzetta AW, Schaefer E, et al. (2003) Identification of a proline-rich Akt substrate as a 14-3-3 binding partner. The Journal of biological chemistry.278(12):10189-94. Epub 2003/01/14.

[50] Oshiro N, Takahashi R, Yoshino K, Tanimura K, Nakashima A, et al. (2007) The proline-rich Akt substrate of 40 kDa (PRAS40) is a physiological substrate of mammalian target of rapamycin complex 1. The Journal of biological chemistry.282(28):20329-39. Epub 2007/05/23.

[51] Wang L, Harris TE, Lawrence JC, Jr. (2008) Regulation of proline-rich Akt substrate of 40 kDa (PRAS40) function by mammalian target of rapamycin complex 1 (mTORC1)-mediated phosphorylation. The Journal of biological chemistry.283(23):15619-27. Epub 2008/03/29.

[52] Kim DH, Sarbassov DD, Ali SM, Latek RR, Guntur KV, et al. (2003) GbetaL, a positive regulator of the rapamycin-sensitive pathway required for the nutrient-sensitive interaction between raptor and mTOR. Molecular cell.11(4):895-904. Epub 2003/04/30.

[53] Frias MA, Thoreen CC, Jaffe JD, Schroder W, Sculley T, et al. (2006) mSin1 is necessary for Akt/PKB phosphorylation, and its isoforms define three distinct mTORC2s. Current biology : CB.16(18):1865-70. Epub 2006/08/22.

[54] Pearce LR, Huang X, Boudeau J, Pawlowski R, Wullschleger S, et al. (2007) Identification of Protor as a novel Rictor-binding component of mTOR complex-2. The Biochemical journal.405(3):513-22. Epub 2007/04/28.

[55] Woo SY, Kim DH, Jun CB, Kim YM, Haar EV, et al. (2007) PRR5, a novel component of mTOR complex 2, regulates platelet-derived growth factor receptor beta expression and signaling. The Journal of biological chemistry.282(35):25604-12. Epub 2007/06/30.

[56] Sarbassov DD, Ali SM, Sengupta S, Sheen JH, Hsu PP, et al. (2006) Prolonged rapamycin treatment inhibits mTORC2 assembly and Akt/PKB. Molecular cell.22(2):159-68. Epub 2006/04/11.

[57] Vander Haar E, Lee SI, Bandhakavi S, Griffin TJ, Kim DH. (2007) Insulin signalling to mTOR mediated by the Akt/PKB substrate PRAS40. Nature cell biology.9(3):316-23. Epub 2007/02/06.

[58] Jacinto E, Facchinetti V, Liu D, Soto N, Wei S, et al. (2006) SIN1/MIP1 maintains rictor-mTOR complex integrity and regulates Akt phosphorylation and substrate specificity. Cell.127(1):125-37. Epub 2006/09/12.
[59] Yang Q, Inoki K, Ikenoue T, Guan KL. (2006) Identification of Sin1 as an essential TORC2 component required for complex formation and kinase activity. Genes & development.20(20):2820-32. Epub 2006/10/18.
[60] Wilkinson MG, Pino TS, Tournier S, Buck V, Martin H, et al. (1999) Sin1: an evolutionarily conserved component of the eukaryotic SAPK pathway. The EMBO journal.18(15):4210-21. Epub 1999/08/03.
[61] Schroder WA, Buck M, Cloonan N, Hancock JF, Suhrbier A, et al. (2007) Human Sin1 contains Ras-binding and pleckstrin homology domains and suppresses Ras signalling. Cellular signalling.19(6):1279-89. Epub 2007/02/17.
[62] Yang Q, Guan KL. (2007) Expanding mTOR signaling. Cell research.17(8):666-81. Epub 2007/08/08.
[63] Thedieck K, Polak P, Kim ML, Molle KD, Cohen A, et al. (2007) PRAS40 and PRR5-like protein are new mTOR interactors that regulate apoptosis. PloS one.2(11):e1217. Epub 2007/11/22.
[64] Tee AR, Fingar DC, Manning BD, Kwiatkowski DJ, Cantley LC, et al. (2002) Tuberous sclerosis complex-1 and -2 gene products function together to inhibit mammalian target of rapamycin (mTOR)-mediated downstream signaling. Proceedings of the National Academy of Sciences of the United States of America.99(21):13571-6. Epub 2002/09/25.
[65] Manning BD, Cantley LC. (2003) United at last: the tuberous sclerosis complex gene products connect the phosphoinositide 3-kinase/Akt pathway to mammalian target of rapamycin (mTOR) signalling. Biochemical Society transactions.31(Pt 3):573-8. Epub 2003/05/30.
[66] Kandt RS, Haines JL, Smith M, Northrup H, Gardner RJ, et al. (1992) Linkage of an important gene locus for tuberous sclerosis to a chromosome 16 marker for polycystic kidney disease. Nature genetics.2(1):37-41. Epub 1992/09/01.
[67] Consortium ECTS. (1993) Identification and characterization of the tuberous sclerosis gene on chromosome 16. Cell.75(7):1305-15. Epub 1993/12/31.
[68] van Slegtenhorst M, de Hoogt R, Hermans C, Nellist M, Janssen B, et al. (1997) Identification of the tuberous sclerosis gene TSC1 on chromosome 9q34. Science.277(5327):805-8. Epub 1997/08/08.
[69] Hodges AK, Li S, Maynard J, Parry L, Braverman R, et al. (2001) Pathological mutations in TSC1 and TSC2 disrupt the interaction between hamartin and tuberin. Human molecular genetics.10(25):2899-905. Epub 2001/12/14.
[70] Garami A, Zwartkruis FJ, Nobukuni T, Joaquin M, Roccio M, et al. (2003) Insulin activation of Rheb, a mediator of mTOR/S6K/4E-BP signaling, is inhibited by TSC1 and 2. Molecular cell.11(6):1457-66. Epub 2003/06/25.
[71] Benvenuto G, Li S, Brown SJ, Braverman R, Vass WC, et al. (2000) The tuberous sclerosis-1 (TSC1) gene product hamartin suppresses cell growth and augments the expression of the TSC2 product tuberin by inhibiting its ubiquitination. Oncogene.19(54):6306-16. Epub 2001/02/15.

[72] Chong-Kopera H, Inoki K, Li Y, Zhu T, Garcia-Gonzalo FR, et al. (2006) TSC1 stabilizes TSC2 by inhibiting the interaction between TSC2 and the HERC1 ubiquitin ligase. The Journal of biological chemistry.281(13):8313-6. Epub 2006/02/09.

[73] Tee AR, Blenis J, Proud CG. (2005) Analysis of mTOR signaling by the small G-proteins, Rheb and RhebL1. FEBS letters.579(21):4763-8. Epub 2005/08/16.

[74] Long X, Lin Y, Ortiz-Vega S, Yonezawa K, Avruch J. (2005) Rheb binds and regulates the mTOR kinase. Current biology : CB.15(8):702-13. Epub 2005/04/28.

[75] Bai X, Ma D, Liu A, Shen X, Wang QJ, et al. (2007) Rheb activates mTOR by antagonizing its endogenous inhibitor, FKBP38. Science.318(5852):977-80. Epub 2007/11/10.

[76] Rosner M, Hofer K, Kubista M, Hengstschlager M. (2003) Cell size regulation by the human TSC tumor suppressor proteins depends on PI3K and FKBP38. Oncogene.22(31):4786-98. Epub 2003/08/02.

[77] Manning BD, Cantley LC. (2007) AKT/PKB signaling: navigating downstream. Cell.129(7):1261-74. Epub 2007/07/03.

[78] Zhao L, Vogt PK. (2010) Hot-spot mutations in p110alpha of phosphatidylinositol 3-kinase (pI3K): differential interactions with the regulatory subunit p85 and with RAS. Cell Cycle.9(3):596-600. Epub 2009/12/17.

[79] Franke TF, Kaplan DR, Cantley LC, Toker A. (1997) Direct regulation of the Akt proto-oncogene product by phosphatidylinositol-3,4-bisphosphate. Science.275(5300):665-8. Epub 1997/01/31.

[80] Martelli AM, Evangelisti C, Chiarini F, Grimaldi C, Cappellini A, et al. (2010) The emerging role of the phosphatidylinositol 3-kinase/Akt/mammalian target of rapamycin signaling network in normal myelopoiesis and leukemogenesis. Biochimica et biophysica acta.1803(9):991-1002. Epub 2010/04/20.

[81] McManus EJ, Collins BJ, Ashby PR, Prescott AR, Murray-Tait V, et al. (2004) The in vivo role of PtdIns(3,4,5)P3 binding to PDK1 PH domain defined by knockin mutation. The EMBO journal.23(10):2071-82. Epub 2004/04/30.

[82] Hay N. (2005) The Akt-mTOR tango and its relevance to cancer. Cancer Cell.8(3):179-83. Epub 2005/09/20.

[83] Toker A, Newton AC. (2000) Cellular signaling: pivoting around PDK-1. Cell.103(2):185-8. Epub 2000/11/01.

[84] Guertin DA, Stevens DM, Thoreen CC, Burds AA, Kalaany NY, et al. (2006) Ablation in mice of the mTORC components raptor, rictor, or mLST8 reveals that mTORC2 is required for signaling to Akt-FOXO and PKCalpha, but not S6K1. Developmental cell.11(6):859-71. Epub 2006/12/05.

[85] Sarbassov DD, Guertin DA, Ali SM, Sabatini DM. (2005) Phosphorylation and regulation of Akt/PKB by the rictor-mTOR complex. Science.307(5712):1098-101. Epub 2005/02/19.

[86] Potter CJ, Pedraza LG, Xu T. (2002) Akt regulates growth by directly phosphorylating Tsc2. Nature cell biology.4(9):658-65. Epub 2002/08/13.

[87] Inoki K, Li Y, Zhu T, Wu J, Guan KL. (2002) TSC2 is phosphorylated and inhibited by Akt and suppresses mTOR signalling. Nature cell biology.4(9):648-57. Epub 2002/08/13.

[88] Dan HC, Sun M, Yang L, Feldman RI, Sui XM, et al. (2002) Phosphatidylinositol 3-kinase/Akt pathway regulates tuberous sclerosis tumor suppressor complex by

phosphorylation of tuberin. The Journal of biological chemistry.277(38):35364-70. Epub 2002/08/09.

[89] Ballif BA, Roux PP, Gerber SA, MacKeigan JP, Blenis J, et al. (2005) Quantitative phosphorylation profiling of the ERK/p90 ribosomal S6 kinase-signaling cassette and its targets, the tuberous sclerosis tumor suppressors. Proceedings of the National Academy of Sciences of the United States of America.102(3):667-72. Epub 2005/01/14.

[90] Gao X, Zhang Y, Arrazola P, Hino O, Kobayashi T, et al. (2002) Tsc tumour suppressor proteins antagonize amino-acid-TOR signalling. Nature cell biology.4(9):699-704. Epub 2002/08/13.

[91] Tee AR, Proud CG. (2002) Caspase cleavage of initiation factor 4E-binding protein 1 yields a dominant inhibitor of cap-dependent translation and reveals a novel regulatory motif. Mol Cell Biol.22(6):1674-83. Epub 2002/02/28.

[92] Huang J, Manning BD. (2008) The TSC1-TSC2 complex: a molecular switchboard controlling cell growth. The Biochemical journal.412(2):179-90. Epub 2008/05/10.

[93] Cai SL, Tee AR, Short JD, Bergeron JM, Kim J, et al. (2006) Activity of TSC2 is inhibited by AKT-mediated phosphorylation and membrane partitioning. The Journal of cell biology.173(2):279-89. Epub 2006/04/26.

[94] Nellist M, Goedbloed MA, de Winter C, Verhaaf B, Jankie A, et al. (2002) Identification and characterization of the interaction between tuberin and 14-3-3zeta. The Journal of biological chemistry.277(42):39417-24. Epub 2002/08/15.

[95] Shumway SD, Li Y, Xiong Y. (2003) 14-3-3beta binds to and negatively regulates the tuberous sclerosis complex 2 (TSC2) tumor suppressor gene product, tuberin. The Journal of biological chemistry.278(4):2089-92. Epub 2002/12/07.

[96] Dong J, Pan D. (2004) Tsc2 is not a critical target of Akt during normal Drosophila development. Genes & development.18(20):2479-84. Epub 2004/10/07.

[97] Wang YH, Huang ML. (2009) Reduction of Lobe leads to TORC1 hypoactivation that induces ectopic Jak/STAT signaling to impair Drosophila eye development. Mechanisms of development.126(10):781-90. Epub 2009/09/08.

[98] Jacinto E, Hall MN. (2003) Tor signalling in bugs, brain and brawn. Nature reviews Molecular cell biology.4(2):117-26. Epub 2003/02/04.

[99] Long X, Ortiz-Vega S, Lin Y, Avruch J. (2005) Rheb binding to mammalian target of rapamycin (mTOR) is regulated by amino acid sufficiency. The Journal of biological chemistry.280(25):23433-6. Epub 2005/05/10.

[100] Smith EM, Finn SG, Tee AR, Browne GJ, Proud CG. (2005) The tuberous sclerosis protein TSC2 is not required for the regulation of the mammalian target of rapamycin by amino acids and certain cellular stresses. The Journal of biological chemistry.280(19):18717-27. Epub 2005/03/18.

[101] Wang X, Proud CG. (2009) Nutrient control of TORC1, a cell-cycle regulator. Trends in cell biology.19(6):260-7. Epub 2009/05/08.

[102] Roccio M, Bos JL, Zwartkruis FJ. (2006) Regulation of the small GTPase Rheb by amino acids. Oncogene.25(5):657-64. Epub 2005/09/20.

[103] Byfield MP, Murray JT, Backer JM. (2005) hVps34 is a nutrient-regulated lipid kinase required for activation of p70 S6 kinase. The Journal of biological chemistry.280(38):33076-82. Epub 2005/07/29.

[104] Nobukuni T, Joaquin M, Roccio M, Dann SG, Kim SY, et al. (2005) Amino acids mediate mTOR/raptor signaling through activation of class 3 phosphatidylinositol 3OH-kinase. Proceedings of the National Academy of Sciences of the United States of America.102(40):14238-43. Epub 2005/09/24.

[105] Findlay GM, Yan L, Procter J, Mieulet V, Lamb RF. (2007) A MAP4 kinase related to Ste20 is a nutrient-sensitive regulator of mTOR signalling. The Biochemical journal.403(1):13-20. Epub 2007/01/27.

[106] Juhasz G, Hill JH, Yan Y, Sass M, Baehrecke EH, et al. (2008) The class III PI(3)K Vps34 promotes autophagy and endocytosis but not TOR signaling in Drosophila. The Journal of cell biology.181(4):655-66. Epub 2008/05/14.

[107] Yan L, Mieulet V, Burgess D, Findlay GM, Sully K, et al. (2010) PP2A T61 epsilon is an inhibitor of MAP4K3 in nutrient signaling to mTOR. Molecular cell.37(5):633-42. Epub 2010/03/17.

[108] Gulati P, Gaspers LD, Dann SG, Joaquin M, Nobukuni T, et al. (2008) Amino acids activate mTOR complex 1 via Ca2+/CaM signaling to hVps34. Cell metabolism.7(5):456-65. Epub 2008/05/08.

[109] Backer JM. (2008) The regulation and function of Class III PI3Ks: novel roles for Vps34. The Biochemical journal.410(1):1-17. Epub 2008/01/25.

[110] Tassa A, Roux MP, Attaix D, Bechet DM. (2003) Class III phosphoinositide 3-kinase--Beclin1 complex mediates the amino acid-dependent regulation of autophagy in C2C12 myotubes. The Biochemical journal.376(Pt 3):577-86. Epub 2003/09/12.

[111] Sancak Y, Peterson TR, Shaul YD, Lindquist RA, Thoreen CC, et al. (2008) The Rag GTPases bind raptor and mediate amino acid signaling to mTORC1. Science.320(5882):1496-501. Epub 2008/05/24.

[112] Kim E, Goraksha-Hicks P, Li L, Neufeld TP, Guan KL. (2008) Regulation of TORC1 by Rag GTPases in nutrient response. Nature cell biology.10(8):935-45. Epub 2008/07/08.

[113] Exton JH. (2002) Phospholipase D-structure, regulation and function. Reviews of physiology, biochemistry and pharmacology.144:1-94. Epub 2002/05/04.

[114] Foster DA. (2007) Regulation of mTOR by phosphatidic acid? Cancer research.67(1):1-4. Epub 2007/01/11.

[115] Fang Y, Vilella-Bach M, Bachmann R, Flanigan A, Chen J. (2001) Phosphatidic acid-mediated mitogenic activation of mTOR signaling. Science.294(5548):1942-5. Epub 2001/12/01.

[116] Hornberger TA, Chu WK, Mak YW, Hsiung JW, Huang SA, et al. (2006) The role of phospholipase D and phosphatidic acid in the mechanical activation of mTOR signaling in skeletal muscle. Proceedings of the National Academy of Sciences of the United States of America.103(12):4741-6. Epub 2006/03/16.

[117] Takahara T, Hara K, Yonezawa K, Sorimachi H, Maeda T. (2006) Nutrient-dependent multimerization of the mammalian target of rapamycin through the N-terminal HEAT repeat region. The Journal of biological chemistry.281(39):28605-14. Epub 2006/07/28.

[118] Park IH, Bachmann R, Shirazi H, Chen J. (2002) Regulation of ribosomal S6 kinase 2 by mammalian target of rapamycin. The Journal of biological chemistry.277(35):31423-9. Epub 2002/06/28.

[119] Lim HK, Choi YA, Park W, Lee T, Ryu SH, et al. (2003) Phosphatidic acid regulates systemic inflammatory responses by modulating the Akt-mammalian target of

rapamycin-p70 S6 kinase 1 pathway. The Journal of biological chemistry.278(46):45117-27. Epub 2003/09/10.

[120] Chen Y, Rodrik V, Foster DA. (2005) Alternative phospholipase D/mTOR survival signal in human breast cancer cells. Oncogene.24(4):672-9. Epub 2004/12/08.

[121] Hui L, Abbas T, Pielak RM, Joseph T, Bargonetti J, et al. (2004) Phospholipase D elevates the level of MDM2 and suppresses DNA damage-induced increases in p53. Mol Cell Biol.24(13):5677-86. Epub 2004/06/17.

[122] Ohguchi K, Banno Y, Nakagawa Y, Akao Y, Nozawa Y. (2005) Negative regulation of melanogenesis by phospholipase D1 through mTOR/p70 S6 kinase 1 signaling in mouse B16 melanoma cells. Journal of cellular physiology.205(3):444-51. Epub 2005/05/17.

[123] Fukami K, Takenawa T. (1992) Phosphatidic acid that accumulates in platelet-derived growth factor-stimulated Balb/c 3T3 cells is a potential mitogenic signal. The Journal of biological chemistry.267(16):10988-93. Epub 1992/06/05.

[124] Sun Y, Fang Y, Yoon MS, Zhang C, Roccio M, et al. (2008) Phospholipase D1 is an effector of Rheb in the mTOR pathway. Proceedings of the National Academy of Sciences of the United States of America.105(24):8286-91. Epub 2008/06/14.

[125] Ha SH, Kim DH, Kim IS, Kim JH, Lee MN, et al. (2006) PLD2 forms a functional complex with mTOR/raptor to transduce mitogenic signals. Cellular signalling.18(12):2283-91. Epub 2006/07/14.

[126] Toschi A, Lee E, Xu L, Garcia A, Gadir N, et al. (2009) Regulation of mTORC1 and mTORC2 complex assembly by phosphatidic acid: competition with rapamycin. Mol Cell Biol.29(6):1411-20. Epub 2008/12/31.

[127] Xu L, Salloum D, Medlin PS, Saqcena M, Yellen P, et al. (2011) Phospholipase D mediates nutrient input to mammalian target of rapamycin complex 1 (mTORC1). The Journal of biological chemistry.286(29):25477-86. Epub 2011/05/31.

[128] Frohman MA, Morris AJ. (1999) Phospholipase D structure and regulation. Chemistry and physics of lipids.98(1-2):127-40. Epub 1999/06/08.

[129] Knizhnik AV, Kovaleva OV, Komelkov AV, Trukhanova LS, Rybko VA, et al. (2012) Arf6 promotes cell proliferation via the PLD-mTORC1 and p38MAPK pathways. Journal of cellular biochemistry.113(1):360-71. Epub 2011/09/20.

[130] Hardie DG. (2007) AMP-activated/SNF1 protein kinases: conserved guardians of cellular energy. Nature reviews Molecular cell biology.8(10):774-85. Epub 2007/08/23.

[131] Kahn BB, Alquier T, Carling D, Hardie DG. (2005) AMP-activated protein kinase: ancient energy gauge provides clues to modern understanding of metabolism. Cell metabolism.1(1):15-25. Epub 2005/08/02.

[132] Shaw RJ. (2009) LKB1 and AMP-activated protein kinase control of mTOR signalling and growth. Acta Physiol (Oxf).196(1):65-80. Epub 2009/02/28.

[133] Sanders MJ, Grondin PO, Hegarty BD, Snowden MA, Carling D. (2007) Investigating the mechanism for AMP activation of the AMP-activated protein kinase cascade. The Biochemical journal.403(1):139-48. Epub 2006/12/07.

[134] Oakhill JS, Steel R, Chen ZP, Scott JW, Ling N, et al. (2011) AMPK is a direct adenylate charge-regulated protein kinase. Science.332(6036):1433-5. Epub 2011/06/18.

[135] Xiao B, Sanders MJ, Underwood E, Heath R, Mayer FV, et al. (2011) Structure of mammalian AMPK and its regulation by ADP. Nature.472(7342):230-3. Epub 2011/03/15.

[136] Hawley SA, Pan DA, Mustard KJ, Ross L, Bain J, et al. (2005) Calmodulin-dependent protein kinase kinase-beta is an alternative upstream kinase for AMP-activated protein kinase. Cell metabolism.2(1):9-19. Epub 2005/08/02.
[137] Zhang Y, Gao X, Saucedo LJ, Ru B, Edgar BA, et al. (2003) Rheb is a direct target of the tuberous sclerosis tumour suppressor proteins. Nature cell biology.5(6):578-81. Epub 2003/05/29.
[138] Inoki K, Ouyang H, Zhu T, Lindvall C, Wang Y, et al. (2006) TSC2 integrates Wnt and energy signals via a coordinated phosphorylation by AMPK and GSK3 to regulate cell growth. Cell.126(5):955-68. Epub 2006/09/09.
[139] Arsham AM, Howell JJ, Simon MC. (2003) A novel hypoxia-inducible factor-independent hypoxic response regulating mammalian target of rapamycin and its targets. The Journal of biological chemistry.278(32):29655-60. Epub 2003/06/05.
[140] Schneider A, Younis RH, Gutkind JS. (2008) Hypoxia-induced energy stress inhibits the mTOR pathway by activating an AMPK/REDD1 signaling axis in head and neck squamous cell carcinoma. Neoplasia.10(11):1295-302. Epub 2008/10/28.
[141] Liu L, Cash TP, Jones RG, Keith B, Thompson CB, et al. (2006) Hypoxia-induced energy stress regulates mRNA translation and cell growth. Molecular cell.21(4):521-31. Epub 2006/02/18.
[142] Brugarolas J, Lei K, Hurley RL, Manning BD, Reiling JH, et al. (2004) Regulation of mTOR function in response to hypoxia by REDD1 and the TSC1/TSC2 tumor suppressor complex. Genes & development.18(23):2893-904. Epub 2004/11/17.
[143] Sofer A, Lei K, Johannessen CM, Ellisen LW. (2005) Regulation of mTOR and cell growth in response to energy stress by REDD1. Mol Cell Biol.25(14):5834-45. Epub 2005/07/01.
[144] DeYoung MP, Horak P, Sofer A, Sgroi D, Ellisen LW. (2008) Hypoxia regulates TSC1/2-mTOR signaling and tumor suppression through REDD1-mediated 14-3-3 shuttling. Genes & development.22(2):239-51. Epub 2008/01/17.
[145] Corradetti MN, Inoki K, Guan KL. (2005) The stress-inducted proteins RTP801 and RTP801L are negative regulators of the mammalian target of rapamycin pathway. The Journal of biological chemistry.280(11):9769-72. Epub 2005/01/06.
[146] Schwarzer R, Tondera D, Arnold W, Giese K, Klippel A, et al. (2005) REDD1 integrates hypoxia-mediated survival signaling downstream of phosphatidylinositol 3-kinase. Oncogene.24(7):1138-49. Epub 2004/12/14.
[147] Bernardi R, Guernah I, Jin D, Grisendi S, Alimonti A, et al. (2006) PML inhibits HIF-1alpha translation and neoangiogenesis through repression of mTOR. Nature.442(7104):779-85. Epub 2006/08/18.
[148] Li Y, Wang Y, Kim E, Beemiller P, Wang CY, et al. (2007) Bnip3 mediates the hypoxia-induced inhibition on mammalian target of rapamycin by interacting with Rheb. The Journal of biological chemistry.282(49):35803-13. Epub 2007/10/12.
[149] Wouters BG, Koritzinsky M. (2008) Hypoxia signalling through mTOR and the unfolded protein response in cancer. Nature reviews Cancer.8(11):851-64. Epub 2008/10/11.
[150] Laplante M, Sabatini DM. (2009) An emerging role of mTOR in lipid biosynthesis. Current biology : CB.19(22):R1046-52. Epub 2009/12/02.

[151] Averous J, Proud CG. (2006) When translation meets transformation: the mTOR story. Oncogene.25(48):6423-35. Epub 2006/10/17.

[152] Fingar DC, Blenis J. (2004) Target of rapamycin (TOR): an integrator of nutrient and growth factor signals and coordinator of cell growth and cell cycle progression. Oncogene.23(18):3151-71. Epub 2004/04/20.

[153] Gingras AC, Raught B, Sonenberg N. (1999) eIF4 initiation factors: effectors of mRNA recruitment to ribosomes and regulators of translation. Annual review of biochemistry.68:913-63. Epub 2000/06/29.

[154] Nielsen FC, Ostergaard L, Nielsen J, Christiansen J. (1995) Growth-dependent translation of IGF-II mRNA by a rapamycin-sensitive pathway. Nature.377(6547):358-62. Epub 1995/09/28.

[155] Rogers GW, Jr., Komar AA, Merrick WC. (2002) eIF4A: the godfather of the DEAD box helicases. Progress in nucleic acid research and molecular biology.72:307-31. Epub 2002/09/11.

[156] Joshi B, Cai AL, Keiper BD, Minich WB, Mendez R, et al. (1995) Phosphorylation of eukaryotic protein synthesis initiation factor 4E at Ser-209. The Journal of biological chemistry.270(24):14597-603. Epub 1995/06/16.

[157] Gingras AC, Raught B, Gygi SP, Niedzwiecka A, Miron M, et al. (2001) Hierarchical phosphorylation of the translation inhibitor 4E-BP1. Genes & development.15(21):2852-64. Epub 2001/11/03.

[158] Wang X, Beugnet A, Murakami M, Yamanaka S, Proud CG. (2005) Distinct signaling events downstream of mTOR cooperate to mediate the effects of amino acids and insulin on initiation factor 4E-binding proteins. Mol Cell Biol.25(7):2558-72. Epub 2005/03/16.

[159] Ferguson G, Mothe-Satney I, Lawrence JC, Jr. (2003) Ser-64 and Ser-111 in PHAS-I are dispensable for insulin-stimulated dissociation from eIF4E. The Journal of biological chemistry.278(48):47459-65. Epub 2003/09/26.

[160] Tomoo K, Matsushita Y, Fujisaki H, Abiko F, Shen X, et al. (2005) Structural basis for mRNA Cap-Binding regulation of eukaryotic initiation factor 4E by 4E-binding protein, studied by spectroscopic, X-ray crystal structural, and molecular dynamics simulation methods. Biochimica et biophysica acta.1753(2):191-208. Epub 2005/11/08.

[161] Herbert TP, Tee AR, Proud CG. (2002) The extracellular signal-regulated kinase pathway regulates the phosphorylation of 4E-BP1 at multiple sites. The Journal of biological chemistry.277(13):11591-6. Epub 2002/01/19.

[162] Wang X, Li W, Parra JL, Beugnet A, Proud CG. (2003) The C terminus of initiation factor 4E-binding protein 1 contains multiple regulatory features that influence its function and phosphorylation. Mol Cell Biol.23(5):1546-57. Epub 2003/02/18.

[163] Beugnet A, Wang X, Proud CG. (2003) Target of rapamycin (TOR)-signaling and RAIP motifs play distinct roles in the mammalian TOR-dependent phosphorylation of initiation factor 4E-binding protein 1. The Journal of biological chemistry.278(42):40717-22. Epub 2003/08/13.

[164] Avruch J, Belham C, Weng Q, Hara K, Yonezawa K. (2001) The p70 S6 kinase integrates nutrient and growth signals to control translational capacity. Progress in molecular and subcellular biology.26:115-54. Epub 2001/09/29.

[165] Roux PP, Blenis J. (2004) ERK and p38 MAPK-activated protein kinases: a family of protein kinases with diverse biological functions. Microbiology and molecular biology reviews : MMBR.68(2):320-44. Epub 2004/06/10.

[166] Reinhard C, Thomas G, Kozma SC. (1992) A single gene encodes two isoforms of the p70 S6 kinase: activation upon mitogenic stimulation. Proceedings of the National Academy of Sciences of the United States of America.89(9):4052-6. Epub 1992/05/01.

[167] Shima H, Pende M, Chen Y, Fumagalli S, Thomas G, et al. (1998) Disruption of the p70(s6k)/p85(s6k) gene reveals a small mouse phenotype and a new functional S6 kinase. The EMBO journal.17(22):6649-59. Epub 1998/11/21.

[168] Price DJ, Grove JR, Calvo V, Avruch J, Bierer BE. (1992) Rapamycin-induced inhibition of the 70-kilodalton S6 protein kinase. Science.257(5072):973-7. Epub 1992/08/14.

[169] Montagne J, Stewart MJ, Stocker H, Hafen E, Kozma SC, et al. (1999) Drosophila S6 kinase: a regulator of cell size. Science.285(5436):2126-9. Epub 1999/09/25.

[170] Radimerski T, Montagne J, Rintelen F, Stocker H, van der Kaay J, et al. (2002) dS6K-regulated cell growth is dPKB/dPI(3)K-independent, but requires dPDK1. Nature cell biology.4(3):251-5. Epub 2002/02/28.

[171] Raught B, Peiretti F, Gingras AC, Livingstone M, Shahbazian D, et al. (2004) Phosphorylation of eucaryotic translation initiation factor 4B Ser422 is modulated by S6 kinases. The EMBO journal.23(8):1761-9. Epub 2004/04/09.

[172] Holz MK, Blenis J. (2005) Identification of S6 kinase 1 as a novel mammalian target of rapamycin (mTOR)-phosphorylating kinase. The Journal of biological chemistry.280(28):26089-93. Epub 2005/05/21.

[173] Pende M, Um SH, Mieulet V, Sticker M, Goss VL, et al. (2004) S6K1(-/-)/S6K2(-/-) mice exhibit perinatal lethality and rapamycin-sensitive 5'-terminal oligopyrimidine mRNA translation and reveal a mitogen-activated protein kinase-dependent S6 kinase pathway. Mol Cell Biol.24(8):3112-24. Epub 2004/04/03.

[174] Tang H, Hornstein E, Stolovich M, Levy G, Livingstone M, et al. (2001) Amino acid-induced translation of TOP mRNAs is fully dependent on phosphatidylinositol 3-kinase-mediated signaling, is partially inhibited by rapamycin, and is independent of S6K1 and rpS6 phosphorylation. Mol Cell Biol.21(24):8671-83. Epub 2001/11/20.

[175] Stolovich M, Tang H, Hornstein E, Levy G, Cohen R, et al. (2002) Transduction of growth or mitogenic signals into translational activation of TOP mRNAs is fully reliant on the phosphatidylinositol 3-kinase-mediated pathway but requires neither S6K1 nor rpS6 phosphorylation. Mol Cell Biol.22(23):8101-13. Epub 2002/11/06.

[176] Ruvinsky I, Sharon N, Lerer T, Cohen H, Stolovich-Rain M, et al. (2005) Ribosomal protein S6 phosphorylation is a determinant of cell size and glucose homeostasis. Genes & development.19(18):2199-211. Epub 2005/09/17.

[177] Yang HS, Jansen AP, Komar AA, Zheng X, Merrick WC, et al. (2003) The transformation suppressor Pdcd4 is a novel eukaryotic translation initiation factor 4A binding protein that inhibits translation. Mol Cell Biol.23(1):26-37. Epub 2002/12/17.

[178] Yang HS, Cho MH, Zakowicz H, Hegamyer G, Sonenberg N, et al. (2004) A novel function of the MA-3 domains in transformation and translation suppressor Pdcd4 is essential for its binding to eukaryotic translation initiation factor 4A. Mol Cell Biol.24(9):3894-906. Epub 2004/04/15.

[179] Peterson TR, Sabatini DM. (2005) eIF3: a connecTOR of S6K1 to the translation preinitiation complex. Molecular cell.20(5):655-7. Epub 2005/12/13.

[180] Shahbazian D, Roux PP, Mieulet V, Cohen MS, Raught B, et al. (2006) The mTOR/PI3K and MAPK pathways converge on eIF4B to control its phosphorylation and activity. The EMBO journal.25(12):2781-91. Epub 2006/06/10.

[181] Harris TE, Chi A, Shabanowitz J, Hunt DF, Rhoads RE, et al. (2006) mTOR-dependent stimulation of the association of eIF4G and eIF3 by insulin. The EMBO journal.25(8):1659-68. Epub 2006/03/17.

[182] Alessi DR, Kozlowski MT, Weng QP, Morrice N, Avruch J. (1998) 3-Phosphoinositide-dependent protein kinase 1 (PDK1) phosphorylates and activates the p70 S6 kinase in vivo and in vitro. Current biology : CB.8(2):69-81. Epub 1998/03/21.

[183] Pullen N, Dennis PB, Andjelkovic M, Dufner A, Kozma SC, et al. (1998) Phosphorylation and activation of p70s6k by PDK1. Science.279(5351):707-10. Epub 1998/02/21.

[184] Schalm SS, Blenis J. (2002) Identification of a conserved motif required for mTOR signaling. Current biology : CB.12(8):632-9. Epub 2002/04/23.

[185] Ali SM, Sabatini DM. (2005) Structure of S6 kinase 1 determines whether raptor-mTOR or rictor-mTOR phosphorylates its hydrophobic motif site. The Journal of biological chemistry.280(20):19445-8. Epub 2005/04/06.

[186] Saitoh M, Pullen N, Brennan P, Cantrell D, Dennis PB, et al. (2002) Regulation of an activated S6 kinase 1 variant reveals a novel mammalian target of rapamycin phosphorylation site. The Journal of biological chemistry.277(22):20104-12. Epub 2002/03/27.

[187] Isotani S, Hara K, Tokunaga C, Inoue H, Avruch J, et al. (1999) Immunopurified mammalian target of rapamycin phosphorylates and activates p70 S6 kinase alpha in vitro. The Journal of biological chemistry.274(48):34493-8. Epub 1999/11/24.

[188] Browne GJ, Proud CG. (2002) Regulation of peptide-chain elongation in mammalian cells. European journal of biochemistry / FEBS.269(22):5360-8. Epub 2002/11/09.

[189] Carlberg U, Nilsson A, Nygard O. (1990) Functional properties of phosphorylated elongation factor 2. European journal of biochemistry / FEBS.191(3):639-45. Epub 1990/08/17.

[190] Wang X, Li W, Williams M, Terada N, Alessi DR, et al. (2001) Regulation of elongation factor 2 kinase by p90(RSK1) and p70 S6 kinase. The EMBO journal.20(16):4370-9. Epub 2001/08/14.

[191] Ryazanov AG, Ward MD, Mendola CE, Pavur KS, Dorovkov MV, et al. (1997) Identification of a new class of protein kinases represented by eukaryotic elongation factor-2 kinase. Proceedings of the National Academy of Sciences of the United States of America.94(10):4884-9. Epub 1997/05/13.

[192] Diggle TA, Seehra CK, Hase S, Redpath NT. (1999) Analysis of the domain structure of elongation factor-2 kinase by mutagenesis. FEBS letters.457(2):189-92. Epub 1999/09/03.

[193] Browne GJ, Proud CG. (2004) A Novel mTOR-Regulated Phosphorylation Site in Elongation Factor 2 Kinase Modulates the Activity of the Kinase and Its Binding to Calmodulin. Molecular and Cellular Biology.24(7):2986-97.

[194] Knebel A, Morrice N, Cohen P. (2001) A novel method to identify protein kinase substrates: eEF2 kinase is phosphorylated and inhibited by SAPK4/p38delta. The EMBO journal.20(16):4360-9. Epub 2001/08/14.
[195] Tsang CK, Liu H, Zheng XF. (2010) mTOR binds to the promoters of RNA polymerase I- and III-transcribed genes. Cell Cycle.9(5):953-7. Epub 2009/12/30.
[196] Dobashi Y, Watanabe Y, Miwa C, Suzuki S, Koyama S. (2011) Mammalian target of rapamycin: a central node of complex signaling cascades. International journal of clinical and experimental pathology.4(5):476-95. Epub 2011/07/09.
[197] Klionsky DJ. (2007) Autophagy: from phenomenology to molecular understanding in less than a decade. Nature reviews Molecular cell biology.8(11):931-7. Epub 2007/08/23.
[198] Levine B, Klionsky DJ. (2004) Development by self-digestion: molecular mechanisms and biological functions of autophagy. Developmental cell.6(4):463-77. Epub 2004/04/08.
[199] Liu JJ, Lin M, Yu JY, Liu B, Bao JK. (2011) Targeting apoptotic and autophagic pathways for cancer therapeutics. Cancer letters.300(2):105-14. Epub 2010/11/03.
[200] Chang YY, Neufeld TP. (2009) An Atg1/Atg13 complex with multiple roles in TOR-mediated autophagy regulation. Molecular biology of the cell.20(7):2004-14. Epub 2009/02/20.
[201] Jung CH, Jun CB, Ro SH, Kim YM, Otto NM, et al. (2009) ULK-Atg13-FIP200 complexes mediate mTOR signaling to the autophagy machinery. Molecular biology of the cell.20(7):1992-2003. Epub 2009/02/20.
[202] Kamada Y, Yoshino K, Kondo C, Kawamata T, Oshiro N, et al. (2010) Tor directly controls the Atg1 kinase complex to regulate autophagy. Mol Cell Biol.30(4):1049-58. Epub 2009/12/10.
[203] Kim J, Kundu M, Viollet B, Guan KL. (2011) AMPK and mTOR regulate autophagy through direct phosphorylation of Ulk1. Nature cell biology.13(2):132-41. Epub 2011/01/25.
[204] Behrends C, Sowa ME, Gygi SP, Harper JW. (2010) Network organization of the human autophagy system. Nature.466(7302):68-76. Epub 2010/06/22.
[205] Hosokawa N, Sasaki T, Iemura S, Natsume T, Hara T, et al. (2009) Atg101, a novel mammalian autophagy protein interacting with Atg13. Autophagy.5(7):973-9. Epub 2009/07/15.
[206] Shang L, Chen S, Du F, Li S, Zhao L, et al. (2011) Nutrient starvation elicits an acute autophagic response mediated by Ulk1 dephosphorylation and its subsequent dissociation from AMPK. Proceedings of the National Academy of Sciences of the United States of America.108(12):4788-93. Epub 2011/03/09.
[207] Joo JH, Dorsey FC, Joshi A, Hennessy-Walters KM, Rose KL, et al. (2011) Hsp90-Cdc37 chaperone complex regulates Ulk1- and Atg13-mediated mitophagy. Molecular cell.43(4):572-85. Epub 2011/08/23.
[208] Itakura E, Mizushima N. (2010) Characterization of autophagosome formation site by a hierarchical analysis of mammalian Atg proteins. Autophagy.6(6):764-76. Epub 2010/07/20.
[209] Jung CH, Seo M, Otto NM, Kim DH. (2011) ULK1 inhibits the kinase activity of mTORC1 and cell proliferation. Autophagy.7(10):1212-21. Epub 2011/07/29.

[210] Dunlop EA, Hunt DK, Acosta-Jaquez HA, Fingar DC, Tee AR. (2011) ULK1 inhibits mTORC1 signaling, promotes multisite Raptor phosphorylation and hinders substrate binding. Autophagy.7(7):737-47. Epub 2011/04/05.

[211] Efeyan A, Sabatini DM. (2010) mTOR and cancer: many loops in one pathway. Current opinion in cell biology.22(2):169-76. Epub 2009/12/01.

[212] Egan DF, Shackelford DB, Mihaylova MM, Gelino S, Kohnz RA, et al. (2011) Phosphorylation of ULK1 (hATG1) by AMP-activated protein kinase connects energy sensing to mitophagy. Science.331(6016):456-61. Epub 2011/01/06.

[213] Lee SB, Kim S, Lee J, Park J, Lee G, et al. (2007) ATG1, an autophagy regulator, inhibits cell growth by negatively regulating S6 kinase. EMBO reports.8(4):360-5. Epub 2007/03/10.

[214] Lee S, Comer FI, Sasaki A, McLeod IX, Duong Y, et al. (2005) TOR complex 2 integrates cell movement during chemotaxis and signal relay in Dictyostelium. Molecular biology of the cell.16(10):4572-83. Epub 2005/08/05.

[215] Feng J, Park J, Cron P, Hess D, Hemmings BA. (2004) Identification of a PKB/Akt hydrophobic motif Ser-473 kinase as DNA-dependent protein kinase. The Journal of biological chemistry.279(39):41189-96. Epub 2004/07/21.

[216] Guertin DA, Sabatini DM. (2007) Defining the role of mTOR in cancer. Cancer Cell.12(1):9-22. Epub 2007/07/07.

[217] Pearce LR, Komander D, Alessi DR. (2010) The nuts and bolts of AGC protein kinases. Nature reviews Molecular cell biology.11(1):9-22. Epub 2009/12/23.

[218] Schaller MD. (2001) Paxillin: a focal adhesion-associated adaptor protein. Oncogene.20(44):6459-72. Epub 2001/10/19.

[219] Etienne-Manneville S, Hall A. (2002) Rho GTPases in cell biology. Nature.420(6916):629-35. Epub 2002/12/13.

[220] Oh WJ, Wu CC, Kim SJ, Facchinetti V, Julien LA, et al. (2010) mTORC2 can associate with ribosomes to promote cotranslational phosphorylation and stability of nascent Akt polypeptide. The EMBO journal.29(23):3939-51. Epub 2010/11/04.

[221] Roberts PJ, Der CJ. (2007) Targeting the Raf-MEK-ERK mitogen-activated protein kinase cascade for the treatment of cancer. Oncogene.26(22):3291-310. Epub 2007/05/15.

[222] Murphy LO, Blenis J. (2006) MAPK signal specificity: the right place at the right time. Trends in biochemical sciences.31(5):268-75. Epub 2006/04/11.

[223] Dalby KN, Morrice N, Caudwell FB, Avruch J, Cohen P. (1998) Identification of regulatory phosphorylation sites in mitogen-activated protein kinase (MAPK)-activated protein kinase-1a/p90rsk that are inducible by MAPK. The Journal of biological chemistry.273(3):1496-505. Epub 1998/01/27.

[224] Anjum R, Blenis J. (2008) The RSK family of kinases: emerging roles in cellular signalling. Nature reviews Molecular cell biology.9(10):747-58. Epub 2008/09/25.

[225] Roux PP, Ballif BA, Anjum R, Gygi SP, Blenis J. (2004) Tumor-promoting phorbol esters and activated Ras inactivate the tuberous sclerosis tumor suppressor complex via p90 ribosomal S6 kinase. Proceedings of the National Academy of Sciences of the United States of America.101(37):13489-94. Epub 2004/09/03.

[226] Ma L, Chen Z, Erdjument-Bromage H, Tempst P, Pandolfi PP. (2005) Phosphorylation and functional inactivation of TSC2 by Erk implications for tuberous sclerosis and cancer pathogenesis. Cell.121(2):179-93. Epub 2005/04/27.

[227] Ma L, Teruya-Feldstein J, Bonner P, Bernardi R, Franz DN, et al. (2007) Identification of S664 TSC2 phosphorylation as a marker for extracellular signal-regulated kinase mediated mTOR activation in tuberous sclerosis and human cancer. Cancer research.67(15):7106-12. Epub 2007/08/03.

[228] Blenis J, Chung J, Erikson E, Alcorta DA, Erikson RL. (1991) Distinct mechanisms for the activation of the RSK kinases/MAP2 kinase/pp90rsk and pp70-S6 kinase signaling systems are indicated by inhibition of protein synthesis. Cell growth & differentiation : the molecular biology journal of the American Association for Cancer Research.2(6):279-85. Epub 1991/06/01.

[229] Chung J, Kuo CJ, Crabtree GR, Blenis J. (1992) Rapamycin-FKBP specifically blocks growth-dependent activation of and signaling by the 70 kd S6 protein kinases. Cell.69(7):1227-36. Epub 1992/06/26.

[230] Roux PP, Shahbazian D, Vu H, Holz MK, Cohen MS, et al. (2007) RAS/ERK signaling promotes site-specific ribosomal protein S6 phosphorylation via RSK and stimulates cap-dependent translation. The Journal of biological chemistry.282(19):14056-64. Epub 2007/03/16.

[231] Magnusson C, Vaux DL. (1999) Signalling by CD95 and TNF receptors: not only life and death. Immunology and cell biology.77(1):41-6. Epub 1999/04/02.

[232] Karin M. (2008) The IkappaB kinase - a bridge between inflammation and cancer. Cell research.18(3):334-42. Epub 2008/02/28.

[233] Glantschnig H, Fisher JE, Wesolowski G, Rodan GA, Reszka AA. (2003) M-CSF, TNFalpha and RANK ligand promote osteoclast survival by signaling through mTOR/S6 kinase. Cell death and differentiation.10(10):1165-77. Epub 2003/09/23.

[234] Lee DF, Kuo HP, Chen CT, Hsu JM, Chou CK, et al. (2007) IKK beta suppression of TSC1 links inflammation and tumor angiogenesis via the mTOR pathway. Cell.130(3):440-55. Epub 2007/08/19.

[235] Dan HC, Adli M, Baldwin AS. (2007) Regulation of mammalian target of rapamycin activity in PTEN-inactive prostate cancer cells by I kappa B kinase alpha. Cancer research.67(13):6263-9. Epub 2007/07/10.

[236] Dan HC, Baldwin AS. (2008) Differential involvement of IkappaB kinases alpha and beta in cytokine- and insulin-induced mammalian target of rapamycin activation determined by Akt. J Immunol.180(11):7582-9. Epub 2008/05/21.

Chapter 2

Sestrins Link Tumor Suppressors with the AMPK-TOR Signaling Network

Andrei V. Budanov

Additional information is available at the end of the chapter

http://dx.doi.org/10.5772/48554

1. Introduction

The strength of the mechanisms involved in the control of health and lifespan determines the rate of aging in any organism. Aging is fueled by the accumulation of damage in a multitude of tissues, causing many age-related diseases including cardio-vascular diseases, neuro-degenerating diseases, metabolic syndrome and cancer[1]. We know that a healthy life-style, good habits, exercise and positive attitude are all factors that support a healthy, long life while the consumption of unhealthy, low nutritional and high caloric diet, bad ecology, bad habits and constitutive stress are known to shorten life and lead to the accumulation of a number of pathologies. However, exposure to low level stresses, for example induced by exercise, increases our resistance to detrimental stress insults, this process is referred to as hermesis[2]. With respect to what is beneficial and what is detrimental for health, we still do not fully understand the underlying processes that support our health and long life nor what allows us to become more resistant to a constantly changing, and sometimes unfriendly, environment.

The causative link between aging and age-related diseases emphasizes how understanding the mechanisms that control aging could aid in the development of approaches for the prevention and treatment of many human diseases. The involvement of similar signaling pathways in the control of aging and defense against different diseases supports this concept. Two protein kinases, Target of Rapamycine (TOR) and AMP-activated protein kinase (AMPK), are central regulators of aging that are often found to be malfunctioned in many human diseases and, according to different animal models, play a role in cancer, diabetes, neurodegeneration and other syndromes[3, 4]. Strikingly, AMPK directly regulates the TOR activity, indicating that these proteins have overlapping functions and are involved in the same pathways[3]. The proteins involved in the AMPK activation and the TOR suppression are potential regulators of longevity and aging. Among the modulators of AMPK and TOR, tumor suppressors p53 and members of the Forkhead Box O (FoxO) family play a central role in defense from stress, determination of lifespan and protection from age-related pathologies via activation of the stress-responsive Sestrin genes.

2. The function of the AMPK –TOR pathway and its role in lifespan regulation

2.1. TOR

The kinase TOR was originally identified as protein that can be inhibited by rapamycin, a macrolid found in the soil of Easter island, named after local name for the island - Rapa Nui[5]. Rapamycin is produced by the bacteria *Streptomyces hygroscopicus* and acts as an antifungal metabolite. Mutagenesis analysis in *Saccharomyces cerevisiae* led to the isolation of strains resistant to rapamycin and the identification of the two genes *TOR1* and *TOR2* that are responsible for this effect[5]. *TOR* genes encode proteins belonging to phosphatidylinositol kinase-related kinase (PIKK) family of Ser/Thr protein kinases[5]. Protein products of *TOR* genes form two complexes called TOR complex-1 (TORC1) and TOR complex-2 (TORC2)[5]. Later TOR orthologs were identified in all studied eukaryotic organisms including mammals, although the mammalian genome contains only one functional *TOR* gene (mammalian *TOR* or *mTOR*)[5]. The mammalian TORC1 (mTORC1) and TORC2 (mTORC2) complexes share several subunits: mTOR itself, lethal with Sec13-protein 8 (mLST8, also known as GβL), DEP-domain containing mTOR-interacting protein (DEPTOR) and Tti1/Tel2[3]. TORC1 contains unique regulatory-associated protein of mTOR (raptor) and proline-rich Akt-substrate 40 kDa (PRAS40)[3]. TORC2 includes the rapamycin-insensitive mTOR companion (rictor), mammalian stress-activated MAP kinase-interacting protein-1 (mSIN1) and protein observed with rictor-1 and -2 (protor1/2)[3, 6]. Raptor and Rictor determine the specificity of mTORC1 and mTORC2 toward their substrates that are responsible for mTOR-dependent processes[5, 6]. Among the two complexes, mTORC1 is sensitive to inhibition by rapamycin, although prolonged rapamycin treatment can also inhibit mTORC2[6]. Rapamycin inhibits mTORC1 via interaction with 12 kDa FK506-binding protein (FKBP12), which in complex with rapamycin, binds and inhibits mTORC1[5] (Fig.1).

mTORC1 and mTORC2 have different substrate specificity, dictated by different subunit composition. Two well-established substrates of mTORC1 are S6 kinase-1 (S6K1) and the eukaryotic translation initiation factor (eIF) 4E (eIF4E) binding protein-1 (4EBP1), involved in regulation of protein synthesis [3] (Fig.1). S6K was originally identified as a kinase phosphorylating ribosomal S6 protein although other substrates involved in the regulation of protein translation were discovered later. Among the targets of S6K1 that support translation initiation and elongation, are eukaryotic elongation factor 2 kinase, (eEF2K), S6K Aly/REF-like target (SKAR), and 80 kDa nuclear cap-binding protein (NCBP1) and eIF4B. eIF4B, activated via S6K-dependent phosphorylation, stimulates the activation of eukaryotic translation initiation factor 4A (eIF4A), an RNA helicase that enhances translation, unwinding structured 5′-untranslated regions of many RNA[6]. 4EBP1 is another regulator of translation which, in its hypo-phosphorylated form, inhibits initiation of cap-dependent translation via interaction with cap-binding protein eIF4E, a component of eIF4F translation initiation complex. When phosphorylated by mTORC1, 4EBP1 dissociates from eIF4E allowing recruitment of translation initiation factor eIF4G and the subsequent stimulation of protein synthesis[3]. mTORC1 also phosphorylates unc-51-like kinase-1 (ULK1/ATG1) and mammalian autophagy-related gene-13 (ATG13), the components of ULK1/ATG13/FLP200(focal adhesion kinase family-interacting protein of 200 kDa) required for the activation of autophagic proteolysis (Fig.1). mTORC1 also regulates other proteins involved in autophagy such as suppressor of autophagy death-associated protein-1 (DAP1) and regulator of early autophagosome formation WIPI2, a mammalian ortholog of yeast Atg18. Additionally, mTORC1 is involved in lysosomal biogenesis through phosphorylation and inhibition of transcription factor EB (TFEB)[3].

The mTORC2 substrates appear to be members of AGC kinase family which includes AKT, serum- and glucocorticoid-induced protein kinase-1 (SGK1), and protein kinase C-α (PKCα), involved in the regulation of metabolism and viability. AKT, phosphorylated by mTORC2 in hydrophobic motif on Ser473, is an important regulator of metabolism and cell viability, while SGK1 controls growth and ion transport, and PKCα is involved in actin cytoskeleton regulation via paxilin and Rho GTPases[3, 7].

The mTOR-containing complexes have different, although in some aspects overlapping, functions[5, 6]. mTORC1 supports many anabolic processes in the cells such as protein and lipid biosynthesis, and ribosomal biogenesis[5]. mTORC1 also influences energy metabolism through the stimulation of mitochondrial respiration and glycolysis[8-11](Fig.1). The importance of mTOR in mitochondrial function is supported at several levels of control including: (i) regulation of mitochondrial biogenesis via the stimulatory effect on Ying-Yang-1 (YY1) - PPAR-γ coactivator-1α (PGC1α) transcriptional complex, involved in transactivation of mitochondrial genes and intensification of mitochondrial respiration[8]; (ii) direct effects on mitochondrial function potentially through interaction with regulatory mitochondrial proteins such as VDAC1 and Bcl-xL, which regulate mitochondrial substrate permeability and mitochondrial integrity[9]; (iii) activation of Hypoxia-Inducible Factor-1 (HIF1), composed of stable HIF1β and inducible HIF1α subunit, the activator of the genes involved in glycolysis, glucose transport and mitochondrial respiration[12]. mTORC1 activates HIF1 via the upregulation of HIF1α translation[13].

Another important function of TOR, critical for the control of metabolism and cell integrity, is the negative regulation of macroautophagy (therein called autophagy)[3, 5] (Fig.1).

Autophagy is the process of double membrane encapsulation and lysosomal degradation of cellular constituents such as organelles, protein aggregates, lipid droplets and portions of cytoplasm[14]. The process of autophagy involves a nucleation step via the formation of a preautophagosomal structure (PAT), continuing to the formation of phagophore and autophagosome vesicles. Finally, the autophagosome fuses with a lysosome allowing lysosomal degradation of the autophagosome content[14]. Autophagy plays three major roles in cells. Firstly, it provides energy through digestion of cellular constituents during starvation and other conditions affecting nutrient availability. This allows cells to survive nutrient limitations and autophagy might be vital for cell survival during stress such as ischemia. Secondly, autophagy regulates cell integrity by removing deposits and aggregates that affect normal cell physiology as well as damaged and malfunctioning organelles, which are the major source of oxidative stress[1]. In agreement, reactive oxygen species (ROS) produced by damaged mitochondria or through other mechanisms stimulate autophagy, results in suppression of oxidative stress[15]. Thirdly, completed autophagy might cause cell death, referred to as type II cell death, although the physiological relevance of this is unclear and disputable[16]. Autophagy is often associated with apoptosis and can be activated by many pro-apoptotic proteins such as p53 upregulated modulator of apoptosis (Puma) and Bcl-2–associated X (Bax) and inhibited by antiapoptotic proteins of the Bcl2 family[17-19]. In some cases, autophagy can be activated in response to pro-apoptotic stimuli as a potential pro-survival control mechanism or as a by-stander of the cell death associated with energy decline. In the other experimental settings, it was shown that autophagy mediated apoptosis in response to genotoxic stress[20]. Nevertheless, autophagy can modulate many effects of stress on cell viability and consequently, can be an important factor in anticancer treatment, which often involves extensive stress response[21].

Hyperactivity of TORC1, which leads to dysregulation of metabolism and inhibition of autophagy, is associated with extensive ROS production[1, 15, 22]. ROS, not being properly decomposed, induces oxidative stress, the major source of cell damage such as DNA-oxidation, lipid peroxidation and protein carbonylation. The accumulation of damage associated with oxidative stress is the driving force of aging, and, accordingly, TORC1 is the critical controller of aging in all eukaryotes from yeast to mammals[5, 6]. This data demonstrates that inhibition of TORC1 via mutagenesis or rapamycin treatment extends lifespan of yeast, worms, flies and mice [3, 23, 24]. Interestingly, two well-established mechanisms of lifespan extension such as caloric restriction and suppression of Insulin/Insulin growth factor-1(IGF1) -dependent signaling pathway control TORC1 activity, indicating that TORC1 inhibition may be critical for lifespan extension and suppression of age-associated pathologies imposed by low-calorie diet and inhibition of Insulin/IGF1-regulated pathway[3].

Stimulation of metabolism, cell growth and ROS by mTORC1 contributes to different pathologies including carcinogenesis, and mTORC1 is often activated in human cancers[3]. Many tumor suppressors found inactivated in cancers such as Tuberoses Sclerosis -1 and -2 (TSC1 and TSC2), liver kinase-B (LKB1), phosphatase and tensin homolog (PTEN), p53 and neurofibromatosis type 1 (NF1) are inhibitors of mTORC1, while proto-oncogenes Ras, PI3K and AKT are mTORC1 activators[3, 5]. Obesity and type II diabetes are associated with chronic mTORC1 activation in metabolically active tissue, and mTORC1 impairs insulin sensitivity, stimulates hyperinsulemia and hyperglycemia[3, 5]. Obesity-associated mTORC1 activation also is a major risk factor for the development of nonalcoholic fatty liver disease (NAFLD), a risk factor of cirrhosis and hepatocellular carcinoma[3]. mTORC1 can also be involved in the pathogenesis of neurodegenerative disorders such as Parkinson-, Alzheimer-, Huntington- diseases, amyotrophic lateral sclerosis and frontotemporal dementia[3, 6]. All of these pathologies share similar etiology defined by the accumulation of toxic protein aggregates, which generate cellular damage, oxidative stress and cause cell death. These inclusions are cleared by autophagy, with mTORC1 potentially contributing to these syndromes via regulation of autophagy and protein synthesis, two processes affecting deposit accumulation[1, 3].

mTORC1 activity is regulated by nutrients (the source of ATP), insulin and growth factors, and amino acids through small GTPases Ras homolog enriched in brain (Rheb) and the members of Ras-related GTP-binding (Rag) protein family RagA, RagB, RagC and RagD (Fig.1). Active GTP-bound Rheb directly interacts with mTORC1 and stimulates its activity through undefined mechanism. The members of Rag family control mTORC1 in a sophisticated manner, forming heterodimers between either RagA or RagB with either RagC and RagD. Interestingly, the RagA and RagB are active in GTP-bound form, whilst RagC and RagD are functional when loaded with GDP. [6]. According to a contemporary model, active Rag complexes directly interact with the mTORC1 subunit raptor directing mTORC1 into the surface of endosomes and late lysosomes, enabling its interaction with activated Rheb[6]. As Rags do not have any membrane-targeting signals, they are delivered to lysosomal surface by Ragulator protein complex, composed of p14, MAPK scaffold protein 1(MP1) and p18[6]. The activity or Rag proteins is regulated by amino acids with Rags being critical transducers of the activating signal from amino acids to mTORC1[3]. As described recently, Rag activation in response to amino acids is mediated by leucyl-tRNA synthetase, which binds Rag proteins and acts as GTPase-activating protein (GAP) for Rags[25]. The other proposed mechanisms of mTORC1 activation by amino acids involve mitogen-activated protein kinase kinase kinase (MAP4K3), inositol polyphosphate monokinase (IPMK) and mammalian vacuolar protein sorting 34 homolog (hVps34), belonging to class 3 PI3K[3, 26]. hVps34 is required for activation of phospholipase-D (PLD) in response to availability of amino acids. Amino acids induce interaction between phosphatidylinositol 3-phosphate and the Phox homology (PX) domain of PLD1, which causes PLD translocation to the lysosomal compartment, required for mTORC1 activation[27].

Rheb GTPase is a critical regulator of mTORC1 in response to insulin, growth factors, energy and stress[1, 6]. Rheb is negatively controlled by the TSC1:TSC2 protein complex where TSC2 is GAP for Rheb, while TSC1 plays a supporting role stabilizing TSC2[28]. The TSC1:TSC2 complex integrates signals from different signaling pathways that positively or negatively modulate the TSC1:TSC2 activity [1]. Insulin and IGF1, the activators of cell growth, stimulate mTORC1 via inhibitory phosphorylation of TSC2 by AKT[3]. Insulin/IGF1 stimulate Insulin/IGF1 receptor (In/IGF1R), which through the engagement of insulin receptor substrate-1 (IRS1) tethers and activates phosphatidylinositol-3-kinase (PI3K), which then converts phosphatidylinositol-4,5-biphosphates (PIP2) into phosphatidylinositol-3,4,5-triphosphates (PIP3). PIP3 induce AKT phosphorylation on Thr308 by phosphoinositide-dependent kinase-1 (PDK1) kinase recruiting both kinases to cytoplasmic membrane via their pleckstrin homology (PH) domains. PI3K also stimulates phosphorylation of AKT on Ser473 by mTORC2 which is required for full AKT activation[3, 7, 15]. The PI3K activity is counteracted by the tumor suppressor PTEN, which is a PIP3 phosphatase[3]. Activated AKT directly phosphorylates TSC2 on multiple sites, causing mTORC1 activation. In parallel AKT also stimulates mTORC1 via phosphorylation of mTORC1 interacting protein PRAS40, an inhibitor of mTORC1, and inhibitory phosphorylation of both TSC2 and PRAS40 cooperates in mTORC1 activation[3]. IGF1 also activates Ras GTPases, activating extracellular-signal-regulated kinase (ERK) and ribosomal S6 kinase (RSK1)[3]. Both ERK and RSK1 directly phosphorylate TSC2, which cause inhibition of its activity and TORC1 activation[3]. Inflammation, accompanied by production of pro-inflammatory cytokines such as tumor necrosis factor-α (TNFα), stimulates mTORC1 via IκB kinase (IKKβ)-mediated phosphorylation of TSC1[3]. The canonical Wnt signaling pathway, the regulator of embriogeneis, provides another important mechanism of mTORC1 regulation. The Wnt pathway inhibits glycogen synthase kinase-3β (GSK3β), which under normal conditions phosphorylates and activates TSC2[3] (Fig.1).

2.2. AMPK

While Insulin, growth factors and nutrients inhibit the TSC1:TSC2 complex and stimulate mTORC1, many stress insults have the opposite effect, activating TSC2 and inhibiting TORC1. Inhibition of mTORC1 under stress conditions allows cells to stop cell growth and proliferation in the unfavorable conditions switching to high-economy mode and supporting stress-relieving measures. Nutrient deficiency and many metabolic derangements cause an accumulation of AMP and ADP, which, in turn, activate AMPK. AMPK inhibits mTORC1 through phosphorylation of TSC2 and raptor[4]. Besides AMP accumulation, AMPK can be activated by different insults such as oxidative stress, DNA-damage or the accumulation of Ca^{2+} potentially through an AMP-independent mechanism. Also some hormones such as leptin and adiponectin are able stimulate AMPK through mechanisms that are yet to be defined[4].

AMPK is a protein complex composed of 3 subunits catalytical AMPKα, (encoded by AMPKα1 and α2 genes scaffold AMPKβ subunit, (encoded by *AMPKβ1* and *β2* genes) and regulatory AMPKγ subunit, (encoded by *AMPKγ1*, *γ2* and *γ3* genes) in mammals. AMPK is activated via phosphorylation of AMPKa subunit on Thr172, although phosphorylation of other sites on AMPKα, β and γ subunits are also involved in AMPK regulation[4]. The upstream AMPK kinase critical for AMPK activation in response to energy deficiency is

LKB1, which constantly phosphorylates AMPKα subunit on Thr172. The most established mechanism of AMPK activation involved binding AMP by AMPKg subunit which stimulates conformational changes in AMPKα subunit making it less accessible for AMPK phosphatases[4, 29]. Several protein phosphatases (PP) have been shown to be involved in the regulation of AMPK phosphorylation including PP2C[30], PP2A[31, 32], PPM1E[33], PP1[33, 34]. LKB activity can be stimulated by oxidative stress via the phosphorylation by ataxia telangiectasia mutated (ATM) kinase, leading to AMPK activation[35]. Other AMPK kinases shown to directly phosphorylate AMPK are Ca^{2+}/Calmodulin-dependent protein kinase II (CaMKII), activated by accumulation of Ca^{2+} ions, and TAK kinase[36], activated in response to treatment with TNF-related apoptosis-inducing ligand (TRAIL) [37](Fig.1). Some proteins such as kinase repressor of Ras-2 (KSR2) can also regulate AMPK phosphorylation working as scaffold protein through regulation of access of either protein kinases or phosphatases to AMPKα subunit[38].

Activated AMPK phosphorylates many targets involved in the regulation of glucose metabolism: 6-phosphofructo-2-kinase/fructose-2,6-biphosphatase 3 (PFKFB3), glycogen synthase-1 (GYS1), glutamine:fructose-6-phosphate amidotransferase (GFAT1), TBC1D1; lipid metabolism: acetyl- CoA Carboxylase-1 and -2 (ACC1 and ACC2), 3-hydroxy-3-methylglutaryl-CoA reductase (HMGR), PLD1; polarity: cytoplasmic linker protein-170 (CLIP170), golgi-specific brefeldin A-resistance guanine nucleotide exchange factor 1 (GBF1), kinesin light chain-2 (KLC2); transcription: (PGC1α, sterol regulatory element-binding protein-1 (SREBP1), FoxOs, Histone-2B, p300 and HDAC4,5,6; and mitosis: protein phosphatase-1 regulatory subunit 12C (PPP1R12C), p21-activated protein kinase (PAK2)[4, 39]. AMPK also contributes to mitochondrial function stimulating mitochondrial biogenesis via phosphorylation of PGC1α co-activator and regulating expression of mitochondrial genes[4]. AMPK regulates cell growth and autophagy in part, through TORC1 inhibition, although as shown recently AMPK can stimulate autophagy through direct phosphorylation of autophagy ULK1 protein. AMPK is also involved in the regulation of cell death in response to genotoxic stress, although the mechanisms are yet to be described[40-42].

Interestingly, lipid biosynthesis and autophagy controlled by mTORC1 via SREBP1 and ULK1, are under direct control by AMPK. AMPK directly phosphorylates and inhibit SREBP1 protein, suppressing lipogenesis[43]. AMPK also phosphorylates and activates ULK1 stimulating autophagy [44]. The redundancy of the mechanisms of regulation of lipid biosynthesis and autophagy though direct and indirect effects of AMPK demonstrates the critical role of AMPK in these processes and the importance of accurate regulation of these processes by mTORC1 and AMPK.

The regulation of metabolism and autophagy by AMPK potentially contributes to lifespan regulation. Accordingly, the inactivation of one of the AMPK subunits (AMP-activated kinase-2 (AAK-2)) in *Caenorhabditis elegans* shortened lifespan by 12%, while animals with increased AAK-2 expression lived 13% longer than their wild type (WT) counterparts[45].

The mechanism of life extension by AMPK involves CRTC-1 and FoxO transcriptional factors[46, 47]. Interestingly, the activity of AAK-2 is also required for protection against oxidative stress [48]. Similar results were obtained in *Drosophila Melanogaster* model, where the inhibition of drosophila AMPK shortened lifespan and increased susceptibility to oxidative stress and starvation[49] In accordance, gain-of-function LKB1 mutant extended lifespan in flies[50]. Although there is no such evidence for mammals, mammalian AMPK presumably plays a similar role in lifespan regulation. This idea is supported by the observation that AMPK activity is decreased in old animals potentiating the aging process[51].

Although the effects of AMPK on the lifespan regulation in mammals are not known, AMPK is involved in protection from different diseases[4, 52]. AMPKα2 subunit controls of glucose metabolism and AMPKα2 mice have pro-diabetic phenotype associated with diminished insulin secretion and glucose intolerance[53]. AMPK can also affect lifespan via the suppression of inflammation, a process associated with aging and many age-related diseases, including cancer[54]. Metformin, the most commonly prescribed anti-diabetic drug, activates AMPK and its activation is required for effect of metformin on glucose production in hepatocytes and, potentially, in glucose uptake in muscle[55]. Resveratrol, the plant-derived polifenol, which prolongs lifespan and improves health conditions of mice kept on high-calorie diet, also activates AMPK, which can potentiate the effects of resveratrol on health and aging [56].

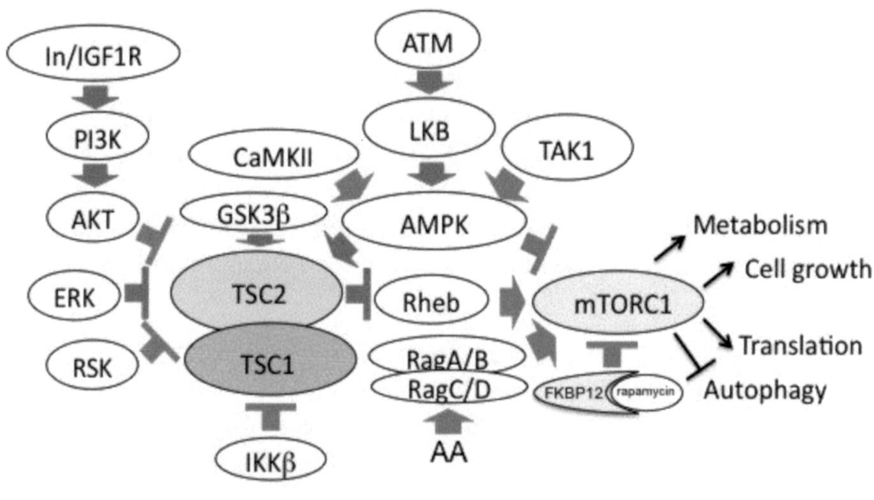

Figure 1. Regulation of the AMPK-mTORC1 axis and the role of mTORC1 in cellular processes. mTORC1 is activated by insulin and IGF1 via stimulation of the PI3K-AKT pathway, followed by inhibitory phosphorylation of TSC2 by AKT. The other signaling pathways stimulate mTORC1 through activation of ERK, RSK and IKKβ kinases in a TSC1:TSC2-dependent manner. TSC1:TSC2 inhibition leads to stimulation of Rheb, an activator of mTORC1. mTORC1 activation also required amino acids (AA) which stimulate mTORC1 via Rag complexes. Many stress insults activate AMPK which inhibits mTORC1 modulating many mTORC1-dependent processes such as metabolism, protein synthesis, cell growth and autophagy.

3. p53 and its role in aging and diseases

Among the proteins involved in the lifespan regulation, the tumor suppressor p53 plays a central role. Originally identified as interactor of human polioma SV40 virus large T antigen, accumulated in transformed cells[57], it was proposed to be involved in cell transformation. Studies further demonstrated that p53 suppressed cell transformation and carcinogenesis[58]. Furthermore, p53 gene is mutated in more than 50% of human tumors, supporting the idea that p53 inactivation is a critical step in carcinogenesis[58]. The patients with Li-Fraumeni syndrome, characterized by predisposition to different form of cancer at early age, often carry a mutant p53 allele[58]. In the following study the tumor suppressive function of p53 was confirmed in mouse knockout model where *p53*-deficeint mice developed cancers and chronic inflammation and the median of survival of *p53*-null mice is six months [59]. The extensive efforts to understand the function of p53 led to characterization of many p53 activities such as the regulation of genomic stability, control of cell cycle, induction cell death and senescence, and suppression of angiogenesis. All these mechanisms potentially contribute to tumor suppressive function of p53, although the mechanisms most critical for tumor suppression are yet to be defined[58].

The vast majority of processes controlled by p53 are exhibited through the regulation of gene expression. Being a transcription factor, p53 directly activates many genes involved in DNA repair such as growth arrest and DNA damage-45 (GADD45) and p53R2; cell cycle arrest and senescence: p21, 14-3-3σ and plasminogen activator inhibitor-1 (PAI-1); cell death: Bax, Puma, apoptosis inducing factor (AIF), Noxa; and inhibition of angiogenesis: trombospondin-1 (TSP-1)[60] (Fig.2). p53 activity is regulated through several mechanisms, many involving protein stabilization. p53 trancriptionally activates its negative regulators murine double minute 2 (MDM2), p53-induced protein with a RING-H2 domain (Pirh2) and constitutively photomorphogenic 1 (COP1), which bind and stimulate p53 degradation working as p53 E3-ubiquitine ligases[61].

The elimination of damaged and modified cells, imposing the threat to the organism, is not the only strategy to fight cancer. It seems reasonable that many functions of p53 in the prevention of carcinogenesis operate via the regulation of metabolism and stress response. Not being properly controlled the derangements of these processes can lead to the accumulation of damage, the major source of mutations[15]. We have described that one of the mechanism involves the regulation of ROS, which being accumulated, might fuel mutagenesis and genomic instability[15]. ROS can also stimulate the cell cycle, migration and angiogenesis, so they can support initiation, promotion and progression of carcinogenesis[62]. Accordingly, our studies showed that inactivation of p53 via different mechanisms such as knockout, knockdown with shRNA, over-expression of Mdm2 or dominant-negative form of p53 led to ROS accumulation causing oxidative DNA-damage, increased rate of mutagenesis and genomic instability[62]. A xenograft study with lung adenocarcinoma A549 cells showed that p53 silencing accelerated tumor growth, and it was reverted by treatment with an antioxidant N-acetylcysteine (NAC)[62]. Moreover, p53-

knockout mice, predisposed to carcinogenesis, were protected from the disease by NAC treatment and had significantly extended lifespan as compared to vehicle-treated controls[62]. A number of p53 targets with antioxidant activities including Sestrins, glutathione peroxidase 1 (GPx1), manganese superoxide dismutase (MnSOD), catalase, aldehyde dehydrogenase 2 (ALDH1), gutaminase 2 (GLT2) and p53-induced nuclear protein 1(INP1)[1, 15] were identified (Fig.2).

Some of the p53-inducible proteins such as TP53-induced glycolysis and apoptosis regulator (TIGAR), an inhibitor of glycolysis, regulate ROS via control of metabolism. TIGAR lowers the fructose-2,6-bisphosphate levels and suppresses activity of phosphofructokinase-1 (PFK1) [63]. It can lead to the re-direction of glycolytic intermediates into the pentose phosphate pathway providing cells with NADPH, the important reducing equivalent for antioxidant reactions in the cell[64]. p53 also coordinates bioenergetic processes such as mitochondrial function regulating mitochondrial respiration via activation of cytochrome C oxidase 2 (SCO2), regulator of complex IV, subunit I of complex IV and apoptosis inducing factor 1 (AIF)[64]. In addition Parkin (PARK2), a gene associated with Parkinson disease, is a p53 target, inactivation of which leads to enhancement of glycolysis, suppression of mitochondrial respiration and ROS accumulation[65]. As a result, p53 may control different metabolic pathway involved in ROS production. On the contrary when stress is too high and damages are irreparable, imposing the threat of mutations and genomic instability, p53 induces ROS production through up-regulation of proapoptotic genes Puma, Bax and PIG3, facilitating cell disorganisation during apoptosis[62, 66] (Fig.2).

The protective effects of p53 can also be mediated by regulation of the AMPK-mTORC1 axis[15]. Elevated activity of mTORC1 is associated with the accumulation of damage and oxidative stress[15, 67], resulting in exacerbated aging and imposing health risks. Overactivation of mTORC1 might be even more detrimental under stress conditions such as genotoxic stress, when the anabolic and catabolic processes should be coordinated to enable the repair and elimination of the damage. Accordingly, it was shown that p53, activated by DNA-damage and via other mechanisms, inhibited mTORC1 and mTORC1-dependent translation[68, 69]. p53 inhibits mTORC1 through activation of genes involved in negative regulation of mTORC1, such as a suppressor of insulin signaling insulin-like growth factor binding protein 3 (IGF-BP3), PTEN, TSC2, AMPKb1, Sestrin1 (Sesn1) and Sestrin2 (Sesn2)[15]. mTORC1 inhibition by p53 is also mediated by stimulation of AMPK phosphorylation on Thr172[70]. The other potential mechanism involves the clearance of epithelial growth factor receptor, the activator of PI3K-AKT-mTORC1 pathway from the surface, disabling the signaling from the receptor[71, 72].

Autophagy is another mechanism imposed by p53 to protect cells from the accumulation of damage [71] (Fig.2). p53 activates autophagy via transcriptional activation of genes involved in the regulation of the AMPK-mTORC1 pathway[70, 73], although other p53 targets are directly involved in the autophagic process or operate through other mechanisms. The list of pro-autophagic genes regulated by p53 includes lysosomal protein damage-regulated autophagy modulator (DRAM), ULK1[74], p53INP1 (which interacts with ATG8 and promote autophagic cell death)[75], Bax, Puma[18] and a new gene with unknown function ISG20L1[76]. Interestingly that autophagy also contributes to p53-induced cell death, potentially providing the ground for elimination of damaged cells, if they are irreparable. The cytoplasmic form of p53 can negatively regulate autophagy, counteracting the effects of the nuclear form of p53[77]. This potential mechanism involves interaction with components of autophagic machinery, such as family kinase interacting protein 200 (FIP200/ATG17)[78].

The effects of p53 on the control of stress response, metabolism, ROS and autophagy connect p53 with the lifespan regulation and longevity. p53 knockout mice develop cancer and die by the age of 6 months, indicating a critical role of p53 in the lifespan regulation through suppression of carcinogenesis[59]. Nevertheless, this model precluded characterization of the role of p53 in aging and longevity. To study the effects of p53 on aging several models were established and these models show different, sometimes contradicting, phenotypes.

In the first model, mice expressed a truncated p53 lacking exons 1-6 (called m allele in *p53*$^{+/m}$ mice). The *p53*^{m} locus produced a 24K C-terminal part of the p53 protein[79]. Interestingly, these mice demonstrated 23% reduction in median of longevity. Although young (3-12 months old) mice did not show any difference compared with WT mice, after 18 months *p53*$^{+/m}$ mice revealed exacerbated aging-related phenotype exhibiting weight loss, lordokyphosis, and an absence of vigor[79]. Tissue analysis demonstrated a decrease in muscle and adipose tissue as well as reduced kidney, liver, spleen and testes mass, typical features of aging. Also, mice showed thickness in both bone density and dermal thickness, and defects in wound healing. Moreover, the mice had reduced survival in response to stress[79]. Surprisingly the frequency of many other pathologies associated with aging including liver diseases, brain atrophy, hair graying and alopecia, skin ulceration, amyloidal deposits and cataract were not increased in this model[79]. The feature reported in the *p53*$^{+/m}$ mice was a decreased predisposition to cancer[79].

As reported in another study, mice with increased levels of expression of natural N-terminally truncated p53 (p44) had an accelerated aging phenotype, deteriorated health and decreased lifespan, characterized by defects in fertility linked with testicular degeneration, lordokyphosis and decrease in bone density, cognitive decline and synaptic deficit early in life[80, 81]. These mice demonstrated overactivated IGF1R signaling and many phenotypes were rescued by IGF1R heterozygosity. p44 also exacerbated a neurodegenerative phenotype in the mouse model of Alzheimer's disease based on the overexpression of human amyloid precursor protein (APP), where p44 facilitated degeneration of memory-forming and memory retrieving areas of the brain[81].

A common phenotype observed in these two models is accelerated aging and decreased susceptibility to carcinogenesis[79, 80]. As it was suggested, p53 is overactivated by short form and stimulated an aging phenotype, it also provided better protection from cancer[79, 80]. An alternative explanation of the effects of truncated p53 on lifespan and aging involves suppression of many p53 activities and downregulation of some critical genes involved in the stress response and metabolism, resulting in an effect on viability, although the expression of some p53 targets was still retained and even increased. Both artificial 24K, and natural p44 forms of p53 lack transactivation domains, which are required for the most of p53 activities including tumor suppression[82]. Both truncated forms bind full-size p53 and counteract many of its activities similar to the effects of N-terminally truncated forms of the other p53 family members p63 and p73 on full size proteins[83]. Accordingly, overexpression of p44 causes accumulation of p53 and disability of full-size p53 to transactivate most of its targets[80, 84, 85]. The truncated p53 retains a full form in cytoplasm, inhibiting the p53 nuclear function [86]. Also, an inhibitory effect of truncated p53 is evident as p44 may be selected in human cancers, supporting carcinogenesis[87]. Thus truncated p53 might compromise p53 activities rather than enhance them. Simultaneously, some p53 functions, for example those involved in ROS production and senescence, might be intact or even increased causing accelerated aging phenotype. A more widespread analysis of p53 targets is required in these models to better understand the impact of truncated p53 in this phenotype.

Other models indicate that tumor suppressive and aging-regulatory functions of p53-dependent might be separated. In one model, a genomic segment containing whole p53 gene was integrated in the mouse genome (p53Tg mice). These mice exhibited increased p53 response to DNA-damage and were able to rescue the cancer-prone phenotype of *p53*-deficient mice. The p53Tg mice were resistant to carcinogenesis, but in contrast to previous models, they did not reveal any signs of accelerated aging. Interestingly, a similar phenotype was observed with *Mdm2* hipomorphic (haploinsufficient) mice, characterized by increased p53 activity, which were cancer resistant but aged normally[88, 89].

MDM2 binds p53 and stimulates protein degradation, inhibiting p53 activity. The Arf tumor suppressor, a product of the INK4A locus, stimulates p53 activity antagonizing MDM2-dependent degradation. Transgenic mice with an extra copy of the Arf gene, along with an extra-copy of p53 gene (super-Arf/p53 (s-Arf/p53) mice) demonstrated increased activity of p53 and enhanced expression of p53-dependent p21 and antioxidant Sesn1 and Sesn2 genes. These mice were resistant to cancer, similar to the p53Tg mice, and fibroblasts from s-Arf/p53 mice were resistant to immortalization and transformation, implying low susceptibility of these mice to carcinogenesis. In contrast to previous models, these mice had an extended average lifespan of 16% and show signs of delayed aging as evident by the test on neuromuscular coordination (tightrope success test) and hair re-growth test. Aging is associated with the accumulation of DNA-damage and oxidative stress, and s-Arf/p53 mice exhibited decreased levels of DNA damage as illustrated by H2AX staining and decreased oxidative stress evident from analysis of ROS in splenocytes, decreased lipid peroxidation and low abundance of carbonylated proteins in liver. The s-Arf/p53 mice were also resistant to oxidative stress, emphasizing the potential role of the mechanisms of stress response in suppression of aging and carcinogenesis[90]. This data is in concordance with previous observations that showed that inactivation of p53 or its upstream regulator ATM decreased lifespan and caused accumulation of oxidative damage in mice[62, 91]. Both *p53*- and *ATM*-null mouse strains were predisposed to cancer, and these phenotypes were prevented by antioxidant NAC treatment[62, 92]. Interestingly, the activity of p53 is decreased with age supporting a concept that p53 might be an important anti-aging factor[93].

Suppression of carcinogenesis was not the primary function of p53 in evolution as p53 is found in the organisms, such as *Caenorhabditis elegans* and *Drosophila Melanogaster,* which do not develop cancer. In the *Drosophila* model, overexpression of p53 in adult flies increased the lifespan of males, but limited lifespan in female flies. Also, the moderate overexpression of p53 during larvae stage extended lifespan in both male and female flies. *p53*-deficient flies were sick and had a decreased lifespan[94]. It is possible that p53 controls the accumulation of damages as well as other functions. Interestingly, the overexpression of dominant-negative form of p53 in flies brain extended their lifespan [94]. This data suggests that p53 can play an opposite role in lifespan regulation and aging in the peripheral organs and in the brain, where it can potentiate hormone production or other processes affecting aging. p53 can also regulate hermesis in response to γ-irradiation[95] and, moreover, p53 also potentiates life extension in response to the mitochondrial stress associated with downregulation of mitochondrial genes[96]. Accordingly, it was reported that the positive and negative effects of p53 on lifespan was dependent on the level of mitochondrial bioenergetic stress[97].

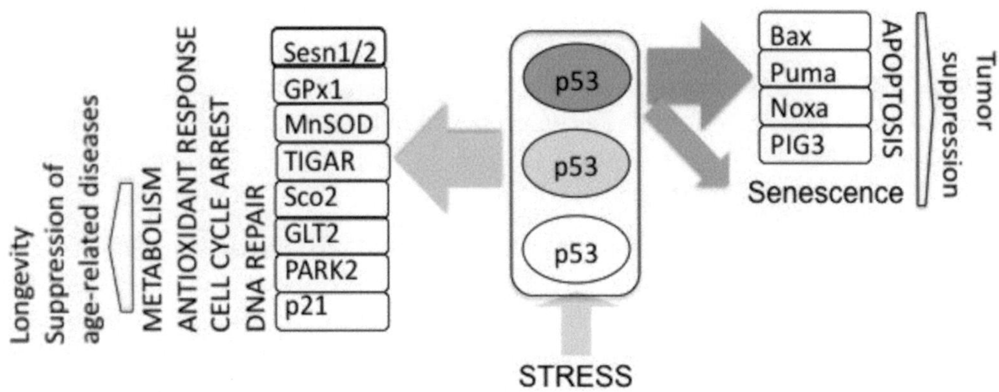

Figure 2. Tumor-suppressor p53 regulates lifespan and suppresses age-related diseases. p53 is activated in response to different stress insults and dependent on the stress intensity triggers different sets of genes either supporting pro-survival or cell death programs. p53 can support longevity and suppress age-related diseases via regulation of DNA-repair, cell cycle, metabolism and antioxidant response. Otherwise p53 eliminates damaged and potentially dangerous cells through activation of apoptosis or senescence, suppressing carcinogenesis.

4. Role of FoxO family in cellular processes and longevity

Another group of proteins playing a critical role in the lifespan regulation and aging are the transcription factors of the FoxO family. Analysis of *Caenorhabditis elegans* mutants, which extended lifespan of the worms, led to the identification of DAF2 and AGE1 genes, the orthologues of the mammalian In/IGF1R and PI3K genes respectively. Simultaneous inactivation of DAF16 suppressed extended lifespan phenotype of the *DAF2*- and *AGE1*-mutants providing a link between DAF2, AGE1 and DAF16. There is only one FoxO gene in invertebrate genome (DAF16 in *Caenorhabditis elegans*; dFoxO in *Drosophila Melanogaster*) while a mammalian genome is composed of four members FoxO1, FoxO3A, FoxO4 and FoxO6[98]. In spite of high sequence similarity and recognition similar sequences in the promoters of target genes, the mammalian FoxO family members have different tissue-specific expression and potentially different, although overlapping, functions in the organism. According to knockout studies, inactivation of FoxO1 is embryonically lethal due to insufficient vascularisation of the embryo. *FoxO3A*-deficient animals are viable, although demonstrate defects in ovarian follicle activation, while *FoxO4*-deficient animals are viable with no significant abnormalities[98].

Insulin/IGF1 signaling inhibits FoxO via activation of the PI3K-AKT pathway(Fig.3), followed by phosphorylation the FoxO proteins by AKT on highly conserved residues. AKT phosphorylation makes FoxOs susceptible for interaction with 14-3-3 proteins, which bind and retain FoxOs in the cytoplasm masking their nuclear localization signal[98]. Thus, AKT phosphorylation invalidates the transcriptional activity of FoxOs, inhibiting FoxO-dependent processes. On the contrary, FoxO can be phosphorylated and activated by Jun N-terminus kinase (JNK) and STE20-like protein kinase 1 (MST1). JNK and MST1 can be activated by different stress insults, most evidently oxidative stress, with activating phosphorylation of FoxOs by JNK and MST1 having predominate inhibitory effects of AKT[98, 99]. Strikingly, prolonged activation of In/IGF1R stimulates ROS production, which leads to JNK activation followed by FoxO phosphorylation and nuclear translocation, counteracting effects of AKT on FoxO suppression. Similar to FoxOs, JNK is an important regulator of longevity[100], extending lifespan in worms and flies by suppressing Insulin/IGF1 signaling pathway [101, 102].

FoxOs impinge on the control of lifespan potentially via transcriptional regulation of genes involved in the stress-response, although the critical targets involved in this process are unknown. Potential candidates are ROS scavengers, such as: MnSOD, Catalase and peroxiredoxin3 (Prx3); regulators of protein synthesis, such as: 4EBP1 and regulators of autophagy, including BCL2/adenovirus E1B 19 kDa protein-interacting protein 3 (BNIP3), LC3 and Garabl12[98]. Interestingly, FoxO can also stimulate autophagy through a mechanism independent of its transcriptional activity[103]. Besides the activation of stress-relieving pathways, FoxOs also inhibit cell cycle though several mechanisms, such as activation of cell cycle inhibitors p27 and p21, and suppression of cell cycle regulators c-Myc and cyclin D[98, 99]. Accordingly, overexpression of FoxO3A causes G2-M delay in fibroblasts[98]. Regulation of the cell cycle by FoxOs might be important for stress-relieving mechanisms, as cells need to restrain proliferation in order to restore homeostasis and avoid accumulation of damages[98].

The activities of FoxOs are not limited to the activation of stress-relieving and pro-survival pathways. FoxOs also activate the expression of proapoptotic proteins Bim, Puma, Fas ligand (FasL) and TRAIL and stimulate cell death under certain conditions[98]. The exact mechanism that discriminates between pro-survival and pro-death programs regulated by FoxOs are unknown, the outcome of FoxOs activation might be dependent on severity of stress and cell type.

The regulation of pro-survival stress-relieving genes and pro-apoptotic genes by FoxOs is reminiscent of the effects p53 on cell homeostasis, which protects under low stress conditions and induces cell death when stress is too strong and causes accumulation of damages within the cell[15]. Strikingly, FoxOs and p53 are able to activate the same targets including MnSOD, catalase, Sesn1, p21 and Puma[15, 98]. It is possible that there is some functional redundancy in the regulation of stress response by p53 and FoxO proteins, ensuring the proper outcome should one of the pathways be disabled. Interestingly, p53 and FoxOs are under mutual regulation. p53 positively regulate FoxO3A via transcriptional activation of FoxO3A gene[104], although p53 also stimulates expression of MDM2, which is involved in FoxO ubiquitination and degradation[105]. Surprisingly, in response to DNA-damage p53 can inhibit FoxO3A via SGK1 kinase activation and subsequent FoxO3A retention in cytoplasm[106]. FoxOs can also regulate p53 in a positive or negative manner. FoxOs stimulate activity of AKT, which negatively regulates p53 via phosphorylation of MDM2[99]. FoxO3A can also impair p53 transactivational function, although can positively regulate p53-dependent cell death in serum starved cells[107]. Otherwise, FoxO3A directly interacts with the ATM kinase, upstream p53 activator, and stimulates ATM phosphorylation on Ser1981, regulating DNA-damage response which might be involved in p53 activation[108]. FoxOs can also upregulate p53 via activation of upstream p53 regulator Arf[109]. This complicated picture illustrates that there is a communication between p53 and FoxOs providing the mutual control of activity determining cell fate (Fig.3).

The antioxidant function of FoxOs is especially important for control of stem cell maintenance. The mice with simultaneous inactivation of FoxO1, FoxO3A and FoxO4 in hematopoietic system had diminished number of hematopoietic stem cells (HSC) in bone marrow, paralleling expansion of myeloid progenitor cells in the blood. *FoxO*-deficient HSC had elevated levels of ROS in comparison to WT control and have strong defects in the ability to restore hematopoietic system of recipient mice, indicating the critical role of FoxO in self-renewal of stem cells. These defects were rescued by treatment with antioxidant NAC, confirming the critical role of FoxO in the regulation of HSC ROS, which is important for regulation of HSC quiescence and regenerating ability[98].

Another function of FoxOs is the control of metabolism. FoxO1 is highly expressed in insulin-responsive tissues and regulates glucose and lipid metabolism, ensuing adaptation to different feeding conditions. In response to the decrease of insulin levels, FoxO1 intensified gluconeogenesis in the liver through regulation of glucose-6-phosphatase (G6Pase) and phosphoenolpyruvate carboxykinase (PEPK). FoxO1 also stimulated transcriptional co-activator PGC1α and synergizes with PGC1α for G6Pase transactivation. The activation of G6Pase and PEPK ensures stable blood glucose levels in fast conditions. FoxO1 also regulates lipid metabolism via activation of an inhibitor of lipoprotein lipase apoliprotein (ApoCIII), which is involved in hypertrigyceridemia development in diabetic patients[98].

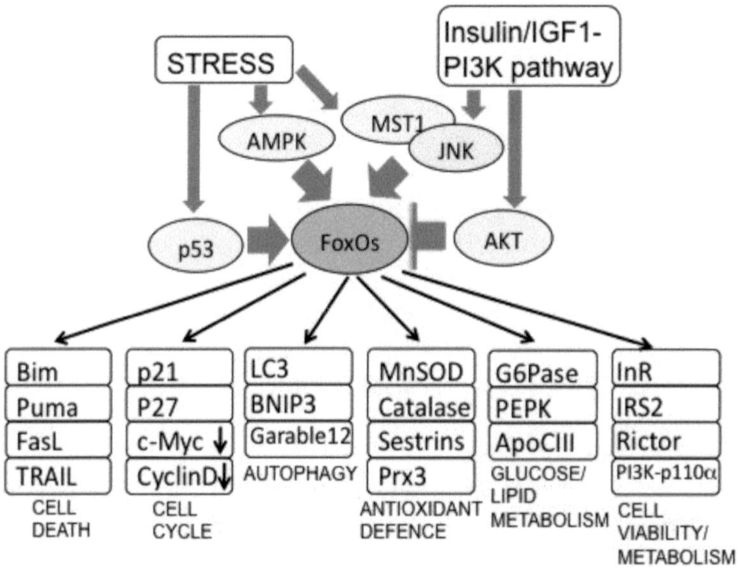

Figure 3. Stress and the insulin/IGF1-PI3K-AKT pathway control cellular processes through regulation of FoxOs. While many stress insults activate FoxOs, the Insulin/IGF1-PI3K-AKT inhibits their activity. Thus FoxO factors integrate the information from different signaling pathways and control the expression of genes involved in regulation of cell proliferation and viability, autophagy, metabolism and cell death. As a result they contribute to regulation of longevity by FoxOs.

The regulation of genes involved in glucose and lipid metabolism underlines the potential role of FoxOs in diabetes which might work in a protective fashion or exacerbate the diabetic phenotype. Insulin resistance and glucose intolerance, the hallmark of type II diabetes, are characterized by the suppression of the PI3K-AKT signaling pathway [110]. This might be due to the elevated activity of mTORC1 which phosphorylates and regulates IRS1 and Grb10 proteins[3]. IRS1 transduces signals from In/IGF1R toward PI3K and its phosphorylation by mTORC1-dependent p70S6K causes its degradation. Grb10 negatively regulates growth factor signaling through binding of IGF1R and its phosphorylation by mTORC1 stabilizes and activates Grb10[111, 112]. FoxOs can modulate insulin signaling through AMPK activation and TORC1 inhibition as well as via transcriptional activation of IRS2, PI3K (p110a) and InR [99] and the activation of these proteins potentially support insulin sensitivity. FoxOs also activate rictor, the critical component of TORC2 complex required for phosphorylation and full activation of AKT [7, 99]. In contrast, the diabetic phenotype caused by InR deficiency was rescued by FoxO1 heterozygosity, where deletion of one FoxO1 allele restored insulin sensitivity[98], indicating that tight control of FoxO activity was required for proper protective function of FoxO factors.

5. Identification and characterization of Sestrins

Sestrins are highly conserved gene gamily found in all multicellular organisms of the animal kingdom. The invertebrate genome contains one Sestrin (Sesn) gene while there are three genes in vertebrates Sesn1, Sesn2 and Sesn3[15]. Sesn1, originally named p53-activated gene #26 (PA26), was identified as a p53-inducibe gene in a screening where p53 was induced in a tetracycline–dependent manner[113]. The human *SESN1* gene is found in 6q21 position[114] and is transcribed into three different mRNA translated into proteins with Mw~46, 55 and 68kD[114]. The Sesn1 mRNAs are transcribed from 3 promoters using an alternative first exon (Exon 1,2 or 3), which is spliced with the common exon 4[114]. All protein products of *SESN1* share the same C-terminal part encoded by exons 4-10. Among the three transcripts only short transcripts 2 and 3 are induced by p53, while transcript 1 is constantly expressed regardless of p53 status[114]. The gene is ubiquitously expressed in all tissues, although at different levels and predominantly in the pancreas, kidney, skeletal muscle, lung, placenta, brain, ovary and testis[114]. Sesn1 is a stress-responsive gene activated in response to genotoxic stress imposed by γ-irradiation, UV-light and doxorubicin treatment in a p53-dependent manner[114]. Sesn1 is induced with kinetics similar to the "classical" p53-inducible genes MDM2 and p21, indicating that this is a direct p53 target[114]. p53-responsive elements were identified within intron 1[115] and intron 2[114] of the Sesn1 gene, although the exact role of either of these elements in Sesn1 activation by p53 *in vivo* requires additional analysis. Besides genotoxic stress, Sesn1 is also activated in response to serum withdrawal[114], indicating the regulation by a transcription factor(s), which are under control by growth factors. Among them, FoxOs are the most prominent candidates, which expression is negatively regulated by insulin and IGF1 through activation of the PI3K-AKT signaling pathway followed by inhibitory phosphorylation of FoxOs by AKT[98, 99]. Accordingly, Sesn1 was identified by microarray analysis and real time PCR as a gene activated by FoxO3A[116] and FoxO1[117, 118] (Fig.4).

Sesn2 was identified by microarray analysis as a gene activated by severe hypoxia in glioblastoma A172 cells [119]. The human *SESN2* gene is located in position of 1p35.3[119] and is transcribed into one mRNA that encodes a polypeptide with Mw~60 kDa[119]. Similar to Sesn1, Sesn2 is expressed in all tissues, but predominantly in the placenta, lung, liver, kidney, pancreas, testis and leucocytes (AVB and Chumakov PM, unpublished). Besides hypoxia, Sesn2 is activated in response to many stress insults including oxidative stress, DNA-damage and metabolic derangements[119]. In spite of the important role of HIF1 in the regulation of hypoxia-inducible genes, activation of Sesn2 by hypoxia was not dependent on HIF1[119]. This is supported by several observations: (i) the kinetics of Sesn2 induction is significantly delayed compared to typical HIF1-dependent genes such as VEGF and RTP801, but similar to induction of HIF1-independent GADD153 gene; (ii) no HIF1-binding sites were found in the promoter or introns of the Sesn2 gene[119]; (iii) Sesn2 was induced in response to hypoxia mimetic deferoxamine mesylate in *HIF1a*-proficient but not *HIF1α*-deficient immortalized astrocytes (ABV, unpublished). Nevertheless, HIF1 can contribute to Sesn2 expression under some conditions. Thus it was showed that HIF1 protected airway epithelium against oxidative stress potentially via the activation of Sesn2[120]. Sesn2 is also activated by NO and hypoxia in a HIF1-dependent manner in macrophages[121], so it is possible that HIF1 plays a role in Sesn2 regulation in tissue-specific manner. Genotoxic stress imposed by γ-irradiation, UV light, doxorubicin, etoposide and camptothecin induces Sesn2 expression in a p53-dependent manner[119, 122]. The activation of two of the three members of Sestrin family by p53 indicates the importance of Sestrins in p53-dependent processes. The p53-binding site was identified by chromatin immunoprecipitation (ChIP) with the paired-end ditag (PET) sequencing strategy in the region 9.6 kb downstream of *SESN2* gene[115]. Oxidative stress activates Sesn2 in a p53-independent manner, although p53, which is also activated by oxidative stress, contributes to transactivation of Sesn2[123]. The mechanism of Sesn2 activation in response to oxidative burst induced by NMDA receptor is described in neurons, where Sesn2 induction is mediated by C/EBPβ transcription factor via –378 to –249 and –249 to –107 regions in *SESN2* promoter[124] (Fig.4A).

Another mechanism of Sesn2 regulation involves nerve growth factor-induced-B member Nur77 (NGFI-Bα/TR3), an orphan nuclear receptor expressed in multiple tissues[125]. Two Nur77 activators 1,1-Bis(3'-indolyl)-1-(*p*-methoxyphenyl)-methane (DIM-C-pPhOCH3) and 1,1-bis(3'-indolyl)-1-(*p*-phenyl)methane (DIM-C-pPhOH) induce Sesn2 and activation of Sesn2 in response to these compounds is inhibited by shRNA against Nur77[125]. Stimulated Nur77 inhibits cell proliferation and induces cell death. Moreover treatment with Nur77 activator DIM-C-pPhOCH3 suppressed growth of human bladder cancer cell line KU7, suggesting the impact of Sesn2 and several other genes co-activated with Sesn2 in suppression of tumor growth and tumor cells' viability [125]. Accordingly we showed that Sesn2 suppressed colony-formation in different cancer cell lines originated from lung, colon, breast and kidney tumors[119] (Fig.4A).

Other stimuli activate Sesn2 via a yet to be defined mechanisms. Sesn2 is activated in response to expression of HIV Tat protein in the brain potentially through induction of inflammation and oxidative stress[126]. Accordingly Sesn2 is also activated in response to β-amyloid peptides associated with oxidative stress in neurons[127]. Impact inflammation in Sesn2 expression might be mediated by NO-production, and accordingly NO is the Sesn2 activator[128]. Sesn2 is also activated in the brain of *Securin*-deficient mice[129]. Securin is a protein, which in complex with Separase, regulates chromosomal separation and metaphase-anaphase transition[129]. Securin deficiency causes genomic instability and might regulate Sesn2 via p53 activation. Sesn2 transcriptional activity is also regulated by the mechanisms involved acetylation/deacetylation of histones, which can be controlled by oxidative stress and other stimuli[130]. In accordance, treatment with the histone deacetylase inhibitor trichostatin A (TSA) induces Sesn2 expression in neurons[130].

Sesn2 modulates cell viability in response to stress, aggravating cell death in response to DNA-damage, induced by UV light and doxorubicin, and serum starvation but supporting cell viability in conditions of H2O2 treatment and hypoxia[119]. It might play an important role in tissue protection in response to ischemia/hypoxia and some other stress insults. According to our data, Sesn2 is activated in the brain in a model of acute ischemia induced by acute hypoxia in a model of stroke, created in rats by permanent middle cerebral artery occlusion (MCAO)[119].

Sesn3 was originally identified *in silico* via search of databases for the sequences sharing homology with the Sesn1 and Sesn2 genes[119, 131]. The human *SESN3* gene is located in position 11q21[119] and is transcribed into 2 mRNA which translated into proteins with Mw~53kDa and ~44kDa, lacking 72 AA at N-terminal part[118]. Similar to other Sestrins, Sesn3 is expressed in all tissues, and increased levels of expression are observed in skeletal muscle, placenta, small intestine, leucocytes, kidney, colon and brain[131]. Sesn3 was identified as a direct target of FoxO3A and FoxO1 transcription factors [117, 118]. FoxO1 directly activates Sesn3 via binding of a 250bp region within 1st intron of human and mouse *SESN3* gene[118] (Fig.4A).

Protein products of Sesrin genes from different organisms display the highest similarity with Sesn1. According to prediction by GLOBE, (http://cubic.bioc.columbia.edu/predictprotein) Sestrins are compact globular domain proteins composed of α-helical regions. Three of these α-helical regions which include helices α3-α8, α9-α10, and α11-α16 are highly conserved among Sestrins and are separated by less conserved hinge regions. According to ProSite analysis (http://www.expasy.ch/prosite) Sestrins contain several Ser/Thr and Tyr phosphorylation sites, mainly located in α-helical regions, including CK2 phosphorylation sites in α8 and α10, three PKC sites in α11, α15 and α16, one cAMP/cGMP-dependent protein kinase phosphorylation site in α10 and one tyrosine phosphorylation site within helix α14. There are also 13 potential tyrosine residues within helices α11-α16, which can be phosphorylated by Tyr kinases[119]. Although these predictions require verification, phosphorylation of several residues was demonstrated in high-throughput screenings, thus S352 of Sesn1 is phosphorylated by ATM kinase, implying the role of Sesn1 in DNA-damage response and metabolism[132]. According to phosphopeptyde database (http://www.phosphosite.org) Sesn2 phosphorylations on Tyr342 and Tyr356 were found in acute myelogenous leukemia indicating involvement of Sesn2 in tyrosine-kinase signaling.

Efforts to characterize Sestrins in the other organisms led to the identification of Sesn1 gene in *Xenopus Laevis*[133]. Although no function was assigned, it was showed that Sesn1 was accumulated in notochord at the onset of neurolation[133]. The reciprocal translocation (6;18)(q21;q21) observed in heterotaxia (abnormal organs arrangement in the body) patients revealed breakpoint region within 1st intron of *Sesn1* gene, which led to propose that Sesn1 might be responsible for the heterotaxia phenotype[131]. These observations were followed by analysis of zebrafish model. Knockdown of Sesn1 in the zebrafish caused lateral disturbances in the heart and gut, providing evidence for a potential role of Sesn1 in the regulation of left-right asymmetry via Nodal signaling pathway[134]. Interestingly, Nodal auto-activation is mediated by a forkhead transcription factor FoxH1 (known as Sur in zebrafish) and Sesn1 is able to interact with FoxH1 *in vitro*[134].

To gain insight into the physiological function of Sestrins we studied the functions of drosophila (d) Sesn (dSesn) in fly model[135]. The analysis of expression has been shown that the dSesn expression is increased in adult flies in comparison to larvae stage, and dSesn is highly expressed in thoracic muscle (analog of skeletal muscle in mammals)[135]. Interestingly, dSesn expression in fly muscles recapitulates the high expression level of the members of the Sestrin family in skeletal muscles in mammals[114, 119, 131]. Overexpression of dSesn in the dorsal wing region produces a bent up wing phenotype and Sesn2 activation in the eyes diminishes the eye size. Both phenotypes were evoked by decreased cell size, while dSesn overexpression did not affect cell number[135]. Knockout of dSesn do not seem to cause any developmental problems indicating no role of dSesn in morphogenesis. Nevertheless, the adult flies accumulated many age related defects, suggesting a role of Sentrins in the regulation of aging (see below)[135]. Interestingly, similar to mammalian Sestrins, dSesn is also under control of p53 and FoxO, although dFoxO appeared to be the predominant transcriptional activator of dSesn[135] (Fig.4B).

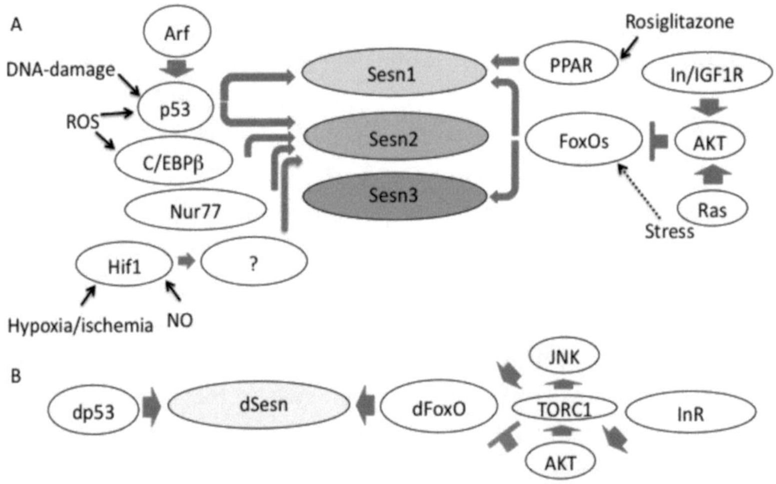

Figure 4. Regulation of Sestrins' expression. (A) Different stress insults regulate Sestrin genes via activation of p53, FoxOs, C/EBPβ and some other transcriptional factors in mammals. On the contrary AKT activated in response to insulin/IGF1 pathway or Ras can suppress activity of FoxOs. **(B)** Similar to mammals, drosophila (d) Sesn is activated by dp53 and dFoxO. Prolonged stimulation of InR stimulates dSesn expression through the TORC1-JNK-dFoxO axis, counteracting an inhibitory effect of AKT activation.

6. Antioxidant function of Sestrins

Identification of Sestrin gene family did not provide any clues toward their functions due to low similarity with any other proteins [1]. To better understand Sestrins' function, an iterative analysis of Sesn2 protein sequence using PSI-BLAST and structural analysis using 3D-PSSM programs were performed. We have observed that a fragment of protein around 75 amino acids in length (corresponding to region amino acids 100-175 of Sesn2) shares sequence and structural homology with *Mycobacterial Tuberculosis* AhpD protein and other related proteins[123]. The homology spans 5 a-helices of conserved region of Sestrins and C-terminal a-helical portion of AhpD[123]. Interestingly, some AhpD family members, such as caroboxymuconolactone decarboxylases, consist of this domain only. AhpD is a critical component *Mycobacterium tuberculosis* hidroperoxide reductase responsible for regeneration of bacterial peroxiredoxin AhpC, which is oxidized during reduction and decomposition of ROS or reactive nitrogen species (RNS). Peroxiredoxins are thiol-containing peroxidases conserved among prokaryotes and eukaryotes which catalytical center contains 2 conserved cysteines, one is a peroxidatic cysteine oxidized to SOH group during reaction with peroxides, and the other is resolving cysteine which forms disulfide bridge with catalytical cysteine. Oxidized cysteines are regenerated by AhpD in *Mycobacterium tuberculosis* or the thioredoxin/thioredoxin-reductase (Trx/TrxR) system in eukaryotes[15, 136]. AhpD contains two critical cysteines, whereas only one of them is conserved in Sestrins[123]. The major difference between prokaryotic and eukaryotic peroxiredoxins is that reactive cysteine of eukaryotic peroxiredoxins can be easily overoxidized to cysteine sulphinic acid (-SO_2H) or sulphonic acid (-SO_3H) forms and special enzymatic system is required for the regeneration of the overoxidized cysteine[136].

The homology between Sestrins and AhpD indicates that Sestrins might be antioxidant proteins regulating mammalian peroxiredoxins. Accordingly, Sesn1- or Sesn2-silenced cells have elevated ROS levels and exhibit oxidative stress as supported by elevated levels of DNA-oxidation and increased mutagenesis[62, 123]. Sesn1- and Sesn2-silenced cells also have higher RNS levels comparatively to control implying the role of Sestrins in RNS metabolism as well. Complementary experiments have been shown that ectopic expression of either Sesn1 or Sesn2 downregulates ROS in different cell lines, indicating that Sestrins are stress-responsive antioxidant proteins[123]. The important role of the conserved cysteine was supported mutation analysis, demonstrating that substitution of the conserved cysteine impairs antioxidant activity of Sestrins. Sestrins co-localize and interact with peroxiredoxin1 (Prx1) and peroxiredoxin2 (Prx2) proteins within the cell and support regeneration of overoxidized peroxiredoxins[123]. However, the following studies showed that sulfiredoxin protein, unrelated to Sestrin family, plays a major role in regeneration of peroxiredoxins in most eukaryotic species and Sestrins do not have intrinsic sulfinil reductase activity[137]. Thus, Sestrins play an indirect role in peroxiredoxin signaling working as auxiliary or regulatory proteins[1]. According to other observations, the important impact of Sestrins on peroxiredoxin-mediated antioxidant response were demonstrated in macrophages and NMDA-stimulated neurons[121, 124].

Being p53-activated proteins, Sesn1 and Sesn2 mediate antioxidant activities of p53, and ectopic expression of Sesn1 and Sesn2 partially restores normal ROS levels, elevated in p53-deficient cells[62]. Sesn1 and Sesn2 also suppress DNA-oxidation and mutagenesis in p53-silenced lung carcinoma A549 cells [62]. FoxO-inducible gene Sesn3 also inhibits ROS accumulation, and AKT stimulates ROS production via FoxO-dependent downregulation of Sesn3[117]. As mentioned, FoxOs, similar to p53, regulate ROS in a pro-oxidant and an anti-oxidant fashion, dependent upon conditions[15, 138]. In response to detrimental genotoxic stress induced by etoposide and doxorubicin, FoxO3A stimulates expression of the pro-apoptotic protein Bim and its induction is associated with oxidative burst and induction of cell death. Simultaneously, FoxO3A stimulates expression of the antioxidant Sesn3 protein, and silencing of Sesn3 accelerates the levels of FoxO3A-induced cell death[138]. It is possible that Sestrins set up a protective mode against misfired induction of cell death by FoxOs and p53 preventing undesirable cell death (Fig.5).

The antioxidant activities of Sestrins play a potential role in carcinogenesis, and inactivation of Sestrins might be desirable for cancer cells, which can exploit the effect of Sestrin deficiency on mild ROS production. ROS are involved in mutagenesis and genomic instability, associated with selection of more malignant cells, stimulation of cell cycle, angiogenesis and epithelial-mesenchymal transition. At the same time, high ROS levels can be detrimental for viability of cancer cells, this feature is exploited by some anticancer treatments[139]. Mutant Ras proteins induce ROS, which are important for cell transformation by the Ras oncogene[140]. Accordingly, expression of Sesn1 and Sesn3 genes are inhibited by Ras, supporting ROS accumulation in response to Ras expression[141]. The expression of both FoxO-dependent genes Sesn1 and Sesn3 were decreased in response to Ras, while Sesn2 was not affected [141]. Ras activates AKT through stimulation of PI3K and potentially inhibit Sesn1 and Sesn3 via suppression of FoxOs[1].

7. Regulation of AMPK-TOR signaling by Sestrins

As antioxidant proteins, Sestrins are potential regulators of many cell signaling pathways which are sensitive to redox status in the cell. One of them is the mTORC1-dependent pathway, which is regulated by ROS on different levels. ROS directly affect activity of mTOR[15] or works upstream via inhibition of different phosphatases, such as PTEN or members of the tyrosine phosphatase family, which catalitical cysteine is sensitive to inhibitory oxidation [142]. Inactivation of these phosphatases can enhance the signaling pathways activated by receptor tyrosine kinases leading to the PI3K-AKT-mTORC1 activation[15]. Ectopic expression of either member of the Sestrin family suppresses mTORC1 activity in different human and mouse cells (Fig.5), as indicated by inhibition of phosphorylation of p70S6K, S6 and 4E-BP proteins[122], similar to effects of rapamycin[122]. In complementary experiments knockdown of either Sesn1 or Sesn2 stimulated mTORC1 activation[122]. Surprisingly, ectopic expression of a redox-deficient mutant of Sesn2 inhibited mTORC1 with the same efficiency as WT Sesn2 protein, indicating that Sestrins regulate mTORC1 in a ROS-independent manner[122].

To gain insight into the mechanism of mTORC1 regulation, Sesn2 was co-expressed with different upstream mTORC1 activators including H-Ras, AKT or Rheb. Sesn2 was able to suppress mTORC1 activity in the cells transfected with H-Ras or AKT constructs, but all effects of Sesn2 were eliminated by co-expression of Rheb. This data indicates that Sestrins regulate mTORC1 downstream of H-Ras and AKT but upstream of Rheb[122]. Rheb-GTP analysis in breast carcinoma MCF7 cells demonstrated that induction of Sesn2 strongly inhibited Rheb-GTP loading, indicating an inhibitory effect of Sestrins on Rheb[122].

Rheb activity is regulated by the TSC1:TSC2 protein complex and Sestrins inhibit Rheb in a TSC2-dependent manner. The following experiments showed that Sestrins regulated TSC1:TSC2 activity not trough regulation of upstream TSC2 kinases AKT and ERK [122]. AMPK is the kinase which directly phosphorylates and activates TSC2 in response to stress and we have shown that either Sesn1 or Sesn2 stimulate AMPK phosphorylation on Thr172 followed TSC2 phosphorylation and activation by AMPK [122] (Fig.5). Moreover, it has been demonstrated that Sesn2 stimulates expression of AMPK subunits in response to DNA-damage[143]. An inhibition of mTORC1 in an AMPK- and TSC2-dependent manner was demonstrated later for Sesn3[118].

To examine whether Sesn2 can be directly involved in TSC2 and AMPK activation, purification and analysis of Sesn2-containing protein complexes were performed in gel-filtration experiments. As shown, Sesn1 and Sesn2 were co-eluted in a high molecular weight fractions (411-1175 kDa), together with the TSC1, TSC2 and AMPK proteins[122]. Immunoprecipitation of protein complexes with anti-Sesn2 antibodies allowed us to co-purify AMPKα1 and AMPKα2 subunits and the TSC1:TSC2 complex with Sesn2, indicating an interaction of Sestrins with the AMPK, TSC1 and TSC2 proteins [122]. Moreover, we observed binding of GST-Sesn2 with AMPKα proteins, supporting the idea that Sestrins activate AMPK via direct protein-protein interactions (AVB, unpublished)[122].

The inhibition of mTORC1 by Sestrins has an impact on many mTORC1-dependent processes including translation, cell growth and proliferation. Accordingly, significant downregulation of CyclinD1 and c-Myc expression was observed in breast carcinoma MCF7 cells in response to Sesn2 induction[122]. The mechanism of inhibition of protein synthesis by Sestrins involves formation of the 4EBP1- eIF-4E complex, which suppresses initiation of translation of the Cap-dependent mRNAs[122]. Being stress-inducible proteins, Sestrins are potential regulators of protein synthesis in response to stress. Accordingly, it has been shown that Sesn1 and Sesn2 play a critical role in inhibition of protein synthesis in response to γ-irradiation in breast epithelial MCF10A cells [144].

Regulation of translation and metabolism via mTORC1 inhibition strongly affects cell growth, proliferation and cell viability. Accordingly, ectopic expression of Sestrins in different cell lines causes a decrease in cell size as compared to GFP control, supporting the inhibitory role of Sestrins on cell growth[122]. Cell growth is linked with cell proliferation, and we showed that Sestrins inhibited cell proliferation in many cell types such as human lung carcinoma H1299, human fibrosarcoma HT1080, human breast carcinoma MCF7 and human immortalized fibroblasts from Li-Fraumeni patient MDA041[119]. Using matched HCT116 cells with normal p53 and p21 status, p53-deficient or p21-deficient cells, we also showed that the inhibition of cell proliferation by Sestrins was p53- and p21- independent (AVB and Chumakov PM, unpublished). Sestrins inhibited cell proliferation as evident by accumulation of cells in the G1 phase of the cell cycle after Sesn2 overexpression[122]. To confirm the importance of mTORC1 in the regulation of cell growth and proliferation Sesn2 was ectopically expressed in *TSC2*-deficient cells, and no effects on cell growth and proliferation were observed in the absence of TSC2 protein[122].

AMPK activation and mTORC1 inhibition also regulates autophagy through phosphorylation of ULK1 kinase and we showed that Sestrins stimulated autophagy in H1299 cells (AVB and Karin M, unpublished). It has been demonstrated that Sesn2 regulates autophagy in response to rapamycin, nutrient-free medium, thapsigargin (an activator of endoplasmic stress), and lithium in human colon carcinoma HCT116 cells [145]. The activation of autophagy in response to these stimuli requires p53, and autophagy was significantly inhibited in HCT116 p53-null cells. The potential explanation for this effect is that expression of Sesn2 and other p53-dependent proteins involved in autophagy such as Sesn1, DRAM, LC3 and ULK1 is supported by p53[15, 20, 74, 146]. Accordingly, silencing of DRAM, another important regulator of autophagy, had similar inhibitory effects on autophagy as Sesn2 knockdown [145] (Fig.5).

The effects of Sestrins on cell physiology is not only limited to regulation of cell proliferation but also involves regulation of cell viability. Sesn2 overexpression in 293 cells stimulates cell death[119]. Sestrins also modulate cell viability under stress condition, protecting from oxidative stress, but supporting cell death in response to genotoxic stress[119, 123, 143, 147]. Cell death in response to γ-irradiation is regulated in an AMPK-dependent manner and Sesn2 plays a major role in regulation of AMPK phosphorylation in response to genotoxic stress[40, 41, 143].

The prominent role of p53 in the regulation of Sesn1 and Sesn2, and FoxOs in the regulation of Sesn3, make Sestrins potential mediators of p53 and FoxO-dependent processes. We showed that silencing of either Sesn1 or Sesn2 released the inhibitory effects of p53 on mTORC1 in different experimental contexts including overexpression of p53 in p53-deficient H1299 cells, stimulation p53 by Nutlin-3 in U2OS cells and activation by the genotoxic drug camptothecin in mouse embryonic fibroblasts[122]. Moreover, Sesn2 regulates mTORC1 activity *in vivo* in mouse liver in response to treatment with the alkylating liver-specific poison diethylnitrosamine[122]. Another group also demonstrated that fangchinoline, bis-benzylisoquinoline alkaloid, which is considered as new antitumor agents, activated Sesn2 expression through p53 and regulates autophagy via activation of AMPK kinase[148]. Interestingly, fangchinoline is able to stimulate cell death through induction of autophagy, explaining the potential role of Sestrins in support of cell death in response to some stimuli[119]. p53 can be inactivated in many cancer cells through interaction with inhibitory proteins, which might be potential targets for anticancer treatment. In lung cancer cell lines p53 is bound to and inactivated by orphan nuclear receptor Nur77/TR3. Nur77 suppression by siRNA released p53, which in turn stimulated Sesn2. It led to AMPK activation and mTORC1 suppression, resulting in inhibition of growth and inducing apoptosis in lung carcinoma cells[149].

The regulation of the AMPK-TORC1 axis by Sestrins is highly conserved in evolution. We showed that similar to mammalian Sestrins, dSesn inhibited TORC1, as indicated by diminished levels of p70S6K phosphorylation, in an AMPK- and TSC2-dependent manner. Inactivation of dSesn led to many abnormalities associated with AMPK-TORC1 dysregulation, such as metabolic derangements and oxidative stress. Interestingly, the effects of dSesn inactivation can be normalized by reconstitution with mammalian Sestrins, while dSesn activates mammalian AMPK and inhibits mTORC1, indicating the highly conservative functions of Sestrins[135].

8. Regulation of TGFβ signaling by Sesn2

The AMPK-TOR axis is not the only signaling pathway modulated by Sestrins. A new role of Sestrins was described in the control of transforming growth factor-β (TGFβ) signaling. TGFβ signaling is regulated by binding of a dimer of TGFβ ligands (composed of TGFβ1,2 3) with TGFβ receptor (TGFβR 1 and 2), stimulating its heterodimerisation and activation of its intrinsic Ser/Thr kinase activity[150, 151]. Cells secrete TGFβ as large latent complex containing one of three latent TGFβ binding proteins LTBP1, LTBP2 and LTBP4 belonging to the fibrillin family of extracellular matrix (ECM) proteins[150]. LTBPs target TGFβ to ECM depositing them for mobilization when activation of TGF-β signaling is required. Activated TGF-βR transduces a signal to proteins of the Smad family, classified as receptor-associated Smads (R-Smads: Smad 1,2,3,5&8), cooperating Smads (Co-Smads: Smad4) and inhibitory Smads (i-Smads: Smad6&7). It was shown that R-Smads, Smad1-5, are substrates of TGFβ receptors, activated by TGFβ, while others are activated by other members of the TGFβ family via interaction with relevant receptors. Phosphorylated Smad2 and Smad3 form heteromeric complexes with Smad4, which translocate to the nucleus where they bind Smad-dependent promoters and activate expression of a number of genes such as α-smooth muscle actin (⟨SMA), connective tissue growth factor (CTGF) and matrix metalloproteinase 2 (MMP2) involved in regulation of cell growth, differentiation and migration[147, 152]. TGFβ also controls other signaling pathways through RhoA, Cdc42, Rac1, Ras, PI3K, PP2A, MEKK1, TAK1 and DAXX proteins. Dysregulation in TGFb-dependent signaling contributes to fibrosis, cancer, cardiovascular and congenital diseases[150]. Sesn2-deficiency leads to activation of TGFβ signaling pathways in lung as well as in mouse lung fibroblasts (MLF) as indicated by increased phosphorylation of Smad2 and Smad3, and elevated expression of TGFb targets such as α-SMA, connective tissue growth factor (CTGF) and MMP2[147]. It has been also shown that inactivation of Sesn2 in MLF activates mTORC1, and TGFβ played a role in this process potentially stimulating the PI3K-AKT pathway[147] (Fig.5). TGFβ pathway is not the only receptor-activated cascade is regulated by Sestins. As reported recently, inactivation of Sesn2 also caused accumulation of platelet-derived growth factor receptor-β (PDGFRβ) in glioblastoma U87 cells. PDGFRβ was accumulated in Sesn2-silenced cell due to impaired ubiquitination and degradation. These cells had increased ROS production and higher rate of autophagy, which can indicate a compromised metabolism[153].

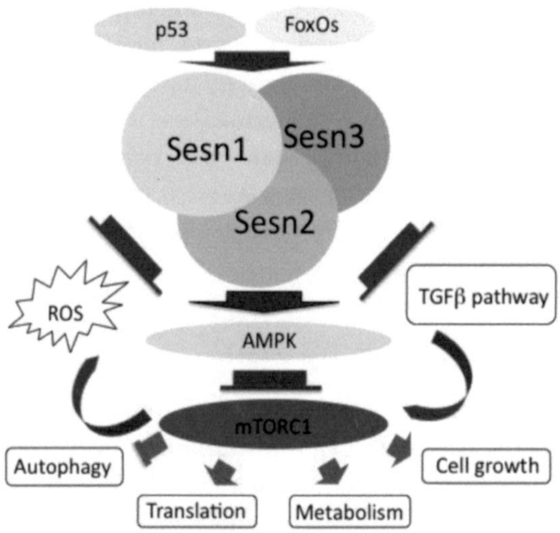

Figure 5. Functions of Sestrins. Sestrins suppress ROS accumulation, inhibit the TGFβ pathway and activate AMPK causing suppression of mTORC1. As a result, Sestrins control many mTORC1-dependent processes such as translation, metabolism, cell growth and autophagy. Inhibition of ROS by Sestrins prevents mutagenesis and genetic instability, the hallmarks of carcinogenesis. Being targets of p53 and FoxOs, Sestrins mediate many p53- and FoxO-regulated processes including regulation of ROS and metabolism potentially contributing to regulation of longevity by these transcriptional factors.

9. Role of Sestrins in aging and diseases

Aging and age-related diseases can be caused by deterioration of the mechanisms controlling stress responses which prevent accumulation of damaged organelles, macromolecular aggregates and ROS in cells through control of anabolic and catabolic processes. Two important functions of mTORC1, such as control of protein synthesis and autophagy are critical for lifespan regulation and fitness, and the pathways, which enhance or suppress mTORC1 activity, may contribute to longevity and health[6]. The members of the Sestrin family are antioxidant proteins involved in suppression of TORC1, so they are potential regulators of aging and longevity.

9.1. Role of Sestrins in aging

The redundancy of the Sestrin family members in mammals complicates the analysis of function of Sestrins in aging and diseases. To gain insight into the role of Sestrins in the regulation of aging, *Drosophila Melanogaster* containing only one Sesn gene (dSesn), was chosen as a convenient model. TORC1 is a critical regulator of aging and lifespan in Drosophila, and activity of TORC1 is elevated in *dSesn*-null flies[135]. Also, we have shown dSesn is induced in response to activation of InR, which stimulate activity of dTOR. dTOR is involved in activation of dSesn through ROS production, which induces JNK followed by activation of dFoxO. AKT, stimulated in response to InR in the same system, is a negative regulator of dFoxO. Thus the signals from AKT and JNK compete for regulation of this transcription factor, with JNK providing the dominant signal. dSesn is induced in response to InR-JNK-dFoxO activation and inhibits TORC1, providing a negative feedback loop toward regulation of InR-AKT-dTOR signaling[135]. Overactivated InR signaling contributes to many age-related pathologies in flies including metabolic derangement and heart and muscle deterioration, so dSesn might have a protective role against these diseases[1, 135].

Accordingly, the *dSesn*-deficient flies have many health-related problems. First, the flies have impaired lipid metabolism and accumulate lipids (Fig.6). The mechanisms of lipid regulation involve two processes: lipogenesis and lipolysis. TOR controls lipolysis through activation of transcriptional factor SREBP. We observed that expression of dSREBP and its targets dFAC, dFAS, dACC and dACS were up-regulated in dSesn-deficient animals, while the expression of the genes involved in lypolisis such as dPGC1α, lip3, CG5966, CG11055 were downregulated. Interestingly, the accumulation of lipids in dSesn-deficient flies was prevented by treatment of flies with either AMPK activators AICAR or metformin, or TOR inhibitor - rapamycin[135].

Second, *dSesn*-null flies demonstrated heart dysfunction manifested in arrhythmia and decreased heart rate due to expansion of diastolic period. This phenotype was largely prevented when flies were treated with AICAR and rapamycin, indicating the role of AMPK-TOR signaling in this process. The activated TOR signaling is associated with ROS accumulation. To examine whether ROS contribute to the phenotype, ROS were suppressed by antioxidant vitamin E or via expression of catalase in heart muscle. Strikingly, both conditions suppressed arrhythmia in *dSesn*-deficient flies but did not prevent the decrease in heart rate, indicating some ROS-independent effects of dSesn on heart protection. We also observed massive disorganization of myofibrils indicated by F-actin staining in *dSesn*-null flies. Thus, dSesn might be important for prevention of heart degeneration associated with activated TOR signaling[135] (Fig.6).

Third, inactivation of dSesn had a detrimental effect on thoracic (skeletal) muscle. The flies were characterized by muscle degeneration as evidenced by loss of sarcomeric structure and diffused sarcomeric boundaries. The muscles exhibited mitochondrial abnormalities such as rounded shape, enlargement and cristae disorganization. Oxidative stress is the typical feature of mitochondrial malfunction and muscle from *dSesn*-null flies showed an increased accumulation of ROS. The detrimental muscle phenotype evoked by dSesn inactivation was prevented by treatment with antioxidant vitamin E, supporting the idea that ROS contribute to muscle degeneration. Deterioration of muscle structure, associated with mitochondrial abnormalities and oxidative stress might be linked to impaired autophagy, the important mechanism for control of muscle cell integrity and function. The defects in autophagy, the controller of muscle integrity, in *dSesn*-deficient flies was evident from accumulation of ubiquitinated protein aggregates, which are cleared via autophagic proteolysis. To examine the potential impact of autophagy on regulation of cardiac and muscle homeostasis we knocked down the ULK1(ATG1) gene, the critical component of the autophagic machinery, which is inhibited by TOR and activated by AMPK. Silencing of ULK1 had effects similar to dSesn inactivation such as cardiac deficiency, muscle degeneration, mitochondrial abnormalities and oxidative stress[135].

The phenotypes observed in young (2-3 weeks old) *dSesn*-deficient flies resembled those in old WT flies, indicating that *dSesn*-null flies in early age have many features of aging animals[135]. Thus dSesn controls processes important for homeostasis, which being improperly regulated can accelerate aging. These processes potentially involve the mechanisms of stress response, which act to repair or remove damaging consequences of stress. Aging and age-related diseases might be a result of unresolved stress which lead to accumulation of damage causing more intense stress, supporting a vicious cycle (Fig.6).

Although the data on the role of Sestrin in aging in vertebrates are scant, there is some evidence that Sestrins might play an important role in protection against aging and age-related diseases in mammals. Strong activation of Sesn1 and Sesn2 was found in s-Arf/p53 mice[90], which demonstrated delayed aging and were protected from carcinogenesis. The activities of AMPK and p53 decline with age as well as the levels of autophagic proteolysis[51, 93, 154]. Sestrins being a link between p53 and AMPK might be suppressed in aging animals, and as a result this dysregulation can weaken the mechanisms protecting their health.

9.2. Sestrins and neurodegenerative diseases

The pathogenesis of many neurodegenerative diseases, such as Alzheimer's, Parkinson's and Huntington's disease are associated with accumulation of protein deposits, which can affect cell physiology and induce oxidative stress and cell death[1]. Inhibition of mTORC1 has a protecting effect by suppressing accumulation of protein deposits, potentially via inhibition of protein translation and activation of autophagy[1, 3]. Sesn2 was activated in human neuroblastoma CHP134 cells in response to amyloid β-peptides, the toxic deposits found in the brain of Alzheimer patients[127]. In another study Sesn2 was found to co-localize with Tau, another protein forming deposits or tangles in neurons, in a subset of neurofibrillary lesions[155]. Pathogenesis of neurodegenerative diseases is associated with oxidative stress and accordingly Sesn2 was activated by ROS in neurons, where Sesn2 plays an antioxidant role[124]. Thus, Sestrins can protect neuronal cells from the toxic effects of neuronal deposits and oxidative stress. The other member of the Sestrin family, Sesn1 was activated in response to the neuroprotective drug rosiglitazone, a member of the thiazolidinedione family of synthetic peroxisome proliferator-activated receptor (PPAR) agonists. Rosiglitazone protects retinal cells from cell death mitigating the effects of ROS and Ca^{2+}, so Sesn1 might be a critical target of this drug involved in regulation of cell viability[156] (Fig.6).

9.3. Sestrins and diabetes

Dysregulation of the AMPK-mTORC1 pathway and ROS metabolism contributes to type II diabetes and Sestrins and their regulator p53 might play a protective role against this disease. According to resent observations, knockin mice where p53 Ser18 (analog of Ser15 in human) was replaced by alanine, showed increased metabolic stress and develop insulin resistance and glucose intolerance, the hallmarks of type II diabetes[157]. Ser18 is the site of phosphorylation of ATM kinase. Inactivation of ATM induces metabolic derangements and development of diabetic phenotype in mice. According to a hyperinsulinemic-euglycemic clamp study, diabetic phenotype of $p53^{S18A}$ mice was evoked by reduction of insulin-stimulated whole-body glycogen synthesis and inefficient suppression of hepatic glucose production by insulin. These mice had decreased levels of expression of Sestrin family members in liver, muscle and white adipose tissue, suggesting that downregulation of Sestrins in the $p53^{S18A}$ mice contributed to the diabetic phenotype. Impressively, downregulation of Sesn2 and Sesn3 genes was also observed in $ATM^{+/-}$ mice where ATM activity was reduced[157]. The fibroblasts from $p53^{S18A}$ mice were characterized by increased ROS levels associated with reduced expression of all members of Sestrin family. Ectopic expression of Sesn2 in the $p53^{S18A}$ fibroblasts restored normal ROS levels, supporting the critical role of Sestrins in ROS regulation in $p53^{S18A}$ mice. To study whether the diabetic phenotype of the $p53^{S18A}$ mice was linked with oxidative stress, associated with a compromised p53 function, the mice were treated with butylated hydroxyanisole (BHA). BHA treatment suppressed diabetic phenotype in the $p53^{S18A}$ mice supporting the role of oxidative stress associated with p53 dysfunction in diabetes[157] (Fig.6).

9.4. Sestrins and respiratory diseases

Antioxidant effects of Sestrins might also be important in protection of respiratory epithelium via control of barrier function. Pollutant-induced inflammation compromises the barrier function, which leads to different respiratory diseases such as asthma, cystic fibrosis, and chronic obstructive pulmonary disease (COPD). The barrier function of the respiratory epithelium is protected by trasncriptional factor HIF1 fortifying an antioxidant defense, and this function is associated with activation of Sesn2, which seems to be a critical HIF1 target involved in this process[120]. Interestingly, according to another work, Sesn2 activity can complicate some aspects of COPD via negative regulation of TGFβ signaling which mitigates emphysema phenotype in mice. Thus, inactivation of Sestrins has some therapeutic potential under some COPD conditions, although more work has to be done to elucidate the exact role of Sestrins in COPD and other respiratory diseases[147].

9.5. Sestrins and cancer

Tumor suppressor p53, the master regulator of Sesn1 and Sesn2, is inactivated in most of human cancers, and p53 inactivation causes downregulation of Sesn1 and Sesn2, which can be responsible for tumor suppressive activities of p53 [62, 114, 119, 123]. Tumor suppressor activity was also recently assigned for the members of the FoxO family. Somatic inactivation of three members of the FoxO family: FoxO1, FoxO3A and FoxO4 in mice stimulated development of lymphomas and hemangiomas[158, 159]. Sesn1 and Sesn3 are FoxO targets, which can potentiate the tumor suppressive effects of FoxOs via regulation of ROS. The potential tumor suppressive activity of Sestrins and their impact on p53 and FoxO-mediated tumor suppression might involve antioxidant defense imposed by Sestrins, which can protect from mutagenesis, genomic instability and angiogenesis, as well as can regulate some other cancer-relevant processes associated with dysregulation of ROS metabolism[62, 141]. The role of Sestrins in many types of cancer is strengthened by the importance of Sestrins in regulation of the LKB1-AMPK-mTORC1 pathway[52, 122]. In agreement with this, it was observed that *Sesn2*-deficient cells are more susceptible to transformation than WT counterparts and Sesn2-silenced A549 tumor xenografts grow faster in nude mice, similar to p53-deficeint cells[62, 122] (Fig.6).

Analysis of human tumors demonstrates that loss of heterozygosity (LOH) in Sesn1 (6q21) found in non-Hodgkin lymphoma, acute lymphoblastic leukemia, bladder carcinoma, ovarian, mammary carcinomas, squamous cell carcinomas of the head and neck, T cell lymphomas[160] and Sesn2 (1p34) loci found in pancreatic adenocarcinoma[161], glioblastoma[162], T-cell lymphomas[160], ovarian cancers [163], thyroid cancers [164], and neuroblastomas[165]. LOH in the Sesn3 locus (11q21) is found in non-Hodgkin lymphoma[166], nasopharyngeal carcinoma[167, 168], pancreatic endocrin tumors[169], and melanomas[170]. Analysis of gene expression have shown that Sesn1 and Sesn2 are downregulated in lung cancers of different origin such as large cell carcinoma, adenocarcinoma, squamos cell carcinoma and small cell lung carcinoma[171-173]. Sesn1 is also found downregulated in breast cancers[174, 175], head and neck cancers[176], brain tumors[177] and T-cell leukemia/lymphoma[177]. Moreover, missense mutation of Sesn2 P87S was recently found in myeloproliferative neoplasm essential thrombocythemia (ET), characterized by increased proliferation of megakariocytes and accumulation of circulated platelets[178]. Another mechanism of inactivation of the members of the Sestrin family was described for endometrial cancers, where Sesn3 is methylated in 20% of cases, supporting the potential role of this gene in tumor suppression [179]. Although more extensive analysis is required to label Sestrins as tumor suppressors, these data clearly indicate the indispensable impact of Sestrins in control of carcinogenesis.

The regulation of the TGFβ pathway by Sestrins can also contribute to carcinogenesis. Although TGFβ can inhibit cell growth and suppress carcinogenesis at early stages, during the late stages of carcinogenesis cells often lose their growth-inhibitory response to TGFβ. Moreover, TGFβ stimulates invasion and metastasis of cancer cells supporting tumor progression. Accordingly, overexpression of TGFβ1 was found in breast, colon, esophageal, gastric, hepatocellular lung and pancreatic cancers. Moreover, high levels of TGFβ correlate with cancer progression, metastasis, angiogenesis and bad prognosis[152]. Inactivation of Sestrins can stimulate TGFβ signaling and potentiate TGFβ-dependent processes contributing to carcinogenesis. The link between Sestrins and TGFβ in human cancers and the impact of TGFβ-dependent pathway in regulation of carcinogenesis by Sestrins has to be addressed in the future studies.

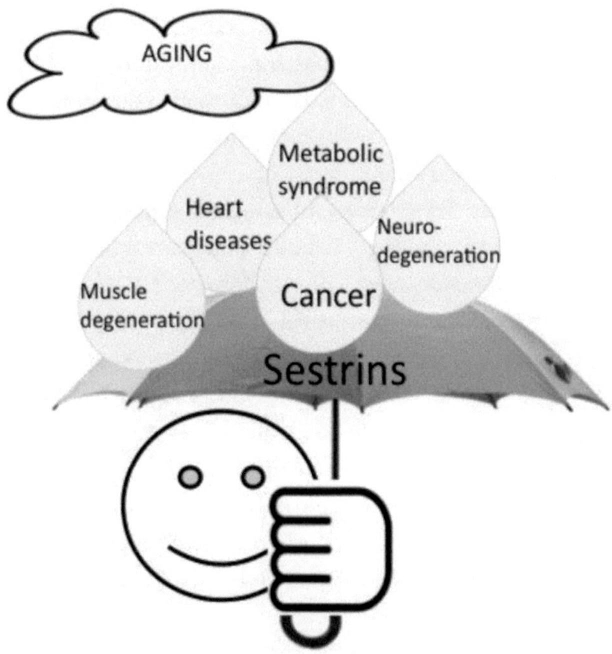

Figure 6. Sestrins protect from aging and age-related diseases. Drosophila Sestrin protect flies from aging, suppressing metabolic derangements, cardiac malfunction and muscle degeneration. In mammals, Sestrins are activated in the mice with delayed aging phenotype, while decreased expression of Sestrins is observed in diabetic mice. Moreover, Sestrins are found downregulated in many cancers. The conservatism of the mechanisms of regulation of longevity and aging between vertebrates and invertebrates via the AMPK-TORC1 pathway support the critical role of Sestrins in regulation of aging at mammals and their protecting activities against age-associated diseases.

Being stress-inducible genes, Sestrins are activated by many anticancer treatments, which involve stress response. Although the stress might be detrimental for cancer cells inducing cell death and senescence, which suppress tumor growth, cancer cells can eventually accumulate mutation in genes critical for the beneficial effects of anti-cancer therapy. Sestrins are important for cell death in response to genotoxic stress[119, 143], so they might be targets for inactivation in response to therapy. Presumably reactivation of Sestrins might be beneficial for treatments involving genotoxic stress. On the contrary, Sestrins might protect against oxidative stress, which also contributes to death of cancer cells, so under some circumstances inactivation of Sestrins might be beneficial for the treatment efficiency. Thus, the detailed characterization of the role of Sestrins in the efficiency of anticancer treatment is very important to set up the best treatment strategy for different forms of cancer.

10. Conclusion

A decade ago we identified a novel Sestrin gene family which happens to be in the intersection of two vital roads controlled by two important guards, p53 and FoxOs, the grants of our well-being and longevity. Sestrins convey the message from them to the AMPK-TORC1 executive branch, responsible for integration of numerous signals from nutrient and energy sources, growth factors, hormones and stress insults to tune up many metabolic, biosynthetic and disposing facilities providing good conditions for the organism well-being. Unfortunately, some hereditary or environmental factors, including an unhealthy life style, can impair the guards and release the malfunctioning machine of TOR signaling leading to non-synchronized anabolic and catabolic process resulting in the accumulation of damage, the major source of our demise. The absence of careful control of these processes also lead to disturbances in different tissues laying the ground for many detrimental age-related diseases, the major threat of developed societies in the 21st century. The restoration of the guards' functions, in part, via enabling Sestrins that are important messengers of their orders, might prove to be a valuable approach to delay or prevent many undesirable manifestations of aging and unhealthy life style. Future experiments on mouse genetic models and detailed analysis of the role of Sestrins in human diseases let us establish the impact of Sestrins in the control of human health and longevity, understand the mechanisms of their action and exploit this knowledge for the development of efficient anti-aging therapies.

Author details

Andrei V. Budanov

Department of Neurosurgery & Department of Biochemistry and Molecular Biology, Massey Cancer Center, Virginia Commonwealth University, Richmond, Virginia, USA

Acknowledgement

This work is supported by the Department of Neurosurgery, Virginia Commonwealth University start up funds given to Andrei V. Budanov. The author thanks Nichola Cruickshanks and Laurence Booth for the help in preparation of the manuscript. The author also thanks Nadushka Pryadilova for the everyday support.

11. References

[1] Budanov AV, Lee JH & Karin M (2010) Stressin' Sestrins take an aging fight. *EMBO Mol Med* 2, 388-400.

[2] Le Bourg E (2009) Hormesis, aging and longevity. *Biochim Biophys Acta* 1790, 1030-1039.

[3] Laplante M & Sabatini DM (2012) mTOR Signaling in Growth Control and Disease. *Cell* 149, 274-293.

[4] Mihaylova MM & Shaw RJ (2011) The AMPK signalling pathway coordinates cell growth, autophagy and metabolism. *Nat Cell Biol* 13, 1016-1023.

[5] Wullschleger S, Loewith R & Hall MN (2006) TOR signaling in growth and metabolism. *Cell* 124, 471-484.

[6] Zoncu R, Efeyan A & Sabatini DM (2011) mTOR: from growth signal integration to cancer, diabetes and ageing. *Nat Rev Mol Cell Biol* 12, 21-35.

[7] Oh WJ & Jacinto E (2011) mTOR complex 2 signaling and functions. *Cell Cycle* 10, 2305-2316.

[8] Cunningham JT, Rodgers JT, Arlow DH, Vazquez F, Mootha VK & Puigserver P (2007) mTOR controls mitochondrial oxidative function through a YY1-PGC-1alpha transcriptional complex. *Nature* 450, 736-740.

[9] Ramanathan A & Schreiber SL (2009) Direct control of mitochondrial function by mTOR. *Proc Natl Acad Sci U S A* 106, 22229-22232.

[10] Schieke SM, Phillips D, McCoy JP, Jr., Aponte AM, Shen RF, Balaban RS & Finkel T (2006) The mammalian target of rapamycin (mTOR) pathway regulates mitochondrial oxygen consumption and oxidative capacity. *J Biol Chem* 281, 27643-27652.

[11] Edinger AL, Linardic CM, Chiang GG, Thompson CB & Abraham RT (2003) Differential effects of rapamycin on mammalian target of rapamycin signaling functions in mammalian cells. *Cancer Res* 63, 8451-8460.

[12] Keith B, Johnson RS & Simon MC (2011) HIF1alpha and HIF2alpha: sibling rivalry in hypoxic tumour growth and progression. *Nat Rev Cancer* 12, 9-22.

[13] Bernardi R, Guernah I, Jin D, Grisendi S, Alimonti A, Teruya-Feldstein J, Cordon-Cardo C, Simon MC, Rafii S & Pandolfi PP (2006) PML inhibits HIF-1alpha translation and neoangiogenesis through repression of mTOR. *Nature* 442, 779-785.

[14] Kroemer G, Marino G & Levine B (2010) Autophagy and the integrated stress response. *Mol Cell* 40, 280-293.

[15] Budanov AV (2011) Stress-responsive sestrins link p53 with redox regulation and mammalian target of rapamycin signaling. *Antioxid Redox Signal* 15, 1679-1690.

[16] Shen S, Kepp O & Kroemer G (2012) The end of autophagic cell death? *Autophagy* 8, 1-3.

[17] Shimizu S, Kanaseki T, Mizushima N, Mizuta T, Arakawa-Kobayashi S, Thompson CB & Tsujimoto Y (2004) Role of Bcl-2 family proteins in a non-apoptotic programmed cell death dependent on autophagy genes. *Nat Cell Biol* 6, 1221-1228.

[18] Yee KS, Wilkinson S, James J, Ryan KM & Vousden KH (2009) PUMA- and Bax-induced autophagy contributes to apoptosis. *Cell Death Differ* 16, 1135-1145.

[19] He C, Bassik MC, Moresi V, Sun K, Wei Y, Zou Z, An Z, Loh J, Fisher J, Sun Q, Korsmeyer S, Packer M, May HI, Hill JA, Virgin HW, Gilpin C, Xiao G, Bassel-Duby R, Scherer PE & Levine B (2012) Exercise-induced BCL2-regulated autophagy is required for muscle glucose homeostasis. *Nature* 481, 511-515.

[20] Crighton D, Wilkinson S, O'Prey J, Syed N, Smith P, Harrison PR, Gasco M, Garrone O, Crook T & Ryan KM (2006) DRAM, a p53-induced modulator of autophagy, is critical for apoptosis. *Cell* 126, 121-134.

[21] Yang ZJ, Chee CE, Huang S & Sinicrope FA (2011) The role of autophagy in cancer: therapeutic implications. *Mol Cancer Ther* 10, 1533-1541.

[22] Chen C, Liu Y, Liu R, Ikenoue T, Guan KL & Zheng P (2008) TSC-mTOR maintains quiescence and function of hematopoietic stem cells by repressing mitochondrial biogenesis and reactive oxygen species. *J Exp Med* 205, 2397-2408.

[23] Bjedov I & Partridge L (2011) A longer and healthier life with TOR down-regulation: genetics and drugs. *Biochem Soc Trans* 39, 460-465.

[24] Harrison DE, Strong R, Sharp ZD, Nelson JF, Astle CM, Flurkey K, Nadon NL, Wilkinson JE, Frenkel K, Carter CS, Pahor M, Javors MA, Fernandez E & Miller RA (2009) Rapamycin fed late in life extends lifespan in genetically heterogeneous mice. *Nature* 460, 392-395.

[25] Han JM, Jeong SJ, Park MC, Kim G, Kwon NH, Kim HK, Ha SH, Ryu SH & Kim S (2012) Leucyl-tRNA Synthetase Is an Intracellular Leucine Sensor for the mTORC1-Signaling Pathway. *Cell* 149, 410-424.

[26] Nobukuni T, Joaquin M, Roccio M, Dann SG, Kim SY, Gulati P, Byfield MP, Backer JM, Natt F, Bos JL, Zwartkruis FJ & Thomas G (2005) Amino acids mediate mTOR/raptor signaling through activation of class 3 phosphatidylinositol 3OH-kinase. *Proc Natl Acad Sci U S A* 102, 14238-14243.

[27] Yoon MS, Du G, Backer JM, Frohman MA & Chen J (2011) Class III PI-3-kinase activates phospholipase D in an amino acid-sensing mTORC1 pathway. *J Cell Biol* 195, 435-447.

[28] Chong-Kopera H, Inoki K, Li Y, Zhu T, Garcia-Gonzalo FR, Rosa JL & Guan KL (2006) TSC1 stabilizes TSC2 by inhibiting the interaction between TSC2 and the HERC1 ubiquitin ligase. *J Biol Chem* 281, 8313-8316.

[29] Wang W & Guan KL (2009) AMP-activated protein kinase and cancer. *Acta Physiol (Oxf)* 196, 55-63.

[30] Tabony AM, Yoshida T, Galvez S, Higashi Y, Sukhanov S, Chandrasekar B, Mitch WE & Delafontaine P (2011) Angiotensin II upregulates protein phosphatase 2Calpha and inhibits AMP-activated protein kinase signaling and energy balance leading to skeletal muscle wasting. *Hypertension* 58, 643-649.

[31] Wang T, Yu Q, Chen J, Deng B, Qian L & Le Y (2010) PP2A mediated AMPK inhibition promotes HSP70 expression in heat shock response. *PLoS One* 5.

[32] Wu Y, Song P, Xu J, Zhang M & Zou MH (2007) Activation of protein phosphatase 2A by palmitate inhibits AMP-activated protein kinase. *J Biol Chem* 282, 9777-9788.

[33] Voss M, Paterson J, Kelsall IR, Martin-Granados C, Hastie CJ, Peggie MW & Cohen PT (2011) Ppm1E is an in cellulo AMP-activated protein kinase phosphatase. *Cell Signal* 23, 114-124.

[34] Rubenstein EM, McCartney RR, Zhang C, Shokat KM, Shirra MK, Arndt KM & Schmidt MC (2008) Access denied: Snf1 activation loop phosphorylation is controlled by availability of the phosphorylated threonine 210 to the PP1 phosphatase. *J Biol Chem* 283, 222-230.

[35] Alexander A, Cai SL, Kim J, Nanez A, Sahin M, MacLean KH, Inoki K, Guan KL, Shen J, Person MD, Kusewitt D, Mills GB, Kastan MB & Walker CL (2010) ATM signals to TSC2 in the cytoplasm to regulate mTORC1 in response to ROS. *Proc Natl Acad Sci U S A* 107, 4153-4158.

[36] Momcilovic M, Hong SP & Carlson M (2006) Mammalian TAK1 activates Snf1 protein kinase in yeast and phosphorylates AMP-activated protein kinase in vitro. *J Biol Chem* 281, 25336-25343.

[37] Herrero-Martin G, Hoyer-Hansen M, Garcia-Garcia C, Fumarola C, Farkas T, Lopez-Rivas A & Jaattela M (2009) TAK1 activates AMPK-dependent cytoprotective autophagy in TRAIL-treated epithelial cells. *EMBO J* 28, 677-685.

[38] Costanzo-Garvey DL, Pfluger PT, Dougherty MK, Stock JL, Boehm M, Chaika O, Fernandez MR, Fisher K, Kortum RL, Hong EG, Jun JY, Ko HJ, Schreiner A, Volle DJ, Treece T, Swift AL, Winer M, Chen D, Wu M, Leon LR, Shaw AS, McNeish J, Kim JK, Morrison DK, Tschop MH & Lewis RE (2009) KSR2 is an essential regulator of AMP kinase, energy expenditure, and insulin sensitivity. *Cell Metab* 10, 366-378.

[39] Banko MR, Allen JJ, Schaffer BE, Wilker EW, Tsou P, White JL, Villen J, Wang B, Kim SR, Sakamoto K, Gygi SP, Cantley LC, Yaffe MB, Shokat KM & Brunet A (2011) Chemical genetic screen for AMPKalpha2 substrates uncovers a network of proteins involved in mitosis. *Mol Cell* 44, 878-892.

[40] Sanli T, Rashid A, Liu C, Harding S, Bristow RG, Cutz JC, Singh G, Wright J & Tsakiridis T (2010) Ionizing radiation activates AMP-activated kinase (AMPK): a target for radiosensitization of human cancer cells. *Int J Radiat Oncol Biol Phys* 78, 221-229.

[41] Sanli T, Storozhuk Y, Linher-Melville K, Bristow RG, Laderout K, Viollet B, Wright J, Singh G & Tsakiridis T (2012) Ionizing radiation regulates the expression of AMP-activated protein kinase (AMPK) in epithelial cancer cells Modulation of cellular signals regulating cell cycle and survival. *Radiother Oncol*.

[42] Cao C, Lu S, Kivlin R, Wallin B, Card E, Bagdasarian A, Tamakloe T, Chu WM, Guan KL & Wan Y (2008) AMP-activated protein kinase contributes to UV- and H2O2-induced apoptosis in human skin keratinocytes. *J Biol Chem* 283, 28897-28908.

[43] Li Y, Xu S, Mihaylova MM, Zheng B, Hou X, Jiang B, Park O, Luo Z, Lefai E, Shyy JY, Gao B, Wierzbicki M, Verbeuren TJ, Shaw RJ, Cohen RA & Zang M (2011) AMPK phosphorylates and inhibits SREBP activity to attenuate hepatic steatosis and atherosclerosis in diet-induced insulin-resistant mice. *Cell Metab* 13, 376-388.

[44] Zhao M & Klionsky DJ (2011) AMPK-dependent phosphorylation of ULK1 induces autophagy. *Cell Metab* 13, 119-120.

[45] Apfeld J, O'Connor G, McDonagh T, DiStefano PS & Curtis R (2004) The AMP-activated protein kinase AAK-2 links energy levels and insulin-like signals to lifespan in C. elegans. *Genes Dev* 18, 3004-3009.

[46] Mair W, Morantte I, Rodrigues AP, Manning G, Montminy M, Shaw RJ & Dillin A (2011) Lifespan extension induced by AMPK and calcineurin is mediated by CRTC-1 and CREB. *Nature* 470, 404-408.

[47] Greer EL, Dowlatshahi D, Banko MR, Villen J, Hoang K, Blanchard D, Gygi SP & Brunet A (2007) An AMPK-FOXO pathway mediates longevity induced by a novel method of dietary restriction in C. elegans. *Curr Biol* 17, 1646-1656.

[48] Lee H, Cho JS, Lambacher N, Lee J, Lee SJ, Lee TH, Gartner A & Koo HS (2008) The Caenorhabditis elegans AMP-activated protein kinase AAK-2 is phosphorylated by LKB1 and is required for resistance to oxidative stress and for normal motility and foraging behavior. *J Biol Chem* 283, 14988-14993.

[49] Tohyama D & Yamaguchi A (2010) A critical role of SNF1A/dAMPKalpha (Drosophila AMP-activated protein kinase alpha) in muscle on longevity and stress resistance in Drosophila melanogaster. *Biochem Biophys Res Commun* 394, 112-118.

[50] Funakoshi M, Tsuda M, Muramatsu K, Hatsuda H, Morishita S & Aigaki T (2011) A gain-of-function screen identifies wdb and lkb1 as lifespan-extending genes in Drosophila. *Biochem Biophys Res Commun* 405, 667-672.

[51] Reznick RM, Zong H, Li J, Morino K, Moore IK, Yu HJ, Liu ZX, Dong J, Mustard KJ, Hawley SA, Befroy D, Pypaert M, Hardie DG, Young LH & Shulman GI (2007) Aging-associated reductions in AMP-activated protein kinase activity and mitochondrial biogenesis. *Cell Metab* 5, 151-156.

[52] Hardie DG (2011) AMP-activated protein kinase: an energy sensor that regulates all aspects of cell function. *Genes Dev* 25, 1895-1908.

[53] Viollet B, Andreelli F, Jorgensen SB, Perrin C, Geloen A, Flamez D, Mu J, Lenzner C, Baud O, Bennoun M, Gomas E, Nicolas G, Wojtaszewski JF, Kahn A, Carling D, Schuit FC, Birnbaum MJ, Richter EA, Burcelin R & Vaulont S (2003) The AMP-activated protein kinase alpha2 catalytic subunit controls whole-body insulin sensitivity. *J Clin Invest* 111, 91-98.

[54] Salminen A, Hyttinen JM & Kaarniranta K (2011) AMP-activated protein kinase inhibits NF-kappaB signaling and inflammation: impact on healthspan and lifespan. *J Mol Med (Berl)* 89, 667-676.

[55] Zhou G, Myers R, Li Y, Chen Y, Shen X, Fenyk-Melody J, Wu M, Ventre J, Doebber T, Fujii N, Musi N, Hirshman MF, Goodyear LJ & Moller DE (2001) Role of AMP-activated protein kinase in mechanism of metformin action. *J Clin Invest* 108, 1167-1174.

[56] Baur JA, Pearson KJ, Price NL, Jamieson HA, Lerin C, Kalra A, Prabhu VV, Allard JS, Lopez-Lluch G, Lewis K, Pistell PJ, Poosala S, Becker KG, Boss O, Gwinn D, Wang M, Ramaswamy S, Fishbein KW, Spencer RG, Lakatta EG, Le Couteur D, Shaw RJ, Navas

P, Puigserver P, Ingram DK, de Cabo R & Sinclair DA (2006) Resveratrol improves health and survival of mice on a high-calorie diet. *Nature* 444, 337-342.

[57] Lane DP & Crawford LV (1979) T antigen is bound to a host protein in SV40-transformed cells. *Nature* 278, 261-263.

[58] Levine AJ (1997) p53, the cellular gatekeeper for growth and division. *Cell* 88, 323-331.

[59] Donehower LA, Harvey M, Slagle BL, McArthur MJ, Montgomery CA, Jr., Butel JS & Bradley A (1992) Mice deficient for p53 are developmentally normal but susceptible to spontaneous tumours. *Nature* 356, 215-221.

[60] Vousden KH & Prives C (2009) Blinded by the Light: The Growing Complexity of p53. *Cell* 137, 413-431.

[61] Harris SL & Levine AJ (2005) The p53 pathway: positive and negative feedback loops. *Oncogene* 24, 2899-2908.

[62] Sablina AA, Budanov AV, Ilyinskaya GV, Agapova LS, Kravchenko JE & Chumakov PM (2005) The antioxidant function of the p53 tumor suppressor. *Nat Med* 11, 1306-1313.

[63] Bensaad K, Tsuruta A, Selak MA, Vidal MN, Nakano K, Bartrons R, Gottlieb E & Vousden KH (2006) TIGAR, a p53-inducible regulator of glycolysis and apoptosis. *Cell* 126, 107-120.

[64] Maddocks OD & Vousden KH (2011) Metabolic regulation by p53. *J Mol Med (Berl)* 89, 237-245.

[65] Zhang C, Lin M, Wu R, Wang X, Yang B, Levine AJ, Hu W & Feng Z (2011) Parkin, a p53 target gene, mediates the role of p53 in glucose metabolism and the Warburg effect. *Proc Natl Acad Sci U S A* 108, 16259-16264.

[66] Polyak K, Xia Y, Zweier JL, Kinzler KW & Vogelstein B (1997) A model for p53-induced apoptosis. *Nature* 389, 300-305.

[67] Blagosklonny MV (2008) Aging: ROS or TOR. *Cell Cycle* 7, 3344-3354.

[68] Horton LE, Bushell M, Barth-Baus D, Tilleray VJ, Clemens MJ & Hensold JO (2002) p53 activation results in rapid dephosphorylation of the eIF4E-binding protein 4E-BP1, inhibition of ribosomal protein S6 kinase and inhibition of translation initiation. *Oncogene* 21, 5325-5334.

[69] Constantinou C & Clemens MJ (2005) Regulation of the phosphorylation and integrity of protein synthesis initiation factor eIF4GI and the translational repressor 4E-BP1 by p53. *Oncogene* 24, 4839-4850.

[70] Feng Z, Zhang H, Levine AJ & Jin S (2005) The coordinate regulation of the p53 and mTOR pathways in cells. *Proc Natl Acad Sci U S A* 102, 8204-8209.

[71] Lemmon MA & Schlessinger J (2010) Cell signaling by receptor tyrosine kinases. *Cell* 141, 1117-1134.

[72] Yu X, Riley T & Levine AJ (2009) The regulation of the endosomal compartment by p53 the tumor suppressor gene. *FEBS J* 276, 2201-2212.

[73] Jing K, Song KS, Shin S, Kim N, Jeong S, Oh HR, Park JH, Seo KS, Heo JY, Han J, Park JI, Han C, Wu T, Kweon GR, Park SK, Yoon WH, Hwang BD & Lim K (2011) Docosahexaenoic acid induces autophagy through p53/AMPK/mTOR signaling and

promotes apoptosis in human cancer cells harboring wild-type p53. *Autophagy* 7, 1348-1358.

[74] Gao W, Shen Z, Shang L & Wang X (2011) Upregulation of human autophagy-initiation kinase ULK1 by tumor suppressor p53 contributes to DNA-damage-induced cell death. *Cell Death Differ* 18, 1598-1607.

[75] Seillier M, Peuget S, Gayet O, Gauthier C, N'Guessan P, Monte M, Carrier A, Iovanna JL & Dusetti NJ (2012) TP53INP1, a tumor suppressor, interacts with LC3 and ATG8-family proteins through the LC3-interacting region (LIR) and promotes autophagy-dependent cell death. *Cell Death Differ*.

[76] Eby KG, Rosenbluth JM, Mays DJ, Marshall CB, Barton CE, Sinha S, Johnson KN, Tang L & Pietenpol JA (2010) ISG20L1 is a p53 family target gene that modulates genotoxic stress-induced autophagy. *Mol Cancer* 9, 95.

[77] Tasdemir E, Maiuri MC, Galluzzi L, Vitale I, Djavaheri-Mergny M, D'Amelio M, Criollo A, Morselli E, Zhu C, Harper F, Nannmark U, Samara C, Pinton P, Vicencio JM, Carnuccio R, Moll UM, Madeo F, Paterlini-Brechot P, Rizzuto R, Szabadkai G, Pierron G, Blomgren K, Tavernarakis N, Codogno P, Cecconi F & Kroemer G (2008) Regulation of autophagy by cytoplasmic p53. *Nat Cell Biol* 10, 676-687.

[78] Morselli E, Shen S, Ruckenstuhl C, Bauer MA, Marino G, Galluzzi L, Criollo A, Michaud M, Maiuri MC, Chano T, Madeo F & Kroemer G (2011) p53 inhibits autophagy by interacting with the human ortholog of yeast Atg17, RB1CC1/FIP200. *Cell Cycle* 10, 2763-2769.

[79] Tyner SD, Venkatachalam S, Choi J, Jones S, Ghebranious N, Igelmann H, Lu X, Soron G, Cooper B, Brayton C, Hee Park S, Thompson T, Karsenty G, Bradley A & Donehower LA (2002) p53 mutant mice that display early ageing-associated phenotypes. *Nature* 415, 45-53.

[80] Maier B, Gluba W, Bernier B, Turner T, Mohammad K, Guise T, Sutherland A, Thorner M & Scrable H (2004) Modulation of mammalian life span by the short isoform of p53. *Genes Dev* 18, 306-319.

[81] Pehar M, O'Riordan KJ, Burns-Cusato M, Andrzejewski ME, del Alcazar CG, Burger C, Scrable H & Puglielli L (2010) Altered longevity-assurance activity of p53:p44 in the mouse causes memory loss, neurodegeneration and premature death. *Aging Cell* 9, 174-190.

[82] Jimenez GS, Nister M, Stommel JM, Beeche M, Barcarse EA, Zhang XQ, O'Gorman S & Wahl GM (2000) A transactivation-deficient mouse model provides insights into Trp53 regulation and function. *Nat Genet* 26, 37-43.

[83] Murray-Zmijewski F, Lane DP & Bourdon JC (2006) p53/p63/p73 isoforms: an orchestra of isoforms to harmonise cell differentiation and response to stress. *Cell Death Differ* 13, 962-972.

[84] Courtois S, Verhaegh G, North S, Luciani MG, Lassus P, Hibner U, Oren M & Hainaut P (2002) DeltaN-p53, a natural isoform of p53 lacking the first transactivation domain, counteracts growth suppression by wild-type p53. *Oncogene* 21, 6722-6728.

[85] Yin Y, Stephen CW, Luciani MG & Fahraeus R (2002) p53 Stability and activity is regulated by Mdm2-mediated induction of alternative p53 translation products. *Nat Cell Biol* 4, 462-467.

[86] Schmid G, Kramer MP, Maurer M, Wandl S & Wesierska-Gadek J (2007) Cellular and organismal ageing: Role of the p53 tumor suppressor protein in the induction of transient and terminal senescence. *J Cell Biochem* 101, 1355-1369.

[87] Melis JP, Hoogervorst EM, van Oostrom CT, Zwart E, Breit TM, Pennings JL, de Vries A & van Steeg H (2011) Genotoxic exposure: novel cause of selection for a functional DeltaN-p53 isoform. *Oncogene* 30, 1764-1772.

[88] Mendrysa SM, McElwee MK, Michalowski J, O'Leary KA, Young KM & Perry ME (2003) mdm2 Is critical for inhibition of p53 during lymphopoiesis and the response to ionizing irradiation. *Mol Cell Biol* 23, 462-472.

[89] Terzian T, Wang Y, Van Pelt CS, Box NF, Travis EL & Lozano G (2007) Haploinsufficiency of Mdm2 and Mdm4 in tumorigenesis and development. *Mol Cell Biol* 27, 5479-5485.

[90] Matheu A, Maraver A, Klatt P, Flores I, Garcia-Cao I, Borras C, Flores JM, Vina J, Blasco MA & Serrano M (2007) Delayed ageing through damage protection by the Arf/p53 pathway. *Nature* 448, 375-379.

[91] Barlow C, Dennery PA, Shigenaga MK, Smith MA, Morrow JD, Roberts LJ, 2nd, Wynshaw-Boris A & Levine RL (1999) Loss of the ataxia-telangiectasia gene product causes oxidative damage in target organs. *Proc Natl Acad Sci U S A* 96, 9915-9919.

[92] Reliene R, Fischer E & Schiestl RH (2004) Effect of N-acetyl cysteine on oxidative DNA damage and the frequency of DNA deletions in atm-deficient mice. *Cancer Res* 64, 5148-5153.

[93] Feng Z, Hu W, Teresky AK, Hernando E, Cordon-Cardo C & Levine AJ (2007) Declining p53 function in the aging process: a possible mechanism for the increased tumor incidence in older populations. *Proc Natl Acad Sci U S A* 104, 16633-16638.

[94] Bauer JH, Poon PC, Glatt-Deeley H, Abrams JM & Helfand SL (2005) Neuronal expression of p53 dominant-negative proteins in adult Drosophila melanogaster extends life span. *Curr Biol* 15, 2063-2068.

[95] Moskalev AA, Plyusnina EN & Shaposhnikov MV (2011) Radiation hormesis and radioadaptive response in Drosophila melanogaster flies with different genetic backgrounds: the role of cellular stress-resistance mechanisms. *Biogerontology* 12, 253-263.

[96] Torgovnick A, Schiavi A, Testi R & Ventura N (2010) A role for p53 in mitochondrial stress response control of longevity in C. elegans. *Exp Gerontol* 45, 550-557.

[97] Ventura N, Rea SL, Schiavi A, Torgovnick A, Testi R & Johnson TE (2009) p53/CEP-1 increases or decreases lifespan, depending on level of mitochondrial bioenergetic stress. *Aging Cell* 8, 380-393.

[98] van der Vos KE & Coffer PJ (2011) The extending network of FOXO transcriptional target genes. *Antioxid Redox Signal* 14, 579-592.

[99] Hay N (2011) Interplay between FOXO, TOR, and Akt. *Biochim Biophys Acta* 1813, 1965-1970.

[100] Wang MC, Bohmann D & Jasper H (2003) JNK signaling confers tolerance to oxidative stress and extends lifespan in Drosophila. *Dev Cell* 5, 811-816.

[101] Oh SW, Mukhopadhyay A, Svrzikapa N, Jiang F, Davis RJ & Tissenbaum HA (2005) JNK regulates lifespan in Caenorhabditis elegans by modulating nuclear translocation of forkhead transcription factor/DAF-16. *Proc Natl Acad Sci U S A* 102, 4494-4499.

[102] Wang MC, Bohmann D & Jasper H (2005) JNK extends life span and limits growth by antagonizing cellular and organism-wide responses to insulin signaling. *Cell* 121, 115-125.

[103] Zhao Y, Yang J, Liao W, Liu X, Zhang H, Wang S, Wang D, Feng J, Yu L & Zhu WG (2010) Cytosolic FoxO1 is essential for the induction of autophagy and tumour suppressor activity. *Nat Cell Biol* 12, 665-675.

[104] Renault VM, Thekkat PU, Hoang KL, White JL, Brady CA, Kenzelmann Broz D, Venturelli OS, Johnson TM, Oskoui PR, Xuan Z, Santo EE, Zhang MQ, Vogel H, Attardi LD & Brunet A (2011) The pro-longevity gene FoxO3 is a direct target of the p53 tumor suppressor. *Oncogene* 30, 3207-3221.

[105] Fu W, Ma Q, Chen L, Li P, Zhang M, Ramamoorthy S, Nawaz Z, Shimojima T, Wang H, Yang Y, Shen Z, Zhang Y, Zhang X, Nicosia SV, Pledger JW, Chen J & Bai W (2009) MDM2 acts downstream of p53 as an E3 ligase to promote FOXO ubiquitination and degradation. *J Biol Chem* 284, 13987-14000.

[106] You H, Jang Y, You-Ten AI, Okada H, Liepa J, Wakeham A, Zaugg K & Mak TW (2004) p53-dependent inhibition of FKHRL1 in response to DNA damage through protein kinase SGK1. *Proc Natl Acad Sci U S A* 101, 14057-14062.

[107] You H, Yamamoto K & Mak TW (2006) Regulation of transactivation-independent proapoptotic activity of p53 by FOXO3a. *Proc Natl Acad Sci U S A* 103, 9051-9056.

[108] Tsai WB, Chung YM, Takahashi Y, Xu Z & Hu MC (2008) Functional interaction between FOXO3a and ATM regulates DNA damage response. *Nat Cell Biol* 10, 460-467.

[109] Bouchard C, Lee S, Paulus-Hock V, Loddenkemper C, Eilers M & Schmitt CA (2007) FoxO transcription factors suppress Myc-driven lymphomagenesis via direct activation of Arf. *Genes Dev* 21, 2775-2787.

[110] Samuel VT & Shulman GI (2012) Mechanisms for insulin resistance: common threads and missing links. *Cell* 148, 852-871.

[111] Hsu PP, Kang SA, Rameseder J, Zhang Y, Ottina KA, Lim D, Peterson TR, Choi Y, Gray NS, Yaffe MB, Marto JA & Sabatini DM (2011) The mTOR-regulated phosphoproteome reveals a mechanism of mTORC1-mediated inhibition of growth factor signaling. *Science* 332, 1317-1322.

[112] Yu Y, Yoon SO, Poulogiannis G, Yang Q, Ma XM, Villen J, Kubica N, Hoffman GR, Cantley LC, Gygi SP & Blenis J (2011) Phosphoproteomic analysis identifies Grb10 as an mTORC1 substrate that negatively regulates insulin signaling. *Science* 332, 1322-1326.

[113] Buckbinder L, Talbott R, Seizinger BR & Kley N (1994) Gene regulation by temperature-sensitive p53 mutants: identification of p53 response genes. *Proc Natl Acad Sci U S A* 91, 10640-10644.

[114] Velasco-Miguel S, Buckbinder L, Jean P, Gelbert L, Talbott R, Laidlaw J, Seizinger B & Kley N (1999) PA26, a novel target of the p53 tumor suppressor and member of the GADD family of DNA damage and growth arrest inducible genes. *Oncogene* 18, 127-137.

[115] Wei CL, Wu Q, Vega VB, Chiu KP, Ng P, Zhang T, Shahab A, Yong HC, Fu Y, Weng Z, Liu J, Zhao XD, Chew JL, Lee YL, Kuznetsov VA, Sung WK, Miller LD, Lim B, Liu ET, Yu Q, Ng HH & Ruan Y (2006) A global map of p53 transcription-factor binding sites in the human genome. *Cell* 124, 207-219.

[116] Tran H, Brunet A, Grenier JM, Datta SR, Fornace AJ, Jr., DiStefano PS, Chiang LW & Greenberg ME (2002) DNA repair pathway stimulated by the forkhead transcription factor FOXO3a through the Gadd45 protein. *Science* 296, 530-534.

[117] Nogueira V, Park Y, Chen CC, Xu PZ, Chen ML, Tonic I, Unterman T & Hay N (2008) Akt determines replicative senescence and oxidative or oncogenic premature senescence and sensitizes cells to oxidative apoptosis. *Cancer Cell* 14, 458-470.

[118] Chen CC, Jeon SM, Bhaskar PT, Nogueira V, Sundararajan D, Tonic I, Park Y & Hay N (2010) FoxOs inhibit mTORC1 and activate Akt by inducing the expression of Sestrin3 and Rictor. *Dev Cell* 18, 592-604.

[119] Budanov AV, Shoshani T, Faerman A, Zelin E, Kamer I, Kalinski H, Gorodin S, Fishman A, Chajut A, Einat P, Skaliter R, Gudkov AV, Chumakov PM & Feinstein E (2002) Identification of a novel stress-responsive gene Hi95 involved in regulation of cell viability. *Oncogene* 21, 6017-6031.

[120] Olson N, Hristova M, Heintz NH, Lounsbury KM & van der Vliet A (2011) Activation of hypoxia-inducible factor-1 protects airway epithelium against oxidant-induced barrier dysfunction. *Am J Physiol Lung Cell Mol Physiol* 301, L993-L1002.

[121] Essler S, Dehne N & Brune B (2009) Role of sestrin2 in peroxide signaling in macrophages. *FEBS Lett* 583, 3531-3535.

[122] Budanov AV & Karin M (2008) p53 target genes sestrin1 and sestrin2 connect genotoxic stress and mTOR signaling. *Cell* 134, 451-460.

[123] Budanov AV, Sablina AA, Feinstein E, Koonin EV & Chumakov PM (2004) Regeneration of peroxiredoxins by p53-regulated sestrins, homologs of bacterial AhpD. *Science* 304, 596-600.

[124] Papadia S, Soriano FX, Leveille F, Martel MA, Dakin KA, Hansen HH, Kaindl A, Sifringer M, Fowler J, Stefovska V, McKenzie G, Craigon M, Corriveau R, Ghazal P, Horsburgh K, Yankner BA, Wyllie DJ, Ikonomidou C & Hardingham GE (2008) Synaptic NMDA receptor activity boosts intrinsic antioxidant defenses. *Nat Neurosci* 11, 476-487.

[125] Cho SD, Lee SO, Chintharlapalli S, Abdelrahim M, Khan S, Yoon K, Kamat AM & Safe S (2010) Activation of nerve growth factor-induced B alpha by methylene-substituted

diindolylmethanes in bladder cancer cells induces apoptosis and inhibits tumor growth. *Mol Pharmacol* 77, 396-404.

[126] Pulliam L, Sun B, Rempel H, Martinez PM, Hoekman JD, Rao RJ, Frey WH, 2nd & Hanson LR (2007) Intranasal tat alters gene expression in the mouse brain. *J Neuroimmune Pharmacol* 2, 87-92.

[127] Kim JR, Lee SR, Chung HJ, Kim S, Baek SH, Kim JH & Kim YS (2003) Identification of amyloid beta-peptide responsive genes by cDNA microarray technology: involvement of RTP801 in amyloid beta-peptide toxicity. *Exp Mol Med* 35, 403-411.

[128] Igwe EI, Essler S, Al-Furoukh N, Dehne N & Brune B (2009) Hypoxic transcription gene profiles under the modulation of nitric oxide in nuclear run on-microarray and proteomics. *BMC Genomics* 10, 408.

[129] Pemberton HN, Franklyn JA, Boelaert K, Chan SY, Kim DS, Kim C, Cheng SY, Kilby MD & McCabe CJ (2007) Separase, securin and Rad21 in neural cell growth. *J Cell Physiol* 213, 45-53.

[130] Soriano FX, Papadia S, Bell KF & Hardingham GE (2009) Role of histone acetylation in the activity-dependent regulation of sulfiredoxin and sestrin 2. *Epigenetics* 4, 152-158.

[131] Peeters H, Debeer P, Bairoch A, Wilquet V, Huysmans C, Parthoens E, Fryns JP, Gewillig M, Nakamura Y, Niikawa N, Van de Ven W & Devriendt K (2003) PA26 is a candidate gene for heterotaxia in humans: identification of a novel PA26-related gene family in human and mouse. *Hum Genet* 112, 573-580.

[132] Matsuoka S, Ballif BA, Smogorzewska A, McDonald ER, 3rd, Hurov KE, Luo J, Bakalarski CE, Zhao Z, Solimini N, Lerenthal Y, Shiloh Y, Gygi SP & Elledge SJ (2007) ATM and ATR substrate analysis reveals extensive protein networks responsive to DNA damage. *Science* 316, 1160-1166.

[133] Hikasa H & Taira M (2001) A Xenopus homolog of a human p53-activated gene, PA26, is specifically expressed in the notochord. *Mech Dev* 100, 309-312.

[134] Peeters H, Voz ML, Verschueren K, De Cat B, Pendeville H, Thienpont B, Schellens A, Belmont JW, David G, Van De Ven WJ, Fryns JP, Gewillig M, Huylebroeck D, Peers B & Devriendt K (2006) Sesn1 is a novel gene for left-right asymmetry and mediating nodal signaling. *Hum Mol Genet* 15, 3369-3377.

[135] Lee JH, Budanov AV, Park EJ, Birse R, Kim TE, Perkins GA, Ocorr K, Ellisman MH, Bodmer R, Bier E & Karin M (2009) Sestrin as a feedback inhibitor of TOR that prevents age-related pathologies. *Science* 327, 1223-1228.

[136] Fourquet S, Huang ME, D'Autreaux B & Toledano MB (2008) The dual functions of thiol-based peroxidases in H2O2 scavenging and signaling. *Antioxid Redox Signal* 10, 1565-1576.

[137] Woo HA, Bae SH, Park S & Rhee SG (2009) Sestrin 2 is not a reductase for cysteine sulfinic acid of peroxiredoxins. *Antioxid Redox Signal* 11, 739-745.

[138] Hagenbuchner J, Kuznetsov A, Hermann M, Hausott B, Obexer P & Ausserlechner MJ (2012) FOXO3-induced reactive oxygen species are regulated by BCL2L11 (Bim) and SESN3. *J Cell Sci*.

[139] Lau AT, Wang Y & Chiu JF (2008) Reactive oxygen species: current knowledge and applications in cancer research and therapeutic. *J Cell Biochem* 104, 657-667.

[140] Irani K, Xia Y, Zweier JL, Sollott SJ, Der CJ, Fearon ER, Sundaresan M, Finkel T & Goldschmidt-Clermont PJ (1997) Mitogenic signaling mediated by oxidants in Ras-transformed fibroblasts. *Science* 275, 1649-1652.

[141] Kopnin PB, Agapova LS, Kopnin BP & Chumakov PM (2007) Repression of sestrin family genes contributes to oncogenic Ras-induced reactive oxygen species up-regulation and genetic instability. *Cancer Res* 67, 4671-4678.

[142] Finkel T (2003) Oxidant signals and oxidative stress. *Curr Opin Cell Biol* 15, 247-254.

[143] Sanli T, Linher-Melville K, Tsakiridis T & Singh G (2012) Sestrin2 modulates AMPK subunit expression and its response to ionizing radiation in breast cancer cells. *PLoS One* 7, e32035.

[144] Braunstein S, Badura ML, Xi Q, Formenti SC & Schneider RJ (2009) Regulation of protein synthesis by ionizing radiation. *Mol Cell Biol* 29, 5645-5656.

[145] Maiuri MC, Malik SA, Morselli E, Kepp O, Criollo A, Mouchel PL, Carnuccio R & Kroemer G (2009) Stimulation of autophagy by the p53 target gene Sestrin2. *Cell Cycle* 8, 1571-1576.

[146] Scherz-Shouval R, Weidberg H, Gonen C, Wilder S, Elazar Z & Oren M (2010) p53-dependent regulation of autophagy protein LC3 supports cancer cell survival under prolonged starvation. *Proc Natl Acad Sci U S A* 107, 18511-18516.

[147] Wempe F, De-Zolt S, Koli K, Bangsow T, Parajuli N, Dumitrascu R, Sterner-Kock A, Weissmann N, Keski-Oja J & von Melchner H (2010) Inactivation of sestrin 2 induces TGF-beta signaling and partially rescues pulmonary emphysema in a mouse model of COPD. *Dis Model Mech* 3, 246-253.

[148] Wang N, Pan W, Zhu M, Zhang M, Hao X, Liang G & Feng Y (2011) Fangchinoline induces autophagic cell death via p53/sestrin2/AMPK signalling in human hepatocellular carcinoma cells. *Br J Pharmacol* 164, 731-742.

[149] Lee SO, Andey T, Jin UH, Kim K, Sachdeva M & Safe S (2011) The nuclear receptor TR3 regulates mTORC1 signaling in lung cancer cells expressing wild-type p53. *Oncogene*.

[150] Santibanez JF, Quintanilla M & Bernabeu C (2011) TGF-beta/TGF-beta receptor system and its role in physiological and pathological conditions. *Clin Sci (Lond)* 121, 233-251.

[151] Krieglstein K, Miyazono K, ten Dijke P & Unsicker K (2012) TGF-beta in aging and disease. *Cell Tissue Res* 347, 5-9.

[152] Bierie B & Moses HL (2006) Tumour microenvironment: TGFbeta: the molecular Jekyll and Hyde of cancer. *Nat Rev Cancer* 6, 506-520.

[153] Liu SY, Lee YJ & Lee TC (2011) Association of platelet-derived growth factor receptor beta accumulation with increased oxidative stress and cellular injury in sestrin 2 silenced human glioblastoma cells. *FEBS Lett* 585, 1853-1858.

[154] Salminen A & Kaarniranta K (2009) Regulation of the aging process by autophagy. *Trends Mol Med* 15, 217-224.

[155] Soontornniyomkij V, Soontornniyomkij B, Moore DJ, Gouaux B, Masliah E, Tung S, Vinters HV, Grant I & Achim CL (2012) Antioxidant Sestrin-2 Redistribution to Neuronal Soma in Human Immunodeficiency Virus-Associated Neurocognitive Disorders. *J Neuroimmune Pharmacol.*

[156] Doonan F, Wallace DM, O'Driscoll C & Cotter TG (2009) Rosiglitazone acts as a neuroprotectant in retinal cells via up-regulation of sestrin-1 and SOD-2. *J Neurochem* 109, 631-643.

[157] Armata HL, Golebiowski D, Jung DY, Ko HJ, Kim JK & Sluss HK (2010) Requirement of the ATM/p53 tumor suppressor pathway for glucose homeostasis. *Mol Cell Biol* 30, 5787-5794.

[158] Paik JH, Kollipara R, Chu G, Ji H, Xiao Y, Ding Z, Miao L, Tothova Z, Horner JW, Carrasco DR, Jiang S, Gilliland DG, Chin L, Wong WH, Castrillon DH & DePinho RA (2007) FoxOs are lineage-restricted redundant tumor suppressors and regulate endothelial cell homeostasis. *Cell* 128, 309-323.

[159] Tothova Z, Kollipara R, Huntly BJ, Lee BH, Castrillon DH, Cullen DE, McDowell EP, Lazo-Kallanian S, Williams IR, Sears C, Armstrong SA, Passegue E, DePinho RA & Gilliland DG (2007) FoxOs are critical mediators of hematopoietic stem cell resistance to physiologic oxidative stress. *Cell* 128, 325-339.

[160] Hartmann S, Gesk S, Scholtysik R, Kreuz M, Bug S, Vater I, Doring C, Cogliatti S, Parrens M, Merlio JP, Kwiecinska A, Porwit A, Piccaluga PP, Pileri S, Hoefler G, Kuppers R, Siebert R & Hansmann ML (2010) High resolution SNP array genomic profiling of peripheral T cell lymphomas, not otherwise specified, identifies a subgroup with chromosomal aberrations affecting the REL locus. *Br J Haematol* 148, 402-412.

[161] Birnbaum DJ, Adelaide J, Mamessier E, Finetti P, Lagarde A, Monges G, Viret F, Goncalves A, Turrini O, Delpero JR, Iovanna J, Giovannini M, Birnbaum D & Chaffanet M (2011) Genome profiling of pancreatic adenocarcinoma. *Genes Chromosomes Cancer* 50, 456-465.

[162] Ohba S, Shimizu K, Shibao S, Miwa T, Nakagawa T, Sasaki H & Murakami H (2011) A glioblastoma arising from the attached region where a meningioma had been totally removed. *Neuropathology* 31, 606-611.

[163] Dimova I, Orsetti B, Negre V, Rouge C, Ursule L, Lasorsa L, Dimitrov R, Doganov N, Toncheva D & Theillet C (2009) Genomic markers for ovarian cancer at chromosomes 1, 8 and 17 revealed by array CGH analysis. *Tumori* 95, 357-366.

[164] Kleer CG, Bryant BR, Giordano TJ, Sobel M & Merino MJ (2000) Genetic Changes in Chromosomes 1p and 17p in Thyroid Cancer Progression. *Endocr Pathol* 11, 137-143.

[165] Mora J, Cheung NK, Kushner BH, LaQuaglia MP, Kramer K, Fazzari M, Heller G, Chen L & Gerald WL (2000) Clinical categories of neuroblastoma are associated with different patterns of loss of heterozygosity on chromosome arm 1p. *J Mol Diagn* 2, 37-46.

[166] Stokke T, DeAngelis P, Smedshammer L, Galteland E, Steen HB, Smeland EB, Delabie J & Holte H (2001) Loss of chromosome 11q21-23.1 and 17p and gain of chromosome 6p

are independent prognostic indicators in B-cell non-Hodgkin's lymphoma. *Br J Cancer* 85, 1900-1913.

[167] Fang Y, Guan X, Guo Y, Sham J, Deng M, Liang Q, Li H, Zhang H, Zhou H & Trent J (2001) Analysis of genetic alterations in primary nasopharyngeal carcinoma by comparative genomic hybridization. *Genes Chromosomes Cancer* 30, 254-260.

[168] Lo KW, Teo PM, Hui AB, To KF, Tsang YS, Chan SY, Mak KF, Lee JC & Huang DP (2000) High resolution allelotype of microdissected primary nasopharyngeal carcinoma. *Cancer Res* 60, 3348-3353.

[169] Stumpf E, Aalto Y, Hoog A, Kjellman M, Otonkoski T, Knuutila S & Andersson LC (2000) Chromosomal alterations in human pancreatic endocrine tumors. *Genes Chromosomes Cancer* 29, 83-87.

[170] Goldberg EK, Glendening JM, Karanjawala Z, Sridhar A, Walker GJ, Hayward NK, Rice AJ, Kurera D, Tebha Y & Fountain JW (2000) Localization of multiple melanoma tumor-suppressor genes on chromosome 11 by use of homozygosity mapping-of-deletions analysis. *Am J Hum Genet* 67, 417-431.

[171] Garber ME, Troyanskaya OG, Schluens K, Petersen S, Thaesler Z, Pacyna-Gengelbach M, van de Rijn M, Rosen GD, Perou CM, Whyte RI, Altman RB, Brown PO, Botstein D & Petersen I (2001) Diversity of gene expression in adenocarcinoma of the lung. *Proc Natl Acad Sci U S A* 98, 13784-13789.

[172] Wachi S, Yoneda K & Wu R (2005) Interactome-transcriptome analysis reveals the high centrality of genes differentially expressed in lung cancer tissues. *Bioinformatics* 21, 4205-4208.

[173] Su LJ, Chang CW, Wu YC, Chen KC, Lin CJ, Liang SC, Lin CH, Whang-Peng J, Hsu SL, Chen CH & Huang CY (2007) Selection of DDX5 as a novel internal control for Q-RT-PCR from microarray data using a block bootstrap re-sampling scheme. *BMC Genomics* 8, 140.

[174] Richardson AL, Wang ZC, De Nicolo A, Lu X, Brown M, Miron A, Liao X, Iglehart JD, Livingston DM & Ganesan S (2006) X chromosomal abnormalities in basal-like human breast cancer. *Cancer Cell* 9, 121-132.

[175] Turashvili G, Bouchal J, Baumforth K, Wei W, Dziechciarkova M, Ehrmann J, Klein J, Fridman E, Skarda J, Srovnal J, Hajduch M, Murray P & Kolar Z (2007) Novel markers for differentiation of lobular and ductal invasive breast carcinomas by laser microdissection and microarray analysis. *BMC Cancer* 7, 55.

[176] Ye H, Yu T, Temam S, Ziober BL, Wang J, Schwartz JL, Mao L, Wong DT & Zhou X (2008) Transcriptomic dissection of tongue squamous cell carcinoma. *BMC Genomics* 9, 69.

[177] Lee J, Kotliarova S, Kotliarov Y, Li A, Su Q, Donin NM, Pastorino S, Purow BW, Christopher N, Zhang W, Park JK & Fine HA (2006) Tumor stem cells derived from glioblastomas cultured in bFGF and EGF more closely mirror the phenotype and genotype of primary tumors than do serum-cultured cell lines. *Cancer Cell* 9, 391-403.

[178] Hou Y, Song L, Zhu P, Zhang B, Tao Y, Xu X, Li F, Wu K, Liang J, Shao D, Wu H, Ye X, Ye C, Wu R, Jian M, Chen Y, Xie W, Zhang R, Chen L, Liu X, Yao X, Zheng H, Yu C, Li Q, Gong Z, Mao M, Yang X, Yang L, Li J, Wang W, Lu Z, Gu N, Laurie G, Bolund L, Kristiansen K, Wang J, Yang H, Li Y & Zhang X (2012) Single-cell exome sequencing and monoclonal evolution of a JAK2-negative myeloproliferative neoplasm. *Cell* 148, 873-885.

[179] Zighelboim I, Goodfellow PJ, Schmidt AP, Walls KC, Mallon MA, Mutch DG, Yan PS, Huang TH & Powell MA (2007) Differential methylation hybridization array of endometrial cancers reveals two novel cancer-specific methylation markers. *Clin Cancer Res* 13, 2882-2889.

Chapter 3

Regulation of Autophagy by Protein Phosphorylation

Björn Stork, Sebastian Alers, Antje S. Löffler and Sebastian Wesselborg

Additional information is available at the end of the chapter

http://dx.doi.org/10.5772/48502

1. Introduction

Macroautophagy (hereafter called autophagy) is an intracellular lysosomal degradation process. Long-lived cytosolic proteins and entire organelles are enveloped by a double membrane. These vesicles are called autophagosomes and are transferred to lysosomes. The enclosed cargo is degraded by lysosomal hydrolases, and the resulting components are transported back to the cytosol and re-used for anabolic and catabolic processes. In recent years it became evident that autophagy is central for cellular homeostasis. Autophagy occurs at basal levels essentially in any cell type, and is actively induced under stress conditions, e.g. nutrient deprivation or infection. Additionally, the involvement of autophagy in human pathologies such as cancerogenesis and neurodegeneration is well-documented and current therapeutic approaches hence target autophagy signaling pathways.

During the past decade the molecular mechanisms for the induction and execution of autophagy have been partially resolved. The discovery of the yeast autophagy-related genes (Atgs) was central for this understanding. To date, 35 yeast Atgs have been identified, many of which have mammalian counterparts. However, autophagy induction is additionally controlled by a complex network of other cellular signaling pathways.

The process of autophagy is mainly regulated by six functional units: 1) the Ulk1-Atg13-FIP200 kinase complex, 2) the PI3K class III complex containing the core proteins Vps34, p150 and Beclin 1, 3) the PI3P-binding Atg2/Atg18 complex, 4) the multi-spanning transmembrane protein Atg9, 5) the ubiquitin-like Atg5/Atg12 system and 6) the ubiquitin-like LC3 conjugation system (reviewed in [1]). These six modules participate in different steps of autophagy execution, i.e. vesicle nucleation, elongation and autophagosome completion. In the following we will summarize the current knowledge about regulatory phosphorylation events occurring during autophagy induction upstream and downstream of the Ulk1-Atg13-FIP200 and PI3K class III "initiator complexes", and during vesicle elongation, e.g. LC3 phosphorylation.

2. The Ulk1-Atg13-FIP200 protein kinase complex

Interestingly, Atg1/Unc-51-like kinase 1 is the only protein kinase among the Atg proteins. In 1993, Tsukada and Ohsumi reported the isolation of different autophagy-defective mutants of *S. cerevisiae* [2]. The apg1 strain was the first identified strain, and subsequently it was discovered that the corresponding gene encodes a serine/threonine protein kinase [3], which was subsequently termed Atg1. During the induction of canonical autophagy in yeast, Atg1 interacts with Atg13, Atg17, Atg29 and Atg31 [4-8]. Apparently a constitutive trimeric complex of Atg17, Atg29 and Atg31 serves as scaffold for the subsequent recruitment of other Atg proteins to the pre-autophagosomal structure (PAS) [9, 10]. In contrast, the interaction between Atg1 and Atg17 is dynamic and mediated by Atg13 [5, 11]. In 2000, Ohsumi and colleagues could nicely demonstrate that the association between Atg1 and Atg13 is negatively regulated by target of rapamycin (TOR) signaling [7]. In their model, nutrient-rich conditions lead to a TOR-mediated hyperphosphorylation of Atg13, which prevents its association with Atg1. In turn, starvation conditions or rapamycin treatment result in an inactivated TOR and a dephosphorylated Atg13. Dephosphorylated Atg13 exhibits a high affinity for Atg1 and induces its kinase activity, ultimately leading to the induction of autophagy [7]. Recently the group could confirm this model by showing that the expression of an Atg13 mutant protein which cannot be phosphorylated by TOR anymore leads to the induction of autophagy under nutrient-rich conditions [12]. Apparently Atg13 mediates the self-association of Atg1, and the appearance of Atg1-Atg1-dimers is correlated with the induction of autophagy [13].

In vertebrates, the situation is a little bit more complex. There exist at least five Atg1 homologs, designated as Unc-51-like kinases 1-4 (Ulk1-4) and STK36 (reviewed in [14-17]). Unc-51 (uncoordinated-51) is the single Atg1 homolog in *C. elegans* [3, 15]. Especially Ulk1 and Ulk2 have been well characterized as the functional homologs of Atg1/Unc-51, and only these two Unc-51-like kinases exclusively exhibit high similarity in both the N-terminal catalytic domain and the rest of the protein, including a central proline/serine-rich (PS) and the C-terminal domain (CTD) [16, 17]. Although overexpression of Ulk3 was able to induce autophagy in the human fibroblast cell line IMR90 [18], only Ulk1 and Ulk2 are capable of interacting with mammalian Atg13 via their conserved CTD [19-22]. Based on an siRNA screen in HEK293 cells, Ulk1 has been proposed as the primary autophagy regulator, since the knockdown of Ulk1 but not that of Ulk2 inhibited the autophagic response upon starvation or rapamycin treatment [23]. Both Ulk1 and Ulk2 are ubiquitously expressed in most adult mammalian tissues [24-26]. Interestingly, in red blood cells only *ulk1* mRNA is significantly up-regulated during terminal erythrocyte differentiation [27]. Accordingly, *ulk1*$^{-/-}$ mice reveal defects in the clearance of mitochondria and RNA-containing ribosomes in reticulocytes during erythrocyte maturation [27]. However, *ulk1*$^{-/-}$ mice are born viable and show normal autophagy induction upon starvation [27], which is in clear contrast to other mouse models deficient for specific Atgs such as Atg5 or Atg7 [28, 29]. Furthermore, *ulk2*$^{-/-}$ mice are likewise viable and autophagy-competent [30, 31]. These observations suggest that Ulk1 and Ulk2 have partially redundant functions and that loss of one kinase can be compensated by the other during non-selective autophagy. However, the ability of Ulk2 to compensate Ulk1-deficiency appears to be cell type-specific and to depend on the type of autophagy. The selective role of Ulk1 for mitophagy described above has recently been confirmed by the observation that Ulk1-mediated phosphorylation of Atg13 at S318 is essential for mitophagy, but not for basal or starvation-induced autophagy [32]. Additionally, only Ulk1 is required for low potassium-induced autophagy in cerebellar granule neurons [31]. Finally, in Ulk1-silenced *ulk2*$^{-/-}$ MEFs or in *ulk1*$^{-/-}$ *ulk2*$^{-/-}$ MEFs autophagy induced by amino acid deprivation is blocked, further supporting the redundant functions of both kinases [30, 31]. Of note, starvation-induced autophagy was not inhibited in *ulk1*$^{-/-}$*ulk2*$^{-/-}$ DT40 B lymphocytes generated in our laboratory, and *ulk1*$^{-/-}$*ulk2*$^{-/-}$ MEFs display autophagy induction upon glucose deprivation [30, 33]. The molecular details of these Ulk1/Ulk2-independent autophagy pathways have to be deciphered in the future.

As described above, the CTD of Ulk1 and Ulk2 can interact with mammalian Atg13. In 2007, mammalian Atg13 has been identified by an *in silico* protein and DNA database screen [34]. Subsequently, the essential role of Atg13 for autophagy has been confirmed in HEK293 cells [19]. Atg17, the other essential component of the yeast Atg1 complex, is conserved in different yeast strains and most filamentous fungi, but primary sequence homologs could not be identified in higher eukaryotes [34]. However, Mizushima and colleagues demonstrated that the focal adhesion kinase (FAK) family interacting protein of 200 kDa (FIP200) is an Ulk1-interacting protein and essential for autophagy induction [35]. FIP200 is a large coiled-coil domain containing protein and regulates diverse cellular functions including cell size, proliferation and migration [35]. FIP200 was initially identified as gene inducing retinoblastoma 1 (RB1) expression in different human cell lines [36] and accordingly termed RB1CC1. Mizushima and colleagues speculated in the original manuscript that FIP200 might represent the functional homolog of yeast Atg17 [35]. Both proteins have multiple coiled-coil domains, enhance the catalytic activity of Atg1/Ulk1, are essential for Atg1/Ulk1 puncta formation, have multiple binding partners and thus scaffolding properties, and are mutually exclusively present in different species [35]. Indeed, several almost simultaneously published articles describe the existence of a mammalian Ulk-Atg13-FIP200 kinase complex, which is directly regulated by the mammalian target of rapamycin complex 1 (mTORC1) [20-22]. The interaction between Ulk1/2 and FIP200 is mediated by Atg13. However, one group described the direct interaction of FIP200 with Ulk [20]. In contrast to the yeast Atg1-Atg13-Atg17 complex, the components of the mammalian Ulk-Atg13-FIP200 complex are constitutively associated, especially independently of nutrient supply [20-22]. However, apparently the phosphorylation status within the Ulk-Atg13-FIP200 complex is considerably altered during autophagy induction (see below).

A fourth component of the Ulk-Atg13-FIP200 complex has recently been characterized. Since it has no obvious homolog in yeast, it was termed Atg101 [37, 38]. Atg101 stably associates with the kinase complex, most likely via direct interaction with Atg13. It appears that Atg101 protects Atg13 from proteasomal degradation [37, 38].

2.1. The Ulk1-Atg13-FIP200 protein kinase complex and protein phosphorylation

In yeast, target of rapamycin complex 1 (TORC1) phosphorylates Atg13 at several serine residues, thus preventing the association of Atg13 with Atg1. In turn, TORC1 inactivation by rapamycin treatment or nutrient deprivation causes Atg13 dephosphorylation, resulting in Atg1-Atg13-Atg17 complex assembly and enhanced Atg1 kinase activity [7, 12]. Regarding TORC1-dependent phospho-sites in Atg13, four serine residues have been clearly identified, i.e. S437, S438, S646, and S649 [12]. Four additional sites were not precisely mapped, but could be deduced from known TORC1 sites or the conservation among *Saccharomyces* species (S348, S496, S535, and S541). As described above, the expression of the corresponding Atg13-8SA mutant was able to induce autophagy through activation of Atg1 even under nutrient-rich conditions [12]. Recently it has been reported that the Ksp1 kinase negatively regulates autophagy in yeast via the TORC1-Atg13 axis [39].

Atg1 itself is phosphorylated at multiple sites [40, 41]. Phosphorylation of T226 and S230 is important for Atg1 kinase activity and its function in autophagy. Both residues are located within the activation loop of the N-terminal kinase domain and apparently become phosphorylated by autophosphorylation [40, 41]. Additional phosphorylation sites have been reported. In one of these studies, a total of 29 constitutive or rapamycin-regulated phospho-sites were identified [40].

As mentioned above, the phosphorylation status within the mammalian Ulk1/2-Atg13-FIP200 complex varies dependent on the cellular energy and nutrient supply. Under normal growth conditions, mTORC1 associates with the complex via the direct interaction between the mTORC1 component raptor and Ulk1/2 [21]. Active mTOR phosphorylates Ulk1/2 and Atg13 and thus suppresses Ulk1/2 kinase activity [20-22]. In a first mass spectrometric approach, Dorsey et al. identified 16 phospho-acceptor sites in Ulk1 under fed conditions [42]. The authors suggested that S341 located in the PS region and S1047 in the CTD represent Ulk1 autophosphorylation sites which are required for protein stability. Upon starvation or rapamycin treatment, mTORC1 dissociates from the Ulk1/2-Atg13-FIP200 complex and the mTOR-dependent phospho-sites of Ulk1 become dephosphorylated. In a SILAC-based approach, Wang and colleagues recently identified 13 serine or threonine residues in Ulk1 phosphorylated under nutrient-rich conditions. Of these residues, S638 and S758 revealed a more than 10-fold decrease of phosphorylation upon starvation [43]. In another study, the mTOR-dependent phosphorylation of Ulk1 at S758 was confirmed [44], and the same phospho-site was also detected in the screen of Dorsey et al. [42]. Interestingly, the total phosphorylation levels of Atg13 were low under nutrient-rich conditions and remained largely unaltered upon nutrient depletion, suggesting that rather Ulk1/2 than Atg13 is the major target of mTOR-dependent autophagy regulation [43]. The dephosphorylated and thus activated Ulk1/2 autophosphorylates and phosphorylates both Atg13 and FIP200, which ultimately leads to the translocation of the complex to the pre-autophagosomal membrane and to autophagy induction [19-23, 35, 45, 46]. Next to the above described autophosphorylation sites mapped for Ulk1 under nutrient-rich conditions, T180 in the activation loop of the kinase domain has been identified as Ulk1 autophosphorylation site [47]. This site is homologous to the site described for yeast Atg1 autophosphorylation [40, 41]. Notably, the functional relevance of Ulk1/2-mediated phosphorylation of both Atg13 and FIP200 remains elusive, and the relevant phospho-sites have not been verified yet. Our group was able to identify five Ulk1-dependent *in vitro* phosphorylation sites in human Atg13, i.e. S48, T170, T331, T428 and T478 [33]. However, expression of the corresponding pan-serine/threonine-to-alanine mutant of Atg13 in *atg13*$^{-/-}$ DT40 B cells did not block autophagy induction upon starvation [33]. Since Ulk1 and Ulk2 are dispensable for autophagy induction in this cellular system, potentially other kinases and Atg13 phospho-acceptor sites might play a role in the regulation of autophagy. As stated above, Ulk1-mediated phosphorylation of S318 in Atg13 solely influences mitophagy and has no impact on starvation-induced autophagy [32]. One might speculate that the Ulk-catalyzed phosphorylation of Atg13 and FIP200 controls the translocation of the kinase complex to pre-autophagosomal structures.

In addition to mTOR, the Ulk1/2-Atg13-FIP200 complex is regulated by other kinases such as PKA, Akt and AMPK, respectively (reviewed in [1, 14, 17]). The cAMP-dependent protein kinase A (PKA) inhibits yeast autophagy by phosphorylation of Atg1 and Atg13. In Atg1, PKA-dependent phosphorylation presumably takes place at S508 and S515, and in Atg13 at S344, S437, and S581 [48, 49]. In mammalian cells, depletion of the type IA regulatory subunit of PKA has been shown to activate mTOR and thus to inhibit autophagy [50]. A direct phosphorylation of Ulk1 at S1043 by PKA has been suggested by Dorsey et al., causing a rather closed and inactive conformation of Ulk1 [42]. A PKA-mediated phosphorylation of mammalian Atg13, in contrast, has not been confirmed yet.

Recently, S774 has been identified as a high-stringency Akt site in Ulk1 [47]. Phosphorylation of Ulk1 at this site was increased by insulin treatment. Notably, this insulin-mediated repression of autophagy was also observed in the presence of rapamycin, suggesting that this inhibition occurs independently of mTOR inhibition. Indeed, synergistic effects of rapamycin and Akt inhibitors on autophagy have been reported [47, 51]. Interestingly, the yeast kinase Sch9, which is a homolog of Akt or p70S6K, has been implicated in the regulation of autophagy. The authors proposed that PKA and Sch9 cooperatively regulate autophagy, and that this is partially independent of TORC1 [52].

Whereas mTOR activity is regulated by a diverse array of positive signals such as high energy levels, normoxia, amino acids and growth factors, the AMP-regulated protein kinase (AMPK) is activated under low energy levels and thus represents the classical energy-sensor of the cell. AMPK is a heterotrimeric kinase, consisting of a catalytic α-subunit and two regulatory β- and γ-subunits, respectively (reviewed in [53]). Additionally, multiple isoforms of each subunit exist, i.e. α1-2, β1-2, and γ1-3 [53]. Phosphorylation of T172 in the catalytic α-subunit is a prerequisite for AMPK activity. In turn, this phosphorylation can be carried out by the ubiquitously expressed and constitutively active LKB1, the Ca^{2+}-activated Ca^{2+}/calmodulin-dependent kinase kinase β (CaMKKβ), or the cytokine-activated TAK1 (transforming growth factor b-activated kinase-1) [14]. An additional level of regulation is mediated by the regulatory β- and γ-subunits. The γ-subunit can bind ATP, ADP and AMP and thus appropriately senses the cellular energy status [53]. The β-subunit contains carbohydrate-binding modules, whose exact functions remain rather elusive. However, it has been speculated that these domains contribute to the subcellular localization of AMPK or targeting the kinase to glycogen-associated substrates [53]. In 2001, it was shown that the yeast AMPK ortholog SNF1 acts as a positive regulator of autophagy, and it has been speculated that this is mediated via Atg1 and Atg13 [71]. Although an initial report described the inhibition of autophagy by the AMPK activator AICAR [54], a positive regulatory role of AMPK for mammalian autophagy has subsequently been confirmed by several groups [55-58]. However, next to energy depletion other stimuli such as the increase of cytosolic Ca^{2+} concentrations, TRAIL-mediated activation of TAK1, and genotoxic stress-induced sestrin1 and sestrin2 expression have been implicated in the AMPK-dependent regulation of autophagy (reviewed in [14, 59-62]). Historically, the AMPK-dependent regulation of autophagy has been proposed to mainly function via the inhibition of mTOR. AMPK regulates the mTORC1 via the direct phosphorylation of two effectors: 1) the upstream regulator tuberous sclerosis complex 2 (TSC2) and 2) the mTORC1-subunit raptor [63-65]. However, in 2010 Behrends et al. first discovered the interaction between AMPK and Ulk1/2 in a global proteomic analysis of the human autophagy network [66]. Subsequently, different groups confirmed the direct interaction between these two kinases [43, 44, 65, 67, 68]. Four of these groups additionally reported the AMPK-mediated phosphorylation of Ulk1. The common theme of these reports is the starvation-induced activation of AMPK, the subsequent phosphorylation and activation of Ulk1, and in turn the induction of autophagy (reviewed in [14, 69]). In contrast, our group was able to identify Ulk1-dependent phosphorylation sites in all three AMPK subunits, suggesting a rather complex level of regulation by mutual phosphorylation [68]. The direct activation of Ulk1 by AMPK represents a valuable model for mTOR-independent autophagy pathways [69, 70]. Furthermore, due to the data obtained in yeast (see above), it has been proposed that this direct autophagy induction pathway most likely arose even earlier in evolution than the mTORC1-mediated regulation [53, 71]. Notably, the direct regulation of Ulk1 by AMPK appears to be rather complex, since the different groups identified different phospho-acceptor sites for AMPK (reviewed in [14, 69]). Kim et al. reported the mTORC1-mediated phosphorylation of S758 in Ulk1 under nutrient-rich conditions, which leads to the inhibition of the AMPK-Ulk1 interaction. Upon glucose starvation, AMPK is activated and 1) inhibits mTORC1 and 2) activates Ulk1 by the phosphorylation at S317 and S778 [44]. Egan et al. characterized Ulk1 both as an AMPK substrate and as 14-3-3-binding protein. However, this group identified four completely different AMPK-sites in Ulk1: S467, S556, T575 and S638 [67]. One of these sites (S556) has later been confirmed as AMPK- and 14-3-3-binding site in another study [47]. Lee et al. earlier showed that the association between Ulk1 and AMPK is important for the induction of autophagy, and mentioned the unpublished observation that purified AMPK could phosphorylate recombinant Ulk1 *in vitro* [65]. Finally and as described above, Shang et al. could identify 13 phospho-acceptor sites in Ulk1 using a SILAC-based approach. In this approach they confirmed the mTOR-site S758 identified by Kim et al., but not their AMPK-sites. However, in contrast to the report by Kim et al., phosphorylation of S758 leads to the association of AMPK and Ulk1 [43]. Notably, the AMPK-sites S556 and S638 in Ulk1 described by Egan et al. were confirmed by Shang et al.. As described above, they observed significant dephosphorylation at S638 and S758 upon starvation. When cells are replenished with growth media, mTOR-mediated phosphorylation of S758 leads to the re-association of Ulk1 and AMPK, and subsequently mTOR and the Ulk1-associated AMPK function to maintain phosphorylation at S638 [43]. In summary, it appears that further studies are necessary to decipher this rather complex "Ulk1 phosphorylation barcode" as well as the exact kinetics of its mTOR- and AMPK-dependent generation. Furthermore, it has to be considered that this barcode might depend on both the type of autophagic stimulus and the type of (organelle-specific) autophagy.

Adding an additional level of complexity, recent reports describe the Ulk1-dependent phosphorylation of AMPK- and mTOR-subunits, respectively. Our group could show that all three AMPK subunits are phosphorylated by Ulk1 and Ulk2, and that thereby AMPK activity is negatively regulated [68]. The phospho-sites include S360/T368, S397, S486/T488 in the α1-subunit, S38, T39, S68 and S173 in the β2-subunit, and S260/T262 and S269 in the γ1-subunit (for some peptides the exact phosphorylation-site could not be narrowed down further). Thus, we propose that Ulk1 is not only necessary for the induction of autophagy, but also is involved in its containment [68]. Finally, two reports describe the Ulk1-dependent phosphorylation of raptor [72, 73]. The common theme here is that this phosphorylation leads to the inhibition of mTORC1 thus inducing autophagy. Dunlop et al. reported that Ulk1 promotes phosphorylation of raptor at S696, T706, S792, S855, S859, S863 and weakly S877 *in vivo*. The direct phosphorylation of the last five residues was confirmed by an *in vitro* kinase assay, with the strongest phosphorylation at S855 and S859, respectively. Collectively, these multiple phosphorylations inhibit mTORC1 activity through hindrance of substrate docking to raptor [72]. These results are in line with the findings by Jung et al. [73]. Collectively, the Ulk1-mediated phosphorylation of AMPK and raptor represent regulatory feedback loops and contribute to the positive and negative regulation of autophagy.

Next to the associated Atg13 and FIP200 and the AMPK and mTORC1 kinase complexes, two additional Ulk1 substrates related to the regulation of autophagy have been identified, i.e. the activating molecule in Beclin1-regulated autophagy 1 (Ambra1; see below) and the myosin light chain kinase (MLCK)-like protein Spaghetti squash activator (Sqa) in *Drosophila*. Regarding Ambra1, Fimia and colleagues showed that Ambra1 tethers the Vps34-Beclin 1-complex (see below) to the cytoskeletal dynein light chains. Upon autophagy induction, Ulk1 phosphorylates Ambra1 and thereby releases the Vps34-Beclin 1 core complex from dynein [74, 75]. Subsequently, this complex translocates to the ER where it contributes to autophagosome formation (see below). The second Ulk1 substrate is the *Drosophila* MLCK-like protein Sqa, whose mammalian ortholog is the zipper interacting protein kinase (ZIPK), which is also termed death-associated protein kinase 3 (DAPK3) [76]. Through the combination of observations obtained in *Drosophila* and mammalian cells, the authors propose a model in which starvation leads to the Atg1/Ulk1-mediated phosphorylation of Sqa/ZIPK at T279/T265 (Sqa/ZIPK sequence). This in turn leads to the phosphorylation of the myosin II regulatory light chain (Spaghetti-Squash, Sqh, in *Drosophila*, and MLC in human). Subsequently, myosin II regulates starvation-induced trafficking of mAtg9 from the trans-Golgi network (TGN) to autophagosomes [76-78]. The role of mAtg9 will be discussed below. Collectively, both models support the view that the cytoskeleton plays a central role for the spatial organization of autophagy-inducing complexes. This is further supported by data showing that the exocyst, a hetero-octameric protein complex normally involved in tethering vesicles to the plasma membrane, serves as an assembly and activation scaffold for components of the autophagic machinery [79, 80]. It could be demonstrated that the small G protein RalB and an Exo84-dependent subcomplex of the exocyst are critical for the recruitment of the Ulk1-Atg13-FIP200 and the Vps34-Beclin 1 initiation complexes as well as the two ubiquitin-like conjugation systems and thus for autophagosome formation [79, 80].

The mutual regulation of AMPK, mTOR and Ulk1/2 and the phosphorylation events upstream and downstream of the Ulk1/2-Atg13-FIP200 kinase complex are depicted in figure 1A and B.

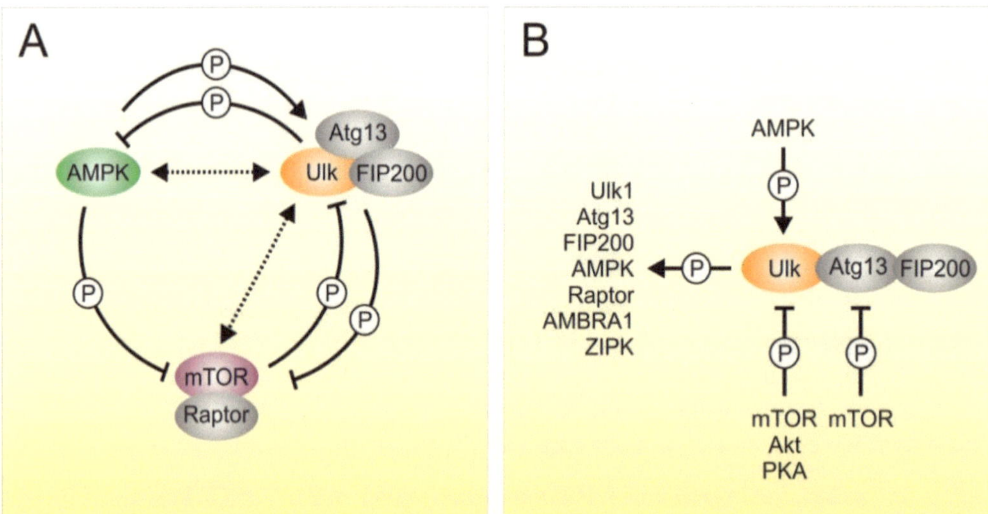

Figure 1. Mutual regulatory phosphorylations of AMPK, mTOR and Ulk1/2 (A) and phosphorylations downstream and upstream of the Ulk1/2-Atg13-FIP200 kinase complex (B). AMBRA1, activating molecule in Beclin1-regulated autophagy 1; AMPK, AMP-regulated protein kinase; Atg, autophagy-related gene; FIP200, focal adhesion kinase family interacting protein of 200 kDa; mTOR, mammalian target of rapamycin; PKA, protein kinase A; Ulk, Unc-51-like kinase; ZIPK, zipper interacting protein kinase. Panel A was modified from supplemental material to reference [68].

3. The PI3K class III complex

In yeast, the class III phosphatidylinositol 3-kinase (PI3K class III) Vps34 participates in both autophagy and vacuolar protein sorting (Vps). Accordingly, two distinct Vps34-containing complexes have been identified [81]. Both complexes share the core components Vps34, Vps15, and Atg6 (Vps30). The first complex (complex I) additionally contains Atg14 and is required for autophagy, while the second complex (complex II) contains Vps38 instead of Atg14 and is important for vacuolar protein sorting via endosomes. It has been shown that the destination-determining factors Atg14 and Vps38 target the Vps34-complexes to either the pre-autophagosomal structure (PAS) or to endosomal membranes, respectively [82]. In mammals, different Vps34-complexes could be identified and characterized (reviewed in [83]). The mammalian PI3K class III core complex contains hVps34, hVps15 (p150), and Beclin 1 (Atg6). This core complex can in turn associate with different regulatory and function-determining proteins. It appears that there are three major sub-complexes, containing either Atg14L or UVRAG (UV-irradiation resistance-associated gene) or a dimer of UVRAG and Rubicon (RUN domain protein as Beclin 1 interacting and cysteine-rich containing), respectively [83, 84].

Atg14L is the putative mammalian homolog of yeast Atg14. Atg14L was identified by a sequence homology screen and has also been termed as Atg14 or Barkor [85-88]. Atg14L contains two coiled-coil domains (CCDs) that are essential for the interaction with the CCDs of Beclin 1 and hVps34, respectively [83]. The interaction between Vps34 and Beclin 1 is not affected by Atg14L. However, Beclin 1 is required for the association of Atg14L with Vps34 [87]. The Atg14L-containing Vps34-Vps15-Beclin 1 complex is essential for the early steps of autophagosome formation and likely represents the equivalent of yeast complex I. Atg14L co-localizes with Atg5 and Atg16L1 on the isolation membrane during autophagy induction [85]. In *atg14*$^{-/-}$ ES cells, starvation does not induce the formation of Atg16L and LC3 puncta or the lipidation of LC3 (see below). Additionally, the bulk degradation of long-lived proteins is suppressed in these cells [86].

UVRAG has been initially identified as Beclin 1-binding protein, and – like Beclin 1 – has been described as tumor suppressor [89]. UVRAG has been suggested as mammalian Vps38 homolog [85, 90], and indeed the binding of Atg14L or UVRAG to Beclin 1 is mutually exclusive [86-88, 90]. The exact role of UVRAG for autophagy induction, however, remains rather controversial. It has been reported that UVRAG expression increases Vps34 activity and that UVRAG and Beclin 1 act together to induce autophagosome formation [89]. However, Mizushima and colleagues could not detect any inhibitory effect of siRNA-mediated UVRAG knockdown on autophagy flux and GFP-LC3 puncta formation [85]. Interestingly, it was recently demonstrated that UVRAG mutations associated with microsatellite unstable colon cancer do not affect autophagy [91]. Notably, UVRAG exhibits a positive regulatory role at later stages of autophagosome maturation independently of Beclin 1. It has been reported that UVRAG interacts with the class C Vps (C-Vps), which is a key component of the endosomal fusion machinery [92]. This UVRAG-C-Vps interaction apparently stimulates Rab7 GTPase activity, which is important for complete autophagosome maturation and autophagsome fusion with late endosomes/lysosomes [83, 92]. In parallel, the UVRAG-C-Vps complex accelerates endosome-endosome fusion, thereby promoting the rapid degradation of endocytic cargo [92].

In 2009, two groups reported the identification and characterization of an additional Beclin 1-associated protein, termed RUN domain protein as Beclin 1 interacting and cysteine-rich containing (Rubicon) [86, 88]. Rubicon is composed of an N-terminal RUN domain, a central CCD and a C-terminal cysteine-rich region. Both reports demonstrated that Rubion-containing Vps34-Beclin 1-complexes are devoid of Atg14L. Since UVRAG is able to bind the core complex independently of Rubicon but Rubicon in turn can only bind to the core complex when UVRAG is bound, it appears that UVRAG mediates the interaction between Rubicon and Beclin 1 [86, 88]. Interestingly, there is no apparent Rubicon homolog in yeast, and there is no sequence homology between Rubicon and Atg14 or Vps38, respectively [86, 88]. Current data show that Rubicon suppresses autophagy, presumably at later stages such as autophagosome maturation. Additionally, Rubicon was shown to decrease Vps34 catalytic activity [88]. However, it has been suggested that the negative regulation of autophagy occurs independently of Beclin 1 and of Rubicon's association with the core complex [83]. In fact, the Rubicon-mediated inhibition of Vps34 kinase activity does not require Beclin 1, and the formation of Rubicon-associated late endosomal/lysosomal structures, which apparently inhibit autophagosome maturation, takes place independently of Beclin 1 [88]. Accordingly, it has been proposed that binding of Rubicon to the Vps34-Beclin 1 core complex rather neutralizes the inhibitory effect of Rubicon [83].

In one of the studies mentioned above, Beclin 1 and interacting proteins were purified from different tissues of Beclin 1-EGFP-transgenic mice [88]. Notably, the protein levels of Beclin 1-EGFP, Vps34, Vps15 and UVRAG were similar and reproducibly higher than those of Atg14L and Rubicon suggesting the existence of a UVRAG-containing core complex. These results could be confirmed for Beclin 1 complexes purified from cultured cells [83, 86, 87]. Interestingly, many previously reported Beclin 1-interacting proteins were not detected in these purifications, indicating that those interactions are rather unstable, transient or specific for certain conditions [88]. These associated proteins include Bcl-2 homologs [93-97], Ambra1 [98], nPIST [99], VMP1 [100], Rab5 [101], FYVE-CENT [102], estrogen receptor [103], MyD88/TRIF [104], SLAM [105], Survivin [106], PINK1 [107], and HMGB1 [108-110]. Additionally Bif1 and IP3Rs have been reported to indirectly bind Beclin 1 via UVRAG and Bcl-2, respectively [111, 112]. Finally, several viral proteins have been reported to bind Beclin 1, such as HSV-1 ICP34.5 [113], γ-herpesvirus viral Bcl-2 [97, 114-117], HIV Nef [118] and the M2 protein of influenza virus [119].

The association between Beclin 1 and anti-apoptotic members of the Bcl-2 family such as Bcl-2, Bcl-xL and viral Bcl-2 is especially interesting, since it represents an important node between apoptosis and autophagy signaling pathways [93-97, 114-117]. Actually, Beclin 1 was initially identified as Bcl-2 interacting protein by a yeast-two-hybrid screen [94], and Beclin 1 contains a BH3-domain which mediates the binding to Bcl-2 family proteins [95, 96]. Independently, several groups subsequently showed that anti-apoptotic Bcl-2, Bcl-xL or viral Bcl-2 proteins can inhibit Beclin 1-dependent autophagy [95, 97, 115]. Especially viral Bcl-2 homologs bind Beclin 1 with high affinity, resulting in an ever stronger inhibition of autophagy compared to cellular Bcl-2 family proteins [115]. Surprisingly, although Beclin 1 represents a BH3-only protein, it does not alter the anti-apoptotic capacity of Bcl-2 [120, 121]. It has been shown that Bcl-2 and Beclin 1 co-localize at both the endoplasmic reticulum (ER) and mitochondria [97]. However, it has been proposed that Bcl-2 exerts its anti-autophagic effect on Beclin 1 especially when targeted to the ER, and not when localized at mitochondria, which suggests an organelle-specific regulation of the autophagic machinery [95, 97]. Recently, the nutrient-deprivation autophagy factor-1 (NAF-1) has been identified as a co-factor that specifically targets Bcl-2 to antagonize the autophagic pathway at the ER

[122]. Nevertheless, an important role of mitochondria-targeted Bcl-2 for the regulation of autophagy has been deciphered by Cecconi and colleagues. They showed that a pool of the positive autophagy regulator Ambra1 can bind to mitochondria- but not to ER-localized Bcl-2. Upon starvation, mitochondria-resident Ambra1 is released from Bcl-2 and can associate with both mitochondrial and ER-localized Beclin 1 [123]. Beclin 1-dependent autophagic processes are thus presumably initiated at both organelles and Bcl-2 proteins accordingly regulate autophagy in two ways, directly by binding Beclin 1 and indirectly by sequestering the positive regulator Ambra1 [123, 124].

Two different models have been proposed to explain the Bcl-2/Bcl-xL-mediated inhibition of Beclin 1-dependent autophagy [97, 125, 126]. First, it could be shown that Bcl-2 interferes with the formation of the autophagy-promoting Vps34/Beclin 1-complex and that Bcl-2 overexpression decreases Vps34 catalytic activity [97]. Second, it has been demonstrated that Beclin 1 forms a dimer and that the Beclin 1 dimer interface is disrupted by UVRAG [125]. Apparently Beclin 1 monomerization activates the lipid kinase activity of Vps34. Bcl-2-like proteins in turn reduce the affinity of UVRAG for Beclin 1 approximately 4-fold and accordingly stabilize the Beclin 1 dimer [125]. Bcl-2 and Bcl-xL obviously bind Beclin 1 with relatively low affinity since several groups could show that cellular Bcl-2 homologs cannot be detected in stable Vps34-Beclin 1-complexes [83, 85, 86, 88, 127]. This in turn suggests that the transient interaction between Bcl-2-homologs and Beclin 1 enables a flexible and dynamic regulation of autophagy induction. Meanwhile, several mechanisms have been proposed how this interaction can be negatively regulated, including the phosphorylation of either Bcl-2 proteins or Beclin 1 (see below), the competitive displacement of Beclin 1 by BH3-only proteins or BH3 mimetics, or the disruption of the Bcl-2/Beclin 1 interaction by membrane-anchored receptors and adaptors such as IP3Rs or MyD88/TRIF, respectively (reviewed in [127]).

3.1. Downstream effectors of the PI3K class III complex

Different downstream effectors of phosphatidylinositol 3-phosphate (PI3P), which is the product of PI3K class III catalytic activity, have been implicated in autophagy regulation. In 2008, Ktistakis and colleagues showed that upon starvation double FYVE domain-containing protein 1 (DFCP1) translocates to a punctate compartment which partially co-localizes with autophagosomal proteins and which is in dynamic equilibrium with the ER [128]. The authors termed these structures omegasomes, since the ring-like structures associated with the underlying ER forming an Ω-like shape [128]. Using electron microscopic tomography two reports could meanwhile confirm the tight connection between the ER and the isolation/phagophore membrane [129, 130]. DFCP1-translocation to omegasomes depends on Vps34 and Beclin 1 function [128]. Interestingly, it appears that there is no yeast homolog of DFCP1 [128]. Live imaging experiments revealed that omegasomes form near Vps34-positive vesicles and provide membrane platforms for the accumulation of autophagy-related proteins, expansion of autophagosomal membranes, and emergence of completed autophagosomes [128]. The omegasome model was recently complemented by data from the labs of Yoshimori and Mizushima [131, 132]. Their results explain how the ER acquires PI3P, which is usually absent from this organelle. They demonstrate that Atg14L localizes close to the omegasome-marker DFCP1 and that knockdown of Atg14L blocks the formation of these structures, indicating that Atg14L is upstream of omegasome formation [131, 132]. Accordingly, the Atg14L-dependent alteration of the ER membrane composition via the recruitment of the PI3K class III complex and the subsequent generation of PI3P represent the basis for isolation membrane formation [1, 132].

The second important PI3P effectors belong to the Atg18 family [1]. In yeast, three members have been identified so far, i.e. Atg18, Atg21 and Ygr223c [1, 133]. These proteins are WD40-repeat containing proteins and bind PI3P and $PI3,5P_2$ through the FRRG-motif [1]. It could be shown that Atg18 is important for autophagy, whereas Atg21 and Ygr223c rather contribute to the Cvt pathway and to micronucleophagy [1, 134-136]. Recently, it could be demonstrated that Atg18 supports the efficient completion of the sequestering autophagic vesicle and facilitates the recruitment of Atg8-PE (see below) to the autophagosome formation site [137]. In mammals, four Atg18 homologs have been identified, i.e. WD-repeat protein interacting with phosphoinositides (WIPI)1-4 [1, 133, 138]. It appears that WIPI1 and WIPI2 share close ancestry with Atg18, and WIPI3 and WIPI4 with Ygr223c [133].

Regarding the hierarchical recruitment of Atgs to the ER subdomain, it has been shown that Atg14L-dependent recruitment of the PI3K class III complex requires the kinase activity of Ulk1, placing the Ulk1-Atg13-FIP200 complex most upstream [131, 132]. Following the association of Ulk1-Atg13-FIP200- and Vps34-Vps15-Beclin 1-Atg14L-complexes to these ER-puncta, the two PI3P-binding proteins DCFP1 and WIPI1 are recruited. Finally, Atg5-Atg12-Atg16L1 complexes and LC3 are recruited and accordingly represent the most downstream components [131]. The Beclin 1-interacting VMP1 also localizes to this site of autophagosome formation, independently of any other known Atg proteins [131]. Interestingly, almost all mammalian Atg proteins except DFCP1 accumulate at the same compartments upon induction of autophagy. However, DFCP1 puncta are always localized adjacently to these Atg-positive structures [131].

Considering all the observations described above, a specialized subdomain of the ER appears to represent the most likely membrane source or the scaffold for autophagosome formation [1]. However, other organelles have been implicated in autophagosomal membrane generation (reviewed in [1, 139]). As described above, Ambra1 was found in complex with mitochondria-resident Beclin 1, where it potentially enhances Beclin 1-dependent autophagy [123]. In 2010, it has been reported that mitochondria supply membranes for autophagosome biogenesis during starvation [140]. The authors observed that the autophagosomal markers Atg5 and LC3 (see below) transiently localize to puncta on mitochondria. In their model, mitochondrial-derived membranes are utilized during autophagy, and autophagosome formation is dependent on ER/mitochondria connections [140]. Apparently these connections are necessary to transfer phosphatidylserine (PS) to the mitochondria, where PS is converted to phosphatidylethanolamine (PE). PE in turn is the target of Atg8-conjugation (see below). One might speculate that these mitochondria-ER connections are identical to DFCP1-positive omegasomes [140]. Alternatively, the mitochondria-ER connections might enable the transport of mito-lipids to the ER, where then autophagosome formation takes place [1]. Finally, it should be noted that other organelles than mitochondria or the ER have been implicated in autophagosome biogenesis, including Golgi complex and endosomes, the nuclear envelope and the plasma membrane (reviewed in [1, 139])

3.2. The PI3K class III complex and protein phosphorylation

The catalytic Vps34 subunit of the PI3K class III complex itself is regulated by protein phosphorylation. It could be shown that cyclin-dependent kinase 1 (Cdk1) and Cdk5 can phosphorylate Vps34 at T159. This phosphorylation interferes with the Vps34-Beclin 1 interaction and thereby reduces Vps34 activity. Additionally, Cdk5 phosphorylates Vps34 at T668. This phosphorylation apparently has a direct negative effect on Vps34 activity, since this residue is located in the catalytic domain of the enzyme. Collectively, these two phosphorylations lead to a reduced PI3P generation and accordingly to a down-regulation of autophagosome formation [141]. Cdk1 plays an important role during mitosis, and Cdk1-mediated phosphorylation of Vps34 explains the observation that autophagy is under strict mitotic control [141-143]. By this means, the input to the autophagic compartment might be reduced during mitosis. In contrast, Cdk5 is a neuronal Cdk and has been shown to play a role in Alzheimer's disease. Abnormal activation of Cdk5 potentially contributes to neurodegeneration by negatively regulating autophagy [141].

Recently, a positively regulating phosphorylation of Vps34 has been reported. It could be demonstrated that protein kinase D (PKD) phosphorylates Vps34 at multiple sites, including T677 in the catalytic domain [144]. These phosphorylations lead to increased Vps34 activity, PI3P generation, and autophagosome formation. In line with this observation, PKD co-localized with LC3-positive structures. In addition, the authors could show that PKD acts downstream of DAPK, and that both DAPK and PKD are required for autophagy induction by oxidative stress [144].

As stated above, one way to abrogate the interaction between Bcl-2 family proteins and Beclin 1 is protein phosphorylation. Interestingly, the association between these two proteins can be disturbed by phosphorylation of either one of the two partners. Zalckvar et al. showed that DAPK phosphorylates Beclin 1 at T119, which is a crucial position within the BH3 domain of Beclin 1 [145, 146]. The authors demonstrated that this phosphorylation promotes the dissociation of Bcl-xL from Beclin 1 and thus the induction of autophagy. Thus, it appears that DAPK regulates the Vps34-Beclin 1 complex by two independent mechanisms: 1) indirectly through phosphorylation of PKD, which phosphorylates and activates Vps34, and 2) directly through the phosphorylation of Beclin 1 [144-146]. In turn, an earlier report described the starvation-induced phosphorylation of Bcl-2 at T69, S70 and S87 by c-Jun N-terminal kinase 1 (Jnk1) [117]. Again these phosphorylations lead to the dissociation of Bcl-2 from Beclin 1 and to the subsequent induction of autophagy. The three residues are located within a non-structured loop between the BH3 and BH4 domain of Bcl-2. Interestingly, this loop is not present in viral Bcl-2 from Kaposi's sarcoma-associated herpesvirus, and accordingly viral Bcl-2 escapes this mode of regulation. Furthermore, the authors could show that Bcl-2 phosphorylation upon starvation is mediated by Jnk1 but not by Jnk2 [117]. The high mobility group box 1 (HMGB1) has also been shown to negatively regulate the association between Bcl-2 family proteins and Beclin 1. Interestingly, two mechanistic pathways have been proposed to explain the HMGB1-mediated regulation [108-110]. First, HMGB1 itself associates with Beclin 1. Starvation-induced production of reactive oxygen species leads to the translocation of HMGB1 to the cytosol. There HMGB1 competes with Bcl-2 for Beclin 1. Apparently, an intramolecular disulfide bridge between C23 and C45 of HMGB1 is central for its interaction with Beclin 1 and its function to sustain autophagy [108-110]. Second, HMGB1 promotes activation of the Erk1/2 pathway, which results in the Erk1/2-mediated phosphorylation of Bcl-2 and the subsequent dissociation from Beclin 1 [108-110].

As discussed above, the Ulk1/2-Atg13-FIP200 kinase complex also (indirectly) regulates the function of the PI3K class III complex. Under starvation conditions, the Ulk1/2-Atg13-FIP200 complex is the most upstream unit and essential for the recruitment of the Atg14L-containing PI3K class III complex [131]. The identification of Ambra1 as a direct Ulk1 substrate might explain this observation. Ambra1 phosphorylation leads to the dissociation of the Vps34-Beclin 1 complex from the dynein motor complex and to its translocation to the ER, where autophagosome nucleation takes place (see above) [74, 75].

Regarding the downstream PI3P effectors, the lipid-binding motif of Atg18 has been identified as potential PKA phosphorylation site [48]. Interestingly, in this evolutionary proteomics approach the autophagy-related proteins Atg1 and Atg13 have additionally been detected as potential PKA substrates. The authors could confirm Atg1 as an *in vivo* PKA substrate (see above), which supports the general validity of this comparative approach [48]. It has been speculated that Atg18 phosphorylation might alter the lipid binding capacity [147].

The above described phosphorylation events regulating the PI3K class III complex are schematically depicted in figure 2.

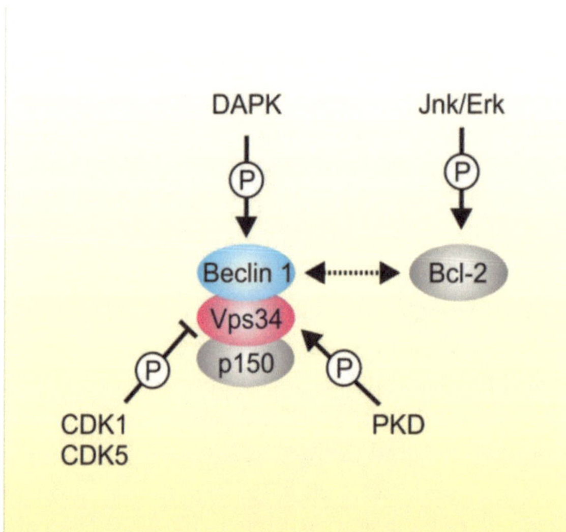

Figure 2. Phosphorylations of the PI3K class III complex. Bcl-2, B-cell CLL/lymphoma 2; CDK, cyclin-dependent kinase; DAPK, death-associated protein kinase; Erk, extracellular signal-regulated kinase; Jnk, c-Jun N-terminal kinase; PKD, protein kinase D; Vps34, vacuolar protein sorting 34.

4. Atg9

Atg9 is a multi-spanning membrane protein which is required for autophagy in several eukaryotic cells (reviewed in [148, 149]). In yeast, Atg9 localizes to the pre-autophagosomal structure (PAS) and to dispersed punctate structures in the yeast cytoplasm [149-151]. There exist two functional Atg9 orthologs in mammals, i.e. Atg9L1 and Atg9L2. Atg9L1 is ubiquitously expressed and is also termed mAtg9 or Atg9A [148]. In mammalian cells, mAtg9 localizes to the TGN, endocytic compartments, and autophagic membranes [78, 149]. Although the dynamic shuttling of Atg9/mAtg9 between these organelles has been well documented, its exact function has not been clarified yet. However, it has been speculated that Atg9 contributes to the regulation of autophagosome size or that it functions as a carrier of lipids for the forming autophagosomes [149].

4.1. Atg9 and protein phosphorylation

Under nutrient-rich conditions, yeast Atg9 localization to the PAS is mediated via its interaction with the peripheral membrane protein Atg11, which is a specific factor for the cytoplasm to vacuole targeting (Cvt) pathway [149, 152]. During autophagy, Atg9 localization to the PAS is independent of Atg11 but requires the physical interaction with Atg17 [149, 153]. This Atg17-dependent PAS localization of Atg9 requires Atg1, but not its kinase activity. This is in accordance with reports stating that Atg1 kinase activity is dispensable for the PAS organization under autophagy-inducing conditions [153-155]. However, Atg1 kinase activity is required for the regulation of the equilibrium between the assembly and disassembly of Atg9 at the PAS [153]. Furthermore, two additional components of the Atg9 cycling complex, i.e. the peripheral membrane protein Atg23 and the type I membrane protein Atg27, are required for efficient Atg9 trafficking during autophagy, but they are not essential [149]. The retrograde transport of Atg9 from the PAS to the peripheral pool involves the Atg1-Atg13 complex, the Atg9-interacting proteins Atg2 and Atg18, and the PI3K class III complex [149, 151].

In mammals, mAtg9 localizes to the TGN and a peripheral endosomal pool under nutrient-rich conditions [78, 149]. During starvation, Atg9 localizes to the peripheral pool and co-localizes with the autophagosomal membrane marker GFP-LC3 (see below) [78, 149]. Additionally, it has been reported that starvation-induced trafficking requires Ulk1 and Atg13 [19, 78]. It has been shown that siRNA-mediated Ulk1 knockdown leads to an Atg9 distribution similar to that of unstarved cells, i.e. localization to the TGN [78]. The Ulk1-mediated phosphorylation of ZIPK/DAPK3 and its contribution to mAtg9 trafficking from TGN to autophagosomes has been described above [76-78]. However, recently Itakura et al. reported that mAtg9 and the Ulk1 complex independently localize to the autophagosome formation site during starvation-induced autophagy [156]. The authors could show that recruitment of mAtg9 to the autophagosome formation site is independent of FIP200, but that mAtg9 recycling requires FIP200 [156]. FIP200-independent localization of mAtg9 to the autophagosome formation site was not only observed for canonical starvation-induced autophagy, but also for mitophagy and *Salmonella* xenophagy [156, 157].

Notably, it could be shown that mAtg9 interacts with the p38-interacting protein (p38IP) and that p38IP is required for starvation-induced mAtg9 trafficking and autophagosome formation [158]. Additionally, the authors could confirm that the MAPK p38 regulates the interaction between mAtg9 and p38IP. The following model has been suggested: in full growth medium, p38IP is found in the mAtg9 pool at peripheral endosomes and is associated with phosphorylated p38, which inhibits autophagy. Upon starvation, p38 is dephosphorylated and binds p38IP with a reduced affinity. Thus, p38 cannot longer block the autophagic process and released p38IP supports mAtg9 trafficking and autophagy [158].

5. Atg12-Atg5 and LC3(Atg8)-PE conjugation systems

In 2007, Ohsumi's group published a hierarchy map of Atgs involved in the yeast PAS organization. The two ubiquitin-like conjugation systems play a role at a late step of autophagosome formation, i.e. expansion and closure of the membrane [1, 10]. Atg12 and Atg8 represent the ubiquitin-like (Ubl) proteins, and E1-, E2- and E3-like enzymatic activities participate in the conjugation of Atg12 to Atg5 and Atg8 to PE, respectively (reviewed in [159]). Within the Atg12-Atg5 conjugation system, Atg12 is activated by the E1-like enzyme Atg7. Following activation, Atg12 is transferred to the E2-like Atg10 and then conjugated to the target protein Atg5. There is no E3-like enzyme involved in the Atg12-Atg5 conjugation system. However, Atg5 interacts with Atg16, and this Atg12-Atg5/Atg16 complex assembles to a multimeric complex consisting of four Atg12-Atg5/Atg16 units [159, 160]. Orthologs of each component of the Atg12-Atg5 conjugation system have been found in mice and humans, and their functions are similar to the yeast counterparts [159]. So far, Atg5 appears the sole target of Atg12 conjugation, and this conjugation is irreversible [159].

Within the Atg8 conjugation system, Atg7 possesses the E1-like activity and Atg3 the E2-like activity. Interestingly, the Atg12-Atg5 conjugate has been proposed to possess E3-like activity, since it accelerates the transfer of Atg8 from Atg3 to PE [159, 161]. Prior to its activation by Atg7, the C-terminal residue R117 of Atg8 is removed by the protease Atg4, leading to the exposure of G116 [162]. In contrast to the Atg12-Atg5 conjugate, the Atg8-conjugation to PE is reversible, and the cleavage is likewise catalyzed by Atg4 [162].

In mammals, there exist at least eight Atg8 orthologs, which can be subdividied into two families: 1) the LC3 subfamily consisting of microtubule-associated proteins 1A/1B light chain 3A (MAP1LC3A), LC3B and LC3C (LC3A exists in two variants generated by alternative splicing), and 2) the GABARAP-GATE16 subfamily consisting of the gamma-aminobutyric acid receptor associated protein (GABARAP), GABARAPL1, Golgi-associated ATPase enhancer of 16 kDa (GATE16, also termed GABARAPL2) and GABARAPL3 [163]. Of these, LC3B is probably the best characterized mammalian Atg8 ortholog. According to Atg8 processing, LC3B is cleaved N-terminally of G120 within six minutes after synthesis, generating a cytosolic LC3-I fragment of 18 kDa which lacks the C-terminal 22 amino acids [164, 165]. Interestingly, there exist four Atg4 orthologs in mammals (Atg4A-D, also termed autophagin-1-4), and it has been demonstrated that these Atg4 homologs have selective preferences toward the different LC3/GABARAP family members [165, 166]. It has been shown that Atg4B (autophagin-1) has the broadest specificity for mammalian Atg8 orthologs [166, 167]. Subsequently, LC3-I is converted to LC-II by conjugation to PE. In SDS-PAGE, LC3-II migrates faster than the I-form and can be detected at an apparent molecular weight of 16 kDa [164, 165]. *In vitro*, the Atg8-like modifiers can also be conjugated to phosphatidylserine (PS). However, *in vivo* PE appears to be the predominant target, indicating that additional factors within this conjugation system ensure selectivity [168]. Again paralleling the process in yeast, LC3-II can be deconjugated by the activity of Atg4 homologs. In 2009, Satoo et al. reported the structure of the Atg4-LC3 complex. It appears that large conformational changes of Atg4 within the regulatory loop and the N-terminal tail are necessary for both the processing of the LC3-proform and the delipidation of LC3-II [169].

Both conjugates, i.e. Atg12-Atg5 and Atg8/LC3-PE, localize at membranes during the autophagic process. Whereas the Atg12-Atg5 conjugate rather localizes to the isolation membrane and is excluded from mature autophagosomes, Atg8/LC3-PE can be detected throughout "the whole life" of an autophagosome, i.e. from biogenesis to fusion with lysosomes/vacuoles [1]. Accordingly, both conjugates are commonly used for the detection of autophagic processes in different assays, including immunoblotting, fluorescence microscopy, fluorescence-activated cell sorting, and immunohistochemistry (reviewed in [170, 171]). It has been confirmed that also the other mammalian Atg8 orthologs localize to the autophagosomal membrane in its lipidated form [165].

Atg8 and its orthologs have at least two central functions during autophagy: biogenesis of the autophagosomal membrane and recognition of target cargo. Ohsumi's group could demonstrate that Atg8 mediates tethering and hemifusion of membranes, and that these two functions contribute to the expansion of autophagosomal membranes [172]. Notably, it could be demonstrated that the size of autophagosomes is directly determined by the amount of Atg8 [173]. Recently, it could be demonstrated that LC3- and GABARAP/GATE16 subfamilies are essential for autophagy but apparently act at different steps of autophagosome biogenesis. It has been suggested that LC3s are involved in the elongation of the phagophore membrane, whereas GABARAPs act at a later stage possibly in the sealing of autophagosomes [163]. Next to the regulation of membrane dynamics during autophagosome biogenesis, LC3 plays an important role in target recognition. In recent years, a new class of cargo-recognition receptors, termed autophagy receptors or adaptors, have been identified and characterized (reviewed in [174-178]). These autophagy receptors are especially important for selective forms of autophagy such as mitophagy and xenophagy, i.e. the autophagic control of intracellular pathogens. The prototype of autophagy receptors is p62 (also termed SQSTM1 or sequestome 1), and it could be shown that p62/SQSTM1 directly binds to Atg8/LC3 to facilitate the degradation of ubiquitinated protein aggregates by autophagy [179, 180]. Three features have been reported to be important for autophagy receptors: 1) direct interaction with LC3 via a so-called LC3-interacting region (LIR), 2) the inherent ability to polymerize or aggregate, and 3) the specific recognition of cargo [175]. The list of autophagy receptors is steadily growing, including p62/SQSTM1 [179, 180], NBR1 [181], NDP52 [182], and optineurin [183]. These four proteins have in common the simultaneous binding of ubiquitin-decorated cargo and LC3/GABARAP [175, 183]. However, there exist additional autophagy receptors which interact with either ubiquitin or LC3/GABARAP or which indirectly associate with ubiquitin and LC3/GABARAP [176]. Examples are the mitochondrial protein NIX, which is a selective autophagy receptor for mitochondrial clearance, or Tecpr1, which binds Atg5 and WIPI-2 [184-186].

5.1. Atg12-Atg5/LC3(Atg8)-PE conjugation systems and protein phosphorylation

Two research groups independently reported the phosphorylation of LC3 [187, 188]. In 2010, Cherra III et al. reported that LC3B is phosphorylated at S12 by PKA. During autophagy induction, this site is dephosphorylated. Apparently, phosphorylation of S12 regulates the incorporation of LC3 into the autophagic vesicle. Notably, this PKA site is not present in Atg8 orthologs of yeast and *Drosophila*, and is also absent in the GABARAP/GATE16 subfamily [187].

Jiang et al. could show that LC3 is phosphorylated at T6 and T29 by PKC. Mutations of these residues significantly reduced LC3 *in vitro* phosphorylation by purified PKC. Notably, HEK293 cells stably expressing LC3 with these sites mutated to A, D or E did not reveal any altered autophagy. The authors suggested that PKC regulates autophagy through a mechanism independent of LC3 phosphorylation [188].

Recently, the regulation of autophagy receptors by phosphorylation emerged as an important theme for the control of selective autophagy. S403 phosphorylation of p62/SQSTM1 leads to increased affinity of the ubiquitin-associated domain of p62 for polyubiquitin chains. This residue is directly phosphorylated by casein kinase 2 (CK2) [189]. Finally, the work of two groups confirmed the importance of the TANK-binding kinase 1 (TBK1) for the xenophagy of *Salmonella*. Ubiquitin-coated *Salmonella* bacteria recruit the autophagy receptor NDP52, which in turn recruits TBK1 to the bacterial loci [182]. The autophagic adaptor optineurin constitutively associates with TBK1, indicating that also optineurin is translocated to the bacteria. The autophagic receptors NDP52 and optineurin bind to LC3 and thereby target the bacterium for autophagosomal degradation. TBK1-mediated phosphorylation of optineurin increases LC3-binding affinity and autophagic clearance of *Salmonella* [183, 190].

Ulk1 itself has been shown to interact with several members of the LC3 and GABARAP/GATE16 subfamily [66, 191]. It has been speculated that these interactions possibly play a role of vesicular transport during axonal elongation [191]. Interestingly, the recruitment of LC3 to the autophagosome formation site is dependent on FIP200 in starvation-induced canonical autophagy [131]. In contrast, recruitment of LC3 to *Salmonella*-containing vacuoles or to depolarized mitochondria is independent of FIP200 [156, 157]. Accordingly, the dependency of LC3 recruitment on the Ulk1 kinase complex appears to be different between starvation-induced autophagy and mitophagy/xenophagy.

The phosphorylations of LC3 and associated autophagy receptors are summarized in figure 3.

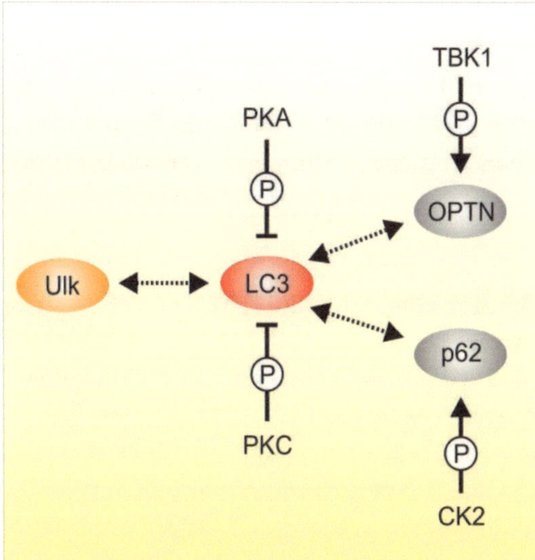

Figure 3. Phosphorylations of LC3 and autophagy receptors. CK2, casein kinase 2; LC3, microtubule-associated proteins 1A/1B light chain 3; OPTN, optineurin; PKA, protein kinase A; PKC, protein kinase C; TBK1, TANK-binding kinase 1; Ulk, Unc-51-like kinase.

6. Conclusion

In recent years, the signal transduction of autophagy has been centered in the focus of many different research areas. Autophagic processes occur at basal levels in any cell. However, under stress conditions, autophagy is dynamically induced and contributes to cellular homeostasis. This dynamic is supported by the network organization of autophagy-relevant proteins [66] and by their rapid and reversible post-translational modifications such as phosphorylation. It is likely that in the future additional phosphorylations (and alternative post-translational modifications) of autophagy proteins will be discovered, which will contribute to our deeper understanding of the autophagic machinery.

Autophagy has been implicated in different human pathologies, including cancer, infectious diseases and neurodegeneration. Accordingly, the modulation of autophagy signaling pathways represents an attractive means of therapeutic intervention. Historically, kinase inhibitors have frequently been used as therapeutic agents, and current clinical trials also target kinases involved in autophagy signaling, e.g. Akt, AMPK, or mTOR. We assume that the development of highly specific and potent Ulk1/2 kinase inhibitors will significantly contribute to the therapeutic success in settings where the blockage of autophagy is desired.

Author details

Björn Stork*, Sebastian Alers, Antje S. Löffler and Sebastian Wesselborg
Institute of Molecular Medicine, University of Düsseldorf, Germany

* Corresponding Author

Acknowledgement

Previous related research of the authors was supported by grants from the Deutsche Forschungsgemeinschaft SFB 773 and GRK 1302, and from the Interdisciplinary Center of Clinical Research, Faculty of Medicine, Tübingen (Nachwuchsgruppe 1866-0-0).

7. References

[1] Mizushima N, Yoshimori T, Ohsumi Y (2011) The role of Atg proteins in autophagosome formation. Annu Rev Cell Dev Biol 27: 107-132

[2] Tsukada M, Ohsumi Y (1993) Isolation and characterization of autophagy-defective mutants of Saccharomyces cerevisiae. FEBS Lett 333: 169-174

[3] Matsuura A, Tsukada M, Wada Y, Ohsumi Y (1997) Apg1p, a novel protein kinase required for the autophagic process in Saccharomyces cerevisiae. Gene 192: 245-250

[4] Funakoshi T, Matsuura A, Noda T, Ohsumi Y (1997) Analyses of APG13 gene involved in autophagy in yeast, Saccharomyces cerevisiae. Gene 192: 207-213

[5] Kabeya Y, Kamada Y, Baba M, Takikawa H, Sasaki M, Ohsumi Y (2005) Atg17 functions in cooperation with Atg1 and Atg13 in yeast autophagy. Mol Biol Cell 16: 2544-2553

[6] Kabeya Y, Kawamata T, Suzuki K, Ohsumi Y (2007) Cis1/Atg31 is required for autophagosome formation in Saccharomyces cerevisiae. Biochem Biophys Res Commun 356: 405-410

[7] Kamada Y, Funakoshi T, Shintani T, Nagano K, Ohsumi M, Ohsumi Y (2000) Tor-mediated induction of autophagy via an Apg1 protein kinase complex. J Cell Biol 150: 1507-1513

[8] Kawamata T, Kamada Y, Suzuki K, Kuboshima N, Akimatsu H, Ota S, Ohsumi M, Ohsumi Y (2005) Characterization of a novel autophagy-specific gene, ATG29. Biochem Biophys Res Commun 338: 1884-1889

[9] Kabeya Y, Noda NN, Fujioka Y, Suzuki K, Inagaki F, Ohsumi Y (2009) Characterization of the Atg17-Atg29-Atg31 complex specifically required for starvation-induced autophagy in Saccharomyces cerevisiae. Biochem Biophys Res Commun 389: 612-615

[10] Suzuki K, Kubota Y, Sekito T, Ohsumi Y (2007) Hierarchy of Atg proteins in pre-autophagosomal structure organization. Genes Cells 12: 209-218

[11] Cheong H, Yorimitsu T, Reggiori F, Legakis JE, Wang CW, Klionsky DJ (2005) Atg17 regulates the magnitude of the autophagic response. Mol Biol Cell 16: 3438-3453

[12] Kamada Y, Yoshino K, Kondo C, Kawamata T, Oshiro N, Yonezawa K, Ohsumi Y (2010) Tor directly controls the Atg1 kinase complex to regulate autophagy. Mol Cell Biol 30: 1049-1058

[13] Yeh YY, Shah KH, Herman PK (2011) An Atg13 protein-mediated self-association of the Atg1 protein kinase is important for the induction of autophagy. J Biol Chem 286: 28931-28939

[14] Alers S, Löffler AS, Wesselborg S, Stork B (2012) Role of AMPK-mTOR-Ulk1/2 in the regulation of autophagy: cross talk, shortcuts, and feedbacks. Mol Cell Biol 32: 2-11

[15] Alers S, Löffler AS, Wesselborg S, Stork B (2012) The incredible ULKs. Cell Commun Signal 10: 7
[16] Chan EY, Tooze SA (2009) Evolution of Atg1 function and regulation. Autophagy 5: 758-765
[17] Mizushima N (2010) The role of the Atg1/ULK1 complex in autophagy regulation. Curr Opin Cell Biol 22: 132-139
[18] Young AR, Narita M, Ferreira M, Kirschner K, Sadaie M, Darot JF, Tavare S, Arakawa S, Shimizu S, Watt FM (2009) Autophagy mediates the mitotic senescence transition. Genes Dev 23: 798-803
[19] Chan EY, Longatti A, McKnight NC, Tooze SA (2009) Kinase-inactivated ULK proteins inhibit autophagy via their conserved C-terminal domains using an Atg13-independent mechanism. Mol Cell Biol 29: 157-171
[20] Ganley IG, Lam du H, Wang J, Ding X, Chen S, Jiang X (2009) ULK1.ATG13.FIP200 complex mediates mTOR signaling and is essential for autophagy. J Biol Chem 284: 12297-12305
[21] Hosokawa N, Hara T, Kaizuka T, Kishi C, Takamura A, Miura Y, Iemura S, Natsume T, Takehana K, Yamada N, Guan JL, Oshiro N, Mizushima N (2009) Nutrient-dependent mTORC1 association with the ULK1-Atg13-FIP200 complex required for autophagy. Mol Biol Cell 20: 1981-1991
[22] Jung CH, Jun CB, Ro SH, Kim YM, Otto NM, Cao J, Kundu M, Kim DH (2009) ULK-Atg13-FIP200 complexes mediate mTOR signaling to the autophagy machinery. Mol Biol Cell 20: 1992-2003
[23] Chan EY, Kir S, Tooze SA (2007) siRNA screening of the kinome identifies ULK1 as a multidomain modulator of autophagy. J Biol Chem 282: 25464-25474
[24] Kuroyanagi H, Yan J, Seki N, Yamanouchi Y, Suzuki Y, Takano T, Muramatsu M, Shirasawa T (1998) Human ULK1, a novel serine/threonine kinase related to UNC-51 kinase of Caenorhabditis elegans: cDNA cloning, expression, and chromosomal assignment. Genomics 51: 76-85
[25] Yan J, Kuroyanagi H, Kuroiwa A, Matsuda Y, Tokumitsu H, Tomoda T, Shirasawa T, Muramatsu M (1998) Identification of mouse ULK1, a novel protein kinase structurally related to C. elegans UNC-51. Biochem Biophys Res Commun 246: 222-227
[26] Yan J, Kuroyanagi H, Tomemori T, Okazaki N, Asato K, Matsuda Y, Suzuki Y, Ohshima Y, Mitani S, Masuho Y, Shirasawa T, Muramatsu M (1999) Mouse ULK2, a novel member of the UNC-51-like protein kinases: unique features of functional domains. Oncogene 18: 5850-5859
[27] Kundu M, Lindsten T, Yang CY, Wu J, Zhao F, Zhang J, Selak MA, Ney PA, Thompson CB (2008) Ulk1 plays a critical role in the autophagic clearance of mitochondria and ribosomes during reticulocyte maturation. Blood 112: 1493-1502
[28] Komatsu M, Waguri S, Ueno T, Iwata J, Murata S, Tanida I, Ezaki J, Mizushima N, Ohsumi Y, Uchiyama Y, Kominami E, Tanaka K, Chiba T (2005) Impairment of starvation-induced and constitutive autophagy in Atg7-deficient mice. J Cell Biol 169: 425-434

[29] Kuma A, Hatano M, Matsui M, Yamamoto A, Nakaya H, Yoshimori T, Ohsumi Y, Tokuhisa T, Mizushima N (2004) The role of autophagy during the early neonatal starvation period. Nature 432: 1032-1036

[30] Cheong H, Lindsten T, Wu J, Lu C, Thompson CB (2011) Ammonia-induced autophagy is independent of ULK1/ULK2 kinases. Proc Natl Acad Sci U S A 108: 11121-11126

[31] Lee EJ, Tournier C (2011) The requirement of uncoordinated 51-like kinase 1 (ULK1) and ULK2 in the regulation of autophagy. Autophagy 7: 689-695

[32] Joo JH, Dorsey FC, Joshi A, Hennessy-Walters KM, Rose KL, McCastlain K, Zhang J, Iyengar R, Jung CH, Suen DF, Steeves MA, Yang CY, Prater SM, Kim DH, Thompson CB, Youle RJ, Ney PA, Cleveland JL, Kundu M (2011) Hsp90-Cdc37 chaperone complex regulates Ulk1- and Atg13-mediated mitophagy. Mol Cell 43: 572-585

[33] Alers S, Löffler AS, Paasch F, Dieterle AM, Keppeler H, Lauber K, Campbell DG, Fehrenbacher B, Schaller M, Wesselborg S, Stork B (2011) Atg13 and FIP200 act independently of Ulk1 and Ulk2 in autophagy induction. Autophagy 7: 1423-1433

[34] Meijer WH, van der Klei IJ, Veenhuis M, Kiel JA (2007) ATG genes involved in non-selective autophagy are conserved from yeast to man, but the selective Cvt and pexophagy pathways also require organism-specific genes. Autophagy 3: 106-116

[35] Hara T, Takamura A, Kishi C, Iemura S, Natsume T, Guan JL, Mizushima N (2008) FIP200, a ULK-interacting protein, is required for autophagosome formation in mammalian cells. J Cell Biol 181: 497-510

[36] Chano T, Ikegawa S, Kontani K, Okabe H, Baldini N, Saeki Y (2002) Identification of RB1CC1, a novel human gene that can induce RB1 in various human cells. Oncogene 21: 1295-1298

[37] Hosokawa N, Sasaki T, Iemura S, Natsume T, Hara T, Mizushima N (2009) Atg101, a novel mammalian autophagy protein interacting with Atg13. Autophagy 5: 973-979

[38] Mercer CA, Kaliappan A, Dennis PB (2009) A novel, human Atg13 binding protein, Atg101, interacts with ULK1 and is essential for macroautophagy. Autophagy 5: 649-662

[39] Umekawa M, Klionsky DJ (2012) The Ksp1 kinase regulates autophagy via the target of rapamycin complex 1 (TORC1) pathway. J Biol Chem 287: 16300-16310

[40] Kijanska M, Dohnal I, Reiter W, Kaspar S, Stoffel I, Ammerer G, Kraft C, Peter M (2010) Activation of Atg1 kinase in autophagy by regulated phosphorylation. Autophagy 6: 1168-1178

[41] Yeh YY, Wrasman K, Herman PK (2010) Autophosphorylation within the Atg1 activation loop is required for both kinase activity and the induction of autophagy in Saccharomyces cerevisiae. Genetics 185: 871-882

[42] Dorsey FC, Rose KL, Coenen S, Prater SM, Cavett V, Cleveland JL, Caldwell-Busby J (2009) Mapping the phosphorylation sites of Ulk1. J Proteome Res 8: 5253-5263

[43] Shang L, Chen S, Du F, Li S, Zhao L, Wang X (2011) Nutrient starvation elicits an acute autophagic response mediated by Ulk1 dephosphorylation and its subsequent dissociation from AMPK. Proc Natl Acad Sci U S A 108: 4788-4793

[44] Kim J, Kundu M, Viollet B, Guan KL (2011) AMPK and mTOR regulate autophagy through direct phosphorylation of Ulk1. Nat Cell Biol 13: 132-141

[45] Chan EY (2009) mTORC1 phosphorylates the ULK1-mAtg13-FIP200 autophagy regulatory complex. Sci Signal 2: pe51

[46] Chang YY, Neufeld TP (2009) An Atg1/Atg13 complex with multiple roles in TOR-mediated autophagy regulation. Mol Biol Cell 20: 2004-2014

[47] Bach M, Larance M, James DE, Ramm G (2011) The serine/threonine kinase ULK1 is a target of multiple phosphorylation events. Biochem J 440: 283-291

[48] Budovskaya YV, Stephan JS, Deminoff SJ, Herman PK (2005) An evolutionary proteomics approach identifies substrates of the cAMP-dependent protein kinase. Proc Natl Acad Sci U S A 102: 13933-13938

[49] Stephan JS, Yeh YY, Ramachandran V, Deminoff SJ, Herman PK (2009) The Tor and PKA signaling pathways independently target the Atg1/Atg13 protein kinase complex to control autophagy. Proc Natl Acad Sci U S A 106: 17049-17054

[50] Mavrakis M, Lippincott-Schwartz J, Stratakis CA, Bossis I (2006) Depletion of type IA regulatory subunit (RIalpha) of protein kinase A (PKA) in mammalian cells and tissues activates mTOR and causes autophagic deficiency. Hum Mol Genet 15: 2962-2971

[51] Takeuchi H, Kondo Y, Fujiwara K, Kanzawa T, Aoki H, Mills GB, Kondo S (2005) Synergistic augmentation of rapamycin-induced autophagy in malignant glioma cells by phosphatidylinositol 3-kinase/protein kinase B inhibitors. Cancer Res 65: 3336-3346

[52] Yorimitsu T, Zaman S, Broach JR, Klionsky DJ (2007) Protein kinase A and Sch9 cooperatively regulate induction of autophagy in Saccharomyces cerevisiae. Mol Biol Cell 18: 4180-4189

[53] Hardie DG (2011) AMP-activated protein kinase: an energy sensor that regulates all aspects of cell function. Genes Dev 25: 1895-1908

[54] Samari HR, Seglen PO (1998) Inhibition of hepatocytic autophagy by adenosine, aminoimidazole-4-carboxamide riboside, and N6-mercaptopurine riboside. Evidence for involvement of amp-activated protein kinase. J Biol Chem 273: 23758-23763

[55] Liang J, Shao SH, Xu ZX, Hennessy B, Ding Z, Larrea M, Kondo S, Dumont DJ, Gutterman JU, Walker CL, Slingerland JM, Mills GB (2007) The energy sensing LKB1-AMPK pathway regulates p27(kip1) phosphorylation mediating the decision to enter autophagy or apoptosis. Nat Cell Biol 9: 218-224

[56] Matsui Y, Takagi H, Qu X, Abdellatif M, Sakoda H, Asano T, Levine B, Sadoshima J (2007) Distinct roles of autophagy in the heart during ischemia and reperfusion: roles of AMP-activated protein kinase and Beclin 1 in mediating autophagy. Circ Res 100: 914-922

[57] Meley D, Bauvy C, Houben-Weerts JH, Dubbelhuis PF, Helmond MT, Codogno P, Meijer AJ (2006) AMP-activated protein kinase and the regulation of autophagic proteolysis. J Biol Chem 281: 34870-34879

[58] Viana R, Aguado C, Esteban I, Moreno D, Viollet B, Knecht E, Sanz P (2008) Role of AMP-activated protein kinase in autophagy and proteasome function. Biochem Biophys Res Commun 369: 964-968

[59] Budanov AV, Karin M (2008) p53 target genes sestrin1 and sestrin2 connect genotoxic stress and mTOR signaling. Cell 134: 451-460

[60] Herrero-Martin G, Hoyer-Hansen M, Garcia-Garcia C, Fumarola C, Farkas T, Lopez-Rivas A, Jaattela M (2009) TAK1 activates AMPK-dependent cytoprotective autophagy in TRAIL-treated epithelial cells. EMBO J 28: 677-685

[61] Hoyer-Hansen M, Bastholm L, Szyniarowski P, Campanella M, Szabadkai G, Farkas T, Bianchi K, Fehrenbacher N, Elling F, Rizzuto R, Mathiasen IS, Jaattela M (2007) Control of macroautophagy by calcium, calmodulin-dependent kinase kinase-beta, and Bcl-2. Mol Cell 25: 193-205

[62] Lee JH, Budanov AV, Park EJ, Birse R, Kim TE, Perkins GA, Ocorr K, Ellisman MH, Bodmer R, Bier E, Karin M (2010) Sestrin as a feedback inhibitor of TOR that prevents age-related pathologies. Science 327: 1223-1228

[63] Gwinn DM, Shackelford DB, Egan DF, Mihaylova MM, Mery A, Vasquez DS, Turk BE, Shaw RJ (2008) AMPK phosphorylation of raptor mediates a metabolic checkpoint. Mol Cell 30: 214-226

[64] Inoki K, Zhu T, Guan KL (2003) TSC2 mediates cellular energy response to control cell growth and survival. Cell 115: 577-590

[65] Lee JW, Park S, Takahashi Y, Wang HG (2010) The association of AMPK with ULK1 regulates autophagy. PLoS One 5: e15394

[66] Behrends C, Sowa ME, Gygi SP, Harper JW (2010) Network organization of the human autophagy system. Nature 466: 68-76

[67] Egan DF, Shackelford DB, Mihaylova MM, Gelino S, Kohnz RA, Mair W, Vasquez DS, Joshi A, Gwinn DM, Taylor R, Asara JM, Fitzpatrick J, Dillin A, Viollet B, Kundu M, Hansen M, Shaw RJ (2011) Phosphorylation of ULK1 (hATG1) by AMP-activated protein kinase connects energy sensing to mitophagy. Science 331: 456-461

[68] Löffler AS, Alers S, Dieterle AM, Keppeler H, Franz-Wachtel M, Kundu M, Campbell DG, Wesselborg S, Alessi DR, Stork B (2011) Ulk1-mediated phosphorylation of AMPK constitutes a negative regulatory feedback loop. Autophagy 7: 696-706

[69] Roach PJ (2011) AMPK -> ULK1 -> autophagy. Mol Cell Biol 31: 3082-3084

[70] Lipinski MM, Hoffman G, Ng A, Zhou W, Py BF, Hsu E, Liu X, Eisenberg J, Liu J, Blenis J, Xavier RJ, Yuan J (2010) A genome-wide siRNA screen reveals multiple mTORC1 independent signaling pathways regulating autophagy under normal nutritional conditions. Dev Cell 18: 1041-1052

[71] Wang Z, Wilson WA, Fujino MA, Roach PJ (2001) Antagonistic controls of autophagy and glycogen accumulation by Snf1p, the yeast homolog of AMP-activated protein kinase, and the cyclin-dependent kinase Pho85p. Mol Cell Biol 21: 5742-5752

[72] Dunlop EA, Hunt DK, Acosta-Jaquez HA, Fingar DC, Tee AR (2011) ULK1 inhibits mTORC1 signaling, promotes multisite Raptor phosphorylation and hinders substrate binding. Autophagy 7: 737-747

[73] Jung CH, Seo M, Otto NM, Kim DH (2011) ULK1 inhibits the kinase activity of mTORC1 and cell proliferation. Autophagy 7: 1212-1221

[74] Di Bartolomeo S, Corazzari M, Nazio F, Oliverio S, Lisi G, Antonioli M, Pagliarini V, Matteoni S, Fuoco C, Giunta L, D'Amelio M, Nardacci R, Romagnoli A, Piacentini M, Cecconi F, Fimia GM (2010) The dynamic interaction of AMBRA1 with the dynein motor complex regulates mammalian autophagy. J Cell Biol 191: 155-168

[75] Fimia GM, Di Bartolomeo S, Piacentini M, Cecconi F (2011) Unleashing the Ambra1-Beclin 1 complex from dynein chains: Ulk1 sets Ambra1 free to induce autophagy. Autophagy 7: 115-117

[76] Tang HW, Wang YB, Wang SL, Wu MH, Lin SY, Chen GC (2011) Atg1-mediated myosin II activation regulates autophagosome formation during starvation-induced autophagy. EMBO J 30: 636-651

[77] Bialik S, Pietrokovski S, Kimchi A (2011) Myosin drives autophagy in a pathway linking Atg1 to Atg9. EMBO J 30: 629-630

[78] Young AR, Chan EY, Hu XW, Kochl R, Crawshaw SG, High S, Hailey DW, Lippincott-Schwartz J, Tooze SA (2006) Starvation and ULK1-dependent cycling of mammalian Atg9 between the TGN and endosomes. J Cell Sci 119: 3888-3900

[79] Bodemann BO, Orvedahl A, Cheng T, Ram RR, Ou YH, Formstecher E, Maiti M, Hazelett CC, Wauson EM, Balakireva M, Camonis JH, Yeaman C, Levine B, White MA (2011) RalB and the exocyst mediate the cellular starvation response by direct activation of autophagosome assembly. Cell 144: 253-267

[80] Farre JC, Subramani S (2011) Rallying the exocyst as an autophagy scaffold. Cell 144: 172-174

[81] Kihara A, Noda T, Ishihara N, Ohsumi Y (2001) Two distinct Vps34 phosphatidylinositol 3-kinase complexes function in autophagy and carboxypeptidase Y sorting in Saccharomyces cerevisiae. J Cell Biol 152: 519-530

[82] Obara K, Sekito T, Ohsumi Y (2006) Assortment of phosphatidylinositol 3-kinase complexes--Atg14p directs association of complex I to the pre-autophagosomal structure in Saccharomyces cerevisiae. Mol Biol Cell 17: 1527-1539

[83] Funderburk SF, Wang QJ, Yue Z (2010) The Beclin 1-VPS34 complex--at the crossroads of autophagy and beyond. Trends Cell Biol 20: 355-362

[84] Matsunaga K, Noda T, Yoshimori T (2009) Binding Rubicon to cross the Rubicon. Autophagy 5: 876-877

[85] Itakura E, Kishi C, Inoue K, Mizushima N (2008) Beclin 1 forms two distinct phosphatidylinositol 3-kinase complexes with mammalian Atg14 and UVRAG. Mol Biol Cell 19: 5360-5372

[86] Matsunaga K, Saitoh T, Tabata K, Omori H, Satoh T, Kurotori N, Maejima I, Shirahama-Noda K, Ichimura T, Isobe T, Akira S, Noda T, Yoshimori T (2009) Two Beclin 1-binding proteins, Atg14L and Rubicon, reciprocally regulate autophagy at different stages. Nat Cell Biol 11: 385-396

[87] Sun Q, Fan W, Chen K, Ding X, Chen S, Zhong Q (2008) Identification of Barkor as a mammalian autophagy-specific factor for Beclin 1 and class III phosphatidylinositol 3-kinase. Proc Natl Acad Sci U S A 105: 19211-19216

[88] Zhong Y, Wang QJ, Li X, Yan Y, Backer JM, Chait BT, Heintz N, Yue Z (2009) Distinct regulation of autophagic activity by Atg14L and Rubicon associated with Beclin 1-phosphatidylinositol-3-kinase complex. Nat Cell Biol 11: 468-476

[89] Liang C, Feng P, Ku B, Dotan I, Canaani D, Oh BH, Jung JU (2006) Autophagic and tumour suppressor activity of a novel Beclin1-binding protein UVRAG. Nat Cell Biol 8: 688-699

[90] Itakura E, Mizushima N (2009) Atg14 and UVRAG: mutually exclusive subunits of mammalian Beclin 1-PI3K complexes. Autophagy 5: 534-536

[91] Knaevelsrud H, Ahlquist T, Merok MA, Nesbakken A, Stenmark H, Lothe RA, Simonsen A (2010) UVRAG mutations associated with microsatellite unstable colon cancer do not affect autophagy. Autophagy 6: 863-870

[92] Liang C, Lee JS, Inn KS, Gack MU, Li Q, Roberts EA, Vergne I, Deretic V, Feng P, Akazawa C, Jung JU (2008) Beclin1-binding UVRAG targets the class C Vps complex to coordinate autophagosome maturation and endocytic trafficking. Nat Cell Biol 10: 776-787

[93] Feng W, Huang S, Wu H, Zhang M (2007) Molecular basis of Bcl-xL's target recognition versatility revealed by the structure of Bcl-xL in complex with the BH3 domain of Beclin-1. J Mol Biol 372: 223-235

[94] Liang XH, Kleeman LK, Jiang HH, Gordon G, Goldman JE, Berry G, Herman B, Levine B (1998) Protection against fatal Sindbis virus encephalitis by beclin, a novel Bcl-2-interacting protein. J Virol 72: 8586-8596

[95] Maiuri MC, Le Toumelin G, Criollo A, Rain JC, Gautier F, Juin P, Tasdemir E, Pierron G, Troulinaki K, Tavernarakis N, Hickman JA, Geneste O, Kroemer G (2007) Functional and physical interaction between Bcl-X(L) and a BH3-like domain in Beclin-1. EMBO J 26: 2527-2539

[96] Oberstein A, Jeffrey PD, Shi Y (2007) Crystal structure of the Bcl-XL-Beclin 1 peptide complex: Beclin 1 is a novel BH3-only protein. J Biol Chem 282: 13123-13132

[97] Pattingre S, Tassa A, Qu X, Garuti R, Liang XH, Mizushima N, Packer M, Schneider MD, Levine B (2005) Bcl-2 antiapoptotic proteins inhibit Beclin 1-dependent autophagy. Cell 122: 927-939

[98] Fimia GM, Stoykova A, Romagnoli A, Giunta L, Di Bartolomeo S, Nardacci R, Corazzari M, Fuoco C, Ucar A, Schwartz P, Gruss P, Piacentini M, Chowdhury K, Cecconi F (2007) Ambra1 regulates autophagy and development of the nervous system. Nature 447: 1121-1125

[99] Yue Z, Horton A, Bravin M, DeJager PL, Selimi F, Heintz N (2002) A novel protein complex linking the delta 2 glutamate receptor and autophagy: implications for neurodegeneration in lurcher mice. Neuron 35: 921-933

[100] Ropolo A, Grasso D, Pardo R, Sacchetti ML, Archange C, Lo Re A, Seux M, Nowak J, Gonzalez CD, Iovanna JL, Vaccaro MI (2007) The pancreatitis-induced vacuole membrane protein 1 triggers autophagy in mammalian cells. J Biol Chem 282: 37124-37133

[101] Ravikumar B, Imarisio S, Sarkar S, O'Kane CJ, Rubinsztein DC (2008) Rab5 modulates aggregation and toxicity of mutant huntingtin through macroautophagy in cell and fly models of Huntington disease. J Cell Sci 121: 1649-1660

[102] Sagona AP, Nezis IP, Bache KG, Haglund K, Bakken AC, Skotheim RI, Stenmark H (2011) A tumor-associated mutation of FYVE-CENT prevents its interaction with Beclin 1 and interferes with cytokinesis. PLoS One 6: e17086

[103] John S, Nayvelt I, Hsu HC, Yang P, Liu W, Das GM, Thomas T, Thomas TJ (2008) Regulation of estrogenic effects by beclin 1 in breast cancer cells. Cancer Res 68: 7855-7863

[104] Shi CS, Kehrl JH (2008) MyD88 and Trif target Beclin 1 to trigger autophagy in macrophages. J Biol Chem 283: 33175-33182

[105] Berger SB, Romero X, Ma C, Wang G, Faubion WA, Liao G, Compeer E, Keszei M, Rameh L, Wang N, Boes M, Regueiro JR, Reinecker HC, Terhorst C (2010) SLAM is a microbial sensor that regulates bacterial phagosome functions in macrophages. Nat Immunol 11: 920-927

[106] Niu TK, Cheng Y, Ren X, Yang JM (2010) Interaction of Beclin 1 with survivin regulates sensitivity of human glioma cells to TRAIL-induced apoptosis. FEBS Lett 584: 3519-3524

[107] Michiorri S, Gelmetti V, Giarda E, Lombardi F, Romano F, Marongiu R, Nerini-Molteni S, Sale P, Vago R, Arena G, Torosantucci L, Cassina L, Russo MA, Dallapiccola B, Valente EM, Casari G (2010) The Parkinson-associated protein PINK1 interacts with Beclin1 and promotes autophagy. Cell Death Differ 17: 962-974

[108] Kang R, Zeh HJ, Lotze MT, Tang D (2011) The Beclin 1 network regulates autophagy and apoptosis. Cell Death Differ 18: 571-580

[109] Kang R, Livesey KM, Zeh HJ, Loze MT, Tang D (2010) HMGB1: a novel Beclin 1-binding protein active in autophagy. Autophagy 6: 1209-1211

[110] Tang D, Kang R, Livesey KM, Cheh CW, Farkas A, Loughran P, Hoppe G, Bianchi ME, Tracey KJ, Zeh HJ, 3rd, Lotze MT (2010) Endogenous HMGB1 regulates autophagy. J Cell Biol 190: 881-892

[111] Takahashi Y, Coppola D, Matsushita N, Cualing HD, Sun M, Sato Y, Liang C, Jung JU, Cheng JQ, Mule JJ, Pledger WJ, Wang HG (2007) Bif-1 interacts with Beclin 1 through UVRAG and regulates autophagy and tumorigenesis. Nat Cell Biol 9: 1142-1151

[112] Vicencio JM, Ortiz C, Criollo A, Jones AW, Kepp O, Galluzzi L, Joza N, Vitale I, Morselli E, Tailler M, Castedo M, Maiuri MC, Molgo J, Szabadkai G, Lavandero S, Kroemer G (2009) The inositol 1,4,5-trisphosphate receptor regulates autophagy through its interaction with Beclin 1. Cell Death Differ 16: 1006-1017

[113] Orvedahl A, Alexander D, Talloczy Z, Sun Q, Wei Y, Zhang W, Burns D, Leib DA, Levine B (2007) HSV-1 ICP34.5 confers neurovirulence by targeting the Beclin 1 autophagy protein. Cell Host Microbe 1: 23-35

[114] E X, Hwang S, Oh S, Lee JS, Jeong JH, Gwack Y, Kowalik TF, Sun R, Jung JU, Liang C (2009) Viral Bcl-2-mediated evasion of autophagy aids chronic infection of gammaherpesvirus 68. PLoS Pathog 5: e1000609

[115] Ku B, Woo JS, Liang C, Lee KH, Hong HS, E X, Kim KS, Jung JU, Oh BH (2008) Structural and biochemical bases for the inhibition of autophagy and apoptosis by viral BCL-2 of murine gamma-herpesvirus 68. PLoS Pathog 4: e25

[116] Sinha S, Colbert CL, Becker N, Wei Y, Levine B (2008) Molecular basis of the regulation of Beclin 1-dependent autophagy by the gamma-herpesvirus 68 Bcl-2 homolog M11. Autophagy 4: 989-997

[117] Wei Y, Pattingre S, Sinha S, Bassik M, Levine B (2008) JNK1-mediated phosphorylation of Bcl-2 regulates starvation-induced autophagy. Mol Cell 30: 678-688

[118] Kyei GB, Dinkins C, Davis AS, Roberts E, Singh SB, Dong C, Wu L, Kominami E, Ueno T, Yamamoto A, Federico M, Panganiban A, Vergne I, Deretic V (2009) Autophagy pathway intersects with HIV-1 biosynthesis and regulates viral yields in macrophages. J Cell Biol 186: 255-268

[119] Gannage M, Dormann D, Albrecht R, Dengjel J, Torossi T, Ramer PC, Lee M, Strowig T, Arrey F, Conenello G, Pypaert M, Andersen J, Garcia-Sastre A, Munz C (2009) Matrix protein 2 of influenza A virus blocks autophagosome fusion with lysosomes. Cell Host Microbe 6: 367-380

[120] Ciechomska IA, Goemans CG, Tolkovsky AM (2009) Why doesn't Beclin 1, a BH3-only protein, suppress the anti-apoptotic function of Bcl-2? Autophagy 5: 880-881

[121] Ciechomska IA, Goemans GC, Skepper JN, Tolkovsky AM (2009) Bcl-2 complexed with Beclin-1 maintains full anti-apoptotic function. Oncogene 28: 2128-2141

[122] Chang NC, Nguyen M, Germain M, Shore GC (2010) Antagonism of Beclin 1-dependent autophagy by BCL-2 at the endoplasmic reticulum requires NAF-1. EMBO J 29: 606-618

[123] Strappazzon F, Vietri-Rudan M, Campello S, Nazio F, Florenzano F, Fimia GM, Piacentini M, Levine B, Cecconi F (2011) Mitochondrial BCL-2 inhibits AMBRA1-induced autophagy. EMBO J 30: 1195-1208

[124] Tooze SA, Codogno P (2011) Compartmentalized regulation of autophagy regulators: fine-tuning AMBRA1 by Bcl-2. EMBO J 30: 1185-1186

[125] Noble CG, Dong JM, Manser E, Song H (2008) Bcl-xL and UVRAG cause a monomer-dimer switch in Beclin1. J Biol Chem 283: 26274-26282

[126] Zhou F, Yang Y, Xing D (2011) Bcl-2 and Bcl-xL play important roles in the crosstalk between autophagy and apoptosis. FEBS J 278: 403-413

[127] He C, Levine B (2010) The Beclin 1 interactome. Curr Opin Cell Biol 22: 140-149

[128] Axe EL, Walker SA, Manifava M, Chandra P, Roderick HL, Habermann A, Griffiths G, Ktistakis NT (2008) Autophagosome formation from membrane compartments enriched in phosphatidylinositol 3-phosphate and dynamically connected to the endoplasmic reticulum. J Cell Biol 182: 685-701

[129] Hayashi-Nishino M, Fujita N, Noda T, Yamaguchi A, Yoshimori T, Yamamoto A (2009) A subdomain of the endoplasmic reticulum forms a cradle for autophagosome formation. Nat Cell Biol 11: 1433-1437

[130] Yla-Anttila P, Vihinen H, Jokitalo E, Eskelinen EL (2009) 3D tomography reveals connections between the phagophore and endoplasmic reticulum. Autophagy 5: 1180-1185

[131] Itakura E, Mizushima N (2010) Characterization of autophagosome formation site by a hierarchical analysis of mammalian Atg proteins. Autophagy 6: 764-776

[132] Matsunaga K, Morita E, Saitoh T, Akira S, Ktistakis NT, Izumi T, Noda T, Yoshimori T (2010) Autophagy requires endoplasmic reticulum targeting of the PI3-kinase complex via Atg14L. J Cell Biol 190: 511-521

[133] Polson HE, de Lartigue J, Rigden DJ, Reedijk M, Urbe S, Clague MJ, Tooze SA (2010) Mammalian Atg18 (WIPI2) localizes to omegasome-anchored phagophores and positively regulates LC3 lipidation. Autophagy 6: 506-522

[134] Barth H, Meiling-Wesse K, Epple UD, Thumm M (2001) Autophagy and the cytoplasm to vacuole targeting pathway both require Aut10p. FEBS Lett 508: 23-28

[135] Barth H, Meiling-Wesse K, Epple UD, Thumm M (2002) Mai1p is essential for maturation of proaminopeptidase I but not for autophagy. FEBS Lett 512: 173-179

[136] Krick R, Henke S, Tolstrup J, Thumm M (2008) Dissecting the localization and function of Atg18, Atg21 and Ygr223c. Autophagy 4: 896-910

[137] Nair U, Cao Y, Xie Z, Klionsky DJ (2010) Roles of the lipid-binding motifs of Atg18 and Atg21 in the cytoplasm to vacuole targeting pathway and autophagy. J Biol Chem 285: 11476-11488

[138] Proikas-Cezanne T, Waddell S, Gaugel A, Frickey T, Lupas A, Nordheim A (2004) WIPI-1alpha (WIPI49), a member of the novel 7-bladed WIPI protein family, is aberrantly expressed in human cancer and is linked to starvation-induced autophagy. Oncogene 23: 9314-9325

[139] Tooze SA, Yoshimori T (2010) The origin of the autophagosomal membrane. Nat Cell Biol 12: 831-835

[140] Hailey DW, Rambold AS, Satpute-Krishnan P, Mitra K, Sougrat R, Kim PK, Lippincott-Schwartz J (2010) Mitochondria supply membranes for autophagosome biogenesis during starvation. Cell 141: 656-667

[141] Furuya T, Kim M, Lipinski M, Li J, Kim D, Lu T, Shen Y, Rameh L, Yankner B, Tsai LH, Yuan J (2010) Negative regulation of Vps34 by Cdk mediated phosphorylation. Mol Cell 38: 500-511

[142] Eskelinen EL, Prescott AR, Cooper J, Brachmann SM, Wang L, Tang X, Backer JM, Lucocq JM (2002) Inhibition of autophagy in mitotic animal cells. Traffic 3: 878-893

[143] Rubinsztein DC (2010) Cdks regulate autophagy via Vps34. Mol Cell 38: 483-484

[144] Eisenberg-Lerner A, Kimchi A (2012) PKD is a kinase of Vps34 that mediates ROS-induced autophagy downstream of DAPk. Cell Death Differ 19: 788-797

[145] Zalckvar E, Berissi H, Eisenstein M, Kimchi A (2009) Phosphorylation of Beclin 1 by DAP-kinase promotes autophagy by weakening its interactions with Bcl-2 and Bcl-XL. Autophagy 5: 720-722

[146] Zalckvar E, Berissi H, Mizrachy L, Idelchuk Y, Koren I, Eisenstein M, Sabanay H, Pinkas-Kramarski R, Kimchi A (2009) DAP-kinase-mediated phosphorylation on the BH3 domain of beclin 1 promotes dissociation of beclin 1 from Bcl-XL and induction of autophagy. EMBO Rep 10: 285-292

[147] Krick R, Tolstrup J, Appelles A, Henke S, Thumm M (2006) The relevance of the phosphatidylinositolphosphat-binding motif FRRGT of Atg18 and Atg21 for the Cvt pathway and autophagy. FEBS Lett 580: 4632-4638

[148] Tooze SA (2010) The role of membrane proteins in mammalian autophagy. Semin Cell Dev Biol 21: 677-682

[149] Webber JL, Tooze SA (2010) New insights into the function of Atg9. FEBS Lett 584: 1319-1326

[150] Lang T, Reiche S, Straub M, Bredschneider M, Thumm M (2000) Autophagy and the cvt pathway both depend on AUT9. J Bacteriol 182: 2125-2133

[151] Reggiori F, Tucker KA, Stromhaug PE, Klionsky DJ (2004) The Atg1-Atg13 complex regulates Atg9 and Atg23 retrieval transport from the pre-autophagosomal structure. Dev Cell 6: 79-90

[152] He C, Song H, Yorimitsu T, Monastyrska I, Yen WL, Legakis JE, Klionsky DJ (2006) Recruitment of Atg9 to the preautophagosomal structure by Atg11 is essential for selective autophagy in budding yeast. J Cell Biol 175: 925-935

[153] Sekito T, Kawamata T, Ichikawa R, Suzuki K, Ohsumi Y (2009) Atg17 recruits Atg9 to organize the pre-autophagosomal structure. Genes Cells 14: 525-538

[154] Cheong H, Nair U, Geng J, Klionsky DJ (2008) The Atg1 kinase complex is involved in the regulation of protein recruitment to initiate sequestering vesicle formation for nonspecific autophagy in Saccharomyces cerevisiae. Mol Biol Cell 19: 668-681

[155] Kawamata T, Kamada Y, Kabeya Y, Sekito T, Ohsumi Y (2008) Organization of the pre-autophagosomal structure responsible for autophagosome formation. Mol Biol Cell 19: 2039-2050

[156] Itakura E, Kishi-Itakura C, Koyama-Honda I, Mizushima N (2012) Structures containing Atg9A and the ULK1 complex independently target depolarized mitochondria at initial stages of Parkin-mediated mitophagy. J Cell Sci 125: 1488-1499

[157] Kageyama S, Omori H, Saitoh T, Sone T, Guan JL, Akira S, Imamoto F, Noda T, Yoshimori T (2011) The LC3 recruitment mechanism is separate from Atg9L1-dependent membrane formation in the autophagic response against Salmonella. Mol Biol Cell 22: 2290-2300

[158] Webber JL, Tooze SA (2010) Coordinated regulation of autophagy by p38alpha MAPK through mAtg9 and p38IP. EMBO J 29: 27-40

[159] Geng J, Klionsky DJ (2008) The Atg8 and Atg12 ubiquitin-like conjugation systems in macroautophagy. 'Protein modifications: beyond the usual suspects' review series. EMBO Rep 9: 859-864

[160] Kuma A, Mizushima N, Ishihara N, Ohsumi Y (2002) Formation of the approximately 350-kDa Apg12-Apg5.Apg16 multimeric complex, mediated by Apg16 oligomerization, is essential for autophagy in yeast. J Biol Chem 277: 18619-18625

[161] Hanada T, Noda NN, Satomi Y, Ichimura Y, Fujioka Y, Takao T, Inagaki F, Ohsumi Y (2007) The Atg12-Atg5 conjugate has a novel E3-like activity for protein lipidation in autophagy. J Biol Chem 282: 37298-37302

[162] Kirisako T, Ichimura Y, Okada H, Kabeya Y, Mizushima N, Yoshimori T, Ohsumi M, Takao T, Noda T, Ohsumi Y (2000) The reversible modification regulates the membrane-binding state of Apg8/Aut7 essential for autophagy and the cytoplasm to vacuole targeting pathway. J Cell Biol 151: 263-276

[163] Weidberg H, Shvets E, Shpilka T, Shimron F, Shinder V, Elazar Z (2010) LC3 and GATE-16/GABARAP subfamilies are both essential yet act differently in autophagosome biogenesis. EMBO J 29: 1792-1802

[164] Kabeya Y, Mizushima N, Ueno T, Yamamoto A, Kirisako T, Noda T, Kominami E, Ohsumi Y, Yoshimori T (2000) LC3, a mammalian homologue of yeast Apg8p, is localized in autophagosome membranes after processing. EMBO J 19: 5720-5728

[165] Kabeya Y, Mizushima N, Yamamoto A, Oshitani-Okamoto S, Ohsumi Y, Yoshimori T (2004) LC3, GABARAP and GATE16 localize to autophagosomal membrane depending on form-II formation. J Cell Sci 117: 2805-2812

[166] Li M, Hou Y, Wang J, Chen X, Shao ZM, Yin XM (2011) Kinetics comparisons of mammalian Atg4 homologues indicate selective preferences toward diverse Atg8 substrates. J Biol Chem 286: 7327-7338

[167] Hemelaar J, Lelyveld VS, Kessler BM, Ploegh HL (2003) A single protease, Apg4B, is specific for the autophagy-related ubiquitin-like proteins GATE-16, MAP1-LC3, GABARAP, and Apg8L. J Biol Chem 278: 51841-51850

[168] Sou YS, Tanida I, Komatsu M, Ueno T, Kominami E (2006) Phosphatidylserine in addition to phosphatidylethanolamine is an in vitro target of the mammalian Atg8 modifiers, LC3, GABARAP, and GATE-16. J Biol Chem 281: 3017-3024

[169] Satoo K, Noda NN, Kumeta H, Fujioka Y, Mizushima N, Ohsumi Y, Inagaki F (2009) The structure of Atg4B-LC3 complex reveals the mechanism of LC3 processing and delipidation during autophagy. EMBO J 28: 1341-1350

[170] Galluzzi L, Aaronson SA, Abrams J, Alnemri ES, Andrews DW, Baehrecke EH, Bazan NG, Blagosklonny MV, Blomgren K, Borner C, Bredesen DE, Brenner C, Castedo M, Cidlowski JA, Ciechanover A, Cohen GM, De Laurenzi V, De Maria R, Deshmukh M, Dynlacht BD, El-Deiry WS, Flavell RA, Fulda S, Garrido C, Golstein P, Gougeon ML, Green DR, Gronemeyer H, Hajnoczky G, Hardwick JM, Hengartner MO, Ichijo H, Jaattela M, Kepp O, Kimchi A, Klionsky DJ, Knight RA, Kornbluth S, Kumar S, Levine B, Lipton SA, Lugli E, Madeo F, Malomi W, Marine JC, Martin SJ, Medema JP, Mehlen P, Melino G, Moll UM, Morselli E, Nagata S, Nicholson DW, Nicotera P, Nunez G, Oren M, Penninger J, Pervaiz S, Peter ME, Piacentini M, Prehn JH, Puthalakath H, Rabinovich GA, Rizzuto R, Rodrigues CM, Rubinsztein DC, Rudel T, Scorrano L, Simon HU, Steller H, Tschopp J, Tsujimoto Y, Vandenabeele P, Vitale I, Vousden KH, Youle RJ, Yuan J, Zhivotovsky B, Kroemer G (2009) Guidelines for the use and interpretation of assays for monitoring cell death in higher eukaryotes. Cell Death Differ 16: 1093-1107

[171] Mizushima N, Yoshimori T, Levine B (2010) Methods in mammalian autophagy research. Cell 140: 313-326

[172] Nakatogawa H, Ichimura Y, Ohsumi Y (2007) Atg8, a ubiquitin-like protein required for autophagosome formation, mediates membrane tethering and hemifusion. Cell 130: 165-178

[173] Xie Z, Nair U, Klionsky DJ (2008) Atg8 controls phagophore expansion during autophagosome formation. Mol Biol Cell 19: 3290-3298

[174] Dikic I, Johansen T, Kirkin V (2010) Selective autophagy in cancer development and therapy. Cancer Res 70: 3431-3434

[175] Johansen T, Lamark T (2011) Selective autophagy mediated by autophagic adapter proteins. Autophagy 7: 279-296

[176] Kirkin V, McEwan DG, Novak I, Dikic I (2009) A role for ubiquitin in selective autophagy. Mol Cell 34: 259-269

[177] Kraft C, Peter M, Hofmann K (2010) Selective autophagy: ubiquitin-mediated recognition and beyond. Nat Cell Biol 12: 836-841

[178] Sumpter R, Jr., Levine B (2010) Autophagy and innate immunity: triggering, targeting and tuning. Semin Cell Dev Biol 21: 699-711

[179] Bjorkoy G, Lamark T, Brech A, Outzen H, Perander M, Overvatn A, Stenmark H, Johansen T (2005) p62/SQSTM1 forms protein aggregates degraded by autophagy and has a protective effect on huntingtin-induced cell death. J Cell Biol 171: 603-614

[180] Pankiv S, Clausen TH, Lamark T, Brech A, Bruun JA, Outzen H, Overvatn A, Bjorkoy G, Johansen T (2007) p62/SQSTM1 binds directly to Atg8/LC3 to facilitate degradation of ubiquitinated protein aggregates by autophagy. J Biol Chem 282: 24131-24145

[181] Kirkin V, Lamark T, Sou YS, Bjorkoy G, Nunn JL, Bruun JA, Shvets E, McEwan DG, Clausen TH, Wild P, Bilusic I, Theurillat JP, Overvatn A, Ishii T, Elazar Z, Komatsu M, Dikic I, Johansen T (2009) A role for NBR1 in autophagosomal degradation of ubiquitinated substrates. Mol Cell 33: 505-516

[182] Thurston TL, Ryzhakov G, Bloor S, von Muhlinen N, Randow F (2009) The TBK1 adaptor and autophagy receptor NDP52 restricts the proliferation of ubiquitin-coated bacteria. Nat Immunol 10: 1215-1221

[183] Wild P, Farhan H, McEwan DG, Wagner S, Rogov VV, Brady NR, Richter B, Korac J, Waidmann O, Choudhary C, Dotsch V, Bumann D, Dikic I (2011) Phosphorylation of the autophagy receptor optineurin restricts Salmonella growth. Science 333: 228-233

[184] Novak I, Kirkin V, McEwan DG, Zhang J, Wild P, Rozenknop A, Rogov V, Lohr F, Popovic D, Occhipinti A, Reichert AS, Terzic J, Dotsch V, Ney PA, Dikic I (2010) Nix is a selective autophagy receptor for mitochondrial clearance. EMBO Rep 11: 45-51

[185] Ogawa M, Sasakawa C (2011) The role of Tecpr1 in selective autophagy as a cargo receptor. Autophagy 7: 1389-1391

[186] Ogawa M, Yoshikawa Y, Kobayashi T, Mimuro H, Fukumatsu M, Kiga K, Piao Z, Ashida H, Yoshida M, Kakuta S, Koyama T, Goto Y, Nagatake T, Nagai S, Kiyono H, Kawalec M, Reichhart JM, Sasakawa C (2011) A Tecpr1-dependent selective autophagy pathway targets bacterial pathogens. Cell Host Microbe 9: 376-389

[187] Cherra SJ, 3rd, Kulich SM, Uechi G, Balasubramani M, Mountzouris J, Day BW, Chu CT (2010) Regulation of the autophagy protein LC3 by phosphorylation. J Cell Biol 190: 533-539

[188] Jiang H, Cheng D, Liu W, Peng J, Feng J (2010) Protein kinase C inhibits autophagy and phosphorylates LC3. Biochem Biophys Res Commun 395: 471-476

[189] Matsumoto G, Wada K, Okuno M, Kurosawa M, Nukina N (2011) Serine 403 phosphorylation of p62/SQSTM1 regulates selective autophagic clearance of ubiquitinated proteins. Mol Cell 44: 279-289

[190] Weidberg H, Elazar Z (2011) TBK1 mediates crosstalk between the innate immune response and autophagy. Sci Signal 4: pe39

[191] Okazaki N, Yan J, Yuasa S, Ueno T, Kominami E, Masuho Y, Koga H, Muramatsu M (2000) Interaction of the Unc-51-like kinase and microtubule-associated protein light chain 3 related proteins in the brain: possible role of vesicular transport in axonal elongation. Brain Res Mol Brain Res 85: 1-12

Fatty Acids Stimulate Glucose Uptake by the PI3K/AMPK/Akt and PI3K/ERK1/2 Pathways

Jing Pu and Pingsheng Liu

Additional information is available at the end of the chapter

http://dx.doi.org/10.5772/52456

1. Introduction

Obesity-driven type II diabetes mellitus has become a major crisis in modern societies. In the United States, over 80% of type II diabetic patients are obese [1]. In the case of Chinese adult diabetic patients, diabetes is also significantly associated with obesity [2]. Previous investigations have focused on looking for obesity-related factors that cause insulin resistance, the failure of the body to respond to insulin, which is the hallmark of type II diabetes. The abnormal plasma fatty acid metabolism associated with diabetes mellitus [3], and the high level of obesity-related plasma free fatty acids (FFAs, also known as non-esterified fatty acids, NEFA) have been identified since the 1950s as major risk factors for insulin resistance.

Natural fatty acids are carboxylic acids with saturated or unsaturated aliphatic tails which have an even number of carbon atoms from 4 to 28. When they are not incorporated into other compounds, like triglyceride or phospholipids, they are known as "free" fatty acids. When metabolized, fatty acids yield a large quantity of ATP, and thus represent an important fuel for the body, particularly for heart and skeletal muscle. They are not only essential dietary nutrients, but also function in many cellular events by activating nuclear receptors, such as the peroxisome proliferator-activated receptors (PPARs), and fatty acid binding proteins (FABPs).

How FFAs induce insulin resistance is not a novel topic in pathological studies on obesity-associated type II diabetes. Many efforts have been made to uncover the underlying molecular mechanisms, but they remain elusive. It seems that FFA-induced insulin resistance occurs not via a single pathway but rather via a complicated network of pathways in organs, tissues, and cells.

1.1. Acute cellular responses to Free Fatty Acids

Major investigatons of the mechanisms of extra FFA-induced insulin resistance have focused on the chronic effects of FFAs. However, plasma FFA concentrations are not consistent and vary widely from hour to hour, displaying waves according to nutritional state and the presence of regulators including hormones (Figure 1). The normal level of postprandial plasma FFAs is about 0.1- 0.4 mmol/L, while in obese individuals this value can reach to 0.2 - 0.6 mmol/L [4]. In healthy people the level of plasma FFAs decreases during the 2 h after a meal until it drops to nearly 0.1 mmol/L, and then rises to a concentration of about 0.3-0.4 mmol/L before the next meal. Such plasma FFA fluctuations also occur in people with metabolic disorders, but display a different pattern. In mild essential hypertensive patients, the plasma FFA concentrations at 3 and 4 h after a meal are significantly higher than that in healthy people (Figure 1, lower panel) [5]. The response of the body to acute variation in plasma FFA concentration is probably associated with the energy balance of the whole body, and requires further investigation to obtain a more in-depth understanding of the pathology of obesity-related metabolic diseases.

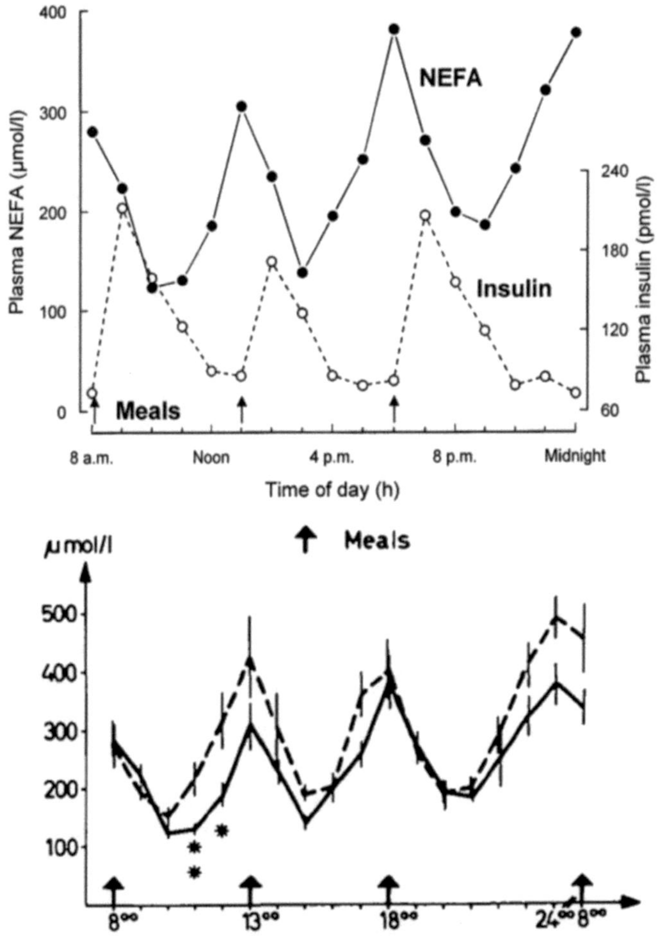

Figure 1. Variation in free fatty acids (•) and insulin (○) concentrations in response to meals in healthy people (upper panel, reprinted from Frayn KN, 1998) [6] and fatty acid levels in mild essential hypertensive patients (---) and normotensive control subjects (——) (lower panel, reprinted from Singer P et al. 1985) [5].

Previous works have reported that FFAs are able to acutely induce several cellular events in various tissues. For example, FFAs can stimulate insulin secretion in pancreatic β-cells [7, 8], leptin secretion in adipocytes [9], and glucose uptake in adipocytes and skeletal muscle cells [10, 11]. All these happen within a short interval after FFA treatment, implying that the FFAs may work as signaling molecules such as hormones, to trigger signal transduction and subsequent physiological events.

During signal transduction, many intracellular signaling proteins work as molecular switches and are activated by GTP binding or phosphorylation. That FFAs acutely stimulate protein phosphorylation suggests that FFAs are able to evoke signal transduction. One study reports that arachidonic acid is able to stimulate the phosphorylation of tyrosine-containing proteins in cultured vascular endothelial and smooth muscle cells [12]; arachidonic acid-induced phosphorylation was rapid and transient, reaching a peak 0.5 min after the addition of arachidonic acid and returning to baseline by 8 min. When cyclooxygenase, lipoxygenase, and epoxygenase pathways were inhibited, phosphorylation was still detected, suggesting it was fatty acid, not its metabolites that triggered the phosphorylation. In addition, increased protein tyrosine phosphorylation was also observed after treatment with oleic, linolenic and γ-linoleic acid. In another work it was reported that unsaturated fatty acids are able to stimulate protein phosphorylation by activating protein kinase C in intact hippocampal slices [13]. Oleic acid stimulated phosphorylation of several proteins of molecular weights 92,000, 58,000, 50,000, 47,000 and 44,000 Da. The 44,000 and 47,000 Da proteins were particularly sensitive to fatty acids and were phosphorylated in a dose- and time-dependent manner. Increased ^{32}P incorporation into the 44,000 Da protein was apparent after 1 min and reached a maximum at 5 min. Phosphorylation of the 47,000 Da protein followed a similar pattern. Studies on fatty acid-stimulated protein phosphorylation have shed light on the role of fatty acids as signal molecules.

1.2. Free Fatty Acid Receptors

During the last decade, a series of free fatty acid receptors (FFARs) has been identified, indicating that like other extracellular signal molecules, FFAs bind to their receptors on the plasma membrane to trigger signal transduction. The FFARs identified belong to a large protein family, the G protein-coupled receptors (GPCRs), which are integral membrane proteins with seven trans-membrane domains. The extracellular parts of the receptors sense external signals and activate heterotrimeric G proteins to transduce signals to downstream molecules. GPCRs are activated by various types of ligands, including ions, nucleotides, amino acids, lipids, peptides, and proteins. It is estimated that more than half of modern drugs target these receptors [14]. The known FFARs include FFAR1 (GPR40), FFAR2 (GPR43), FFAR3 (GPR41), GPR84, GPR119 and GPR120 (Table 1).

Protein	Tissue Expression	Ligand	Function	Synthetic Agonist	G protein-coupling
GPR 40 (FFAR1)	Pancreatic β -cell [15, 16], intestinal tract [17], muscle[16], brain, monocytes [18]	Medium- and long- C8-C22 [18, 15]	Insulin secretion [15]; incretin secretion [17]	Thiazolidinedione [16], GW9508, MEDICA16 [18]	$G_{q/11}$, G_i [15, 16]
GPR 41 (FFAR3)	Adipose tissue [9], sympathetic ganglia [19], enteroendocrine cells [20]	Short C2-C4 [9]	Leptin secretion [9]; PYY secretion [20]	/	$G_{i/o}$ [19, 21]
GPR 43 (FFAR2)	Leukocyte, spleen, bone marrow, adipose tissue [22]	Short C2-C4 [21]	5-HT secretion; PYY secretion [23]; inhibition of lipolysis [24]	/	$G_{q/11}$, $G_{i/o}$ [21]
GPR 84	Immune cell, bone marrow, leukocyte, lung, lymph node, spleen [25, 26]	Medium C9-14C [26]	Amplify IL-12 p40 [27]	/	$G_{i/o}$ [26]
GPR 119	Brain, gastrointestinal tract, pancreas [28]	Ethanolamide [28], Lysophosphatidyl choline [29]	Insulin secretion [29]; food intake; body weight [28]	PSN632408, PSN37569 [30], AR23145 [31]	G_s [29]
GPR 120	Intestinal tract, Macrophage, lung, adipose tissue [32, 33]	Medium- and long- C10-C22 [32]	GLP-1 secretion [32]	NCG21 [34], GW9508 [35]	$G_{q/11}$ [32]

Table 1. Characteristic of FFARs.

It has been reported that GPR40 is activated by medium- and long-chain FFAs [18, 15, 16]. GPR40 is abundantly expressed in the pancreas, and is especially enriched in pancreatic β-cells. When activated by FFAs, GPR40 activates G-protein, which transduces the signal leading to stimulation of insulin secretion. Using Chinese hamster ovary (CHO) cells in which GPR40 is stably expressed, Itoh et al. found that free fatty acids are able to stimulate the formation of inositol 1,4,5-trisphosphate, intracellular Ca^{2+} mobilization, and the phosphorylation of extracellular signal-regulated kinase (ERK) 1/2 [15]. Furthermore, in 2006 Feng et al. reported that fatty acids, especially linoleic acid, are able to stimulate insulin secretion in rat β-cells by reducing the voltage-gated K^+ current via GPR40 and the cAMP-protein kinase A system [36].

Unlike GPR40, the physiological ligands of GPR41 and GPR43 are short chain fatty acids (SCFAs), including acetate (C2), propionate (C3), butyrate (C4), and valerate (C5). SCFAs are generated by bacterial fermentation of undigested carbohydrates from ingested dietary fiber in the gut. Subsequently SCFAs are released in the bloodstream and accumulate to micromolar concentrations.

GPR41 is expressed abundantly in adipose tissue, enteroendocrine cells, and sympathetic ganglia. SCFAs activate GPR41 and stimulate leptin expression in mouse adipocytes and mouse primary-cultured adipocytes. Acute oral administration of propionate increases circulating leptin levels in mice [9]. Overexpression of exogenous GPR41 and knockdown of GPR41 by RNAi regulates leptin production positively and negatively. Given that leptin is a potent anorexigenic hormone that reduces food intake, propionate may inhibit food intake by increasing leptin release. The analysis of GPR41-deficient mice showed that GPR41 is expressed in enteroendocrine cells, and GPR41 deficiency is associated with reduced expression of PYY [20]. GPR41 is also abundantly expressed in sympathetic ganglia in mice and humans [19]. Studies using GPR41-/- mice and co-culturing of fetal-isolated cardiomyocytes with primary-cultured sympathetic neurons have shown that propionate promotes sympathetic outflow via GPR41, reduces intracellular cAMP concentrations and promotes ERK1/2 phosphorylation, phenomena which were not observed in sympathetic neurons from GPR41−/− mice. GPR41-mediated rise in beat rate was effectively blocked by Gallein ($G\beta_\gamma$ blocker) and pertussis toxin (PTX) treatments, whereas NF023 ($G_{\alpha(i/o)}$ blocker) had no inhibitory effects. Knockdown of PLCβ 2/3 or ERK1/2 by RNAi significantly inhibits the propionate-induced rise in the beat rate of cardiomyocytes. These results indicate that GPR41 activation of sympathetic neurons may involve $G\beta_\gamma$, PLCβ, and MAPK.

GPR43 is highly expressed in immune cells, spleen, and bone marrow, and is also detected at low levels in the placenta, lung, liver, and adipose tissues [22]. A study on adipocytes showed that acetate and propionate can reduce lipolytic activity and thus plasma FFA level in a mouse *in vivo* model. This inhibition of lipolysis is abolished in adipocytes isolated from GPR43 knockout animals [24]. Similar to GPR41, GPR43 activation is also coupled to intracellular Ca^{2+} release, ERK1/2 activation, and a reduction in cAMP accumulation. Unlike GPR41, however, which signals via the $G_{i/o}$ family, GPR43 signals via both the $G_{i/o}$ and G_q pathways [21].

GPR84 mRNA is expressed mainly in bone marrow, leukocytes, the spleen and lung [25, 26]. GPR84 functions as a receptor for medium-chain FFAs with carbon chain lengths of 9–14. Capric acid (C10:0), undecanoic acid (C11:0), and lauric acid (C12:0) are the most potent agonists of GPR84. A functional study conducted in GPR84-/- mice revealed that primary stimulation of T cells with anti-CD3 results in increased IL-4, but not IL-2 or IFN-γ production, compared to wild-type mice [27]. Wang et al. reported that medium-chain FFAs act through GPR84 to amplify the stimulation of IL-12 p40 production by lipopolysaccharides in monocytes/macrophages [26]. Medium-chain FFAs induce Ca^{2+} mobilization and inhibit cAMP production. The activation of GPR84 by medium-chain FFAs is primarily coupled to a PTX-sensitive $G_{i/o}$ pathway [26].

GPR119 in humans and rodents is expressed predominantly in the pancreas and gastrointestinal tract and also in the rodent brain [28]. The lipid signaling agent oleoylethanolamide (OEA) is an endogenous ligand of GPR119. OEA is a peripherally acting agent that reduces food intake and body weight gain in rat feeding models, suggesting that GPR119 might mediate the OEA-induced reduction of food intake [28]. Lysophosphatidyl choline (LPC) is another bioactive lipid mediator that activates GPR119 to stimulate insulin release from pancreatic islets, via G_s activation which leads to cAMP production [29].

GPR120 is highly expressed in the human and mouse intestinal tract, as well as in adipocytes, taste buds, and lungs [32, 33]. GRP120 activation by saturated FFAs with a carbon chain length of 14–18, and by unsaturated FFAs with a chain length of 16–22 has been detected [32]. Activated by medium- and long- chain fatty acids, GPR120 increases insulin secretion indirectly by stimulating the secretion of glucagon-like peptide-1 (GLP-1), the most potent insulinotropic incretin, which is coupled to the elevation of Ca^{2+} and activation of the ERK cascade [32]. In addition, GPR120 is also reported to function as an ω-3 FA receptor in proinflammatory macrophages and mature adipocytes that mediates the potent anti-inflammatory effects of DHA and EPA by inhibiting both the TLR and TNF-α inflammatory signaling pathways [37]. Chronic tissue inflammation is another important mechanism causing insulin resistance, so the effect of GPR120 on insulin sensitivity as well as on the stimulation of insulin-secretion will make it an attractive drug target for diabetes-therapeutic agents.

The discovery of FFARs developed our understanding of the role of FFAs as signal molecules. Cells expressing FFARs, such as pancreatic β-cells, adipocytes, and macrophages sense FFAs and make various corresponding responses to control metabolic homeostasis (Figure 2). FFARs have thus attracted considerable attention due to their potential as valuable drug targets.

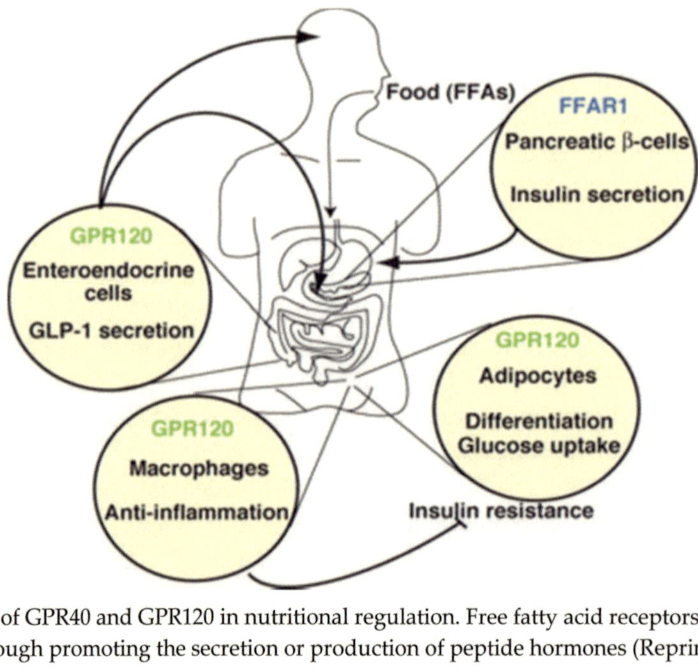

Figure 2. Roles of GPR40 and GPR120 in nutritional regulation. Free fatty acid receptors control metabolism through promoting the secretion or production of peptide hormones (Reprinted from Hara et al., 2011) [38].

In addition to the functions described above, FFAs are also able to acutely stimulate glucose uptake in adipocytes and skeletal muscle cells, which is directly associated with metabolic homeostasis. A few reports indicate that fatty acids have acute effects on glucose uptake, but conclusions have been inconsistent and the underlying molecular mechanisms controlling these responses are still elusive. For example, alpha-lipoic acid has been shown to enhance basal glucose uptake both in normal and ob/ob mice [10], while palmitic acid (PA) treatment was reported to inhibit insulin-stimulated but not basal glucose uptake [11].

Although both adipocytes and skeletal muscle cells are able to ingest glucose by stimulation of FFAs, skeletal muscle consumes more than 70% of the plasma glucose, suggesting that whole body plasma glucose concentration is tightly associated to the sensitivity of muscle tissue to insulin [39, 40]. We therefore focused on the molecular mechanism of fatty acid-induced glucose uptake in skeletal muscle cells [41].

2. Mechanism study on Free Fatty Acid acute stimulation of glucose uptake

2.1. Palmitate stimulates glucose uptake, GLUT4 translocation, and phosphorylation of Akt, AMPK, and ERK1/2 in L6 cells

A rat skeletal muscle cell line L6 with stable expression of myc-tagged GLUT4 (L6) was used to study the acute effects of fatty acids. When L6 cells were treated with palmitic acid (PA), the most abundant free fatty acid in the blood, glucose uptake increased rapidly in a time-dependent manner, beginning from 5 min, and reaching a peak at 20 min (Figure 3, lower panel). By incubating intact PA-treated L6-GLUT4myc cells with myc antibody to detect plasma membrane-located GLUT4, we found that PA stimulates GLUT4 translocation from the cytosol to the plasma membrane (Figure 3, upper panel). The stimulatory effects of PA on glucose uptake and GLUT4 translocation are similar to those of insulin.

Fluorescence imaging shows GLUT4 translocation to the cell surface after L6-GLUT4myc (L6) cells are treated with (upper right panel) or without (upper left panel) PA or insulin (upper middle panel). The lower panel shows that glucose uptake increases in a time-dependent manner when L6 cells are treated with PA.

Akt plays an important role in insulin-stimulated GLUT4 translocation and glucose uptake. Akt, also known as protein kinase B (PKB), is a serine/threonine-specific protein kinase. Akt possesses a protein domain known as the PH domain, which binds to phosphoinositides. Binding to PIP3, and phosphorylated from PIP2 by PI3 Kinase (PI3K) via its PH domain, Akt can be phosphorylated by phosphoinositide dependent kinase 1 (PDK1) at threonine 308 and/or the mammalian target of rapamycin complex 2 (mTORC2) at serine 473. In the insulin signaling pathway, the insulin receptor (IR) is activated and tyrosine is phosphorylated after binding to insulin, subsequently activating hte IRS-1/PI3K/PDK/Akt cascade, and finally increasing the level of GLUT4 in the plasma membrane (Figure 4).

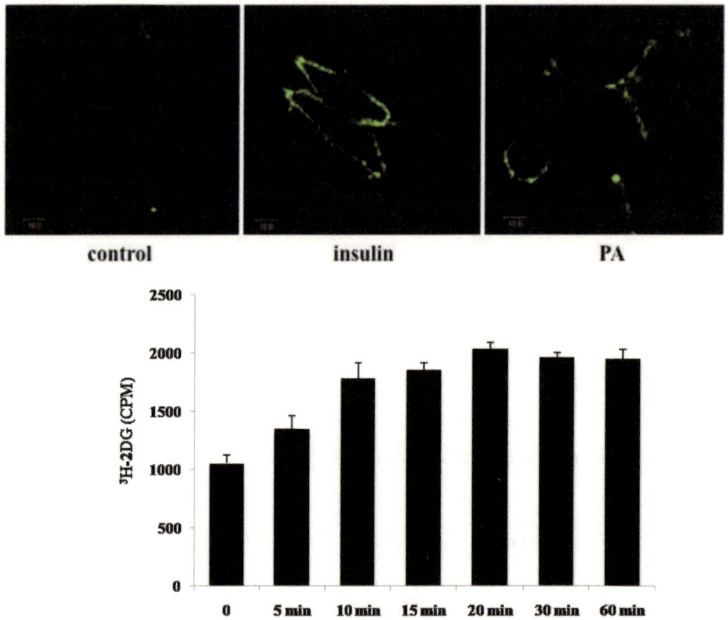

Figure 3. Palmitate stimulates GLUT4 translocation and glucose uptake [41].

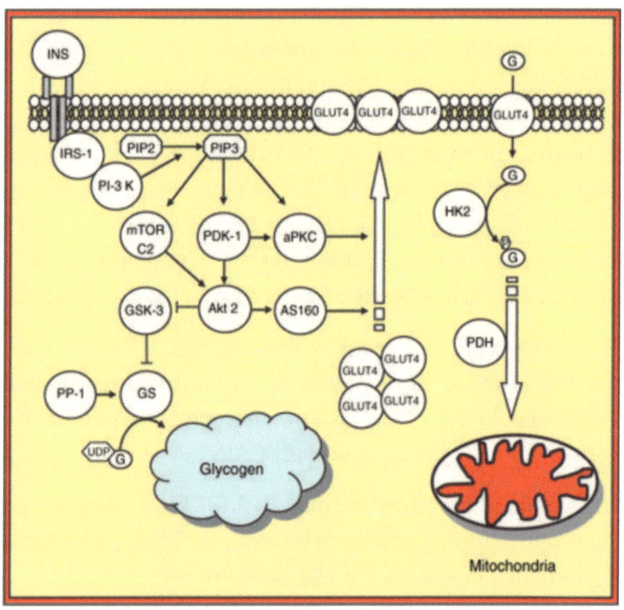

Figure 4. Insulin signaling pathway for glucose uptake stimulation (Reprinted from Frøsig and Richter, 2009) [42].

In our study, PA stimulated Akt phosphorylation at serine 473 in a time- and dose-dependent manner (Figure 5). During PA treatment, Akt phosphorylation was detected after 10 min, peaked at 45 min, then decreased dramatically after 1 h, and became nondetectable after 3 h. When treated with different concentrations of PA, Akt phosphorylation increased with PA concentration, beginning from 0.2 mM. Such time- and dose-dependent responses to PA treatment in cells match the characteristics of signal transduction, and so it is possible that a signal transduction cascade initiated by PA leads to the activation of Akt. To further verify the stimulatory effect of PA on Akt activation, we treated rat skeletal muscle tissue with PA. Rats were anesthetized and perfused with 2 mM PA. Skeletal muscle strips were collected and then incubated *in vitro* with PA. Similar to the results from cells, Akt phosphorylation also increased in PA-treated skeletal muscle tissue, suggesting that this acute response of PA may be physiologically relevant.

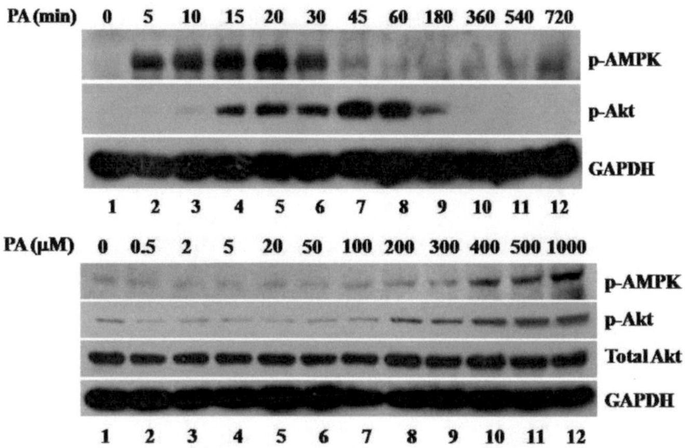

Figure 5. Palmitate acutely stimulates AMPK and Akt phosphorylation in a time- and dose-dependent manner [41].

To investigate the putative PA-mediated signaling pathway, we tested the activity of other molecules and found that AMP-activated protein kinase (AMPK) and extracellular signal-related kinase (ERK1/2) can also be activated by acute PA treatment. AMPK is a heterotrimeric complex composed of a catalytic α subunit and regulatory β and γ subunits, which together make a functional enzyme that plays a role in cellular energy homeostasis [43]. AMPK is activated by an elevated AMP/ATP ratio and undergoes a conformational change of its γ subunit to expose the active site (Thr172) on the catalytic subunit α that is phosphorylated by the upstream kinase AMPK kinase (AMPKK) [44]. Upon activation, AMPK decreases energy consumption by inhibiting fatty acid and protein synthesis and enhances energy production by stimulating fatty acid oxidation and glucose transport to increase cellular energy levels. While it is known that AMPKα is phosphorylated at Thr258 and Ser485, its upstream kinases still need further study [45]. ERK1/2 belongs to the mitogen-activated protein kinase (MAPK) family, a widely conserved family of serine/threonine protein kinases. The ERK1/2 (p44/42 MAPK) signaling pathway responds to various extracellular stimuli including mitogens, growth factors, and cytokines [46]. Upon activation by MEK1 and MEK2 by phosphorylation of its Thr202 and Tyr204 residues, respectively, ERK1/2 phosphorylates downstream targets, forming a signal cascade.

Similar to Akt, AMPK in L6 cells is also activated acutely by PA. AMPK phosphorylation (Thr172) starts as early as 5 min after PA treatment and reaches a peak at 20 min. After 1 h, the signal cannot be detected (Figure 5, upper panel). In addition, PA-induced phosphorylation of AMPK is also dose-dependent. Unlike Akt and AMPK, ERK1/2 is phosphorylated for a shorter duration, increasing after 5 min and returning to basal level after 15 min (Figure 6).

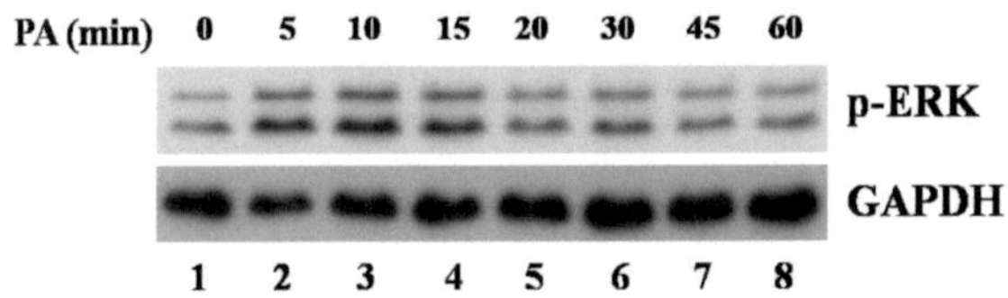

Figure 6. Palmitate acutely stimulates ERK1/2 phosphorylation in a time-dependent manner [41].

2.2. Akt, AMPK and ERK1/2 are involved in PA-stimulated glucose uptake

To test if Akt, AMPK, and ERK1/2 are involved in PA-stimulated glucose uptake, tools such as inhibitors, dominant negative constructs, and short interference RNA (siRNA) were used to inhibit their protein activity or expression levels. Western blotting and glucose uptake assay results showed that all of these proteins participate in signal transduction.

We applied API-2, an Akt selective inhibitor, to block Akt activity. As a result, API-2 abolished Akt phosphorylation as well as significantly decreasing PA-induced glucose uptake (Figure 7, left panel). In addition, siRNA duplexes were nucleofected into L6 cells; compared to the negative control (N.C.), total Akt expression level was efficiently down-regulated. Glucose uptake assays showed that PA-induced glucose uptake decreased when Akt expression decreased due to RNAi (Figure 7, right panel). Together, these data suggest that PA induces glucose uptake in skeletal muscle cells via Akt activation.

To study the role of AMPK in PA-induced glucose uptake, we used AMPK inhibitor Compound C, an myc-tagged AMPK dominant negative (AMPK-DN) plasmid, and siRNA targeting AMPK catalytic subunits α1 and α2. Since AMPK and Akt activation was observed sequentially in PA-treated cells, we also examined the relationship between AMPK and Akt. AMPK inhibitor Compound C suppressed AMPK activity and decreased PA-induced Akt phosphorylation and glucose uptake (Figure 8, left panel). Similar results were obtained when AMPK-DN was nucleofected into L6 cells. Furthermore, an siRNA duplex mixture targeting AMPK α decreases PA-stimulated Akt phosphorylation in L6 cells (Figure 8, right panel), consistent with the inhibitor and AMPK-DN experiments.

In contrast, when AMPK agonist AICAR was used to stimulate AMPK phosphorylation, Akt was also stimulated rapidly in a time-dependent manner (Figure 9), suggesting that it is possible to stimulate Akt via AMPK activation in L6 cells. These data suggest that PA-stimulated AMPK phosphorylation may contribute to regulating Akt activity and is involved in PA-induced glucose uptake.

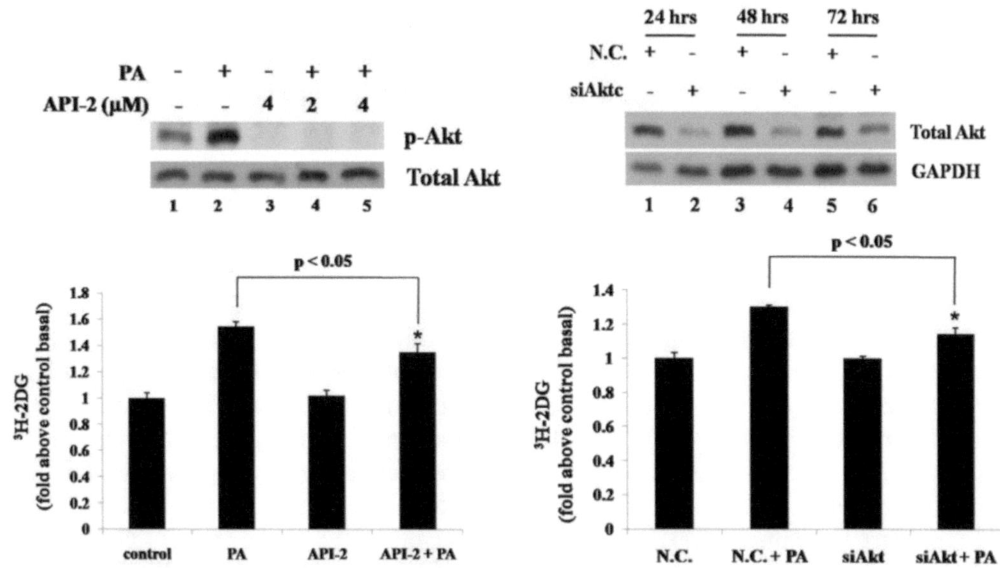

Figure 7. PA-induced glucose uptake is decreased when Akt activity is blocked by an Akt inhibitor (left panel) or RNAi (right panel) [41].

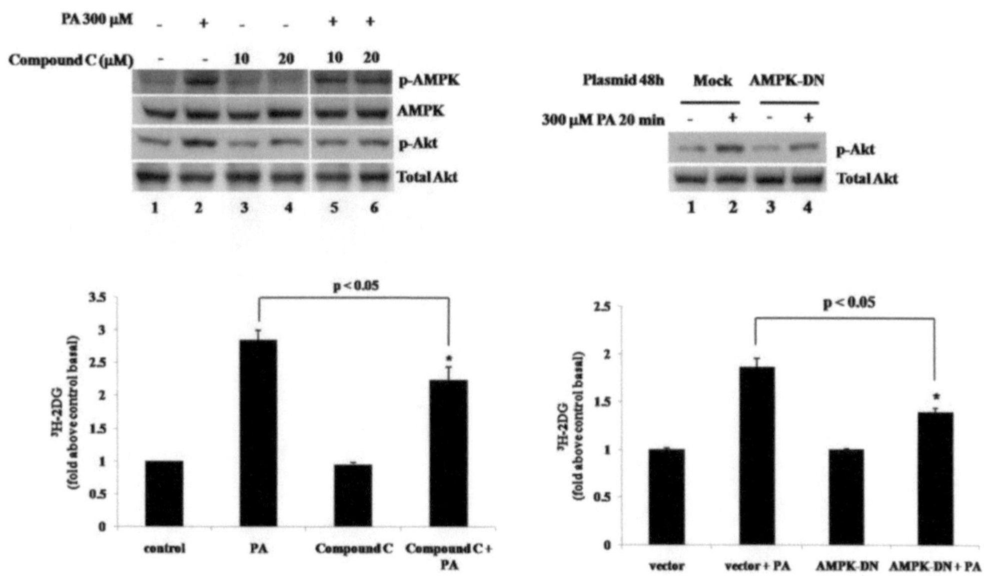

Figure 8. PA-induced glucose uptake and Akt phosphorylation is decreased when AMPK activity is reduced by an AMPK inhibitor (left panel) or AMPK dominant-negative construct (right panel) [41].

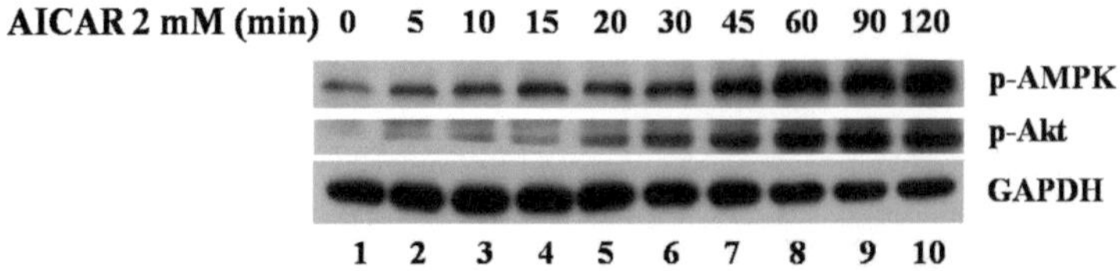

Figure 9. AMPK agonist AICAR stimulates Akt phosphorylation in a time-dependent manner [41].

The role of ERK1/2 in PA-stimulated signal transduction was examined by using the MEK1/2 inhibitors PD98056 and U0126. While both inhibitors decreased basal and PA-induced ERK1/2 phosphorylation, U0126 was more potent (Figure 10, upper left). When ERK1/2 activity was inhibited by U0126, PA-induced glucose uptake was reduced significantly (Figure 10, upper right). These data suggest that PA-stimulated ERK1/2 phosphorylation may contribute to PA-induced glucose uptake. To determine the relationship between ERK1/2 and the AMPK/Akt pathway, AMPK α1/α2 siRNA transfected cells were used to test ERK1/2 activity; ERK1/2 phosphorylation increased at the same rate as in N.C. cells after PA treatment (Figure 10, lower left). In addition, the Akt inhibitor API-2 did not affect PA-induced ERK1/2 phosphorylation, and MEK1/2 inhibitors PD98056 and U0126 did not affect PA-induced Akt phosphorylation (Figure 10, lower right). These data suggest that ERK1/2 contributes to PA-stimulated signal transduction independently from the AMPK/Akt pathway, consistent with the partial decrease in PA-induced glucose uptake by inhibition of either Akt, AMPK, or ERK1/2.

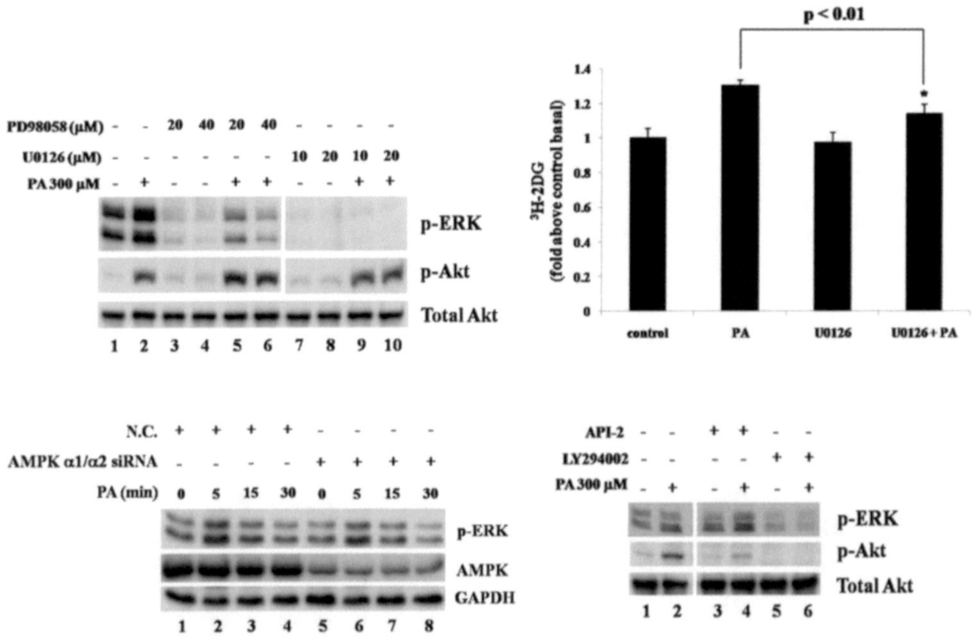

Figure 10. MEK1/2 inhibitors decrease PA-induced ERK1/2 phosphorylation and glucose uptake, but do not affect Akt activity; AMPK and Akt activity inhibition does not affect ERK1/2, while PI3K inhibitor does [41].

Having shown that the two pathways work independently in PA-induced glucose uptake in L6 cells, we investigated signaling molecules upstream of the intersection. When we used PI3 Kinase (PI3K) -specific inhibitor LY294002 to treat L6 cells, PA-induced glucose uptake was totally abolished (Figure 11, upper panel), suggesting that PI3K may control these two pathways. Indeed, LY294002 could abolish PA-stimulated AMPK, Akt, and ERK1/2 phosphorylation (Figure 10, lower right and Figure 11, lower panel). Results from the above experiments indicate that, in skeletal muscle cell lines and tissues, acute PA-stimulated glucose uptake occurs via activation of the PI3K/AMPK/Akt and PI3K/ERK1/2 pathways leading to GLUT4 translocation (Figure 12).

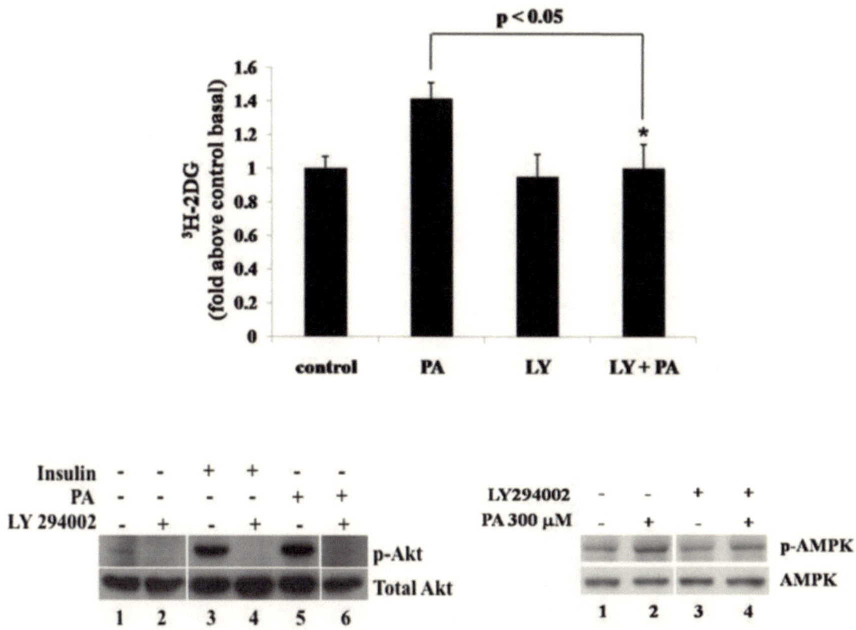

Figure 11. PI3K-specific inhibition abolishes PA-induced glucose uptake and phosphorylation of Akt and AMPK [41].

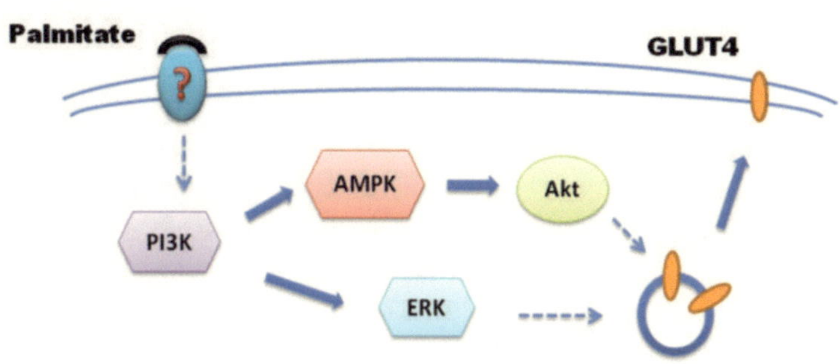

Figure 12. Schematic diagram of PA-induced signal pathway stimulation of acute glucose uptake in skeletal muscle cells [41].

2.3. Palmitate stimulates Akt phosphorylation via binding to the plasma membrane

As shown in Figure 12, how PA activates PI3K is still unknown. According to our current understanding of signal transduction, we speculate that PA may bind to a protein on the cell plasma membrane to trigger signal transduction. We performed fatty acid binding assays to test this hypothesis.

L6 cells were incubated with PA at low temperature (4°C) to facilitate PA binding to the cell surface while preventing its internalization, then washed with buffer to remove unbound PA, or with BSA solution to remove not only unbound but also some membrane-bound PA by competitive binding, Cells were then transferred to 37°C to recover cellular activity. The amount of PA which binds to the cell surface was measured by adding trace amounts of ^{3}H-labeled PA to the solution. Results showed that after washing, with either buffer or BSA solution, very little PA remained (Figure 13, upper panel). When these cells were transferred to 37°C, Western blot results showed that Akt phosphorylation took place at a similar level to that in cells kept at 37°C, and increased in a time-dependent manner in buffer-washed cells, while p-Akt was not detectable in BSA solution-washed cells (Figure 13, lower panel). These results suggest that the amount of cell surface-bound PA was sufficient to activate Akt; intracellular PA accumulation was not required. Moreover, based on lipid analysis by TLC, fatty acids were the main component of total lipids during cell treatment with fatty acid and the 10 min incubation at 37°C. These results indicate that it is fatty acids rather than their metabolites that trigger signal transduction .

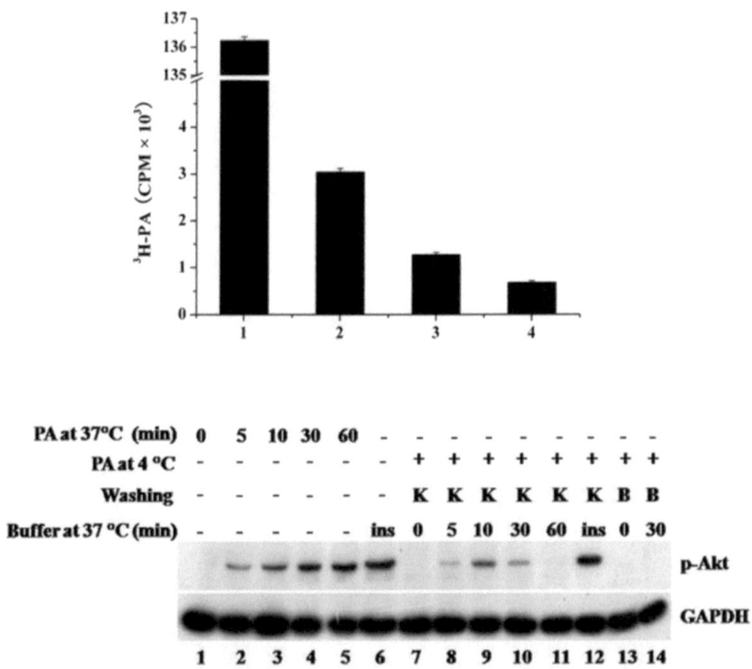

Figure 13. Cell plasma-bound PA stimulates Akt phosphorylation [41].

3. Future work

Could the postulated cell membrane protein which binds to FFAs and triggers signal transduction to stimulate glucose uptake in skeletal muscle cells be a G-protein coupled receptor? FFA binding assays suggest that PA initiates signal transduction via a protein(s) on the cell surface, and meanwhile in the FFA-stimulated signal cascade ERK1/2 pathways were involved, which also appeared in some known FFAR signal pathways. Therefore, a GPCR on the plasma membrane of skeletal muscle cells may be the FFA receptor we have postulated.

PA is a long-chain fatty acid with 16 carbons. We tested other long-chain fatty acids such as C18:1 (oleic acid), C18:2 (Linoleic acid), and C18:0 (Stearic acid) in addition to PA to examine their effects of stimulating AMPK and Akt phosphorylation. All of these fatty acids activated AMPK and Akt in a time- and dose-dependent manner. It is thus likely that our postulated FFAR may function using long-chain FFAs as its ligands.

The known long-chain FFARs include GPR40 and GPR120, both of which are related to insulin secretion. Oh et al. found that GPR120 agonists DHA and GW9508 enhance glucose uptake by activating the PI3K-Akt pathway and GLUT4 translocation in 3T3-L1 adipocytes. The stimulatory effect of DHA and GW9508 was blocked when GPR120 or $G_{\alpha q/11}$ was depleted by siRNA knockdown [37], indicating that FFAs stimulate glucose uptake in adipocytes via the FFA receptor GPR120. However, neither GPR120 nor GPR40 is expressed in muscles. In the Oh *et al.* study, DHA and GW9508 did not enhance glucose uptake in L6 skeletal muscle cells. We therefore conclude that known long-chain FFARs GPR40 and GPR120 are not our postulated FFA receptor. In 2005, Gaël Jean-Baptiste *et al.* described the GPCRs expressed in skeletal muscle tissue, but none of them are FFA receptors [47]. Our postulated receptor might therefore be a novel FFAR whose function is to stimulate glucose uptake in skeletal muscle tissue. Like GPR40 and GPR120, our postulated FFAR is also related to metabolic homeostasis, and so it is likely to be a potential drug target for the treatment of diabetes. Identification of this FFAR is one of our goals.

Another significant implication of our results is that PA plays two opposing roles in skeletal muscle. Under chronic treatment it inhibits insulin-stimulated glucose uptake by blocking Akt phosphorylation, while it enhances glucose uptake by activating Akt when cells are exposed to PA for a short time. What is the relationship between the long-term and short-term effects of FFAs on glucose uptake? Our results show that phosphorylation of Akt is only stimulated when the concentration of PA reached a certain level (at or above 0.2 mmol/L in C2C12 cells). We thus conclude that phosphorylation of Akt may require high concentrations of fatty acids under physiological situations. Akt phosphorylation is not detectable 3 h after fatty acid treatment (Figure 5, upper panel). In addition, when fatty acids are withdrawn, the Akt phosphorylation signal disappears after 3 h in C2C12 cells (data not shown), suggesting that fatty acid-induced phosphorylation and dephosphorylation of Akt can be completed within one cycle of a postprandial FFA wave. It is therefore possible that

Akt phosphorylation and dephosphorylation occur again and again as the concentration of FFA increases and decreases. Plasma FFA concentration starts to rise from 2 h after a meal (Figure 1) and continues to rise until the next meal due to the release of FFA from adipocytes during fasting. Based on our findings, when increasing plasma FFA reaches a certain level it stimulates Akt phosphorylation and glucose uptake. In obesity patients, elevated plasma FFA probably reaches the FFA level triggering Akt phosphorylation earlier during a plasma FFA wave, leading to abnormal glucose uptake. Many abnormal fatty acid cycles may contribute to the development of insulin resistance by disturbing glucose homeostasis. This Yin-Yang balance of PA in skeletal muscle is likely to be physiologically significant, and the possibility of its involvement in the development of insulin resistance needs to be investigated further.

4. Conclusion

Free fatty acids (FFAs) function as signal molecules by activating their receptors in the cell plasma membrane to evoke signal transduction by a series of protein phosphorylation events, eventually leading to physiological events. Some of the known cell responses to FFAs are directly or indirectly related to metabolic homeostasis, so the study of FFA-triggered signal transduction will help us to understand the development of metabolic disorders and to design strategies for therapy. FFA receptors have become attractive drug targets for metabolic diseases. We have investigated the mechanism of long-chain fatty acid palmitate-induced glucose uptake in skeletal muscle cells and found that the two independent PI3K/AMPK/Akt and PI3K/ERK1/2 pathways are responsible for this process. Our results also provide supporting evidence that palmitate triggers signal transduction via a cell surface protein(s) that is probably a novel FFA receptor whose identity still remains to be determined.

Author details

Jing Pu
Cell Biology and Metabolism Program, Eunice Kennedy Shriver National Institute of Child Health and Human Development, National Institutes of Health, Bethesda, MD, USA

Pingsheng Liu*
National Laboratory of Biomacromolecules, Institute of Biophysics, Chinese Academy of Sciences, Beijing, China

Acknowledgement

This work was supported by grants from the Ministry of Science and Technology of China (2006CB911001 and 2009CB919003), and the National Natural Science Foundation of China (30871229).

* Corresponding Author

5. References

[1] Bloomgarden Z.T. (2000). American Diabetes Association Annual Meeting, 1999: diabetes and obesity. Diabetes Care, 23, 118-124.

[2] Yang W., Lu J., Weng J., Jia W., Ji L., Xiao J., Shan Z., Liu J., Tian H. & Ji Q. (2010). Prevalence of diabetes among men and women in China. New England Journal of Medicine, 362, 1090-1101.

[3] Bierman E.L., Dole V.P. & Roberts T.N. (1957). An abnormality of nonesterified fatty acid metabolism in diabetes mellitus. Diabetes, 6, 475.

[4] Golay A., Swislocki Alm, Chen Ydi, Jaspan Jb & Reaven Gm (1986). Effect of obesity on ambient plasma glucose, free fatty acid, insulin, growth hormone, and glucagon concentrations. Journal of Clinical Endocrinology & Metabolism, 63, 481-484.

[5] Singer P., Godicke W., Voigt S., Hajdu I. & Weiss M. (1985). Postprandial hyperinsulinemia in patients with mild essential hypertension. Hypertension, 7, 182-186.

[6] Frayn K.N. (1998). Non-esterified fatty acid metabolism and postprandial lipaemia. Atherosclerosis, 141, S41-S46.

[7] Nunez Ea (1997). Biological complexity is under the 'strange attraction'of non-esterified fatty acids. Prostaglandins, leukotrienes and essential fatty acids, 57, 107-110.

[8] Haber Ep, Ximenes Hma, Procopio J., Carvalho Cro, Curi R. & Carpinelli Ar (2003). Pleiotropic effects of fatty acids on pancreatic β -cells. Journal of cellular physiology, 194, 1-12.

[9] Xiong Y., Miyamoto N., Shibata K., Valasek M. A., Motoike T., Kedzierski R. M. & Yanagisawa M. (2004). Short-chain fatty acids stimulate leptin production in adipocytes through the G protein-coupled receptor GPR41. Proc Natl Acad Sci U S A, 101, 1045-50.

[10] Eason Rc, Archer He, Akhtar S. & Bailey Cj (2002). Lipoic acid increases glucose uptake by skeletal muscles of obese-diabetic ob/ob mice. Diabetes, Obesity and Metabolism, 4, 29-35.

[11] Hardy R.W., Ladenson J.H., Henriksen E.J., Holloszy J.O. & Mcdonald J.M. (1991). Palmitate stimulates glucose transport in rat adipocytes by a mechanism involving translocation of the insulin sensitive glucose transporter (GLUT4). Biochemical and biophysical research communications, 177, 343-349.

[12] Buckley B. J. & Whorton A. R. (1995). Arachidonic acid stimulates protein tyrosine phosphorylation in vascular cells. Am J Physiol, 269, C1489-95.

[13] Chen S. G. & Murakami K. (1995). Synergistic activation by cis-fatty acid and diacylglycerol of protein kinase C and protein phosphorylation in hippocampal slices. Neuroscience, 68 1017-26.

[14] Wise A., Gearing K. & Rees S. (2002). Target validation of G-protein coupled receptors. Drug Discov Today, 7, 235-46.

[15] Itoh Y., Kawamata Y., Harada M., Kobayashi M., Fujii R., Fukusumi S., Ogi K., Hosoya M., Tanaka Y. & Uejima H. (2003). Free fatty acids regulate insulin secretion from pancreatic β cells through GPR40. Nature, 422, 173-176.

[16] Kotarsky K., Nilsson N.E., Flodgren E., Owman C. & Olde B. (2003). A human cell surface receptor activated by free fatty acids and thiazolidinedione drugs. Biochemical and biophysical research communications, 301, 406-410.

[17] Edfalk S., Steneberg P. & Edlund H. (2008). Gpr40 is expressed in enteroendocrine cells and mediates free fatty acid stimulation of incretin secretion. Diabetes, 57, 2280-7.

[18] Briscoe C.P., Tadayyon M., Andrews J.L., Benson W.G., Chambers J.K., Eilert M.M., Ellis C., Elshourbagy N.A., Goetz A.S. & Minnick D.T. (2003). The orphan G protein-coupled receptor GPR40 is activated by medium and long chain fatty acids. Journal of Biological Chemistry, 278, 11303-11311.

[19] Kimura I., Inoue D., Maeda T., Hara T., Ichimura A., Miyauchi S., Kobayashi M., Hirasawa A. & Tsujimoto G. (2011). Short-chain fatty acids and ketones directly regulate sympathetic nervous system via G protein-coupled receptor 41 (GPR41). Proc Natl Acad Sci U S A, 108, 8030-5.

[20] Samuel B. S., Shaito A., Motoike T., Rey F. E., Backhed F., Manchester J. K., Hammer R. E., Williams S. C., Crowley J., Yanagisawa M. & Gordon J. I. (2008). Effects of the gut microbiota on host adiposity are modulated by the short-chain fatty-acid binding G protein-coupled receptor, Gpr41. Proc Natl Acad Sci U S A, 105, 16767-72.

[21] Le Poul E., Loison C., Struyf S., Springael J. Y., Lannoy V., Decobecq M. E., Brezillon S., Dupriez V., Vassart G., Van Damme J., Parmentier M. & Detheux M. (2003). Functional characterization of human receptors for short chain fatty acids and their role in polymorphonuclear cell activation. J Biol Chem, 278, 25481-9.

[22] Brown A. J., Goldsworthy S. M., Barnes A. A., Eilert M. M., Tcheang L., Daniels D., Muir A. I., Wigglesworth M. J., Kinghorn I., Fraser N. J., Pike N. B., Strum J. C., Steplewski K. M., Murdock P. R., Holder J. C., Marshall F. H., Szekeres P. G., Wilson S., Ignar D. M., Foord S. M., Wise A. & Dowell S. J. (2003). The Orphan G protein-coupled receptors GPR41 and GPR43 are activated by propionate and other short chain carboxylic acids. J Biol Chem, 278, 11312-9.

[23] Karaki S., Mitsui R., Hayashi H., Kato I., Sugiya H., Iwanaga T., Furness J. B. & Kuwahara A. (2006). Short-chain fatty acid receptor, GPR43, is expressed by enteroendocrine cells and mucosal mast cells in rat intestine. Cell Tissue Res, 324, 353-60.

[24] Ge H., Li X., Weiszmann J., Wang P., Baribault H., Chen J. L., Tian H. & Li Y. (2008). Activation of G protein-coupled receptor 43 in adipocytes leads to inhibition of lipolysis and suppression of plasma free fatty acids. Endocrinology, 149, 4519-26.

[25] Wittenberger T., Schaller H. C. & Hellebrand S. (2001). An expressed sequence tag (EST) data mining strategy succeeding in the discovery of new G-protein coupled receptors. J Mol Biol, 307, 799-813.

[26] Wang J., Wu X., Simonavicius N., Tian H. & Ling L. (2006). Medium-chain fatty acids as ligands for orphan G protein-coupled receptor GPR84. J Biol Chem, 281, 34457-64.

[27] Venkataraman C. & Kuo F. (2005). The G-protein coupled receptor, GPR84 regulates IL-4 production by T lymphocytes in response to CD3 crosslinking. Immunol Lett, 101, 144-53.

[28] Overton H. A., Babbs A. J., Doel S. M., Fyfe M. C., Gardner L. S., Griffin G., Jackson H. C., Procter M. J., Rasamison C. M., Tang-Christensen M., Widdowson P. S., Williams G. M. & Reynet C. (2006). Deorphanization of a G protein-coupled receptor for oleoylethanolamide and its use in the discovery of small-molecule hypophagic agents. Cell Metab, 3, 167-75.

[29] Soga T., Ohishi T., Matsui T., Saito T., Matsumoto M., Takasaki J., Matsumoto S., Kamohara M., Hiyama H., Yoshida S., Momose K., Ueda Y., Matsushime H., Kobori M. & Furuichi K. (2005). Lysophosphatidylcholine enhances glucose-dependent insulin secretion via an orphan G-protein-coupled receptor. Biochem Biophys Res Commun, 326, 744-51.

[30] Overton H.A., Babbs A.J., Doel S.M., Fyfe M.C.T., Gardner L.S., Griffin G., Jackson H.C., Procter M.J., Rasamison C.M. & Tang-Christensen M. (2006). Deorphanization of a G protein-coupled receptor for oleoylethanolamide and its use in the discovery of small-molecule hypophagic agents. Cell metabolism, 3, 167-175.

[31] Chu Z. L., Jones R. M., He H., Carroll C., Gutierrez V., Lucman A., Moloney M., Gao H., Mondala H., Bagnol D., Unett D., Liang Y., Demarest K., Semple G., Behan D. P. & Leonard J. (2007). A role for beta-cell-expressed G protein-coupled receptor 119 in glycemic control by enhancing glucose-dependent insulin release. Endocrinology, 148, 2601-9.

[32] Hirasawa A., Tsumaya K., Awaji T., Katsuma S., Adachi T., Yamada M., Sugimoto Y., Miyazaki S. & Tsujimoto G. (2004). Free fatty acids regulate gut incretin glucagon-like peptide-1 secretion through GPR120. Nature medicine, 11, 90-94.

[33] Gotoh C., Hong Y.H., Iga T., Hishikawa D., Suzuki Y., Song S.H., Choi K.C., Adachi T., Hirasawa A. & Tsujimoto G. (2007). The regulation of adipogenesis through GPR120. Biochemical and biophysical research communications, 354, 591-597.

[34] Sun Q., Hirasawa A., Hara T., Kimura I., Adachi T., Awaji T., Ishiguro M., Suzuki T., Miyata N. & Tsujimoto G. (2010). Structure-activity relationships of GPR120 agonists based on a docking simulation. Mol Pharmacol, 78, 804-10.

[35] Briscoe C. P., Peat A. J., Mckeown S. C., Corbett D. F., Goetz A. S., Littleton T. R., Mccoy D. C., Kenakin T. P., Andrews J. L., Ammala C., Fornwald J. A., Ignar D. M. & Jenkinson S. (2006). Pharmacological regulation of insulin secretion in MIN6 cells through the fatty acid receptor GPR40: identification of agonist and antagonist small molecules. Br J Pharmacol, 148, 619-28.

[36] Feng D.D., Luo Z., Roh S., Hernandez M., Tawadros N., Keating D.J. & Chen C. (2006). Reduction in voltage-gated K+ currents in primary cultured rat pancreatic β-cells by linoleic acids. Endocrinology, 147, 674-682.

[37] Oh D.Y., Talukdar S., Bae E.J., Imamura T., Morinaga H., Fan W.Q., Li P., Lu W.J., Watkins S.M. & Olefsky J.M. (2010). GPR120 is an omega-3 fatty acid receptor mediating potent anti-inflammatory and insulin-sensitizing effects. Cell, 142, 687-698.

[38] Hara T., Hirasawa A., Ichimura A., Kimura I. & Tsujimoto G. (2011). Free fatty acid receptors FFAR1 and GPR120 as novel therapeutic targets for metabolic disorders. Journal of pharmaceutical sciences.

[39] Defronzo Ra, Jacot E., Jequier E., Maeder E., Wahren J. & Felber Jp (1981). The effect of insulin on the disposal of intravenous glucose. Results from indirect calorimetry and hepatic and femoral venous catheterization. Diabetes, 30, 1000.

[40] Shulman G.I., Rothman D.L., Jue T., Stein P., Defronzo R.A. & Shulman R.G. (1990). Quantitation of muscle glycogen synthesis in normal subjects and subjects with non-insulin-dependent diabetes by 13C nuclear magnetic resonance spectroscopy. New England Journal of Medicine, 322, 223-228.

[41] Pu J., Peng G., Li L., Na H., Liu Y. & Liu P. (2011). Palmitic acid acutely stimulates glucose uptake via activation of Akt and ERK1/2 in skeletal muscle cells. J Lipid Res, 52, 1319-27.

[42] Frøsig C. & Richter E.A. (2009). Improved insulin sensitivity after exercise: focus on insulin signaling. Obesity, 17, S15-S20.

[43] Carling D. (2004). The AMP-activated protein kinase cascade–a unifying system for energy control. Trends in biochemical sciences, 29, 18-24.

[44] Hawley S.A., Davison M., Woods A., Davies S.P., Beri R.K., Carling D. & Hardie D.G. (1996). Characterization of the AMP-activated protein kinase kinase from rat liver and identification of threonine 172 as the major site at which it phosphorylates AMP-activated protein kinase. Journal of Biological Chemistry, 271, 27879.

[45] Woods A., Vertommen D., Neumann D., Türk R., Bayliss J., Schlattner U., Wallimann T., Carling D. & Rider M.H. (2003). Identification of phosphorylation sites in AMP-activated protein kinase (AMPK) for upstream AMPK kinases and study of their roles by site-directed mutagenesis. Journal of Biological Chemistry, 278, 28434.

[46] Roux P.P. & Blenis J. (2004). ERK and p38 MAPK-activated protein kinases: a family of protein kinases with diverse biological functions. Microbiology and Molecular Biology Reviews, 68, 320-344.

[47] Jean-Baptiste G., Yang Z., Khoury C., Gaudio S. & Greenwood M.T. (2005). Peptide and non-peptide G-protein coupled receptors (GPCRs) in skeletal muscle. Peptides, 26, 1528-1536.

Section 2

Protein Phosphorylation in Transcription, pre-mRNA Splicing and DNA Damage

Chapter 5

RNA Polymerase II Phosphorylation and Gene Expression Regulation

Olga Calvo and Alicia García

Additional information is available at the end of the chapter

http://dx.doi.org/10.5772/48490

1. Introduction

RNA polymerases (RNAPs) are among the most important cellular enzymes. They are present in all living organisms from Bacteria and Archaea to Eukarya and are responsible for DNA-dependent transcription. Although in Bacteria and Archaea there is only one RNAP, Eukarya possess up to three RNAPs in animals (I, II and III) and five in plants (IV and V) [1-2]. All of the RNAPs are evolutionarily related and have common structural and functional properties. The minimally conserved structural organization is represented by the bacterial enzyme, which contains only 4 subunits ($\alpha, \alpha', \beta, \beta'$), whereas Archaea and Eukarya RNAPs are composed of 12 subunits (Rpb1-Rpb12) [3]. In prokaryotes, one RNAP transcribes all of the genes into all of the RNAs, however, in eukaryotes, this is achieved by three RNAPs. RNAPI transcribes genes that encode for 18S and 28S ribosomal RNAs; RNAPIII transcribes short genes, such as tRNAs and 5S ribosomal RNA, and RNAPII transcribes all protein-coding genes and genes for small noncoding RNAs (e.g., small nuclear RNAs (snRNAs) that are involved in splicing). The largest catalytic subunits of all three eukaryotic polymerases share homology among themselves and with the largest subunit of bacterial polymerase [4]. Solely the largest subunit of RNAPII (Rpb1) contains an unusual evolutionarily conserved carboxy-terminal domain (CTD) [5], which is subjected to numerous post-translational modifications of extraordinary importance in gene expression regulation [6-8].RNAPII transcription plays a central role in gene expression and is highly regulated at many steps, such as initiation, elongation and termination. Furthermore, phosphorylation of the Rpb1 CTD is known to regulate all of the transcription steps and coordinate these steps with other nuclear events. Prior to mRNA biosynthesis, RNAPII proceeds through several steps, such as promoter recognition, preinitiation complex (PIC) assembly, open complex formation, initiation and promoter escape. This sequence of events is initiated by the binding of gene-specific activators and coactivators, which results in the recruitment of basal transcription machinery (i.e., general transcription factors (GTFs):

TFIIA, TFIIB, TFIID, TFIIE, TFIIF, and TFIIH) and RNAPII to promoters [9-11]. Basal transcription factors position RNAPII on promoters to form the PIC but also function at later steps, such as promoter melting and initiation site selection. Thereafter, initiation proceeds, and RNAPII leaves the promoter during promoter clearance and proceeds into processive transcript elongation. Finally, when the gene has been fully transcribed, transcriptional termination occurs, and RNAPII is released and recycled to reinitiate a new round of transcription [12-14].

During its passage across a gene, RNAPII must overcome challenges. Initially, the polymerase needs to escape from the promoter, and the synthesis of the pre-mRNAs must be tightly coupled to its subsequent processing (i.e., capping, splicing, and polyadenylation). Then, initiation factors must be exchanged for elongation factors [15], which are thought to increase the transcription rate and RNAPII processivity. In fact, recently, there has been an extraordinary increase in the number of proteins known to influence transcription elongation by avoiding transcriptional arrest, facilitating chromatin passage and mRNA processing [16-21], allowing mRNA packaging into a mature ribonucleoprotein (mRNP) and controlling mRNP quality and mRNA export [13, 22-28]. Therefore, the discovery of all of these factors has provided further evidence that the elongation phase is also highly regulated in eukaryotic cells and strictly coordinated with other nuclear processes [12-14].

2. RNAPII CTD phosphorylation: The CTD code

During the last two decades, gene expression studies have provided further evidence that many steps in gene expression, originally considered distinct and independent, are, in fact, highly coordinated, linked and regulated in a complex web of connections [29-30]. The central coordinator that directs this regulatory network (i.e., from transcription initiation to termination and with pre-mRNA processing) in combination with many other nuclear functions is RNAPII, and the carboxy-terminal domain (CTD) of its largest subunit is of remarkable importance. CTD phosphorylation regulates and coordinates the entire transcription cycle with pre-mRNA processing, mRNA transport and with chromatin remodeling and modification [13]. The CTD, therefore, has a critical integrating role in essentially all of the mRNA biogenesis steps, thus, it is subject to a dynamic regulation during the transcription cycle (i.e., [21, 31-32]). Therefore, RNAPII phosphorylation is one of the key processes in the regulation of transcription specifically and gene expression in general; consequently, deciphering the mechanisms that underlie RNAPII phosphorylation regulation has become one of the most studied issues in the field of gene expression.

RNAPII is comprised of 12 subunits (Rpb1-12) that are structurally and functionally conserved from yeast to mammals [33-34]. In 1985, the largest subunit of RNAPII, Rpb1, from mouse and *Saccharomyces cerevisiae,* was cloned [4, 35], and its sequence revealed that it contained a highly conserved carboxy-terminal domain (CTD). This domain has been extensively studied since then and, although it is a simple repetition in tandem of the heptapeptide consensus sequence Tyr1-Ser2-Pro3-Thr4-Ser5-Pro6-Ser7 (YSPTSPS); Figure 1), the CTD has an extremely complex functionality. The consensus sequence is present in animals, plants, yeast, and in many protists [5, 36-37], and it has been hypothesized that the CTD structure has originated through amplifications of a repetitive DNA sequence and that the number of repeats appears directly correlated with genomic complexity (Figure 1A; [38]). For example, mouse and human CTDs contain 52 repeats [35, 39-40]; the Drosophila CTD contains 45 repeats [41]; 25-27 repeats are found in the yeast CTD (Figure 1A; [4]); and 15 repeats are found in protozoan CTDs [5, 38]. Although the CTD is completely dispensable for *in vitro* transcription, it is required for efficient RNA processing [17, 42]. In fact, the CTD is essential for cell viability because its deletion is lethal in mice, *Drosophila* and yeast, and partial truncations or site-specific mutations cause specific growth defects [5, 42].

Human RNAPII-CTD				*Saccharomyces cerevisiae* RNAPII-CTD	
1	YSPTSPA	28	YSPTSPS	1	YSPTSPA
2	YEPRSPGG	29	YSPTSPS	2	YSPTSPS
3	YTPQSPS	30	YSPTSPS	3	YSPTSPS
4	YSPTSPS	31	YSPSSPR	4	YSPTSPS
5	YSPTSPS	32	YTPQSPT	5	YSPTSPS
6	YSPTSPN	33	YTPSSPS	6	YSPTSPS
7	YSPTSPS	34	YSPSSPS	7	YSPTSPS
8	YSPTSPS	35	YSPTSPK	8	YSPTSPS
9	YSPTSPS	36	YTPTSPS	9	YSPTSPS
10	YSPTSPS	37	YSPSSPE	10	YSPTSPS
11	YSPTSPS	38	YTPTSPK	11	YSPTSPS
12	YSPTSPS	39	YSPTSPK	12	YSPTSPS
13	YSPTSPS	40	YSPTSPK	13	YSPTSPS
14	YSPTSPS	41	YSPTSPT	14	YSPTSPS
15	YSPTSPS	42	YSPTTPK	15	YSPTSPS
16	YSPTSPS	43	YSPTSPT	16	YSPTSPA
17	YSPTSPS	44	YSPTSPV	17	YSPTSPS
18	YSPTSPS	45	YTPTSPK	18	YSPTSPS
19	YSPTSPS	46	YSPTSPT	19	YSPTSPS
20	YSPTSPS	47	YSPTSPK	20	YSPTSPS
21	YSPTSPS	48	YSPTSPT	21	YSPTSPN
22	YSPTSPN	49	YSPTSPKGST	22	YSPTSPS
23	YSPTSPN	50	YSPTSPG	23	YSPTSPG
24	YTPTSPS	51	YSPTSPT	24	YSPGSPA
25	YSPTSPS	52	YSLTSPAISPDDSDEEN	25	YSPKQDEQKHNENENSR
26	YSPTSPN				
27	YTPTSPN				

Consensus sequence:	$Y_1S_2P_3T_4S_5P_6S_7$
Main phosphorylation sites:	$Y_1S_2P_3T_4S_5P_6S_7$
Other phosphorylation sites:	$Y_1S_2P_3T_4S_5P_6S_7$

Figure 1. Human and *Saccharomyces cerevisiae* Rpb1-CTDs.

Original studies showed that two RNAPII forms can be differentiated in SDS-PAGE gels because of the different mobility of Rpb1 [43]. These two forms were termed RNAPIIA and RNAPIIO, and they differ in the extent of CTD phosphorylation. RNAPIIA is hypophosphorylated [44], and RNAPIIO is hyperphosphorylated [45]. Moreover, both forms, IIA and IIO, are functionally distinct because the IIA form is preferentially recruited to the promoter and associated with preinitiation complexes [46], whereas RNAPIIO functions during elongation, is highly phosphorylated [44] and thus requires de-phosphorylation to stimulate its recruitment into the PIC complexes and to reinitiate a new round of transcription [47]. We currently know that this earlier two-step transcription cycle model that is based on the two RNAPII forms is overly simple. Different phosphorylated forms of RNAPII are specific and characteristic of the different steps that occur during the transcription cycle [48], and the correct progression of RNAPII through the transcription cycle is dependent on changes in the CTD phosphorylation status. Differential CTD phosphorylation promotes the exchange of initiation and elongation factors during promoter clearance [15], the exchange of elongation and 3'-end processing factors at termination [49], as well as RNAPII recycling [50] and, moreover, links pre-mRNA processing and other nuclear events with transcription [17, 42]. Therefore, the CTD phosphorylation cycle is very complex. It is widely known that the three serines (i.e., Ser2, Ser5, and Ser7) [7, 51], the tyrosine [52-53] and the threonine [54] in each repeat can be phosphorylated. Additionally, both proline residues can be isomerized by a prolyl isomerase [55]. Moreover, glycosylation of serines and threonine can also occur [8], and in human cells, the CTD can be methylated at some of the degenerate repeat sites [56]. The multitude of possible CTD modifications, especially Ser phosphorylations, in combination with the numerous repetitions, gives rise to a wide range of variations (i.e., phosphorylation patterns) that have been termed the "CTD code" (Figure 2) [6-8].

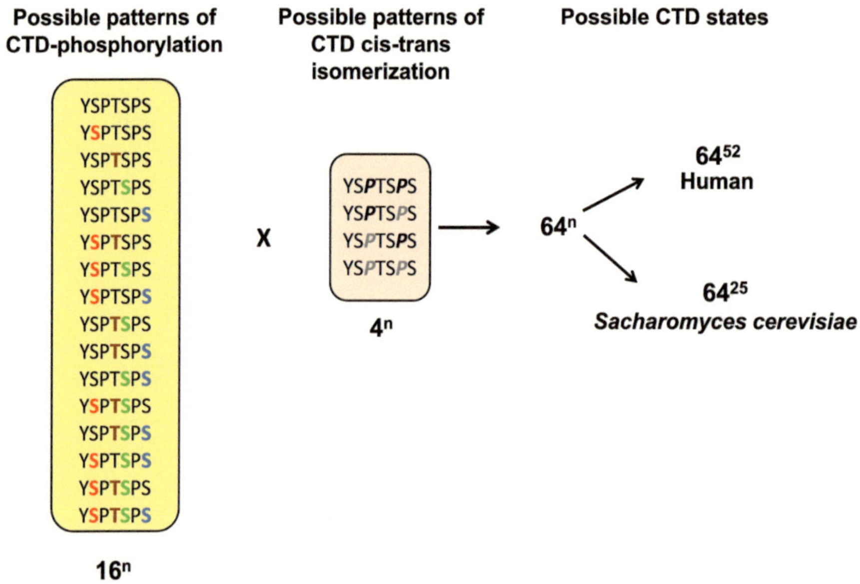

Figure 2. The CTD Code. Only Ser (S) and Thr (T) phosphorylation sites have been considered. CTD glycosylation has not been considered [57] because this modification is mutually exclusive of phosphorylation [8]. n: number of consensus repetitions.

The RNAPII CTD code determines and coordinates the timely sequential recruitment of required specific factors during the transcription cycle. Therefore, the CTD functions as a scaffold that coordinates mRNA biogenesis, such as transcription initiation [58], promoter clearance [59], elongation [60], and termination [31, 61-62], as well as RNA processing [17, 21, 30] and snRNA and snoRNA gene expression [63-65] by recruiting the appropriate set of factors when required during active transcription. These factors recognize CTD phosphorylation patterns either indirectly or directly by contacting phosphorylated residues. Among the CTD-associated factors are export and histone modifier factors and DNA repair factors [21].

2.1. Ser2P and Ser5P, and to a lesser extent, Ser7P, are the main determinants of the CTD code

To determine precisely which serine residues are phosphorylated in a particular repeat has been challenging because of the numbers of phospho-acceptor amino acid residues and consensus motif repetitions (Figure 1). However, studies involving chromatin immunoprecipitation with specific monoclonal antibodies have provided evidence that differential phosphorylation of the Ser residues coincides with the temporal and spatial recruitment of different factors [8, 32, 48, 66-67]. In fact, these antibodies have been largely used to decipher and characterize the role of CTD phosphorylation during the transcription cycle and in gene expression regulation [8, 32, 68]. Antibodies that selectively recognize either Ser2 or Ser5 phosphorylation (i.e., Ser2P or Ser5P, respectively) were the first residues to be described [66]; phosphorylation of these two residues has been extensively studied, and they have been considered as the two main determinants of the CTD code [6]. It is widely known that CTD phosphorylation switch from Ser5 to Ser2 during the course of transcription and is subject to a dynamic regulation during the whole transcription cycle [69-71]. The level of Ser5 phosphorylation peaks early in the transcription cycle and remains constant or decreases as RNAPII progresses to the 3′ end of the gene (Figure 3); [48, 67, 72]). In contrast, Ser2 phosphorylation is the predominant modification in the coding and 3′-end gene regions and occurs simultaneously with productive elongation [31, 48, 73]. On the other hand, de-phosphorylation of Ser5 occurs during the initiation-elongation transition and throughout the entire elongation step, whereas Ser2 de-phosphorylation occurs at the end of transcription to recycle the polymerase and reinitiate a new round of transcription. Therefore, reversible phosphorylation/de-phosphorylation of the CTD plays a significant role in modulating the transcription cycle [31-32].

Most recently, the use of new anti-CTD monoclonal antibodies has demonstrated that Ser7, which is the most degenerate position of the CTD [41], can be phosphorylated during the transcription of snRNA genes and protein-coding genes [64, 68, 74]. Subsequently, this mark increases the complexity of the CTD code [7-8]. Ser7 phosphorylation is mediated by the same kinase [74-75], although, at least in *Saccharomyces cerevisiae,* Ser7P appears not to be dephosphorylated by the same Ser5 phosphatase (see below) [76].The first study on Ser7 phosphorylation provided further evidence that this modification is functionally important for transcription and processing of snRNAs [8, 64] and hypothesized that the CTD code could be gene-transcription dependent. In mammals, Ser7P peaks at the promoter region of snRNA genes but is enhanced toward the 3′ end of protein-coding genes [68]. Recent genome-wide distribution studies in yeast have provided further evidence that Ser7P in protein coding genes occurs early during transcription initiation and is maintained during the entire transcription cycle. In fact, Ser7P is not only maintained, but it is also generated *de novo* during transcription elongation. Additionally, it has been hypothesized that Ser7 phosphorylation could facilitate elongation and suppress cryptic transcription [77].

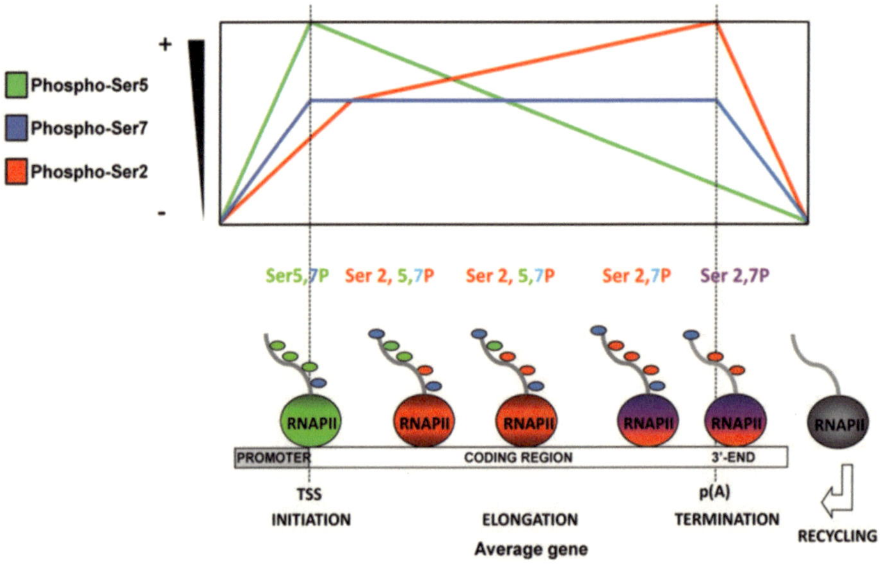

Figure 3. **RNAPII CTD phosphorylation profile in *Sacharomyces cerevisiae*.** During transcription initiation and promoter escape RNAPII CTD is phosphorylated on Ser5 (Ser5P) [48, 78]. Concurrently, Ser7 is phosphorylated (Ser7P), establishing a bivalent mark at both protein-coding and noncoding genes [74-76]. Shortly after promoter dissociation, Ser5P is rapidly removed while phosphorylated Ser2 (Ser2P) and Ser7P continue to accumulate [70, 77]. Finally, all CTD marks are rapidly removed at the end of transcription, and the hypophosphorylated RNAPII (in grey) is ready to assemble into the pre-initiation complex and re-initiate transcription [73, 79-80]. Small circles represent phosphorylated serine residues (green cirlces for Ser5P, blue circles for Ser7P and red circles for Ser2P). Differently colored big circles represent the distinct phosphorylated forms of RNAPII during initiation, elongation and termination. TSS: transcription start site; p(A): polyadenylation site.

2.2. Tyrosine 1 and Threonine 4 can also be phosphorylated

Tyrosine 1 (Tyr1) is evolutionarily conserved and present in all of the 52 repeats of the mammalian CTD, and in all of the 26-27 repeats of the yeast CTD. Although, it is well known that Tyr1 is susceptible to phosphorylation by tyrosine kinases *in vivo* [52-53] and that Tyr1 mutations are lethal in yeast [81], the function of this modification is unknown. Additionally, threonine 4 (Thr4) is also subjected to phosphorylation, at least in mammalian and in yeast cells [54, 82], and recently it has been demonstrated that phosphorylation of the Thr4 residues is required specifically for histone mRNA 3' end processing, which facilitates the recruitment of 3' processing factors to histone genes, and is evolutionarily conserved from yeast to human [54].

In mammals, there is an important degeneracy at some positions in the CTD, mainly in most of the carboxy-terminal repeats. Thus, the last repeat of the CTD is followed by a conserved 10 amino acid extension (Figure 1; [5]) that contains a constitutive site for the casein kinase (CK) II site [83]. Though deletion of this extension results in degradation of the CT, and effects in transcription and pre-mRNA processing [83-84], mutation of the CKII target site does not affect RNAPII CTD stability. Additionally, this extension is required for the phosphorylation of Tyr1 by c-Abl in mammals and it has been suggested that Tyr1 phosphorylation could be involved in functions specific of these higher eukaryotes [85]. Finally, non-consensus residues, such as lysine and arginine, are also present in the CTD, and they could be potentially modified by acetylation, ubiquitylation, sumoylation (lysine residues) and methylation (lysine and arginine residues) [86]. Therefore, the possibilities of CTD modifications are enormous, and only some of the modifications have been demonstrated to influence, while interacting with numerous factors, different aspects of gene expression.

3. Modifying enzymes: Kinases and phosphatases

Most of what is known concerning CTD-protein interactions, and in particular RNAPII CTD modifying enzymes, is derived from animal and yeast models, especially *Saccharomyces cerevisiae*, since the consensus sequence and repetitive structure of the CTD in addition to the CTD-modifying enzymes are highly conserved across a wide range of organisms. A number of kinases and phosphatases that target the CTD have been described and extensively studied (Tables 1 and 2, and reference therein). Recent genome-wide distribution studies of the CTD modifications in yeast have provided further evidence that complex interplay exists between these enzymes (i.e., kinases, phosphatases and isomerase), which coordinate a universal RNAPII CTD cycle [69]. These modifying enzymes alter specific serine residues within the CTD repeats and have distinct and specific functions along the transcription cycle. Although the catalytic mechanisms of CTD kinases and phosphatases are known, the basis for their specificity remains incompletely understood [87-88].

Below, in figure 4, we will highlight the most relevant features and functions of CTD kinases and phosphatases, with special emphasis on the budding yeast enzymes because extensive studies on RNAPII CTD phosphorylation have been performed on that organism, and most of these enzyme complexes are evolutionarily conserved.

3.1. RNAPII CTD kinases

The CTD is phosphorylated by members of the cyclin-dependent kinase (CDK) family, which usually consists of a catalytic and a cyclin subunit. Although CDKs are cell cycle regulators, several members of this family have direct functions in RNAPII activity regulation [39, 88]. All these kinases are members of multiprotein transcription regulatory complexes and, in mammals, the best known are Cdk7/CycH, Cdk8/CycC and Cdk9/CycT; recently, Cdk12/CycK has been characterized as a new CTD kinase [89]. These kinases are evolutionarily conserved, and the following four complexes with kinase activity have been identified in the well-known yeast model *Saccharomyces cerevisae*: Kin28/Ccl1, Srb10/Srb11, Bur1/Bur2 and Ctk1/Ctk2 (Table 1).

KINASES	SPECIFICITY	FUNCTION	REFERENCES
ySrb10 / Srb11 **hCdk8 / CycC**	CTD-Ser2 CTD-Ser5 **Other substrates** Bdf1 and Taf2, Med2 Gcn4, Msn2, Ste12, Gal4	*TFIIH inhibition* *PIC inhibition / activation* *Scaffold complex formation* *SAGA-dependent transcription*	[90-94]
yKin28 / Ccl1-Tfb3 **hCdk7 / CycH**	CTD-Ser5 CTD-Ser7 **Other substrates** Med4 Rgr1/Med14	*Promoter scape* *Scaffold complex formation* *Capping complex recruitment* *Bur1 activity stimulation* *Set1/COMPASS recruitment* *Elongation factor Paf1C recruitment* *SAGA complex recruitment* *snRNA 3′ processing* *Promoter-pausing* *Gene looping*	[64, 72, 74-76, 90, 94-100]
yBur1 / Bur2 **hCdk9 / CycT**	CTD-Ser2 CTD-Ser5 CTD-Ser7 CTD-Thr4 **Other Substrates** hDSIF (ySpt5), Rad6/Bre1	*Ctk1 activity stimulation* *Elongation* *PAF complex recruitment* *H3K4 methylation* *H2B monoubiquitination* Histone genes 3′-end processing	[54, 99, 101-104]
yCtk1 / Ctk2-Ctk3 **hCdk12 / CycK**	CTD-Ser2 **Other Substrates** Rps2	*RNAPII release from basal initiation factors* *3′-processing factors recruitment* *Transcription termination* *Spt6 recruitment* *H3K36 methylation* *Translation elongation*	[16, 49, 89, 105-112]

Table 1. RNAPII CTD kinases. Mammalian and *Saccharomyces cerevisiae* kinases are shown.

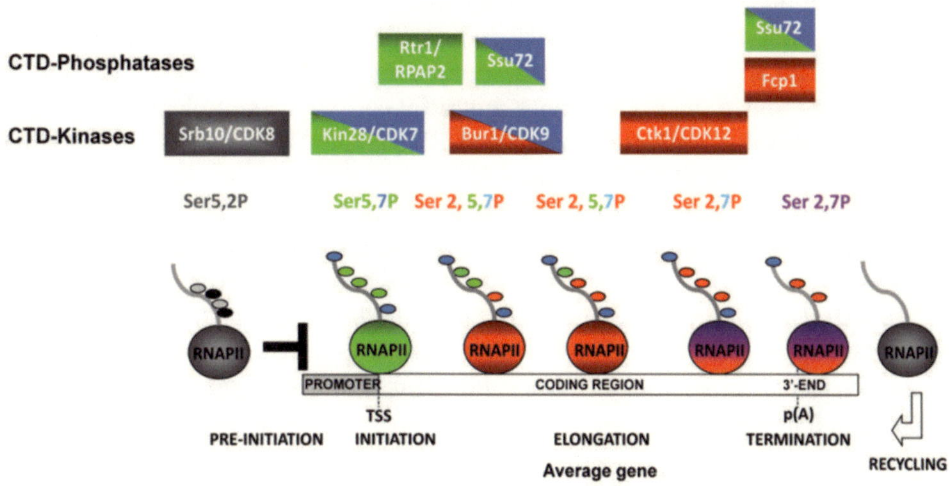

Figure 4. The levels of CTD phosphorylation are precisely modulated during the whole transcription cycle by the action of evolutionary conserved kinases and phosphatases. The level of Ser5 phosphorylation peaks early in the transcription cycle due to the action of Kin28 (Cdk7 in human) and remains constant or decreases as RNAPII progresses to the 3′ end of the gene [48, 67, 72]. In contrast, Ser2 phosphorylation is the predominant modification in the gene body and towards the 3′ end, and occurs concurrently with productive elongation [31, 48]. Ctk1 is the principal kinase responsible for Ser2 phosphorylation in the body of the genes [16, 73]. In addition to Ctk1, the Bur1/Bur2 kinase complex phosphorylates Ser2 when RNAPII is near the promoter and stimulates Ser2 phosphorylation by Ctk1 during elongation [99]. Several CTD-phosphatases have been shown to specifically de-phosphorylate Ser5P (Ssu72 and Rtr1), Ser2P (Fcp1) and Ser7 (Ssu72) to promote the initiation-elongation transition, elongation, termination, and RNAPII recycling [50, 73, 79, 167, 182]. Srb10 was demonstrated to phosphorylate the RNAPII CTD prior to PIC assembly, negatively regulating transcription initiation [92].

3.1.1. Pre-initiation and Initiation RNAPII CTD kinases

Cdk8/CycC and Srb10/Srb11

Human Cdk8/CycC and yeast Srb10/Srb11 are part of the CDK-module of Mediator [113], a large complex of 25-30 proteins that is structured in 4 sub-complexes or modules that act as a molecular bridge between DNA-binding transcription factors and RNAPII [114-115]. Mediator is required for the expression of nearly all RNAPII transcribed genes [116]. Cdk8/Srb10 is part of the CDK-module (Cdk8, cyclin C, MED12 and MED13 in mammals; Srb8, 9, 10 and 11 in yeast), which dynamically associates with Mediator [93, 117]. Although Cdk8/Srb10 can phosphorylate Ser2 and Ser5 of the CTD repeats *in vitro* [90, 92-94, 109, 113], the *in vivo* relevance of Cdk8/Srb10 remains to be defined. In fact, several studies have provided evidence that Srb10/11 can have both negative [116] and positive [118] effects on gene expression *in vivo*. Srb10 was demonstrated to phosphorylate the RNAPII CTD prior to PIC assembly, negatively regulating transcription initiation (Figure 4; [92]). Notably, human Cdk8 represses transcription via phosphorylation and inactivation of the cyclin H subunit of

TFIIH, which is the Cdk7 partner [90]. However, subsequent work showed that Srb10 functions in association with Kin28 (hCdk7) to promote RNAPII re-initiation [94]. Following PIC formation and an initial round of transcription, it is thought that subsequent rounds of RNAPII binding and promoter clearance are facilitated via a "scaffold complex" that is composed of a subset of Mediator subunits and GTFs (except TFIIB and TFIIF) that remains bound at the promoter [119]. Therefore, Kin28 and Srb10 have overlapping positive functions in promoting transcription and in the formation of the scaffold complex [94]. Srb10 phosphorylates two subunits of the general transcription factor TFIID (Bdf1 and Taf2) at the PIC; however, the role of these phosphorylation events has not yet been defined. Moreover, Srb10 phosphorylates and inactivates some transcription factors [120-122] by triggering their nuclear export or degradation [123-124] and phosphorylates and enhances the activity of others (Table 1). In summary, the *in vivo* relevance of RNAPII phosphorylation by Cdk8/Srb10 and its role in gene expression have yet to be elucidated.

Cdk7/CycH and Kin28/Ccl1-Tfb3

The Cdk7/cyclin H complex in mammals and its homolog in *Saccharomyces cerevisiae*, Kin28/Ccl1, are part of the TFIIH general transcription factor. In yeast, Kin28 is found associated with a third subunit (Tfb3) to form a trimer, called TFIIK (Kin28-Ccl1-Tfb3) within TFIIH [125]. Mammalian Cdk7 was isolated as a RNAPII CTD kinase that possesses Cdk-activating kinase (CAK) activity [126-128], whereas in yeast, Kin28 lacks this activity [129]. The CAK activity is fulfilled by a different kinase, Cak1 [130-131]. Cdk7 and Kin28 are both essential for cell viability [132], and the *in vivo* function of Kin28 has been extensively studied in yeast. Cdk7/Kin28 is the primary kinase that phosphorylates the CTD within a transcription initiation complex (Figure 4). Cdk7/Kin28 has been demonstrated to phosphorylate both Ser5 and Ser7 *in vitro* and *in vivo* [72, 74-76, 92]. Phosphorylation on Ser5 by Cdk7/Kin28 is thought to disrupt the stable interactions between the CTD and PIC components, thereby permitting the polymerase to release from the promoter and commence productive transcript elongation [92, 133-134]. Ser5 phosphorylation by Cdk7/Kin28 is required for the recruitment of the mRNA-capping complex [72, 135-137] and nuclear cap-binding complex (CBC) [100] to nascent transcripts and for co-transcriptional recruitment of elongation factor Paf1C [138], histone H3-lysine 4 methyltransferase complex (SET1/COMPASS) [98], and histone acetyltransferase complex SAGA [97].

Additionally, yeast Kin28 phosphorylates two subunits of Mediator (i.e., Med4 and Rgr1/Med14), and although the functionally of these modifications is unknown, it has been demonstrated that Mediator significantly enhances the phosphorylation of RNAPII CTD by Kin28 [94, 96]. In fact, *in vitro* assembly of TFIIH into a pre-initiation complex requires Mediator [139], and following transcription initiation, phosphorylation of Ser5 by Kin28 parallels with the release of Mediator from the CTD of RNAPII as promoter clearance occurs [80].

As discussed above, in yeast, Kin28 and Srb10 have overlapping functions in promoting transcription, PIC dissociation and subsequent scaffold complex formation [94]. Genetic analysis has provided further evidence that Kin28 and Srb10 are not redundant because only

Kin28 is essential for growth, and Srb10 is much less processive in terms of phosphorylation than Kin28 [140]. It is clear that Kin28 is the primary kinase responsible for the high level of phosphorylation of RNAPII during initiation [48, 67, 94, 141]. In fact, one essential role of Kin28 that Srb10 does not have is the stimulation of pre-mRNA processing. However, what appears clear, at least in yeast, is that PIC dissociation is dependent on the kinase activities of Kin28 and Srb10. Additionally, another function of RNAPII CTD Ser5 phosphorylation by Kin28 is the enhancement of Bur1/Bur2 recruitment and Ser2 CTD phosphorylation near the promoters [99]. Moreover, it has recently been demonstrated that TFIIH kinase places bivalent marks on the CTD, thereby phosphorylating Ser7 during transcription initiation [74-75].

3.1.2. RNAPII CTD elongating kinases

Cdk9/CycT and Cdk12/CycK

Eukaryotic organisms possess many factors that regulate transcriptional elongation; among these factors is Cdk9 kinase, which is the catalytic subunit of the positive transcription elongation factor b (P-TEFb) that controls the elongation phase of transcription by RNAPII in mammals and *Drosophila melanogaster* [12]. Cdk9 is the major Ser2 kinase, but it also contributes to Ser5 phosphorylation *in vitro* and *in vivo* during the initiation-elongation transition and the polymerase release of promoter-proximal pausing [109, 142]. Cdk9 activity is also required for efficient coupling of transcription with pre-mRNA processing [108]. Additionally, very recently, it has been shown that Thr4 is phosphorylated by Cdk9 [54].

In higher eukaryotes, the transcription factor P-TEFb not only regulates CTD phosphorylation, but it also inhibits the action of transcriptional repressors and is required for the association of several elongation factors with the transcribing polymerase. P-TEFb also targets DRB sensitivity-inducing factor (DSIF) and negative elongation factor (NELF) [142-144] (Table 1). Thus, P-TEFb promotes transcription by the following two different mechanisms: inhibiting the action of transcriptional repressors and phosphorylating the CTD during transcription elongation. Until recently, it was believed that Cdk9 was the only CTD Ser2 kinase in higher eukaryotes. In fact, Cdk9 can reconstitute the activity of both *S. cerevisiae* Ser2 CTD kinases, Bur1 and Ctk1. However, it has recently been demonstrated that *Drosophila* have one ortholog of yeast Ctk1, Cdk12, whereas humans have two, Cdk12 and Cdk13; only Cdk12 has been clearly demonstrated to be an elongating CTD kinase [89, 145]. Notably and similarly, fission yeast *Schizosaccharomyces pombe* has the following two Ser2 elongating kinases: Lsk1 (ScCtk1) and Cdk9 (ScBur1) [146].

Bur1/Bur2

Bur1 kinase and its cyclin, Bur2, form an essential CDK in *S. cerevisiae* involved in transcription elongation [147-148]. Although Bur1 and Ctk1 kinase complexes appear to functionally reconstitute the activity of P-TEFb in yeast [149], Bur1 is more related in sequence and functionally to mammalian P-TEFb than Ctk1 [147, 149], and as we have discussed, it is clear that Cdk12 is the functional equivalent of yeast Ctk1 [89, 145]. Bur1 can phosphorylate Ser2 and Ser5 [99, 147, 150] [151], and although it was first demonstrated to show some preference for Ser5 and to be less active than Ctk1 or Kin28 [147], later studies provided evidence that Bur1 interacts with the RNAPII CTD and phosphorylates at Ser2. In fact, Bur1 phosphorylates elongating RNAPII molecules that have been previously phosphorylated at Ser5 and are located near the promoter during early transcription elongation (Figure 4, and [99]. Thus, it has been hypothesized that Bur1/Bur2 is recruited to RNAPII, whose repeats are phosphorylated on Ser5 to enhance phosphorylation on Ser2 by Ctk1. Consistent with it, Bur1 produces the Ser2 phosphorylated residues that remains when Ctk1 is inactivated [152]. Bur1 also stimulates transcription elongation as its mammalian homologue P-TEFb [150, 152], and mutations on *BUR1* cause sensitivity to drugs that are known to affect transcription elongation (e.g., 6-azauracil) [147, 150]. More recently, a chemical-genomic analysis has provided further evidence that Bur1 also phosphorylates Ser7 in the body of the genes [77].

Bur1 shares another function with the mammalian and *Schizosaccharomyces pombe* Cdk9 [142, 153]. Bur1 kinase activity is important for the *in vivo* phosphorylation of the elongation factor Spt5 (mammalian DSIF) [102, 154]. Spt5 contains a carboxy-terminal domain that consists of approximately 15 repeats (CTR) that are similar to the RNAPII CTD [102], which is subject to phosphorylation. The Spt5-CTR is required for efficient elongation by RNAPII and for chromatin modifications in transcribed regions (see below). Thus, Spt5 phosphorylation mediates, at least in part, Bur1 kinase roles on transcription elongation and histone modifications [154].

Ctk1/Ctk2-Ctk3

Ctk1 was originally identified as the kinase subunit of the yeast CTDK-I complex that catalyzes phosphorylation of the RNAPII CTD [155]. Ctk2 is the cyclin, and the Ctk3 function remains unknown. Ctk1 is the principal kinase that is responsible for CTD-Ser2P during transcription elongation, which is coincident with reduced Ser5P [73, 156]. Although Ctk1 is not directly involved in transcription elongation [16, 18, 157], it associates with RNAPII throughout elongation [49], and the kinase activity of Ctk1 is required for the association of polyadenylation and termination factors [16] and histone modification factors [158]. Additionally, Ctk1 interacts genetically as well as biochemically with the TREX complex [159], which couples transcription elongation to mRNA export [160]. Moreover, Ctk1 promotes the dissociation of basal transcription factors from elongating RNAPII, early during transcription, however, kinase activity is not required [105].

In addition to its functions in transcribing gene coding proteins, Ctk1 is involved in RNAPI transcription, interacts with RNAPI *in vivo* [161], and it is required for the integrity of the rDNA tandem array [162]. All of these studies suggest that Ctk1 might participate in the regulation of distinct nuclear transcriptional machineries. Additionally, it has been demonstrated that Ctk1 is required for DNA damage-induced transcription [163], and notably, that Ctk1 has a role in the fidelity of translation elongation in the cytoplasm [110, 164].

3.2. RNAPII CTD phosphatases

Dynamic de-phosphorylation of Ser2P and Ser5P make a significant contribution to changes in CTD phosphorylation patterns during the transcription cycle and is essential for RNAPII recycling [8, 31]. Dephosphrylation is achieved by several CTD phosphatases (Table 2). Initially, only one phosphatase was identified, Fcp1, which is required for Ser2P de-phosphorylation, transcription elongation and RNAPII recycling to initiate new rounds of transcription [47, 165]. Two other CTD phosphatase were later identified in yeast, Ssu72, a component of the mRNA 3'-end processing machinery [79, 88, 166] and Rtr1 [167]. In mammals, in addition to Fcp1, there are other CTD phosphatases, i.e., the small phosphatase SCP1 [168] and RPAP2, which is the human homolog of Rtr1 [169]. Briefly, Fcp1 dephosphorylates Ser2P [73]; Ssu72 dephosphorylates Ser5P and Ser7P [50, 69]; and Rtr1 in yeast and SCP1 in mammals specifically dephosphorylate Ser5P [79, 167-168].

Rtr1 / RPAP2

Chromatin immunoprecipitation studies have provided further evidence that the increase in Ser2P occurs as transcription progresses through the gene and follows Ser5P de-phosphorylation. Rtr1 in yeast was identified as the RNAPII CTD phosphatase driven the Ser5-Ser2P transition at the 5′ regions of the transcribed genes. Rtr1 genetically interacts with the RNAPII machinery, and Rtr1 deletion provokes global Ser5P accumulation in whole-cell extracts and Ser5P association throughout the coding regions [167, 171]. RPAP2 was identified in a systematic analysis carried out to determine the composition and organization of the soluble RNAPII machinery [169], and as in the case of Rtr1, Ser5P levels increase *in vivo* when RPAP2 is knocked down. Additionally, RPAP2 depletion affects snRNA gene expression as it does mutations of the Ser7 residue [64]. In fact, Ser7P recruits the 3′-end processing Integrator complex and RPAP2 to drive Ser5 de-phosphorylation of RNAPII CTD during the transcription of snRNA genes [170, 183]. Recently, a model has been proposed in which RPAP2 recruitment to snRNA genes through CTD-Ser7P triggers a cascade of events that are critical for proper gene expression [170].

PHOSPHATASES	SPECIFICITY	FUNCTION	REFERENCES
yRtr1 **hRpap2**	CTD-Ser5P	*Promote Ser5P to Ser2P transition* *Association of Integrator with snRNA genes*	[167, 169-171]
ySsu72 **hSsu72**	CTD-Ser5P, Ser7P CTD-Ser5P	*Transcription initiation/elongation* *Transcription termination and 3′-end processing* *Facilitate Fcp1 activity* *Gene looping and RNAPII recycling*	[50, 69, 79, 166, 172-176]
y/h Fcp1	CTD-Ser2P	*Positive regulator of RNAPII transcription* *Transcription elongation* *Transcription termination and RNAPII recycling*	[47, 73, 165, 177-182]
hSCP1	CTD-Ser5P	*Transition from initiation / capping to processive transcript elongation.*	[168]

Table 2. RNAPII CTD phosphatases. Human and *Saccharomyces cerevisiae* phosphatases are shown.

Ssu72

Ssu72 was first described as a Ser5P phosphatase and recently as a Ser7P phosphatase [50, 69]. In fact, Ssu72 was originally identified as functionally interacting with the general transcription factor TFIIB [184-185]. Afterward, it was demonstrated that Ssu72 is part of the cleavage and polyadenylation factor (CPF) with a role at the 3′-end of genes [166, 175]. In fact, Ssu72 is crucial for transcription-coupled 3′-end processing and termination of protein-coding genes [175, 186-187]. Later, Ssu72 was characterized as a Ser5P phosphatase [79] and a potential tyrosine phosphatase [188] and, most recently, it has been demonstrated that Ssu72 is also a Ser7 phosphatase [50, 69]. A genome-wide distribution analysis of Ssu72 has demonstrated two peaks of association (Figure 4): a low peak at the 5′-end of genes and a higher peak at the cleavage and polyadenylation site or immediately after it [50]. In agreement with it, Ssu72 dephosphorylates RNAPII CTD following cleavage and polyadenylation and recycles the terminating RNAPII, giving rise to a hypophosphorylated polymerase. In fact, inactivation of Ssu72 leads to the accumulation of Ser7P marks that avoids RNAPII recruitment to the PIC, and therefore inhibits transcription initiation, which results in cell death [50]. In other words, Ssu72 is critical for transcription termination, 3′-end processing and RNAPII recycling to restart a new round of transcription. Additionally, it has been shown that Ssu72 has a function in gene looping [172]. In a screen looking for mammalian retinoblastoma tumor suppressors, a human homolog of yeast Ssu72 was identified. As in yeast, mammalian Ssu72 associates with TFIIB and the yeast cleavage/polyadenylation factor Pta1, and exhibits intrinsic phosphatase activity [176]. The crystal complex structure that is formed by human symplekin (Pta1 in yeast), hSsu72 and a CTD phosphopeptide has been elucidated, and hSsu72 was demonstrated to have a function in coupling transcription to pre-mRNA 3'-end processing [187].

Fcp1 / SCP1

Fcp1 was the first discovered CTD phosphatase and is highly conserved among eukarya [177, 189-191]. It directly de-phosphorylates RNAPII, and its activity is stimulated *in vitro* by TFIIF and inhibited by TFIIB [73, 177-178]. Fcp1 is essential for cell viability and for transcription in yeast [177-178] and preferentially dephosphorylates Ser2P [73, 192]. Fcp1 has two essential domains: an FCP homologous domain near the amino-terminus and a downstream BRCA1 carboxy-terminal (BRCT) domain [87]. Higher eukaryotes have additional small CTD phosphatases (SCPs) that contain only the FCPH domain characteristic of the Fcp1 proteins. However, SCP1 preferentially catalyzes Ser5P de-phosphorylation and is especially active on RNAPII molecules that have been phosphorylated by TFIIH [168].

Gene transcription is decreased in cells lacking Fcp1 function, and *fcp1* mutants exhibited a general accumulation of hyperphosphorylated RNAPII in whole-cell extracts, and specifically in the gene coding regions [178]. Fcp1 also has the ability to stimulate RNAPII transcript elongation *in vitro* independent of its phosphatase activity [182], which suggests that it associates with and modulates elongating RNAPII. In agreement with this, chromatin immunoprecipitation studies have demonstrated that Fcp1 associates with the promoter and coding region of active genes *in vivo* [73]. Recent genome-wide studies have provided further evidence that Fcp1 associates with genes from promoter to 3′-end regions, showing the highest association of Fcp1 with the cleavage and polyadenylation site. This association occurs after Bur1 and Ctk1 have dissociated, which permits Fcp1 to completely dephosphorylate all the remaining Ser2P residues ([50], Figure 4). Fcp1 is also responsible for de-phosphorylation of RNAPII following its release from DNA [165]. Fcp1 association with genes at the cleavage polyadenylation site overlaps with Ssu72 association, whereas this overlapping does not exist at the 5′ and coding regions (Figure 4). This fact indicates that CTD de-phosphorylation may be coupled at the 3′-ends, and it has been hypothesized that Ssu72 activity may be important for Fcp1 function, thereby coupling Ser2P de-phosphorylation to the removal of Ser5P and Ser7P [69].

4. Other factors influencing RNAPII CTD phosphorylation

Although many factors can have effects on CTD phosphorylation, we will highlight the following two that we believe are of significant relevance: the prolyl isomerases hPin1/yEss1 and the structure of the RNAPII itself. In addition, we will describe the role of ySub1 in CTD phosphorylation, because it has been extensively studied by us.

4.1. hPin1 / yEss1

The CTD can adopt either cis- or trans-conformations, which can significantly affect its modification, especially its phosphorylation. Peptidyl prolyl isomerases (PPIases) are enzymes that accelerate the rates of rotation about the peptide bond preceding proline and are important for protein folding and regulation of dynamic cellular processes [193-194]. Pin1 in mammals and Ess1 in *S. cerevisiae* are RNAPII CTD PPIases. Phosphorylated Ser2 and Ser5 match with the pSer-Pro sequence that is recognized by Pin1, and the CTD appears to be its principal target of regulation [195-196]. Pin1 has specificity for phosphorylated Ser/Thr-Pro sequences, and it modulates RNAPII activity during cell cycle at least in part by regulating RNAPII CTD phosphorylation levels [195]. Yeast Ess1 physically interacts with the CTD [55, 197], and it preferentially binds and isomerizes *in vitro* Ser5P residues [198]. Although Pin1 stimulates RNAPII CTD hyperphosphorylation, which results in transcription repression and inhibition of mRNA splicing [195-196], *in vivo* studies have proposed that Ess1 promotes RNAPII CTD de-phosphorylation. In any case, both isomerases have important functions in transcription. Therefore, initiation-elongation transition is inhibited by Pin1 [196], whereas Ess1 affects multiple steps, such as initiation, elongation, 3′-end processing, and termination [197, 199-201]. In fact, it has been demonstrated that Ess1 promotes Ssu72-dependent function by creating the CTD structural conformation that is recognized by Ssu72 [202], and recently it has been confirmed that isomerization is a key regulator of RNAPII CTD de-phosphorylation at the end of genes [69].

4.2. RNAPII structure and Rpb1-CTD localization

The structure of the complete 12-subunit RNAPII (Rpb1-12) is known [203-204]. Rpb4 and Rpb7 subunits form a conserved sub-complex that is conserved in all three eukaryotic RNA polymerases and archaea RNAP [205-206]. Crystal structures of the Rpb4/7 heterodimer in the context of the complete RNAPII complex localized it in the proximity of the Rpb1-CTD [203, 207], and biochemical and genetic studies suggest that Rpb4/7 might have a function in the recruitment of some CTD-binding proteins to transcribing RNAPII. Moreover, it is possible that this sub-complex, Rpb4/7, would regulate the access of CTD modifying enzymes during the whole transcription cycle [203, 207, 209-212]. Actually, structural studies have provided further evidence that the CTD extends from the RNAPII core enzyme near the RNA exit channel [204], where it is ideally located to bind and be affected by the action of a multitude of factors, among them kinases, phosphatases and isomerases. In fact, in yeast, the isopropylisomerase Ess1 and the phosphatase Fcp1 are associated with Rpb7 and Rpb4, respectively [55, 87, 208].

4.3. The ssDNA binding protein Sub1 as a general regulator of transcription

Sub1 is an ssDNA binding protein that has been implicated in several steps of mRNA metabolism, such as initiation, transcription termination and 3'-end processing [186, 213-215]. Sub1 was originally described as a transcriptional stimulatory protein that is homologous to the human positive coactivator PC4, which physically interacts with activators and components of the RNAPII basal transcription machinery [216-220]. Sub1 genetically and physically interacts with TFIIB [214-215, 221], and several functions have been proposed for Sub1 that include stimulating PIC recruitment and promoter escape. In fact, most recently, using a quantitative proteomic screen to identify promoter-bound PIC components, Sub1 was identified as a functional PIC component that is associated with RNAPII complexes [225]. In addition, we have recently demonstrated that Sub1 globally regulates RNAPII CTD phosphorylation (Figure 5, [222]) and that it is a *bona fide* elongation factor that influences transcription elongation rates (García and Calvo, unpublished results). Although it has been broadly studied, and several functions have been hypothesized for Sub1 [213, 215, 222-225]; however, the exact mechanism by which Sub1 functions in transcription remains unclear. Sub1 globally regulates RNAPII-CTD phosphorylation during the entire transcription cycle by modulating, albeit differentially, the activity and recruitment of CTD modifying enzymes [222, 224]. We have proposed a model showing how Sub1 might function to globally regulate RNAPII CTD phosphorylation (Figure 5). In wild-type cells (*wt*), non-phosphorylated Sub1 joins the promoter (possibly via TFIIB; [214-215, 221]), contacting the promoter via its DNA binding domain. At that point, Sub1 interacts with the Cdk8-Mediator complex, helping to maintain the PIC in a stable but inactive conformation. Sub1 is then phosphorylated (possibly by the action of kinases at the PIC, similarly to PC4, its human homolog), losing its DNA binding capacity and promoting clearance of TFIIB [214-215, 226]. The PIC next changes conformation such that Kin28 can be activated, and with the help of Srb10 promotes PIC dissociation into the scaffold complex as well as the recruitment of elongating kinases Ctk1 and Bur1. In contrast, in the absence of Sub1 (*sub1Δ*), Srb10 activity and recruitment are decreased, while Kin28 recruitment and activity increases, in agreement with TFIIH being negatively regulated by Cdk8-containing Mediator complexes [90, 227]. As a result, Ser5P levels are increased, and consequently Bur1 and Ctk1 association with chromatin is also enhanced [99, 228]. Furthermore, in *sub1Δ* cells there is a reduction on Fcp1 phosphatase levels and its association with chromatin, which induces an additional increase in Ser2P, impairing RNAPII recycling after transcription termination. Thus, a decrease in RNAPII recruitment is observed in cells lacking Sub1 [224]. Additionally, Sub1 also influences Spt5 elongation factor phosphorylation by Bur1 (García and Calvo, unpublished results). We currently do not understand the biochemical basis for these effects. We have not found evidence that Sub1 associates with any of the CTD kinases or evidence that Sub1 influences the CTD kinase activities by influencing post-translational modifications of the kinases. Therefore, we currently consider two possible explanations for the effects of Sub1 on the activities of the CTD kinases. One explanation is that Sub1 enhances the association (or dissociation) of an unidentified, common regulator with the kinases, whereas the other is that Sub1 in some manner influences kinase accessibility to the CTD.

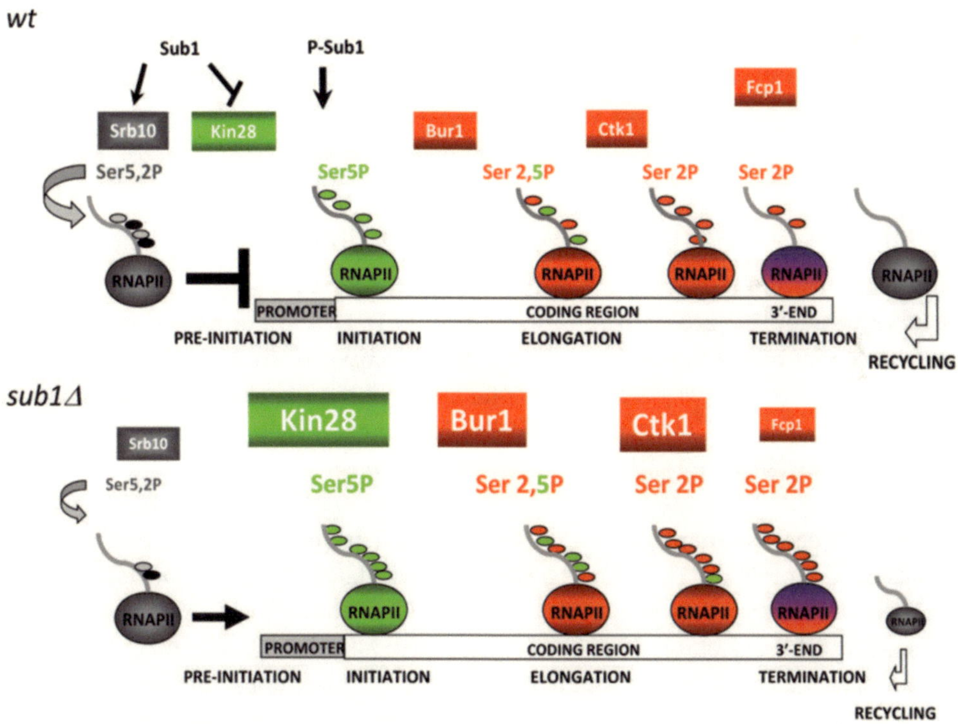

Figure 5. Model showing how Sub1 might function to globally regulate RNAPII CTD phosphorylation [222] . Different font sizes in the figure text indicate the increase or decrease of the corresponding CTD modifying enzymes in *sub1Δ* versus *wt* cells.

5. RNAPII CTD phosphorylation and pre-mRNA processing

The CTD is an unordered structure that extends from the RNAPII core enzyme, near the RNA exit channel [204, 209]. This localization is convenient to interact with a plethora of factors, such as the CTD-modifying enzymes and binding factors involved in distinct nuclear processes, for example, components of the RNA processing machinery [32, 88]. Furthermore, its length and the ability to adopt numerous conformations permit it to interact with different factors at the same time [31-32], and it is currently clear that these interactions depends on the CTD phosphorylation patterns during the transcription cycle [8, 21].

As transcription progresses the nascent RNA is capped to protect the 5′ end, intron sequences are removed, and a polyadenylated tail is added to the 3′ end. Coupling mRNA processing to transcription increases processing efficiency and allows multiple regulatory pathways to guarantee that only correctly modified mRNAs are exported. For more than a decade, numerous studies have provided evidence that the CTD serves as a scaffold for the assembly of an enormous variety of protein complexes to coordinate not only transcription of non-coding and protein-coding genes [8, 58-62, 64-65], but also pre-mRNA processing [21, 31-32]: capping [42, 135, 137], splicing [229], and 3′-end cleavage and polyadenylation [42]. All of these functions are achieved through the recognition and reading of the CTD code during the transcription cycle [6-8, 31]. Thus, co-transcriptional CTD-mediated processing of nascent RNA plays a crucial role in both recruitment of RNA processing machineries and regulation of their activities. Indeed, a functional CTD is not required for *in vitro* transcription by RNAPII, but it is essential for efficient pre-mRNA processing [42, 230-231].

Capping

The capping reaction consists in the addition of an inverted 7-methylguanosine cap to the first RNA residue by a 5'-5' triphosphate bridge. It is a characteristic of all RNAPII transcripts and is added to the 5′-end of nascent transcripts when they are only 25-50 bases long. The capping complex contains the following three enzymatic activities: RNA 5'-triphosphatase, guanylyl transferase and RNA (guanine-7) methyltransferase [17, 67]. In yeast, these activities are achieved by three enzymes (i.e., Cet1, Ceg1 and Abd1, respectively), whereas in metazoans, these activities are performed by two enzymes (i.e., HCE and MT) because guanylyl transferase and RNA 5'-triphosphatase are two functionally domains of HCE protein [17]. Following Ser5 phosphorylation by TFIIH, the mRNA capping complex binds directly and specifically to Ser5P residues through the Ceg1 subunit in yeast or the guanylyl transferase domain in metazoans [48, 67, 78, 95, 137]. Furthermore, phosphorylated CTD interaction with the capping complex allosterically stimulates the capping enzyme activity and in response, enhances early transcription [136, 232]. Because the CTD is located near the RNA exit channel, its interaction with the capping complex permits its positioning for rapid processing of the mRNA 5′-end as the nascent transcript emerges from the polymerase. This is thought to protect the RNA from degradation and promote RNAPII to proceed into productive transcription elongation. In fact, by coupling capping and early transcription, only capped RNA will be elongated [67, 136, 232-233].

3′-end processing

Not only capping and transcription are linked at the 5′-end regions of protein coding-genes, but also polyadenylation and transcription termination at the 3′-end regions. In brief, 3′-end processing consists of the following two-step reaction: endonucleolytic cleavage of the pre-mRNA and subsequent addition of a poly(A) tail [17]. Both enzymatic reactions require a functional CTD [42, 230]. In fact, deletion of the CTD or absence of CTD phosphorylation negatively affects 3′-end processing [16, 30, 106, 157, 234]. Furthermore, the CTD binds 3′-end processing factors and stimulates cleavage/polyadenylation *in vivo* and *in vitro* [42, 230]. The cleavage is achieved by a complex that consists of CstF, CPSF, CF1, and CF2 in higher eukaryotes and CF1A, CF1B, and CFII in yeast, whereas the polyadenylation reaction is performed by a poly(A) polymerase in both cases [17] . Cleavage/polyadenylation factors CPSF and CstF can specifically bind to CTD affinity columns and are copurified with RNAPII [42]. In yeast, several 3′-end factors preferentially binds phosphorylated CTD [72, 106-107, 235]. Furthermore, yeast 3'-end processing factors are recruited depending on Ser2 phosphorylation by Ctk1 when RNAPII reaches the 3′-end regions of the transcribed genes. Therefore, regulation of CTD phosphorylation as the polymerase transcribes facilitates coordination of the assembly of the 3′-end processing machinery with transcription [16]. Additionally, the polyadenylation signals are required for proper transcription termination in mammals and yeast [236-237]. In fact, Rtt103, which is a 3'-end mRNA processing factor, interacts with the CTD phosphorylated on Ser2 and recruits a 5′-3′ RNA exonuclease, thereby promoting the release of RNAPII from the DNA [238-239]. In summary, Ser5 phosphorylation by TFIIH kinase (Kin28/Cdk7) is required to recruit the RNA-capping machinery to RNAPII [48, 67, 72], whereas Ser2 phosphorylation is required for the recruitment of 3′-end processing complexes and for transcription termination [16, 30, 106, 238-239] (Figure 7). However, it is unknown whether phosphorylation of Ser5 and Ser2 of all of the repeats or only some of the repeats is required to enhance capping and cleavage/polyadenylation, respectively.

Ser7 phosphorylation has been functionally related with 3′-end processing of snRNA in higher eukaryotes. Human snRNA genes, contrary to protein-coding genes, are not polyadenylated, and instead of a poly(A) signal, they contain a conserved 3′ box RNA-processing element that is recognized by the snRNA gene-specific Integrator RNA 3′ end-processing complex. This complex binds to RNAPII CTD and links transcription and 3′-end processing [63-64, 240-241]. Therefore, in metazoans, Ser7P, in combination with Ser2P, is a major determinant for the recruitment of the Integrator complex to snRNA genes during its transcription [64, 240-241]. In yeast, the Integrator-like complex recruitment depends on Ser7 phosphorylation, the promoter elements and the specialized PIC that binds those elements [74]. After promoter escape, the RNA processing complex travels with the elongating phosphorylated polymerase up to the 3′-end box at the end of the snRNA transcription unit, where it associates with the nascent transcript in a co-transcriptional-dependent manner.

Splicing

As in the case of capping and cleavage/polyadenylation, a number of studies performed *in vivo* and *in vitro* during the last decades have demonstrated the existence of a functional interaction between the transcriptional machinery and the splicing apparatus [21, 242]. However, this functional interaction and the underlying mechanism are less accurately understood. The most complex pre-mRNA processing reaction is splicing, which is carried out by a large complex, the spliceosome, consisting of at least 150 protein components and five snRNAs [242]. The first indication of a coupling between transcription and splicing came from studies demonstrating that truncation of the CTD severely altered splicing *in vitro* [42]. Later it was shown that the CTD directly affects splicing, and that a phosphorylated CTD is required for the efficient splicing reaction [231, 243]. These data provided evidence that an elongating RNAPII with phosphorylated CTD is an active component of the splicing reaction. A number of physical links between the phosphorylated CTD and the splicing apparatus have been established, and chromatin immunoprecipitation analysis have shown that the direct binding of the splicing machinery to the nascent RNA is responsible in a large part for the co-transcriptional splicing in yeast and mammals [244-245]. Hyperphosphorylated, but not hypophosphorylated RNAPII, has been found associated with splicing factors and detected in active spliceosomes [246-248]. For instance, in yeast, the splicing factor Prp40 binds to phosphorylated CTD [249]; in mammals, Spt6 binds selectively to the CTD-Ser2P [112], and the spliceosome-associated protein CA150 interacts with phosphorylated CTD while interacting with the SF1 splicing factor [250-251]. Therefore, all these studies led to the idea that the phosphorylated CTD acts as a scaffold, binding multiple splicing factors, and directly enhancing the spliceosome assembly. Corroborating this idea, a recent study identified a splicing factor, U2AF65, that interacts directly with the CTD to activate splicing and likely plays a role in spliceosome assembly [242, 252]. Another recent study provided evidence that coupling transcription and splicing through CTD phosphorylation can be a regulatory point in the control of gene expression. For instance, it has been described that a set of inducible genes can be actively transcribed by RNAPII phosphorylated on Ser5, but not on Ser2, under non-inducing conditions, giving rise to a full length unspliced transcript. However, after induction, Cdk9 is recruited, phosphorylates the CTD on Ser2 and the generated transcript is properly spliced [253]. This fact strongly implicates Ser2P as a key in the integration of splicing and transcription. In addition to constitutive splicing, functional links between the CTD and alternative splicing have also been provided [86]. Thus, it has been suggested that the CTD may regulate the choice of alternative exons by increasing the local concentration of splicing factors [229], and that possibility participate in the physical modulation of alternative splicing.

6. RNAPII CTD phosphorylation coordinates transcription to other nuclear processes

6.1. Coupling the CTD code and the histone code

The nucleosome is the basic element of chromatin and consists of a histone octamer composed of two copies of histone 2A (H2A), H2B, H3 and H4, wrapped by 146 bp of DNA [254]. The histones carry numerous post-translational modifications, and some of these are associated with transcription. In fact, a general view is that histone post-translational modifications draw parallel with either positive or negative transcriptional states. Numerous discoveries have led to the idea that such modifications regulate transcription either directly by causing structural changes to chromatin (e.g., histone acetylation) or indirectly by recruiting protein complexes (e.g., histone methylation) [255-257]. Therefore, chromatin not only plays an essential role in packaging the DNA, but also in regulating gene expression. Most histone modifications reside in their amino- and carboxy-terminal tails, and a few of them in their globular domains. As in the case of CTD phosphorylation, where Ser5P triggers Ser2 phosphorylation, some histone modifications mark the deposition of another, thus creating a complex epigenetic signal code, the "histone code", that governs chromatin organization and DNA-dependent processes such as transcription. Therefore, the histone code is responsible for an active or inactive chromatin state with respect to transcription, because it coordinates the recruitment of various chromatin modifying and remodeling complexes to regulate chromatin structure and, consequently, transcription [258-259]. Because this review focuses on RNAPII CTD phosphorylation, only certain histone modifications, which are functionally related to the CTD code and transcription, will be discussed. There are excellent reviews that discuss all the histone modifications and their roles in different nuclear processes [255, 258, 260-261].

Lysine is a key substrate residue because it undergoes many exclusive modifications important for transcription regulation (i.e., acetylation, methylation, ubiquitination and SUMOylation [255, 261]. The lysine residues can be mono-, di- or trimethylated, and each level of modification can result in distinct biological effects. In brief, with respect to transcription, acetylation activates and sumoylation appears to be repressive, and both modifications may mutually interfere. On the other hand, methylation can have distinct effects; thus, lysine 4 in histone H3 (H3K4me3) is trimethylated at the 5′-ends of genes during activation, whereas trimethylation of H3K9 occurs in transcriptionally silent regions. Arginine residues of H3 and H4 can also be mono- or dimethylated, which activate transcription. Serine/threonine phosphorylation of H3 in specific sites also marks activated transcription, and ubiquitination of H2B and H2A are associated with active and repressed transcription, respectively (reviewed by [255-257]. All histone modifications are removable by specific enzymes (e.g., histone deacetylases (HDACs), phosphatases, and ubiquitin proteases ([255-257], and references therein). In fact HDACs play important regulatory roles during active transcription [262].

Methylation of H3K4 and K36 are the most well characterized histone modifications with roles in active transcription [263], and whose functions are directly linked to RNAPII CTD phosphorylation (Figure 6). H3K4 is methylated by the Set1/COMPASS complex, while K36 is mediated by the Set2 complex. The profile of H3K4 tri-methylation (H3K4me3) strongly correlates with the distribution pattern of the RNAPII CTD-Ser5P. It is mainly found around the transcriptional start site (TSS) contributing to transcription initiation, elongation and RNA processing [264]. Set1 recruitment and H3K4 tri-methylation usually peaks at the promoter and 5′ region of a gene, depending on Kin28/Cdk7 activity (Figure 7) and Paf1 complex, a RNAPII-associated complex [265], and contributes to transcription initiation, elongation and RNA processing [264] [98]. H3K4 mono and di-methylation tend to expand along the coding regions compared to try-methylation. On the other hand, H3K36 methylation by Set2 is observed across the entire coding region with an increase toward the

3′-ends of actively transcribed genes. Ctk1 also regulates H3K4 methylation [158, 266]. Thereby, differently phosphorylated CTD by Kin28 and Ctk1 is responsible for the characteristic distribution of H3K4 tri-methylation in the coding region [158]. In contrast to Set1, the recruitment of Set2 and H3K36 methylation depends on a CTD-Ser2P/Ser5P double mark (Figure 6), and therefore, on Ctk1 kinase activity [158, 266]. Interestingly, the other Ser2 kinase complex, Bur1/2, also promotes Set2 recruitment and assists H3-K36 methylation, particularly at the 5′ ends of genes and is required for the histone 2B ubiquitination activity of the Rad6/Bre1 complex [101, 103, 152].

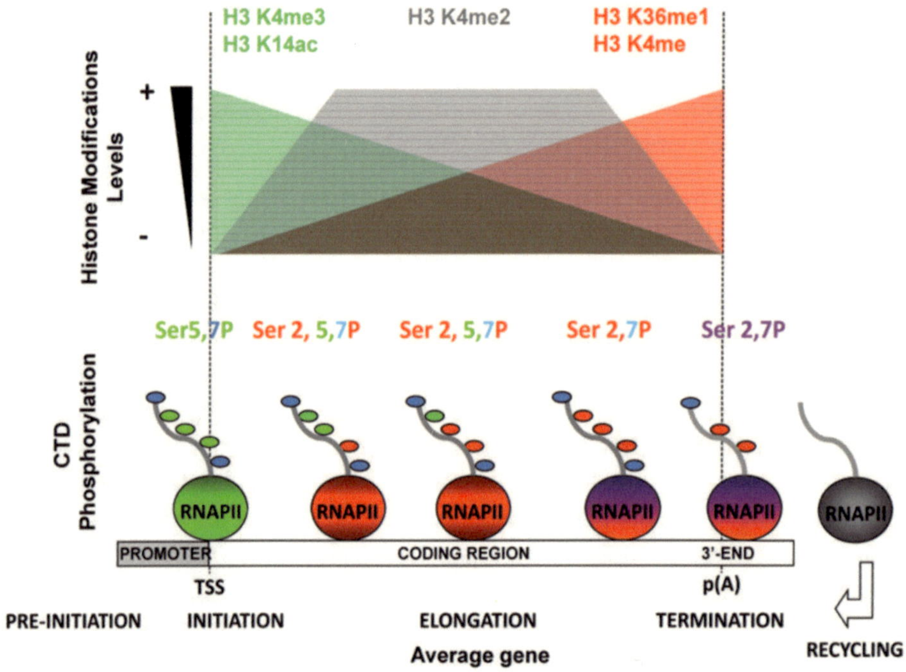

Figure 6. Histone H3 tri-, di-, and mono-methylation and acetylation during RNAPII transcription in *S. cerevisiae.*

H3 acetylation / deacetylation is also relevant during active transcription. Thus, histone acetyl and deacetyl transferase complexes (HAT and HDACs, respectively) are recruited to the transcriptional machinery during elongation through the interaction with RNAPII. Indeed, they modulate histone occupancy in the coding regions of actively transcribed genes, and this depends on CTD phosphorylation status [267-268]. HAT acetylates nucleosomes promoting nucleosomes eviction and allowing RNAPII to pass through. Afterward, the nucleosomes are immediately reassembled behind the polymerase and HDACs are co-transcriptionally recruited to rapidly and efficiently deacetylate the reassembled nucleosomes behind the polymerase. Altogether, this avoids cryptic transcription and maintains active transcription [262]. Methylation of histone H3 by Set1 and Set2 is required for deacetylation of nucleosomes in coding regions by the histone deacetylase complexes (HDACs) Set3C and Rpd3C(S), respectively. HDACs' recruitment is triggered by H3K4 methylation at promoters and within coding regions to restrict hyperactetylated histones to promoters and to maintain transcription activity. Set1-H3K4me2 can be recognized by two different HDACs, RPD3S or SET3C [264]. The Set1-SET3C pathway preferentially affects actively transcribed genes with promoters configured for efficient initiation/re-initiation [269]. In contrast, Set1-RPD3S pathway is active at loci subjected to cryptic and weak transcription encompassing repressed promoters of coding genes. Related to this, phosphorylation of the CTD by Kin28/Cdk7 is important for the initial recruitment of the Rpd3S and Set3 HDACs to coding sequences ([268], Figure 7). In fact, it has been reported that Set3C and Rpd3C(S) are co-transcriptionally recruited in the absence of Set1 and Set2, but stimulated by the CTD kinase Kin28/Cdk7. Hence, the Rpd3C(S) and Set3C co-transcriptional recruitment is stimulated by CTD Ser5P to achieve the deacetylation of H3 residues. This, together with evidence that the RNAPII CTD recruits additional chromatin modifying complexes, histone chaperones and elongation factors, suggest that phosphorylated RNAPII is crucial in coordinating the activities of the many factors required for regulating histone dynamics and consequently transcription elongation at actively transcribing genes ([262], and references therein).

6.2. Transport

In addition to the complexes involved in mRNA processing, several other proteins bind to the RNAs as soon as their 5′-end emerges from the RNAPII, packaging them into a messenger ribonucleoparticle (mRNP). This set of interactions of packaging and export factors play a dual function of protecting the RNA from degradation and preparing it to be exported. Although interactions between the CTD and many mRNA processing factors have been characterized, this is not the case for mRNA packaging and export factors. However, packaging and export seems to be also coupled to transcription through RNAPII CTD interactions because defects in transcription elongation, splicing, and 3′-end processing affect export [270]. In yeast, mRNA export is linked to transcription through the TREX (transcription export) complex, which is composed of the THO complex (Tho2, Hpr1, Mft1, and Thp2) and the evolutionally conserved RNA export proteins, Sub2 (UAP56 in human) and Yra1 (REF/Aly in human), and a novel protein termed Tex1 [271-272]. Deletions of the individual THO components causes defects on transcription, transcription-dependent hyper-recombination, and on mRNA export [160, 273]. In addition, the Sub2/Yra1 complex is directly recruited to the actively transcribed regions via the THO complex [272, 274]. Although it has been shown that the TREX complex and Ctk1 are functionally related [159], recruitment of the TREX complex to transcribed genes is not dependent on Ctk1 in yeast [16], and the association of the human TREX complex to transcript might be coupled to transcription indirectly through splicing [275]. Then, the potential role of the CTD and CTD phosphorylation in this process remains unclear, however in a very recent study, the mRNA export factor Yra1 was identified as a CTD phosphorylated-binding protein [276]. Then, this study provides strong support for the idea that the phosphorylated CTD is directly involved in the cotranscriptional recruitment of export factors to active genes. In summary, many aspects of the mRNA metabolism from the 5' capping to the export occur co-transcriptionally and are coordinated through transcription, with the RNAPII CTD and its phosphorylation being the main coordinator in most cases (Figure 7).

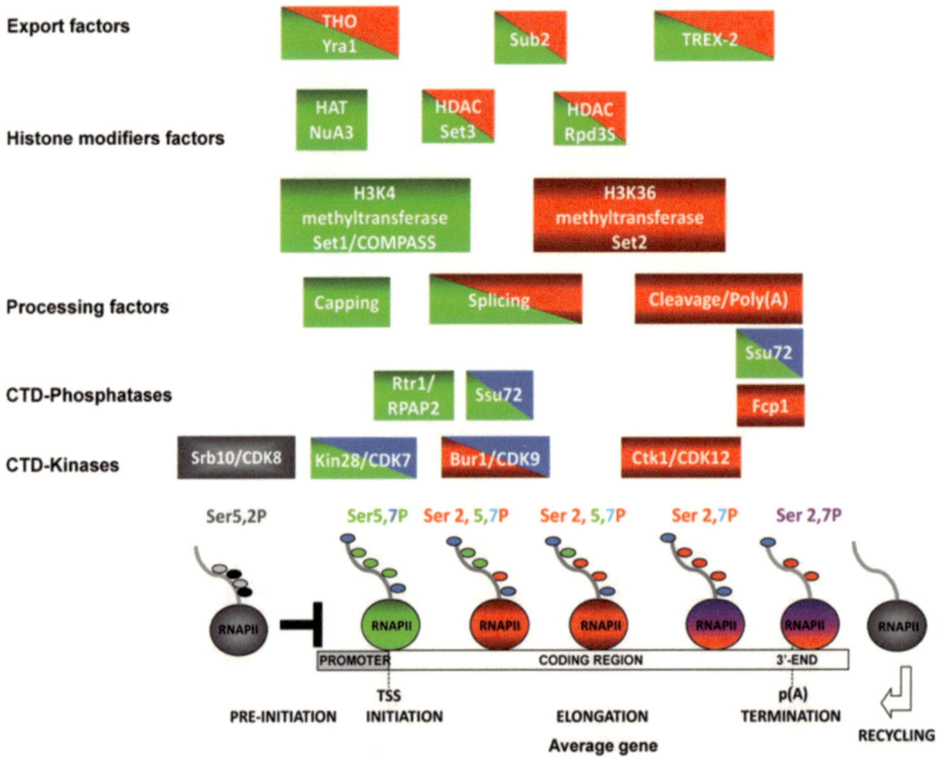

Figure 7. RNAPII CTD phosphorylation/ de-phosphorylation is co-transcriptionally connected and coordinated with other nuclear processes: pre-mRNA processing; histone modifications and mRNA export. The main complexes required for co-transcriptional processes occurring during the expression of a regular protein coding-gene are shown. See text for details.

7. RNAPII CTD phosphorylation and transcription regulation

The levels of CTD phosphorylation/de-phosphorylation are precisely modulated during the entire transcription cycle, which regulates the association of many important factors with initiating and elongating RNAPII, such as transcription and pre-mRNA processing factors, chromatin modifiers and mRNA export factors [21]. The interplay of all of these factors is essential to regulating transcription and, consequently, gene expression. Subsequently, in a regular protein-coding gene, the following set of coordinated nuclear events must occur for it to be properly transcribed in a functional mRNA before it is exported to the cytoplasm and translated (Figure 7). Unphosphorylated RNAPII is recruited to the pre-initiation complex (PIC); then, after its binding to the promoters, it is phosphorylated on Ser5 by yKin28 (hCdk7). Ser5 phosphorylation is required for RNAPII dissociation from the PIC and consequently promotes transcription initiation. Simultaneously, Ser5 phosphorylation targets capping and splicing factor recruitment, the Set1 methyltransferase complex, and the Set3C and Rpd3S histone deacetylase complexes. During early elongation, Ser5P levels are decreased, whereas Ser2P levels increase due to the kinase activity of yBur1 (hCdk9) near the promoters, and by the kinase activity of yCtk1 (hCdk12) at the forward coding and 3'-ends, which leads to the recruitment of the histone methyltransferase Set2 and the activation of the Rpd3S complex, which prevents cryptic transcription within the genes. When RNAPII arrives at and recognizes the termination site, the 3'-end-processing factors that are associated with the CTD achieve cleavage and polyadenylation of the nascent mRNA, which also requires proper phosphorylation of the polymerase. During the termination process, the CTD is de-phosphorylated by Ssu72 and Fcp1, and the polymerase is recycled to initiate a new round of transcription. All along the gene, packaging and export factors (TREX complexes) are incorporated into the transcriptional machinery protecting the transcript from degradation and preparing it for export to the cytoplasm.

8. Therapeutic potential

Cellular differentiation, morphogenesis, development and adaptability of all organisms are subjected to proper gene expression and, therefore, variations in gene regulation can have profound effects on protein function, challenging the viability of the organisms. Currently, it is clear that RNAPII phosphorylation has an important role on gene expression, and therefore, in all the processes mentioned above. Consequently, over the last decade CTD phosphorylation has attracted the attention of biomedical research, especially due to the fact that the CTD kinase Cdk9 has been involved in several physiological cell processes, whose deregulation may be associated with cancer, and also due to the fact that Cdk9 activity is required for human immunodeficiency virus type 1 (HIV-1) replication. Related to it, many studies have shown the enormous potential of Cdk9 kinase inhibition as a treatment of several kinds of tumors, HIV infection, and cardiac hypertrophy.

The human immunodeficiency virus type 1 (HIV-1) requires host cell factors for all steps of the viral replication, among them the transcription elongation factor P-TEFb. Transcription of HIV-1 viral genes is achieved by host RNAPII and is induced by a viral trans-activator protein, Tat. When bound to the TAR viral RNA region, Tat activates HIV-1 transcription by early recruiting of host transcriptional activators including P-TEFb, which phosphorylates RNAPII CTD promoting viral transcript elongation [280]. Thus, treatment with drugs that inhibit Cdk9, such as flavopiridol, has been used as a retroviral therapy on AIDS patients [281]. Therefore, from the point of view of basic research, the study of the functions of Cdk9 and RNAPII CTD phosphorylations are of great interest in understanding the mechanisms that regulate HIV replication, which consequently lead to progress on AIDS biomedical research. Further evidence has been provided of a deregulated Cdk9 function in several tumors such as lymphoma, neuroblastoma, primary neuroectodermal tumor, rhabidomiosarcoma or prostate cancer [282-284]. The Cdk9 inhibition by chemotherapeutic agents, such as flavopiridol or CY-202, has shown to reduce transcription in malignant cells, mainly affecting the short half-lives RNAs. Most of these RNAs code for anti-apoptotic proteins, for instance onco-protein Mcl-1, which is necessary in tumor proliferation maintenance. Unfortunately, they only have a modest activity in patients although promising studies continue at present [285]. Cardiac hypertrophy consists of an increased size of cardiomyocytes, associated to some cardiac diseases as hypertension or diminished heart function. Hypertrophy is a physiological response to a stress stimulus that results in an increase of the cell size, and that may eventually produce a heart failure. Increased cell size produces increased mRNAs transcription, which requires Cdk9 activity. Thus, it has been shown that therapy with Cdk9 inhibitors benefits patients with cardiovascular disorders [286].

9. Concluding remarks

The primary function of the RNAPII CTD phosphorylation in eukaryotes is the integration of transcription with distinct nuclear processes. Thus, CTD phosphorylation operates as a fine-tuning regulatory mechanism during the whole transcription cycle and is consequently of extraordinary importance for proper gene expression. Since the late 1980's, an overwhelming number of laboratories have tried to decipher the mechanism underlying the creation of a CTD code and how this code is translated during transcription to coordinate mRNA processing, export and chromatin modifications. Although great progress has been achieved, most recently due to wide-genomic analysis techniques, a number of issues remained unsolved. For instance, it is very challenging to determine the exact phosphorylation state of specific residues within specific repeats during each step of transcription, as well as to determine the exact number of repeats that are phosphorylated within the CTD at every step of transcription, and how this is related to CTD specific roles in gene expression. Moreover, it needs to be determined if phosphorylation of the repeats with non-consensus sequences is regulated in the same manner as the consensus repeats, and if this is achieved by the same set of CTD modifying enzymes. In addition, other residues such as lysine and arginine can be potentially modified; therefore, further increasing the complexity of the CTD, and suggesting that if they are transcriptionally modified, may further elucidate the CTD functions or discover new ones. Finally, detailed understanding of RNAPII CTD phosphorylation is very relevant and will add insight into the processes that alter gene expression, such as HIV infection and cancer, and will help to investigate if other human CTD modifying enzymes, in addition to Cdk9, may be good candidates for therapy. In conclusion, research has made much progress, but further progress is still needed, and the new massive techniques in genomics and proteomics will help to advance complete understanding much faster.

Author details

Olga Calvo and Alicia García
Instituto de Biología Funcional y Genómica, Consejo Superior de Investigaciones Científicas / Universidad de Salamanca, Spain

Acknowledgement

This work was supported by a grant from the Spanish Ministerio de Ciencia e Innovación (BFU 2009-07179) to OC. AG was supported by a fellowship from the Junta de Castilla y León. The IBFG acknowledges support from "Ramón Areces Foundation".

10. References

[1] Jun SH, Reichlen MJ, Tajiri M, Murakami KS (2011) Archaeal RNA polymerase and transcription regulation. Crit Rev Biochem Mol Biol. 46: 27-40.

[2] Werner F, Grohmann D (2011) Evolution of multisubunit RNA polymerases in the three domains of life. Nat Rev Microbiol. 9: 85-98.

[3] Grohmann D, Werner F (2011) Cycling through transcription with the RNA polymerase F/E (RPB4/7) complex: structure, function and evolution of archaeal RNA polymerase. Res Microbiol. 162: 10-18.

[4] Allison LA, Moyle M, Shales M, Ingles CJ (1985) Extensive homology among the largest subunits of eukaryotic and prokaryotic RNA polymerases. Cell. 42: 599-610.

[5] Corden JL (1990) Tails of RNA polymerase II. Trends Biochem Sci. 15: 383-387.

[6] Buratowski S (2003) The CTD code. Nat Struct Biol. 10: 679-680.

[7] Corden JL (2007) Transcription. Seven ups the code. Science. 318: 1735-1736.

[8] Egloff S, Murphy S (2008) Cracking the RNA polymerase II CTD code. Trends Genet. 24: 280-288.

[9] Hahn S, Young ET (2011) Transcriptional regulation in Saccharomyces cerevisiae: transcription factor regulation and function, mechanisms of initiation, and roles of activators and coactivators. Genetics. 189: 705-736.

[10] Sikorski TW, Buratowski S (2009) The basal initiation machinery: beyond the general transcription factors. Curr Opin Cell Biol. 21: 344-351.

[11] Thomas MC, Chiang CM (2006) The general transcription machinery and general cofactors. Crit Rev Biochem Mol Biol. 41: 105-178.

[12] Saunders A, Core LJ, Lis JT (2006) Breaking barriers to transcription elongation. Nat Rev Mol Cell Biol. 7: 557-567.

[13] Selth LA, Sigurdsson S, Svejstrup JQ (2010) Transcript Elongation by RNA Polymerase II. Annu Rev Biochem. 79: 271-293.

[14] Shilatifard A, Conaway RC, Conaway JW (2003) The RNA polymerase II elongation complex. Annu Rev Biochem. 72: 693-715.

[15] Pokholok DK, Hannett NM, Young RA (2002) Exchange of RNA polymerase II initiation and elongation factors during gene expression in vivo. Mol Cell. 9: 799-809.

[16] Ahn SH, Kim M, Buratowski S (2004) Phosphorylation of serine 2 within the RNA polymerase II C-terminal domain couples transcription and 3' end processing. Mol Cell. 13: 67-76.

[17] Hirose Y, Manley JL (2000) RNA polymerase II and the integration of nuclear events. Genes Dev. 14: 1415-1429.

[18] Mason PB, Struhl K (2005) Distinction and relationship between elongation rate and processivity of RNA polymerase II in vivo. Mol Cell. 17: 831-840.

[19] Orphanides G, Reinberg D (2000) RNA polymerase II elongation through chromatin. Nature. 407: 471-475.

[20] Orphanides G, Reinberg D (2002) A unified theory of gene expression. Cell. 108: 439-451.

[21] Perales R, Bentley D (2009) "Cotranscriptionality": the transcription elongation complex as a nexus for nuclear transactions. Mol Cell. 36: 178-191.

[22] Carmody SR, Wente SR (2009) mRNA nuclear export at a glance. J Cell Sci. 122: 1933-1937.

[23] Chanarat S, Seizl M, Strasser K (2011) The Prp19 complex is a novel transcription elongation factor required for TREX occupancy at transcribed genes. Genes Dev. 25: 1147-1158.

[24] Gonzalez-Aguilera C, Tous C, Babiano R, de la Cruz J, Luna R, Aguilera A (2011) Nab2 functions in the metabolism of RNA driven by polymerases II and III. Mol Biol Cell. 22: 2729-2740.

[25] Iglesias N, Stutz F (2008) Regulation of mRNP dynamics along the export pathway. FEBS Lett. 582: 1987-1996.

[26] Komili S, Silver PA (2008) Coupling and coordination in gene expression processes: a systems biology view. Nat Rev Genet. 9: 38-48.

[27] Kruk JA, Dutta A, Fu J, Gilmour DS, Reese JC (2011) The multifunctional Ccr4-Not complex directly promotes transcription elongation. Genes Dev. 25: 581-593.

[28] Svejstrup JQ (2007) Elongator complex: how many roles does it play? Curr Opin Cell Biol. 19: 331-336.

[29] Maniatis T, Reed R (2002) An extensive network of coupling among gene expression machines. Nature. 416: 499-506.

[30] Proudfoot NJ, Furger A, Dye MJ (2002) Integrating mRNA processing with transcription. Cell. 108: 501-512.

[31] Buratowski S (2009) Progression through the RNA polymerase II CTD cycle. Mol Cell. 36: 541-546.

[32] Phatnani HP, Greenleaf AL (2006) Phosphorylation and functions of the RNA polymerase II CTD. Genes Dev. 20: 2922-2936.

[33] Cramer P (2002) Multisubunit RNA polymerases. Curr Opin Struct Biol. 12: 89-97.

[34] Cramer P (2002) Common structural features of nucleic acid polymerases. Bioessays. 24: 724-729.

[35] Corden JL, Cadena DL, Ahearn JM, Jr., Dahmus ME (1985) A unique structure at the carboxyl terminus of the largest subunit of eukaryotic RNA polymerase II. Proc Natl Acad Sci U S A. 82: 7934-7938.

[36] Liu P, Greenleaf AL, Stiller JW (2008) The essential sequence elements required for RNAPII carboxyl-terminal domain function in yeast and their evolutionary conservation. Mol Biol Evol. 25: 719-727.

[37] Liu P, Kenney JM, Stiller JW, Greenleaf AL (2010) Genetic organization, length conservation, and evolution of RNA polymerase II carboxyl-terminal domain. Mol Biol Evol. 27: 2628-2641.

[38] Chapman RD, Heidemann M, Hintermair C, Eick D (2008) Molecular evolution of the RNA polymerase II CTD. Trends Genet. 24: 289-296.

[39] Prelich G (2002) RNA polymerase II carboxy-terminal domain kinases: emerging clues to their function. Eukaryot Cell. 1: 153-162.

[40] Wintzerith M, Acker J, Vicaire S, Vigneron M, Kedinger C (1992) Complete sequence of the human RNA polymerase II largest subunit. Nucleic Acids Res. 20: 910.

[41] Allison LA, Wong JK, Fitzpatrick VD, Moyle M, Ingles CJ (1988) The C-terminal domain of the largest subunit of RNA polymerase II of Saccharomyces cerevisiae, Drosophila melanogaster, and mammals: a conserved structure with an essential function. Mol Cell Biol. 8: 321-329.

[42] McCracken S, Fong N, Yankulov K, Ballantyne S, Pan G, Greenblatt J, Patterson SD, Wickens M, Bentley DL (1997) The C-terminal domain of RNA polymerase II couples mRNA processing to transcription. Nature. 385: 357-361.

[43] Schwartz LB, Roeder RG (1975) Purification and subunit structure of deoxyribonucleic acid-dependent ribonucleic acid polymerase II from the mouse plasmacytoma, MOPC 315. J Biol Chem. 250: 3221-3228.

[44] Cadena DL, Dahmus ME (1987) Messenger RNA synthesis in mammalian cells is catalyzed by the phosphorylated form of RNA polymerase II. J Biol Chem. 262: 12468-12474.

[45] Zhang J, Corden JL (1991) Phosphorylation causes a conformational change in the carboxyl-terminal domain of the mouse RNA polymerase II largest subunit. J Biol Chem. 266: 2297-2302.

[46] Lu H, Flores O, Weinmann R, Reinberg D (1991) The nonphosphorylated form of RNA polymerase II preferentially associates with the preinitiation complex. Proc. Natl. Acad. Sci. U S A. 88: 10004-10008.

[47] Cho H, Kim TK, Mancebo H, Lane WS, Flores O, Reinberg D (1999) A protein phosphatase functions to recycle RNA polymerase II. Genes Dev. 13: 1540-1552.

[48] Komarnitsky P, Cho EJ, Buratowski S (2000) Different phosphorylated forms of RNA polymerase II and associated mRNA processing factors during transcription. Genes Dev. 14: 2452-2460.

[49] Kim M, Ahn SH, Krogan NJ, Greenblatt JF, Buratowski S (2004) Transitions in RNA polymerase II elongation complexes at the 3' ends of genes. EMBO J. 23: 354-364.

[50] Zhang DW, Mosley AL, Ramisetty SR, Rodriguez-Molina JB, Washburn MP, Ansari AZ (2012) Ssu72 Phosphatase-dependent Erasure of Phospho-Ser7 Marks on the RNA Polymerase II C-terminal Domain Is Essential for Viability and Transcription Termination. J Biol Chem. 287: 8541-8551.

[51] Palancade B, Bensaude O (2003) Investigating RNA polymerase II carboxyl-terminal domain (CTD) phosphorylation. Eur J Biochem. 270: 3859-3870.

[52] Baskaran R, Chiang GG, Mysliwiec T, Kruh GD, Wang JY (1997) Tyrosine phosphorylation of RNA polymerase II carboxyl-terminal domain by the Abl-related gene product. J Biol Chem. 272: 18905-18909.

[53] Baskaran R, Dahmus ME, Wang JY (1993) Tyrosine phosphorylation of mammalian RNA polymerase II carboxyl-terminal domain. Proc Natl Acad Sci U S A. 90: 11167-11171.

[54] Hsin JP, Sheth A, Manley JL (2011) RNAPII CTD phosphorylated on threonine-4 is required for histone mRNA 3' end processing. Science. 334: 683-686.

[55] Wu X, Wilcox CB, Devasahayam G, Hackett RL, Arevalo-Rodriguez M, Cardenas ME, Heitman J, Hanes SD (2000) The Ess1 prolyl isomerase is linked to chromatin remodeling complexes and the general transcription machinery. EMBO J. 19: 3727-3738.
[56] Sims RJ, 3rd, Rojas LA, Beck D, Bonasio R, Schuller R, Drury WJ, 3rd, Eick D, Reinberg D (2011) The C-terminal domain of RNA polymerase II is modified by site-specific methylation. Science. 332: 99-103.
[57] Kelly WG, Dahmus ME, Hart GW (1993) RNA polymerase II is a glycoprotein. Modification of the COOH-terminal domain by O-GlcNAc. J Biol Chem. 268: 10416-10424.
[58] Kim YJ, Bjorklund S, Li Y, Sayre MH, Kornberg RD (1994) A multiprotein mediator of transcriptional activation and its interaction with the C-terminal repeat domain of RNA polymerase II. Cell. 77: 599-608.
[59] Corden JL (1993) RNA polymerase II transcription cycles. Curr Opin Genet Dev. 3: 213-218.
[60] Corden JL, Patturajan M (1997) A CTD function linking transcription to splicing. Trends Biochem Sci. 22: 413-416.
[61] Gudipati RK, Villa T, Boulay J, Libri D (2008) Phosphorylation of the RNA polymerase II C-terminal domain dictates transcription termination choice. Nat Struct Mol Biol. 15: 786-794.
[62] Vasiljeva L, Kim M, Mutschler H, Buratowski S, Meinhart A (2008) The Nrd1-Nab3-Sen1 termination complex interacts with the Ser5-phosphorylated RNA polymerase II C-terminal domain. Nat Struct Mol Biol. 15: 795-804.
[63] Egloff S, Murphy S (2008) Role of the C-terminal domain of RNA polymerase II in expression of small nuclear RNA genes. Biochem Soc Trans. 36: 537-539.
[64] Egloff S, O'Reilly D, Chapman RD, Taylor A, Tanzhaus K, Pitts L, Eick D, Murphy S (2007) Serine-7 of the RNA polymerase II CTD is specifically required for snRNA gene expression. Science. 318: 1777-1779.
[65] Jacobs EY, Ogiwara I, Weiner AM (2004) Role of the C-terminal domain of RNA polymerase II in U2 snRNA transcription and 3' processing. Mol Cell Biol. 24: 846-855.
[66] Patturajan M, Schulte RJ, Sefton BM, Berezney R, Vincent M, Bensaude O, Warren SL, Corden JL (1998) Growth-related changes in phosphorylation of yeast RNA polymerase II. J Biol Chem. 273: 4689-4694.
[67] Schroeder SC, Schwer B, Shuman S, Bentley D (2000) Dynamic association of capping enzymes with transcribing RNA polymerase II. Genes Dev. 14: 2435-2440.
[68] Chapman RD, Heidemann M, Albert TK, Mailhammer R, Flatley A, Meisterernst M, Kremmer E, Eick D (2007) Transcribing RNA polymerase II is phosphorylated at CTD residue serine-7. Science. 318: 1780-1782.
[69] Bataille AR, Jeronimo C, Jacques PE, Laramee L, Fortin ME, Forest A, Bergeron M, Hanes SD, Robert F (2012) A universal RNA polymerase II CTD cycle is orchestrated by complex interplays between kinase, phosphatase, and isomerase enzymes along genes. Mol Cell. 45: 158-170.
[70] Kim H, Erickson B, Luo W, Seward D, Graber JH, Pollock DD, Megee PC, Bentley DL (2010) Gene-specific RNA polymerase II phosphorylation and the CTD code. Nat Struct Mol Biol. 17: 1279-1286.

[71] Mayer A, Lidschreiber M, Siebert M, Leike K, Soding J, Cramer P (2010) Uniform transitions of the general RNA polymerase II transcription complex. Nat Struct Mol Biol. 17: 1272-1278.

[72] Rodriguez CR, Cho EJ, Keogh MC, Moore CL, Greenleaf AL, Buratowski S (2000) Kin28, the TFIIH-associated carboxy-terminal domain kinase, facilitates the recruitment of mRNA processing machinery to RNA polymerase II. Mol Cell Biol. 20: 104-112.

[73] Cho EJ, Kobor MS, Kim M, Greenblatt J, Buratowski S (2001) Opposing effects of Ctk1 kinase and Fcp1 phosphatase at Ser 2 of the RNA polymerase II C-terminal domain. Genes Dev. 15: 3319-3329.

[74] Akhtar MS, Heidemann M, Tietjen JR, Zhang DW, Chapman RD, Eick D, Ansari AZ (2009) TFIIH kinase places bivalent marks on the carboxy-terminal domain of RNA polymerase II. Mol Cell. 34: 387-393.

[75] Glover-Cutter K, Larochelle S, Erickson B, Zhang C, Shokat K, Fisher RP, Bentley DL (2009) TFIIH-associated Cdk7 kinase functions in phosphorylation of C-terminal domain Ser7 residues, promoter-proximal pausing, and termination by RNA polymerase II. Mol Cell Biol. 29: 5455-5464.

[76] Kim M, Suh H, Cho EJ, Buratowski S (2009) Phosphorylation of the yeast Rpb1 C-terminal domain at serines 2, 5, and 7. J Biol Chem. 284: 26421-26426.

[77] Tietjen JR, Zhang DW, Rodriguez-Molina JB, White BE, Akhtar MS, Heidemann M, Li X, Chapman RD, Shokat K, Keles S, Eick D, Ansari AZ (2010) Chemical-genomic dissection of the CTD code. Nat Struct Mol Biol. 17: 1154-1161.

[78] Ghosh A, Shuman S, Lima CD (2011) Structural insights to how mammalian capping enzyme reads the CTD code. Mol Cell. 43: 299-310.

[79] Krishnamurthy S, He X, Reyes-Reyes M, Moore C, Hampsey M (2004) Ssu72 Is an RNA polymerase II CTD phosphatase. Mol Cell. 14: 387-394.

[80] Svejstrup JQ, Li Y, Fellows J, Gnatt A, Bjorklund S, Kornberg RD (1997) Evidence for a mediator cycle at the initiation of transcription. Proc Natl Acad Sci U S A. 94: 6075-6078.

[81] West ML, Corden JL (1995) Construction and analysis of yeast RNA polymerase II CTD deletion and substitution mutations. Genetics. 140: 1223-1233.

[82] Zhang J, Corden JL (1991) Identification of phosphorylation sites in the repetitive carboxyl-terminal domain of the mouse RNA polymerase II largest subunit. J Biol Chem. 266: 2290-2296.

[83] Chapman RD, Palancade B, Lang A, Bensaude O, Eick D (2004) The last CTD repeat of the mammalian RNA polymerase II large subunit is important for its stability. Nucleic Acids Res. 32: 35-44.

[84] Fong N, Bird G, Vigneron M, Bentley DL (2003) A 10 residue motif at the C-terminus of the RNA pol II CTD is required for transcription, splicing and 3' end processing. EMBO J. 22: 4274-4282.

[85] Baskaran R, Escobar SR, Wang JY (1999) Nuclear c-Abl is a COOH-terminal repeated domain (CTD)-tyrosine (CTD)-tyrosine kinase-specific for the mammalian RNA polymerase II: possible role in transcription elongation. Cell Growth Differ. 10: 387-396.

[86] Munoz MJ, de la Mata M, Kornblihtt AR (2010) The carboxy terminal domain of RNA polymerase II and alternative splicing. Trends Biochem Sci. 35: 497-504.

[87] Kamenski T, Heilmeier S, Meinhart A, Cramer P (2004) Structure and mechanism of RNA polymerase II CTD phosphatases. Mol Cell. 15: 399-407.

[88] Meinhart A, Kamenski T, Hoeppner S, Baumli S, Cramer P (2005) A structural perspective of CTD function. Genes Dev. 19: 1401-1415.

[89] Bartkowiak B, Liu P, Phatnani HP, Fuda NJ, Cooper JJ, Price DH, Adelman K, Lis JT, Greenleaf AL (2010) CDK12 is a transcription elongation-associated CTD kinase, the metazoan ortholog of yeast Ctk1. Genes Dev. 24: 2303-2316.

[90] Akoulitchev S, Chuikov S, Reinberg D (2000) TFIIH is negatively regulated by cdk8-containing mediator complexes. Nature. 407: 102-106.

[91] Hallberg M, Polozkov GV, Hu GZ, Beve J, Gustafsson CM, Ronne H, Bjorklund S (2004) Site-specific Srb10-dependent phosphorylation of the yeast Mediator subunit Med2 regulates gene expression from the 2-microm plasmid. Proc Natl Acad Sci U S A. 101: 3370-3375.

[92] Hengartner CJ, Myer VE, Liao SM, Wilson CJ, Koh SS, Young RA (1998) Temporal regulation of RNA polymerase II by Srb10 and Kin28 cyclin-dependent kinases. Mol Cell. 2: 43-53.

[93] Larschan E, Winston F (2005) The Saccharomyces cerevisiae Srb8-Srb11 complex functions with the SAGA complex during Gal4-activated transcription. Mol Cell Biol. 25: 114-123.

[94] Liu Y, Kung C, Fishburn J, Ansari AZ, Shokat KM, Hahn S (2004) Two cyclin-dependent kinases promote RNA polymerase II transcription and formation of the scaffold complex. Mol Cell Biol. 24: 1721-1735.

[95] Fabrega C, Shen V, Shuman S, Lima CD (2003) Structure of an mRNA capping enzyme bound to the phosphorylated carboxy-terminal domain of RNA polymerase II. Mol Cell. 11: 1549-1561.

[96] Guidi BW, Bjornsdottir G, Hopkins DC, Lacomis L, Erdjument-Bromage H, Tempst P, Myers LC (2004) Mutual targeting of mediator and the TFIIH kinase Kin28. J Biol Chem. 279: 29114-29120.

[97] Govind CK, Zhang F, Qiu H, Hofmeyer K, Hinnebusch AG (2007) Gcn5 promotes acetylation, eviction, and methylation of nucleosomes in transcribed coding regions. Mol Cell. 25: 31-42.

[98] Ng HH, Robert F, Young RA, Struhl K (2003) Targeted recruitment of Set1 histone methylase by elongating Pol II provides a localized mark and memory of recent transcriptional activity. Mol Cell. 11: 709-719.

[99] Qiu H, Hu C, Hinnebusch AG (2009) Phosphorylation of the Pol II CTD by KIN28 enhances BUR1/BUR2 recruitment and Ser2 CTD phosphorylation near promoters. Mol Cell. 33: 752-762.

[100] Wong CM, Qiu H, Hu C, Dong J, Hinnebusch AG (2007) Yeast cap binding complex impedes recruitment of cleavage factor IA to weak termination sites. Mol Cell Biol. 27: 6520-6531.

[101] Laribee RN, Krogan NJ, Xiao T, Shibata Y, Hughes TR, Greenblatt JF, Strahl BD (2005) BUR kinase selectively regulates H3 K4 trimethylation and H2B ubiquitylation through recruitment of the PAF elongation complex. Curr Biol. 15: 1487-1493.

[102] Liu Y, Warfield L, Zhang C, Luo J, Allen J, Lang WH, Ranish J, Shokat KM, Hahn S (2009) Phosphorylation of the transcription elongation factor Spt5 by yeast Bur1 kinase stimulates recruitment of the PAF complex. Mol Cell Biol. 29: 4852-4863.

[103] Wood A, Schneider J, Dover J, Johnston M, Shilatifard A (2005) The Bur1/Bur2 complex is required for histone H2B monoubiquitination by Rad6/Bre1 and histone methylation by COMPASS. Mol Cell. 20: 589-599.

[104] Zhou Z, Lin IJ, Darst RP, Bungert J (2009) Maneuver at the transcription start site: Mot1p and NC2 navigate TFIID/TBP to specific core promoter elements. Epigenetics. 4: 1-4.

[105] Ahn SH, Keogh MC, Buratowski S (2009) Ctk1 promotes dissociation of basal transcription factors from elongating RNA polymerase II. EMBO J. 28: 205-212.

[106] Licatalosi DD, Geiger G, Minet M, Schroeder S, Cilli K, McNeil JB, Bentley DL (2002) Functional interaction of yeast pre-mRNA 3' end processing factors with RNA polymerase II. Mol Cell. 9: 1101-1111.

[107] Meinhart A, Cramer P (2004) Recognition of RNA polymerase II carboxy-terminal domain by 3'-RNA-processing factors. Nature. 430: 223-226.

[108] Ni Z, Schwartz BE, Werner J, Suarez JR, Lis JT (2004) Coordination of transcription, RNA processing, and surveillance by P-TEFb kinase on heat shock genes. Mol Cell. 13: 55-65.

[109] Ramanathan Y, Rajpara SM, Reza SM, Lees E, Shuman S, Mathews MB, Pe'ery T (2001) Three RNA polymerase II carboxyl-terminal domain kinases display distinct substrate preferences. J Biol Chem. 276: 10913-10920.

[110] Rother S, Strasser K (2007) The RNA polymerase II CTD kinase Ctk1 functions in translation elongation. Genes Dev. 21: 1409-1421.

[111] Wood A, Shukla A, Schneider J, Lee JS, Stanton JD, Dzuiba T, Swanson SK, Florens L, Washburn MP, Wyrick J, Bhaumik SR, Shilatifard A (2007) Ctk complex-mediated regulation of histone methylation by COMPASS. Mol Cell Biol. 27: 709-720.

[112] Yoh SM, Cho H, Pickle L, Evans RM, Jones KA (2007) The Spt6 SH2 domain binds Ser2-P RNAPII to direct Iws1-dependent mRNA splicing and export. Genes Dev. 21: 160-174.

[113] Liao SM, Zhang J, Jeffery DA, Koleske AJ, Thompson CM, Chao DM, Viljoen M, van Vuuren HJ, Young RA (1995) A kinase-cyclin pair in the RNA polymerase II holoenzyme. Nature. 374: 193-196.

[114] Kornberg RD (2005) Mediator and the mechanism of transcriptional activation. Trends Biochem Sci. 30: 235-239.

[115] Taatjes DJ (2010) The human Mediator complex: a versatile, genome-wide regulator of transcription. Trends Biochem Sci. 35: 315-322.

[116] Holstege FC, Jennings EG, Wyrick JJ, Lee TI, Hengartner CJ, Green MR, Golub TR, Lander ES, Young RA (1998) Dissecting the regulatory circuitry of a eukaryotic genome. Cell. 95: 717-728.

[117] Knuesel MT, Meyer KD, Bernecky C, Taatjes DJ (2009) The human CDK8 subcomplex is a molecular switch that controls Mediator coactivator function. Genes Dev. 23: 439-451.

[118] Carlson M (1997) Genetics of transcriptional regulation in yeast: connections to the RNA polymerase II CTD. Annu. Rev. Cell Dev. Biol. 13: 1-23.

[119] Yudkovsky N, Ranish JA, Hahn S (2000) A transcription reinitiation intermediate that is stabilized by activator. Nature. 408: 225-229.

[120] Hirst M, Kobor MS, Kuriakose N, Greenblatt J, Sadowski I (1999) GAL4 is regulated by the RNA polymerase II holoenzyme-associated cyclin-dependent protein kinase SRB10/CDK8. Mol Cell. 3: 673-678.

[121] Vincent O, Kuchin S, Hong SP, Townley R, Vyas VK, Carlson M (2001) Interaction of the Srb10 kinase with Sip4, a transcriptional activator of gluconeogenic genes in Saccharomyces cerevisiae. Mol Cell Biol. 21: 5790-5796.

[122] Galbraith MD, Donner AJ, Espinosa JM (2010) CDK8: a positive regulator of transcription. Transcription. 1: 4-12.

[123] Chi Y, Huddleston MJ, Zhang X, Young RA, Annan RS, Carr SA, Deshaies RJ (2001) Negative regulation of Gcn4 and Msn2 transcription factors by Srb10 cyclin-dependent kinase. Genes Dev. 15: 1078-1092.

[124] Nelson C, Goto S, Lund K, Hung W, Sadowski I (2003) Srb10/Cdk8 regulates yeast filamentous growth by phosphorylating the transcription factor Ste12. Nature. 421: 187-190.

[125] Keogh MC, Cho EJ, Podolny V, Buratowski S (2002) Kin28 is found within TFIIH and a Kin28-Ccl1-Tfb3 trimer complex with differential sensitivities to T-loop phosphorylation. Mol Cell Biol. 22: 1288-1297.

[126] Roy R, Adamczewski JP, Seroz T, Vermeulen W, Tassan JP, Schaeffer L, Nigg EA, Hoeijmakers JH, Egly JM (1994) The MO15 cell cycle kinase is associated with the TFIIH transcription-DNA repair factor. Cell. 79: 1093-1101.

[127] Serizawa H, Makela TP, Conaway JW, Conaway RC, Weinberg RA, Young RA (1995) Association of Cdk-activating kinase subunits with transcription factor TFIIH. Nature. 374: 280-282.

[128] Shiekhattar R, Mermelstein F, Fisher RP, Drapkin R, Dynlacht B, Wessling HC, Morgan DO, Reinberg D (1995) Cdk-activating kinase complex is a component of human transcription factor TFIIH. Nature. 374: 283-287.

[129] Cismowski MJ, Laff GM, Solomon MJ, Reed SI (1995) KIN28 encodes a C-terminal domain kinase that controls mRNA transcription in Saccharomyces cerevisiae but lacks cyclin-dependent kinase-activating kinase (CAK) activity. Mol Cell Biol. 15: 2983-2992.

[130] Espinoza FH, Farrell A, Nourse JL, Chamberlin HM, Gileadi O, Morgan DO (1998) Cak1 is required for Kin28 phosphorylation and activation in vivo. Mol Cell Biol. 18: 6365-6373.

[131] Kaldis P, Sutton A, Solomon MJ (1996) The Cdk-activating kinase (CAK) from budding yeast. Cell. 86: 553-564.

[132] Simon M, Seraphin B, Faye G (1986) KIN28, a yeast split gene coding for a putative protein kinase homologous to CDC28. EMBO J. 5: 2697-2701.

[133] Akoulitchev S, Makela TP, Weinberg RA, Reinberg D (1995) Requirement for TFIIH kinase activity in transcription by RNA polymerase II. Nature. 377: 557-560.

[134] Jiang Y, Yan M, Gralla JD (1996) A three-step pathway of transcription initiation leading to promoter clearance at an activation RNA polymerase II promoter. Mol Cell Biol. 16: 1614-1621.

[135] Cho EJ, Takagi T, Moore CR, Buratowski S (1997) mRNA capping enzyme is recruited to the transcription complex by phosphorylation of the RNA polymerase II carboxy-terminal domain. Genes Dev. 11: 3319-3326.

[136] Ho CK, Shuman S (1999) Distinct roles for CTD Ser-2 and Ser-5 phosphorylation in the recruitment and allosteric activation of mammalian mRNA capping enzyme. Mol Cell. 3: 405-411.

[137] McCracken S, Fong N, Rosonina E, Yankulov K, Brothers G, Siderovski D, Hessel A, Foster S, Shuman S, Bentley DL (1997) 5'-Capping enzymes are targeted to pre-mRNA by binding to the phosphorylated carboxy-terminal domain of RNA polymerase II. Genes Dev. 11: 3306-3318.

[138] Qiu H, Hu C, Wong CM, Hinnebusch AG (2006) The Spt4p subunit of yeast DSIF stimulates association of the Paf1 complex with elongating RNA polymerase II. Mol Cell Biol. 26: 3135-3148.

[139] Ranish JA, Yudkovsky N, Hahn S (1999) Intermediates in formation and activity of the RNA polymerase II preinitiation complex: holoenzyme recruitment and a postrecruitment role for the TATA box and TFIIB. Genes Dev. 13: 49-63.

[140] Borggrefe T, Davis R, Erdjument-Bromage H, Tempst P, Kornberg RD (2002) A complex of the Srb8, -9, -10, and -11 transcriptional regulatory proteins from yeast. J Biol Chem. 277: 44202-44207.

[141] Valay JG, Simon M, Dubois MF, Bensaude O, Facca C, Faye G (1995) The KIN28 gene is required both for RNA polymerase II mediated transcription and phosphorylation of the Rpb1p CTD. J Mol Biol. 249: 535-544.

[142] Wada T, Takagi T, Yamaguchi Y, Watanabe D, Handa H (1998) Evidence that P-TEFb alleviates the negative effect of DSIF on RNA polymerase II-dependent transcription in vitro. EMBO J. 17: 7395-7403.

[143] Wada T, Orphanides G, Hasegawa J, Kim DK, Shima D, Yamaguchi Y, Fukuda A, Hisatake K, Oh S, Reinberg D, Handa H (2000) FACT relieves DSIF/NELF-mediated inhibition of transcriptional elongation and reveals functional differences between P-TEFb and TFIIH. Mol Cell. 5: 1067-1072.

[144] Yamaguchi Y, Takagi T, Wada T, Yano K, Furuya A, Sugimoto S, Hasegawa J, Handa H (1999) NELF, a multisubunit complex containing RD, cooperates with DSIF to repress RNA polymerase II elongation. Cell. 97: 41-51.

[145] Bartkowiak B, Greenleaf AL (2011) Phosphorylation of RNAPII: To P-TEFb or not to P-TEFb? Transcription. 2: 115-119.

[146] Viladevall L, St Amour CV, Rosebrock A, Schneider S, Zhang C, Allen JJ, Shokat KM, Schwer B, Leatherwood JK, Fisher RP (2009) TFIIH and P-TEFb coordinate transcription with capping enzyme recruitment at specific genes in fission yeast. Mol Cell. 33: 738-751.

[147] Keogh MC, Podolny V, Buratowski S (2003) Bur1 kinase is required for efficient transcription elongation by RNA polymerase II. Mol Cell Biol. 23: 7005-7018.

[148] Yao S, Neiman A, Prelich G (2000) BUR1 and BUR2 encode a divergent cyclin-dependent kinase-cyclin complex important for transcription in vivo. Mol Cell Biol. 20: 7080-7087.

[149] Wood A, Shilatifard A (2006) Bur1/Bur2 and the Ctk complex in yeast: the split personality of mammalian P-TEFb. Cell Cycle. 5: 1066-1068.

[150] Murray S, Udupa R, Yao S, Hartzog G, Prelich G (2001) Phosphorylation of the RNA polymerase II carboxy-terminal domain by the Bur1 cyclin-dependent kinase. Mol Cell Biol. 21: 4089-4096.

[151] Lindstrom DL, Hartzog GA (2001) Genetic interactions of Spt4-Spt5 and TFIIS with the RNA polymerase II CTD and CTD modifying enzymes in Saccharomyces cerevisiae. Genetics. 159: 487-497.

[152] Chu Y, Simic R, Warner MH, Arndt KM, Prelich G (2007) Regulation of histone modification and cryptic transcription by the Bur1 and Paf1 complexes. EMBO J. 26: 4646-4656.

[153] Pei Y, Shuman S (2003) Characterization of the Schizosaccharomyces pombe Cdk9/Pch1 protein kinase: Spt5 phosphorylation, autophosphorylation, and mutational analysis. J Biol Chem. 278: 43346-43356.

[154] Zhou K, Kuo WH, Fillingham J, Greenblatt JF (2009) Control of transcriptional elongation and cotranscriptional histone modification by the yeast BUR kinase substrate Spt5. Proc. Natl. Acad. Sci. U S A. 106: 6956-6961.

[155] Sterner DE, Lee JM, Hardin SE, Greenleaf AL (1995) The yeast carboxyl-terminal repeat domain kinase CTDK-I is a divergent cyclin-cyclin-dependent kinase complex. Mol Cell Biol. 15: 5716-5724.

[156] Jones JC, Phatnani HP, Haystead TA, MacDonald JA, Alam SM, Greenleaf AL (2004) C-terminal repeat domain kinase I phosphorylates Ser2 and Ser5 of RNA polymerase II C-terminal domain repeats. J Biol Chem. 279: 24957-24964.

[157] Skaar DA, Greenleaf AL (2002) The RNA polymerase II CTD kinase CTDK-I affects pre-mRNA 3' cleavage/polyadenylation through the processing component Pti1p. Mol Cell. 10: 1429-1439.

[158] Xiao T, Shibata Y, Rao B, Laribee RN, O'Rourke R, Buck MJ, Greenblatt JF, Krogan NJ, Lieb JD, Strahl BD (2007) The RNA polymerase II kinase Ctk1 regulates positioning of a 5' histone methylation boundary along genes. Mol Cell Biol. 27: 721-731.

[159] Hurt E, Luo MJ, Rother S, Reed R, Strasser K (2004) Cotranscriptional recruitment of the serine-arginine-rich (SR)-like proteins Gbp2 and Hrb1 to nascent mRNA via the TREX complex. Proc Natl Acad Sci U S A. 101: 1858-1862.

[160] Jimeno S, Rondon AG, Luna R, Aguilera A (2002) The yeast THO complex and mRNA export factors link RNA metabolism with transcription and genome instability. EMBO J. 21: 3526-3535.

[161] Bouchoux C, Hautbergue G, Grenetier S, Carles C, Riva M, Goguel V (2004) CTD kinase I is involved in RNA polymerase I transcription. Nucleic Acids Res. 32: 5851-5860.

[162] Grenetier S, Bouchoux C, Goguel V (2006) CTD kinase I is required for the integrity of the rDNA tandem array. Nucleic Acids Res. 34: 4996-5006.

[163] Ostapenko D, Solomon MJ (2003) Budding yeast CTDK-I is required for DNA damage-induced transcription. Eukaryot Cell. 2: 274-283.

[164] Hampsey M, Kinzy TG (2007) Synchronicity: policing multiple aspects of gene expression by Ctk1. Genes Dev. 21: 1288-1291.

[165] Kong SE, Kobor MS, Krogan NJ, Somesh BP, Sogaard TM, Greenblatt JF, Svejstrup JQ (2005) Interaction of Fcp1 phosphatase with elongating RNA polymerase II holoenzyme, enzymatic mechanism of action, and genetic interaction with elongator. J Biol Chem. 280: 4299-4306.

[166] Dichtl B, Blank D, Ohnacker M, Friedlein A, Roeder D, Langen H, Keller W (2002) A role for SSU72 in balancing RNA polymerase II transcription elongation and termination. Mol Cell. 10: 1139-1150.

[167] Mosley AL, Pattenden SG, Carey M, Venkatesh S, Gilmore JM, Florens L, Workman JL, Washburn MP (2009) Rtr1 is a CTD phosphatase that regulates RNA polymerase II during the transition from serine 5 to serine 2 phosphorylation. Mol Cell. 34: 168-178.

[168] Yeo M, Lin PS, Dahmus ME, Gill GN (2003) A novel RNA polymerase II C-terminal domain phosphatase that preferentially dephosphorylates serine 5. J Biol Chem. 278: 26078-26085.

[169] Jeronimo C, Forget D, Bouchard A, Li Q, Chua G, Poitras C, Therien C, Bergeron D, Bourassa S, Greenblatt J, Chabot B, Poirier GG, Hughes TR, Blanchette M, Price DH, Coulombe B (2007) Systematic analysis of the protein interaction network for the human transcription machinery reveals the identity of the 7SK capping enzyme. Mol Cell. 27: 262-274.

[170] Egloff S, Zaborowska J, Laitem C, Kiss T, Murphy S (2012) Ser7 phosphorylation of the CTD recruits the RPAP2 Ser5 phosphatase to snRNA genes. Mol Cell. 45: 111-122.

[171] Gibney PA, Fries T, Bailer SM, Morano KA (2008) Rtr1 is the Saccharomyces cerevisiae homolog of a novel family of RNA polymerase II-binding proteins. Eukaryot Cell. 7: 938-948.

[172] Ansari A, Hampsey M (2005) A role for the CPF 3'-end processing machinery in RNAPII-dependent gene looping. Genes Dev. 19: 2969-2978.

[173] Ganem C, Devaux F, Torchet C, Jacq C, Quevillon-Cheruel S, Labesse G, Facca C, Faye G (2003) Ssu72 is a phosphatase essential for transcription termination of snoRNAs and specific mRNAs in yeast. EMBO J. 22: 1588-1598.

[174] Pappas DL, Jr., Hampsey M (2000) Functional interaction between Ssu72 and the Rpb2 subunit of RNA polymerase II in Saccharomyces cerevisiae. Mol Cell Biol. 20: 8343-8351.

[175] Steinmetz EJ, Brow DA (2003) Ssu72 protein mediates both poly(A)-coupled and poly(A)-independent termination of RNA polymerase II transcription. Mol Cell Biol. 23: 6339-6349.

[176] St-Pierre B, Liu X, Kha LC, Zhu X, Ryan O, Jiang Z, Zacksenhaus E (2005) Conserved and specific functions of mammalian ssu72. Nucleic Acids Res. 33: 464-477.

[177] Archambault J, Chambers RS, Kobor MS, Ho Y, Cartier M, Bolotin D, Andrews B, Kane CM, Greenblatt J (1997) An essential component of a C-terminal domain phosphatase that interacts with transcription factor IIF in Saccharomyces cerevisiae. Proc Natl Acad Sci U S A. 94: 14300-14305.

[178] Kobor MS, Archambault J, Lester W, Holstege FC, Gileadi O, Jansma DB, Jennings EG, Kouyoumdjian F, Davidson AR, Young RA, Greenblatt J (1999) An unusual eukaryotic protein phosphatase required for transcription by RNA polymerase II and CTD dephosphorylation in S. cerevisiae. Mol Cell. 4: 55-62.
[179] Licciardo P, Ruggiero L, Lania L, Majello B (2001) Transcription activation by targeted recruitment of the RNA polymerase II CTD phosphatase FCP1. Nucleic Acids Res. 29: 3539-3545.
[180] Lin PS, Dubois MF, Dahmus ME (2002) TFIIF-associating carboxyl-terminal domain phosphatase dephosphorylates phosphoserines 2 and 5 of RNA polymerase II. J Biol Chem. 277: 45949-45956.
[181] Lin PS, Marshall NF, Dahmus ME (2002) CTD phosphatase: role in RNA polymerase II cycling and the regulation of transcript elongation. Prog Nucleic Acid Res Mol Biol. 72: 333-365.
[182] Mandal SS, Cho H, Kim S, Cabane K, Reinberg D (2002) FCP1, a phosphatase specific for the heptapeptide repeat of the largest subunit of RNA polymerase II, stimulates transcription elongation. Mol Cell Biol. 22: 7543-7552.
[183] Ni Z, Olsen JB, Guo X, Zhong G, Ruan ED, Marcon E, Young P, Guo H, Li J, Moffat J, Emili A, Greenblatt JF (2011) Control of the RNA polymerase II phosphorylation state in promoter regions by CTD interaction domain-containing proteins RPRD1A and RPRD1B. Transcription. 2: 237-242.
[184] Sun ZW, Hampsey M (1996) Synthetic enhancement of a TFIIB defect by a mutation in SSU72, an essential yeast gene encoding a novel protein that affects transcription start site selection in vivo. Mol Cell Biol. 16: 1557-1566.
[185] Wu WH, Pinto I, Chen BS, Hampsey M (1999) Mutational analysis of yeast TFIIB. A functional relationship between Ssu72 and Sub1/Tsp1 defined by allele-specific interactions with TFIIB. Genetics. 153: 643-652.
[186] He X, Khan AU, Cheng H, Pappas DL, Jr., Hampsey M, Moore CL (2003) Functional interactions between the transcription and mRNA 3' end processing machineries mediated by Ssu72 and Sub1. Genes Dev. 17: 1030-1042.
[187] Xiang K, Nagaike T, Xiang S, Kilic T, Beh MM, Manley JL, Tong L (2010) Crystal structure of the human symplekin-Ssu72-CTD phosphopeptide complex. Nature. 467: 729-733.
[188] Meinhart A, Silberzahn T, Cramer P (2003) The mRNA transcription/processing factor Ssu72 is a potential tyrosine phosphatase. J Biol Chem. 278: 15917-15921.
[189] Chambers RS, Dahmus ME (1994) Purification and characterization of a phosphatase from HeLa cells which dephosphorylates the C-terminal domain of RNA polymerase II. J Biol Chem. 269: 26243-26248.
[190] Chambers RS, Kane CM (1996) Purification and characterization of an RNA polymerase II phosphatase from yeast. J Biol Chem. 271: 24498-24504.
[191] Kimura M, Ishihama A (2004) Tfg3, a subunit of the general transcription factor TFIIF in Schizosaccharomyces pombe, functions under stress conditions. Nucleic Acids Res. 32: 6706-6715.

[192] Hausmann S, Shuman S (2002) Characterization of the CTD phosphatase Fcp1 from fission yeast. Preferential dephosphorylation of serine 2 versus serine 5. J Biol Chem. 277: 21213-21220.

[193] Lu KP, Finn G, Lee TH, Nicholson LK (2007) Prolyl cis-trans isomerization as a molecular timer. Nat Chem Biol. 3: 619-629.

[194] Lu KP, Zhou XZ (2007) The prolyl isomerase PIN1: a pivotal new twist in phosphorylation signalling and disease. Nat Rev Mol Cell Biol. 8: 904-916.

[195] Xu YX, Hirose Y, Zhou XZ, Lu KP, Manley JL (2003) Pin1 modulates the structure and function of human RNA polymerase II. Genes Dev. 17: 2765-2776.

[196] Xu YX, Manley JL (2007) Pin1 modulates RNA polymerase II activity during the transcription cycle. Genes Dev. 21: 2950-2962.

[197] Morris DP, Phatnani HP, Greenleaf AL (1999) Phospho-carboxyl-terminal domain binding and the role of a prolyl isomerase in pre-mRNA 3'-End formation. J Biol Chem. 274: 31583-31587.

[198] Gemmill TR, Wu X, Hanes SD (2005) Vanishingly low levels of Ess1 prolyl-isomerase activity are sufficient for growth in Saccharomyces cerevisiae. J Biol Chem. 280: 15510-15517.

[199] Hani J, Schelbert B, Bernhardt A, Domdey H, Fischer G, Wiebauer K, Rahfeld JU (1999) Mutations in a peptidylprolyl-cis/trans-isomerase gene lead to a defect in 3'-end formation of a pre-mRNA in Saccharomyces cerevisiae. J Biol Chem. 274: 108-116.

[200] Wilcox CB, Rossettini A, Hanes SD (2004) Genetic interactions with C-terminal domain (CTD) kinases and the CTD of RNA Pol II suggest a role for ESS1 in transcription initiation and elongation in Saccharomyces cerevisiae. Genetics. 167: 93-105.

[201] Wu X, Rossettini A, Hanes SD (2003) The ESS1 prolyl isomerase and its suppressor BYE1 interact with RNA pol II to inhibit transcription elongation in Saccharomyces cerevisiae. Genetics. 165: 1687-1702.

[202] Krishnamurthy S, Ghazy MA, Moore C, Hampsey M (2009) Functional interaction of the Ess1 prolyl isomerase with components of the RNA polymerase II initiation and termination machineries. Mol Cell Biol. 29: 2925-2934.

[203] Armache KJ, Kettenberger H, Cramer P (2003) Architecture of initiation-competent 12-subunit RNA polymerase II. Proc Natl Acad Sci U S A. 100: 6964-6968.

[204] Cramer P, Bushnell DA, Kornberg RD (2001) Structural basis of transcription: RNA polymerase II at 2.8 angstrom resolution. Science. 292: 1863-1876.

[205] Grohmann D, Klose D, Klare JP, Kay CW, Steinhoff HJ, Werner F (2010) RNA-binding to archaeal RNA polymerase subunits F/E: a DEER and FRET study. J Am Chem Soc. 132: 5954-5955.

[206] Young RA (1991) RNA polymerase II. Annual Review of Biochemistry. 60: 689-715.

[207] Bushnell DA, Kornberg RD (2003) Complete, 12-subunit RNA polymerase II at 4.1-A resolution: implications for the initiation of transcription. Proc Natl Acad Sci U S A. 100: 6969-6973.

[208] Kimura M, Suzuki H, Ishihama A (2002) Formation of a carboxy-terminal domain phosphatase (Fcp1)/TFIIF/RNA polymerase II (pol II) complex in Schizosaccharomyces pombe involves direct interaction between Fcp1 and the Rpb4 subunit of pol II. Mol Cell Biol. 22: 1577-1588.

[209] Armache KJ, Mitterweger S, Meinhart A, Cramer P (2005) Structures of complete RNA polymerase II and its subcomplex, Rpb4/7. J Biol Chem. 280: 7131-7134.
[210] Cai G, Imasaki T, Takagi Y, Asturias FJ (2009) Mediator structural conservation and implications for the regulation mechanism. Structure. 17: 559-567.
[211] Cai G, Imasaki T, Yamada K, Cardelli F, Takagi Y, Asturias FJ (2010) Mediator head module structure and functional interactions. Nat Struct Mol Biol. 17: 273-279.
[212] Sampath V, Balakrishnan B, Verma-Gaur J, Onesti S, Sadhale PP (2008) Unstructured N terminus of the RNA polymerase II subunit Rpb4 contributes to the interaction of Rpb4.Rpb7 subcomplex with the core RNA polymerase II of Saccharomyces cerevisiae. J Biol Chem. 283: 3923-3931.
[213] Calvo O, Manley JL (2001) Evolutionarily conserved interaction between CstF-64 and PC4 links transcription, polyadenylation, and termination. Mol Cell. 7: 1013-1023.
[214] Henry NL, Bushnell DA, Kornberg RD (1996) A yeast transcriptional stimulatory protein similar to human PC4. J Biol Chem. 271: 21842-21847.
[215] Knaus R, Pollock R, Guarente L (1996) Yeast SUB1 is a suppressor of TFIIB mutations and has homology to the human co-activator PC4. EMBO J. 15: 1933-1940.
[216] Ge H, Roeder RG (1994) Purification, cloning, and characterization of a human coactivator, PC4, that mediates transcriptional activation of class II genes. Cell. 78: 513-523.
[217] Kaiser K, Stelzer G, Meisterernst M (1995) The coactivator p15 (PC4) initiates transcriptional activation during TFIIA-TFIID-promoter complex formation. EMBO J. 14: 3520-3527.
[218] Kretzschmar M, Kaiser K, Lottspeich F, Meisterernst M (1994) A novel mediator of class II gene transcription with homology to viral immediate-early transcriptional regulators. Cell. 78: 525-534.
[219] Malik S, Guermah M, Roeder RG (1998) A dynamic model for PC4 coactivator function in RNA polymerase II transcription. Proc. Natl. Acad. Sci. U S A. 95: 2192-2197.
[220] Werten S, Stelzer G, Goppelt A, Langen FM, Gros P, Timmers HT, Van der Vliet PC, Meisterernst M (1998) Interaction of PC4 with melted DNA inhibits transcription. EMBO J. 17: 5103-5111.
[221] Rosonina E, Willis IM, Manley JL (2009) Sub1 functions in osmoregulation and in transcription by both RNA polymerases II and III. Mol Cell Biol. 29: 2308-2321.
[222] Garcia A, Rosonina E, Manley JL, Calvo O (2010) Sub1 globally regulates RNA polymerase II C-terminal domain phosphorylation. Mol Cell Biol. 30: 5180-5193.
[223] Calvo O, Manley JL (2003) Strange bedfellows: polyadenylation factors at the promoter. Genes Dev. 17: 1321-1327.
[224] Calvo O, Manley JL (2005) The transcriptional coactivator PC4/Sub1 has multiple functions in RNA polymerase II transcription. EMBO J. 24: 1009-1020.
[225] Sikorski TW, Ficarro SB, Holik J, Kim T, Rando OJ, Marto JA, Buratowski S (2011) Sub1 and RPA Associate with RNA Polymerase II at Different Stages of Transcription. Mol Cell. 44: 397-409.
[226] Ge H, Zhao Y, Chait BT, Roeder RG (1994) Phosphorylation negatively regulates the function of coactivator PC4. Proc Natl Acad Sci U S A. 91: 12691-12695.

[227] Ohkuni K, Yamashita I (2000) A transcriptional autoregulatory loop for KIN28-CCL1 and SRB10-SRB11, each encoding RNA polymerase II CTD kinase-cyclin pair, stimulates the meiotic development of S. cerevisiae. Yeast. 16: 829-846.

[228] Donner AJ, Ebmeier CC, Taatjes DJ, Espinosa JM (2010) CDK8 is a positive regulator of transcriptional elongation within the serum response network. Nat. Struct. Mol. Biol. 17: 194-201.

[229] de la Mata M, Kornblihtt AR (2006) RNA polymerase II C-terminal domain mediates regulation of alternative splicing by SRp20. Nat Struct Mol Biol. 13: 973-980.

[230] Hirose Y, Manley JL (1998) RNA polymerase II is an essential mRNA polyadenylation factor. Nature. 395: 93-96.

[231] Hirose Y, Tacke R, Manley JL (1999) Phosphorylated RNA polymerase II stimulates pre-mRNA splicing. Genes Dev. 13: 1234-1239.

[232] Cho EJ, Rodriguez CR, Takagi T, Buratowski S (1998) Allosteric interactions between capping enzyme subunits and the RNA polymerase II carboxy-terminal domain. Genes Dev. 12: 3482-3487.

[233] Kim HJ, Jeong SH, Heo JH, Jeong SJ, Kim ST, Youn HD, Han JW, Lee HW, Cho EJ (2004) mRNA capping enzyme activity is coupled to an early transcription elongation. Mol Cell Biol. 24: 6184-6193.

[234] Fong N, Bentley DL (2001) Capping, splicing, and 3' processing are independently stimulated by RNA polymerase II: different functions for different segments of the CTD. Genes Dev. 15: 1783-1795.

[235] Barilla D, Lee BA, Proudfoot NJ (2001) Cleavage/polyadenylation factor IA associates with the carboxyl-terminal domain of RNA polymerase II in Saccharomyces cerevisiae. Proc Natl Acad Sci U S A. 98: 445-450.

[236] Bauren G, Belikov S, Wieslander L (1998) Transcriptional termination in the Balbiani ring 1 gene is closely coupled to 3'-end formation and excision of the 3'-terminal intron. Genes Dev. 12: 2759-2769.

[237] Birse CE, Minvielle-Sebastia L, Lee BA, Keller W, Proudfoot NJ (1998) Coupling termination of transcription to messenger RNA maturation in yeast. Science. 280: 298-301.

[238] Kim M, Krogan NJ, Vasiljeva L, Rando OJ, Nedea E, Greenblatt JF, Buratowski S (2004) The yeast Rat1 exonuclease promotes transcription termination by RNA polymerase II. Nature. 432: 517-522.

[239] West S, Gromak N, Proudfoot NJ (2004) Human 5' --> 3' exonuclease Xrn2 promotes transcription termination at co-transcriptional cleavage sites. Nature. 432: 522-525.

[240] Baillat D, Hakimi MA, Naar AM, Shilatifard A, Cooch N, Shiekhattar R (2005) Integrator, a multiprotein mediator of small nuclear RNA processing, associates with the C-terminal repeat of RNA polymerase II. Cell. 123: 265-276.

[241] Egloff S, Szczepaniak SA, Dienstbier M, Taylor A, Knight S, Murphy S (2010) The integrator complex recognizes a new double mark on the RNA polymerase II carboxyl-terminal domain. J Biol Chem. 285: 20564-20569.

[242] David CJ, Boyne AR, Millhouse SR, Manley JL (2011) The RNA polymerase II C-terminal domain promotes splicing activation through recruitment of a U2AF65-Prp19 complex. Genes Dev. 25: 972-983.

[243] Millhouse S, Manley JL (2005) The C-terminal domain of RNA polymerase II functions as a phosphorylation-dependent splicing activator in a heterologous protein. Mol Cell Biol. 25: 533-544.

[244] Listerman I, Sapra AK, Neugebauer KM (2006) Cotranscriptional coupling of splicing factor recruitment and precursor messenger RNA splicing in mammalian cells. Nat Struct Mol Biol. 13: 815-822.

[245] Moore MJ, Schwartzfarb EM, Silver PA, Yu MC (2006) Differential recruitment of the splicing machinery during transcription predicts genome-wide patterns of mRNA splicing. Mol Cell. 24: 903-915.

[246] Kim E, Du L, Bregman DB, Warren SL (1997) Splicing factors associate with hyperphosphorylated RNA polymerase II in the absence of pre-mRNA. J Cell Biol. 136: 19-28.

[247] Mortillaro MJ, Blencowe BJ, Wei X, Nakayasu H, Du L, Warren SL, Sharp PA, Berezney R (1996) A hyperphosphorylated form of the large subunit of RNA polymerase II is associated with splicing complexes and the nuclear matrix. Proc Natl Acad Sci U S A. 93: 8253-8257.

[248] Yuryev A, Patturajan M, Litingtung Y, Joshi RV, Gentile C, Gebara M, Corden JL (1996) The C-terminal domain of the largest subunit of RNA polymerase II interacts with a novel set of serine/arginine-rich proteins. Proc Natl Acad Sci U S A. 93: 6975-6980.

[249] Morris DP, Greenleaf AL (2000) The splicing factor, Prp40, binds the phosphorylated carboxyl-terminal domain of RNA polymerase II. J Biol Chem. 275: 39935-39943.

[250] Carty SM, Goldstrohm AC, Sune C, Garcia-Blanco MA, Greenleaf AL (2000) Protein-interaction modules that organize nuclear function: FF domains of CA150 bind the phosphoCTD of RNA polymerase II. Proc Natl Acad Sci U S A. 97: 9015-9020.

[251] Goldstrohm AC, Albrecht TR, Sune C, Bedford MT, Garcia-Blanco MA (2001) The transcription elongation factor CA150 interacts with RNA polymerase II and the pre-mRNA splicing factor SF1. Mol Cell Biol. 21: 7617-7628.

[252] David CJ, Manley JL (2011) The RNA polymerase C-terminal domain: a new role in spliceosome assembly. Transcription. 2: 221-225.

[253] Hargreaves DC, Horng T, Medzhitov R (2009) Control of inducible gene expression by signal-dependent transcriptional elongation. Cell. 138: 129-145.

[254] Luger K (2003) Structure and dynamic behavior of nucleosomes. Curr Opin Genet Dev. 13: 127-135.

[255] Berger SL (2007) The complex language of chromatin regulation during transcription. Nature. 447: 407-412.

[256] Cho EJ (2007) RNA polymerase II carboxy-terminal domain with multiple connections. Exp. Mol. Med. 39: 247-254.

[257] Hampsey M, Reinberg D (2003) Tails of intrigue: phosphorylation of RNA polymerase II mediates histone methylation. Cell. 113: 429-432.

[258] Jenuwein T, Allis CD (2001) Translating the histone code. Science. 293: 1074-1080.

[259] Strahl BD, Allis CD (2000) The language of covalent histone modifications. Nature. 403: 41-45.

[260] Kouzarides T (2007) SnapShot: Histone-modifying enzymes. Cell. 128: 802.

[261] Kouzarides T (2007) Chromatin modifications and their function. Cell. 128: 693-705.

[262] Spain MM, Govind CK (2011) A role for phosphorylated Pol II CTD in modulating transcription coupled histone dynamics. Transcription. 2: 78-81.

[263] Kouzarides T (2002) Histone methylation in transcriptional control. Curr Opin Genet Dev. 12: 198-209.

[264] Pinskaya M, Morillon A (2009) Histone H3 lysine 4 di-methylation: a novel mark for transcriptional fidelity? Epigenetics. 4: 302-306.

[265] Krogan NJ, Dover J, Wood A, Schneider J, Heidt J, Boateng MA, Dean K, Ryan OW, Golshani A, Johnston M, Greenblatt JF, Shilatifard A (2003) The Paf1 complex is required for histone H3 methylation by COMPASS and Dot1p: linking transcriptional elongation to histone methylation. Mol Cell. 11: 721-729.

[266] Kizer KO, Phatnani HP, Shibata Y, Hall H, Greenleaf AL, Strahl BD (2005) A novel domain in Set2 mediates RNA polymerase II interaction and couples histone H3 K36 methylation with transcript elongation. Mol Cell Biol. 25: 3305-3316.

[267] Drouin S, Laramee L, Jacques PE, Forest A, Bergeron M, Robert F (2010) DSIF and RNA polymerase II CTD phosphorylation coordinate the recruitment of Rpd3S to actively transcribed genes. PLoS Genet. 6: e1001173.

[268] Govind CK, Qiu H, Ginsburg DS, Ruan C, Hofmeyer K, Hu C, Swaminathan V, Workman JL, Li B, Hinnebusch AG (2010) Phosphorylated Pol II CTD recruits multiple HDACs, including Rpd3C(S), for methylation-dependent deacetylation of ORF nucleosomes. Mol Cell. 39: 234-246.

[269] Kim T, Buratowski S (2009) Dimethylation of H3K4 by Set1 recruits the Set3 histone deacetylase complex to 5' transcribed regions. Cell. 137: 259-272.

[270] Brodsky AS, Silver PA (2000) Pre-mRNA processing factors are required for nuclear export. RNA. 6: 1737-1749.

[271] Rondon AG, Jimeno S, Aguilera A (2010) The interface between transcription and mRNP export: from THO to THSC/TREX-2. Biochim Biophys Acta. 1799: 533-538.

[272] Strasser K, Masuda S, Mason P, Pfannstiel J, Oppizzi M, Rodriguez-Navarro S, Rondon AG, Aguilera A, Struhl K, Reed R, Hurt E (2002) TREX is a conserved complex coupling transcription with messenger RNA export. Nature. 417: 304-308.

[273] Rondon AG, Jimeno S, Garcia-Rubio M, Aguilera A (2003) Molecular evidence that the eukaryotic THO/TREX complex is required for efficient transcription elongation. J Biol Chem. 278: 39037-39043.

[274] Zenklusen D, Vinciguerra P, Wyss JC, Stutz F (2002) Stable mRNP formation and export require cotranscriptional recruitment of the mRNA export factors Yra1p and Sub2p by Hpr1p. Mol Cell Biol. 22: 8241-8253.

[275] Masuda S, Das R, Cheng H, Hurt E, Dorman N, Reed R (2005) Recruitment of the human TREX complex to mRNA during splicing. Genes Dev. 19: 1512-1517.

[276] MacKellar AL, Greenleaf AL (2011) Cotranscriptional association of mRNA export factor Yra1 with C-terminal domain of RNA polymerase II. J Biol Chem. 286: 36385-36395.

[277] Krogan NJ, Kim M, Tong A, Golshani A, Cagney G, Canadien V, Richards DP, Beattie BK, Emili A, Boone C, Shilatifard A, Buratowski S, Greenblatt J (2003) Methylation of histone H3 by Set2 in Saccharomyces cerevisiae is linked to transcriptional elongation by RNA polymerase II. Mol Cell Biol. 23: 4207-4218.

[278] Lunde BM, Reichow SL, Kim M, Suh H, Leeper TC, Yang F, Mutschler H, Buratowski S, Meinhart A, Varani G (2010) Cooperative interaction of transcription termination factors with the RNA polymerase II C-terminal domain. Nat Struct Mol Biol. 17: 1195-1201.

[279] Stewart M (2010) Nuclear export of mRNA. Trends Biochem Sci. 35: 609-617.

[280] Ammosova T, Berro R, Jerebtsova M, Jackson A, Charles S, Klase Z, Southerland W, Gordeuk VR, Kashanchi F, Nekhai S (2006) Phosphorylation of HIV-1 Tat by CDK2 in HIV-1 transcription. Retrovirology. 3: 78.

[281] Coley W, Kehn-Hall K, Van Duyne R, Kashanchi F (2009) Novel HIV-1 therapeutics through targeting altered host cell pathways. Expert Opin Biol Ther. 9: 1369-1382.

[282] Bellan C, De Falco G, Lazzi S, Micheli P, Vicidomini S, Schurfeld K, Amato T, Palumbo A, Bagella L, Sabattini E, Bartolommei S, Hummel M, Pileri S, Tosi P, Leoncini L, Giordano A (2004) CDK9/CYCLIN T1 expression during normal lymphoid differentiation and malignant transformation. J Pathol. 203: 946-952.

[283] Lee DK, Duan HO, Chang C (2001) Androgen receptor interacts with the positive elongation factor P-TEFb and enhances the efficiency of transcriptional elongation. J Biol Chem. 276: 9978-9984.

[284] Simone C, Giordano A (2007) Abrogation of signal-dependent activation of the cdk9/cyclin T2a complex in human RD rhabdomyosarcoma cells. Cell Death Differ. 14: 192-195.

[285] Shapiro GI (2006) Cyclin-dependent kinase pathways as targets for cancer treatment. J Clin Oncol. 24: 1770-1783.

[286] Krystof V, Chamrad I, Jorda R, Kohoutek J (2010) Pharmacological targeting of CDK9 in cardiac hypertrophy. Med Res Rev. 30: 646-666.

Chapter 6

The Prp4 Kinase: Its Substrates, Function and Regulation in Pre-mRNA Splicing

Martin Lützelberger and Norbert F. Käufer

Additional information is available at the end of the chapter

http://dx.doi.org/10.5772/48270

1. Introduction

The genome of fission yeast *Schizosaccharomyces pombe* encodes about 107 predicted protein kinases, of which 17 are known to be essential for cell growth. These include the cell cycle regulator Cdc2 as well as several kinases which coordinate cell growth, cell polarity and cell morphogenesis within the cell cycle [1]. Another one of these essential kinases is Prp4. The study of precursor mRNA processing (*prp*) mutants in fission yeast identified Prp4 as the first kinase being involved in the regulation of pre-mRNA splicing in fungi and mammals. Interestingly, all eukaryotic organisms whose genome has been sequenced to date contain a counterpart of Prp4, with the exception of the *hemiascomycetes* to which the other yeast model organism *Saccharomyces cerevisiae* belongs. Here we review the discovery of Prp4 kinase, its genetic interactions and biochemical properties, its substrate specificity *in vitro* and *in vivo*, as well as the molecular consequences of these interactions. We compare and discuss results reported from the counterparts of Prp4 and its substrates in other organisms. We propose a model how Prp4 might be involved in the quality control of pre-mRNA splicing by acting at different "checkpoints" during the recognition of introns and the activation of pre-catalytic spliceosomal complexes.

2. Discovery of Prp4 kinase

More than 25 years ago we and others suggested that the introns found in fission yeast *Schizosaccharomyces pombe* represent a different type than those found in budding yeast *Saccharomyces cerevisiae*. The suggestion was mainly based on the observation that the simian virus 40 (SV40) small T antigen transcript displaying a 66 nt intron was accurately spliced and small T antigen proteins were synthesized in *S. pombe*, but not in *S. cerevisiae* [2]. We used fission yeast and generated temperature-sensitive (ts) mutants in order to screen for those which indicate a defect in pre-mRNA splicing at the restrictive temperature. For these screens we constructed an artificial reporter gene using the naturally intron-less *ura4* gene encoding a carboxylase involved in uracil synthesis. The insertion of introns into the *ura4* gene led to the discovery that introns in *S. pombe* are recognized independently of their exon context. This indicated already at that time that introns in *S. pombe* are recognized by a mechanism now called "intron definition" [3–5]. The ts mutants were transformed with a plasmid containing a 108 bp intronic sequence within the *ura4* gene. Then, the mutant strains were compared for the presence of mRNA and pre-mRNA of the *ura4-108I* transcript under growing (permissive, 25 °C) and non-growing (restrictive, 36 °C) conditions, respectively. Out of hundreds of ts mutants, there were three which showed spliced (mRNA) and unspliced (pre-mRNA) transcripts of the *ura4-I108* reporter gene at the permissive temperature, but when shifted to the restrictive temperature a time dependent decrease of mRNA was observed, while pre-mRNA remained stable. This indicated that the *ura4-108I* gene was still transcribed, but the artificial intron was not removed under this condition. In addition, the natural introns of the *cdc2* transcripts were also not removed in these mutants at the restrictive temperature.

Further genetic analysis revealed that two of this mutants belonged to a complementation group of three already existing pre-mRNA processing mutants, called $prp1^{ts}$, $prp2^{ts}$ and $prp3^{ts}$, which were isolated as described in [6]. One mutant allele, however, defined a new complementation group, and therefore was called $prp4\text{-}73^{ts}$ [7]. The $prp4^{+}$ gene was isolated by functional complementation of the $prp4\text{-}73^{ts}$ mutant allele at the restrictive temperature using a genomic library. The construction of a null-allele by replacing the $prp4^{+}$ gene in the genome via homologous recombination with an auxotrophic marker gene revealed that *prp4* is essential for growth [8]. The polypeptide sequence derived from the $prp4^{+}$ gene showed all signature sequences predicting a serine/protein kinase, according to the classification system of Hanks and Hunter [9]. Based on this classification system primers were designed for the T-Loop region of the *prp4* gene, taking into consideration the differences in codon usage of fission yeast and mammalian cells. These primers were used to produce PCR products from a HeLa cDNA library. The PCR products were then used as probes to screen a mouse cDNA library. With this approach cDNAs from human and mouse were obtained. Both show an open reading frame (ORF) encoding a C-terminal kinase domain and an N-terminal domain of unknown function, which consists of about 150 amino acids [10]. Throughout the kinase domain the fission yeast and mammalian sequences share 53 % identical amino acids. The N-termini, however, share less than 20 % identical amino acids. The two mammalian primary amino acid sequences are 98 % identical.

Chimeric mouse/fission yeast gene constructs were used to investigate by functional complementation, whether the mouse kinase is active in *S. pombe*. The mouse kinase domain complemented the $prp4\text{-}73^{ts}$ allele only when the N-terminus of the fission yeast *prp4* gene was fused to it [10]. Meanwhile, identification and characterization of mammalian counterparts of Prp4 by other groups revealed that it has an extented N-terminal region [12–14]. When compared with the sequences of Prp4 homologs in the database, this region shows variable length within different organisms, with fission yeast displaying the shortest N-terminal region [15]. In addition, all eukaryotic organisms whose genome is known contain a counterpart of Prp4 kinase, with the remarkable exception of the *hemiascomycetes* to which the budding yeast *S. cerevisiae* belongs. Therefore, we use for comparison the Prp4 counterpart found in the

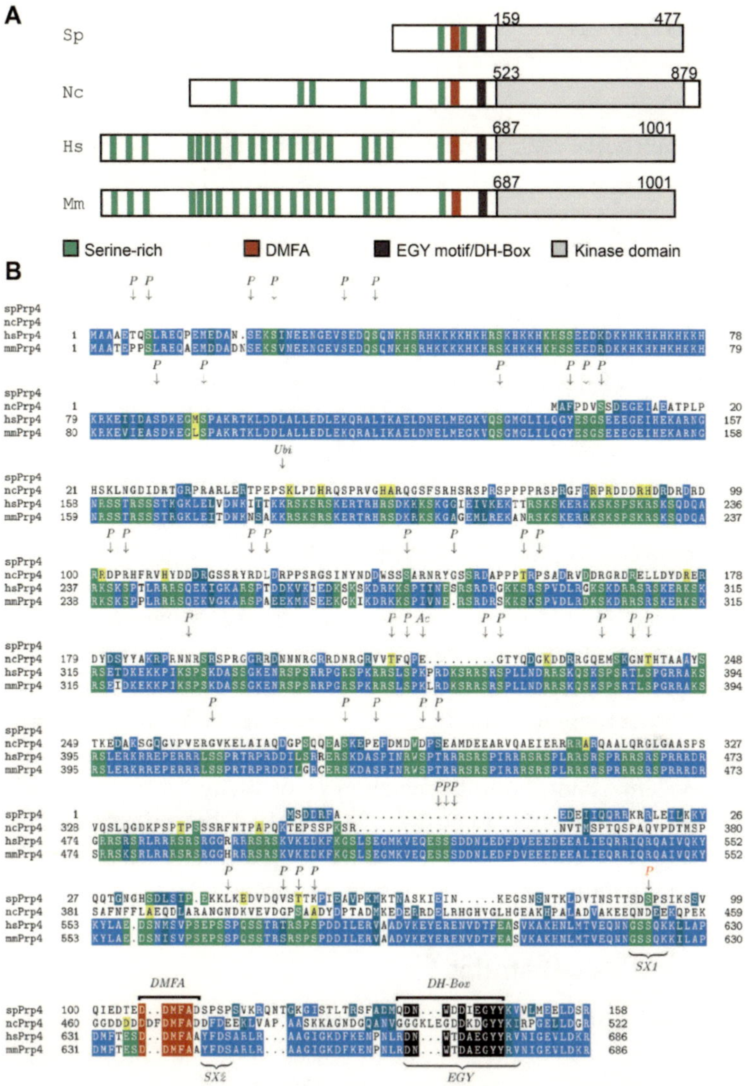

Figure 1. Structure of the Prp4 kinase. **(A)** Schematic representation of the Prp4 homologs from *S. pombe*, *N. crassa*, *M. musculus* and *H. sapiens*. Numbers on top indicate positions of the kinase domain and total length of the proteins, respectively. **(B)** ClustalX alignment of the N-terminus of Prp4 kinase homologs. Serine-rich elements matching the search pattern [SPRKEQLG]X_{0-1}S are highlighted in green. Sequence motifs of spPrp4, which were characterized previously in reference [10], are marked with braces underneath the alignment. The highly conserved DMFA motif and the DYRK homology box (DH-Box) are marked with lines. Amino acid residues of the human Prp4 kinase altered by post-translational modification, such as phosphorylation (P), acetylation (Ac) or ubiquitinylation (Ubi), are marked with arrows (↓). Positions were retrieved from the GeneBank entry of human Prp4 kinase. The phosphorylated S92 of spPrp4 is shown in red. GeneBank accession numbers of the aligned sequences are for spPrp4: CAA20718, ncPrp4: XP001728078, mmPrp4: AAM19102 and hsPrp4: Q13523. Sequences were aligned with ClustalX using default parameters. Shading and labeling of the alignment was done with TEXshade [11].

filamentous fungus *Neurospora crassa*. The N-terminal domain of Prp4 in *S. pombe, N. crassa, M. musculus* and *H. sapiens* comprises 158, 522 and 686 amino acids, respectively (Figure 1).

A mutational analysis of the N-terminus of the fission yeast kinase, testing the effect of the mutations by functional complementation led to the discovery of three short elements, essential for functioning of the kinase. Two elements, SDSPSI and SPSPSV at position 90–95 and 112–117, respectively, were called the serine elements (SX1 and SX2). The third element EGY at position 144–147 is located proximal to the kinase domain [10]. In all Prp4 counterparts this sequence is highly conserved (Figure 1). Alignment analyses led to the classification of Prp4 as a dual specificity tyrosine-regulated kinase (DYRK) family member. The element (EGY), called DH-box in these analyses, is part of the signature which assigns the Prp4 kinases to the third subfamily of the DYRK family [16]. Based on our sequence comparison there is one more highly conserved element in the N-terminal region close to the kinase domain. The sequence DDMFA at position 106–110 is highly conserved in all Prp4 sequences and may represent together with the DH-Box a signature in the N-terminus, indicating the archetypal Prp4 kinase (Figure 1). One serine element (SX2) is located next to DDMFA and shows no conservation between the *N. crassa* and the mammalian sequence at that position. The same is true for the other serine element (SX1). Neither the fungal nor the mammalian sequence is conserved in this position. However, in the *N. crassa* and the mammalian sequence serine elements similar to those in the N-terminus of the fission yeast sequence were found. Particularly, the mammalian sequence shows serine elements containing prolines, for example, SVPSEPSSP or SRSPSPD proximal to the kinase domain. In the extended N-terminal sequence serine elements of iterated serine/proline and serine/arginine dipeptides such as SRRSRSP are prevalent. Phosphoproteome analysis of fission yeast indicated that element SX1 is phosphorylated at the serine in position 92 which is followed by a proline [17]. Several of the serine elements in the mammalian sequence are phosphorylated. The phosphorylated serines were frequently found next to a proline or an arginine (Figure 1).

3. Prp4 kinase and its substrates

Both protein kinases, that is the fission yeast Prp4 kinase and the chimeric mouse Prp4 kinase, consisting of the mouse kinase domain preceded by the *S. pombe* Prp4 N-terminus, phosphorylated *in vitro* the arginine/serine-rich (RS) domain of the mammalian protein ASF/SF2 [10]. This protein belongs to the SR superfamily of splicing factors. SR proteins consist of one or two N-terminal RNA-binding domains (RBDs) and a C-terminal arginine/serine-rich (RS) domain. Members of the SR protein superfamily in mammals are involved in constitutive splicing and are specific modulators of alternative splicing. They serve as well as chaperones to couple splicing with transcription and RNA export. The versatile functions of SR proteins are modulated by reversible phosphorylation [18]. In fission yeast two SR proteins have been identified [19, 20]. Srp1 contains one RBD at the N-terminus followed by three serine elements, which we called RS1, RS2 and RS3, respectively, containing a various number of SR and SP dipeptides. Phosphoproteome analysis of fission yeast revealed several phosphorylated serines in these three RS elements (Figure 2). Srp2 contains two N-terminal RBDs and two SR and SP dipeptide displaying elements in the C-terminus, which we called SR1 and SR2. Again, phosphoprotein analysis detected phosphorylated serines in these elements (Figure 2). An extensive mutational analysis of both (SR1 and SR2) elements by replacing the serines with other amino acids and testing the effect of the mutations *in vivo*, revealed that when in both elements the serines were mutated, the GFP-Srp2 fusion protein failed to enter the nucleus and was found instead in distinct dots distributed in the cell [20].

Over the last ten years then, it has been shown that Srp1 and Srp2 are authentic targets of the kinase Dsk1 and that the phosphorylation status influences the distribution of Srp1 and Srp2 between cytoplasm and nucleus. For example, efficient localization of Srp2 in the nucleus requires Dsk1 kinase activity [21]. Dsk1 is the ortholog of the human SR protein-specific kinase 1 (SRPK1). While Dsk1 was detected in the cytoplasm and nucleus, Prp4 is localized predominantly in the nucleus [22]. As mentioned above, initial experiments showed that Prp4 kinase of fission yeast phosphorylated the human SR protein ASF/SF2 *in vitro*. Other experiments indicated, that overexpression of ASF/SF2 leads to the partial suppression of the splicing defect of intron containing genes in a *prp4-73*^{ts} background at the restrictive temperature [10, 19]. Based on these observations we checked whether Prp4 kinase phosphorylates *in vitro* Srp1 and/or Srp2. Notably, Srp2, representing the SR family member displaying two RBDs, was phosphorylated by Prp4, but Srp1 displaying one RBD was not (Figure 2). In contrast, Dsk1 kinase phosphorylated Srp1 as well as Srp2, however, which peptides are phosphorylated has not been determined so far [23, 24]. Therefore, we used and combined mutants in which serines were replaced with other amino acids at different positions in the SR1 and SR2 elements of Srp2, and produced the mutant proteins in bacteria followed by affinity purification. In order to determine which serines become phosphorylated *in vitro* by these kinases, the Srp2 mutant proteins were then employed in kinase assays using either bacterially produced Prp4 or Dsk1 kinase, respectively. Intriguingly, both kinases appear *in vitro* to phosphorylate the same dipeptides. In the SR1 element only one serine at position 188 followed by a proline is phosphorylated by both kinases. In the SR2 element we do not know which serines are phosphorylated. However, phosphoproteome analysis *in vivo* revealed that all of them are phosphorylated [17]. Consistently, our analysis shows that both kinases phosphorylate the SR2 element *in vitro*, as well as two serines to the left and right of SR2 displaying the tripeptides RSR and PSP, respectively (Figure 2).

4. Function of Prp4 in pre-mRNA splicing

We began to address the role of Prp4 kinase in spliceosome assembly *in vivo* by monitoring the co-transcriptional recruitment of spliceosomal and non-spliceosomal components including Srp2 using ChIP (Chromatin Immuno Precipitation, [25]). Varying the kinase activity with an ATP analog in a fission yeast strain expressing an (analog-sensitive) asPrp4 kinase indicates that recruitment of Srp2 to nascent intron containing transcripts depends on Prp4 kinase activity (D. Eckert and N. F. Käufer, unpublished results). It has been shown that Srp2 promotes the splicing of reporter genes by binding to purine-rich exonic splicing enhancer (ESE) sequences [26]. Based on these observations, we hypothesize that phosphorylation within the SR elements of Srp2 by Prp4 kinase in the nucleus may serve to target Srp2 to ESE containing pre-mRNAs, thereby modulating their splicing efficiency. Human Prp4 kinase phosphorylates *in vitro* the serine/arginine rich domain of the SR protein ASF/SF2 and has

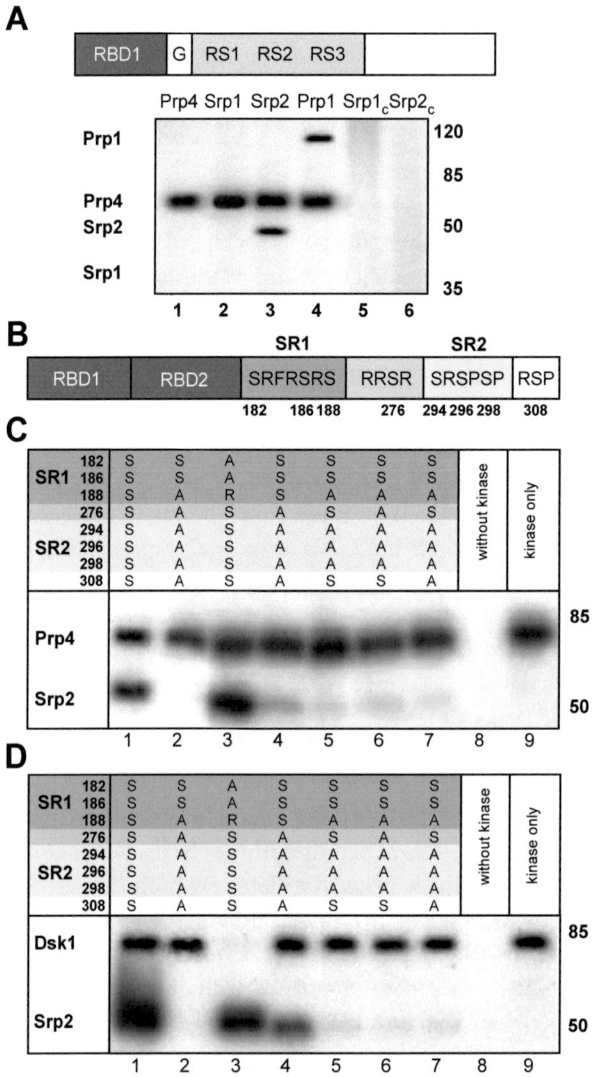

Figure 2. Phosphorylation of SR proteins by Prp4 kinase *in vitro*. **(A)** Schematic representation of Srp1 from fission yeast. Srp1 consists of an N-terminal RNA-binding domain (RBD1), followed by a glycine-rich domain (G) and a domain containing three arginine/serine-rich elements (RS1–3). In order to test whether Srp1 or Srp2 are phosphorylated by Prp4 kinase, recombinant proteins purified from *E. coli* were incubated in the presence of $\gamma[^{32}P]$ATP and separated by SDS-PAGE. Phosphorylated proteins were detected by auto-radiography. Prp1, which has been previously identified as a substrate of Prp4 kinase served as a positive control. Lanes 5 & 6: negative control without addition of the kinase. **(B)** Schematic representation of Srp2 from fission yeast. Srp2 consists of two N-terminal RNA-binding domains (RBD1, RBD2) and a C-terminal domain containing two serine/arginine-rich elements (SR1, SR2). Numbers below indicate positions of the serine residues within the SR elements. **(C)** *In vitro* kinase assay of recombinant Srp2 proteins, mutated within the SR elements as indicated in the table, with recombinant Prp4 kinase. **(D)** *In vitro* kinase assay of mutated Srp2 proteins with recombinant Dsk1 kinase.

been shown to co-localize in HeLa cells with SR family members, including ASF/SF2, in molecular structures called speckles [13]. In addition, Clk1 (Cdc2-like kinase 1) as well as SRPK1, a protein kinase phosphorylating SR-rich domains in SR proteins, have been shown to phosphorylate *in vitro* several of the serines within the SRSP elements that are located in the extended N-terminus of hsPrp4 (Figure 1, ↓, P). Phosphorylation of the serine elements in this region may be in mammalian cells part of the process to move and target hsPrp4 kinase to the location of its action [13]. In mammals the SR protein ASF/SF2 is involved in the regulation of alternatively spliced genes. Intriguingly, based on results with human immunodeficiency virus type 1 (HIV-1), it has been proposed that the interaction of hsPrp4 kinase with the HIV-1 Gag polyprotein may lead to the down-regulation of alternative splicing through reduced phosphorylation of ASF/SF2 by hsPrp4 at late stages of infection to support production of unspliced viral genomic RNA [27].

We took advantage of the powerful genetic system available with fission yeast and produced an epistasis map, particularly, by screening for genetic interactions with the *prp4-73*^{ts} allele. With this approach we identified Prp8/U5-220K and Brr2/U5-200K [29, 30]. Both proteins are highly conserved between yeast and human and play key regulatory roles in the activation of spliceosomes. Prp8/U5-220K interacts directly with the splice sites and branch region of pre-mRNAs [31]. Brr2/U5-200K belongs to the DEAD/DEXH-box family of ATP-dependent RNA helicases containing two helicase domains. Brr2/U5-200K has been implicated in the unwinding of U4/U6 molecules as a prerequisite for the snRNA rearrangements necessary for the activation of a spliceosome [32]. As mentioned above, we started to investigate with ChIP analysis the association of spliceosomal and non-spliceosomal proteins with nascent transcripts. Brr2, represents a specific U5 snRNP protein. The recruitment of Brr2 to nascent intron containing transcripts appears to be strongly influenced by active Prp4 kinase. (D. Eckert and N. F. Käufer, unpublished results). Genetic interactions with the *prp4-73*^{ts} allele indicate by no means that the interaction partner is a substrate of Prp4 kinase. However, the multiple genetic interactions we determined between Prp8, Brr2, Prp1 and Prp4 kinase, and among themselves, unambiguously pointed to Prp8, Brr2 and Prp1 as a structural center of the spliceosome which is targeted by Prp4 kinase [15, 29, 30]. While there is no indication that Prp4 kinase is a stable spliceosomal component, Prp8, Brr2 and Prp1 have been determined as *bona fide* spliceosomal components on all accounts present together in pre-catalytic spliceosomes. We identified Prp1 as a physiological substrate of Prp4 kinase in fission yeast by demonstrating that *in vivo* Prp1 was not phosphorylated in the genetic background of *prp4-73*^{ts} at the restrictive temperature. In addition, immunoprecipitated (IP) and recombinant Prp4 kinase phosphorylated recombinant Prp1 *in vitro* [33].

To avoid confusion, we discuss here shortly the nomenclature of the orthologs of Prp1 in the literature and suggest a standardization. The ortholog of Prp1 in *S. cerevisiae* is called Prp6, whereas the ortholog in human is called hsPrp6 or U5-102K, referring to a protein with a molecular weight of 102 kDa, which is associated with the spliceosomal snRNP U5 in mammalian cells. Prp1 (Prp6/U5-102K) is a protein consisting of multiple direct repeats called tetra-tricopeptide repeats (TPRs), which are listed as HATs (half a TPR) in UniProtKB (Q12381, PRP1_SCHPO; P19735, PRP6_YEAST; Q872D2_NEUCS ; O94906, PRP6_HUMAN). In this report, we analysed Prp1 of fission yeast and its homologs in other eukaryotes

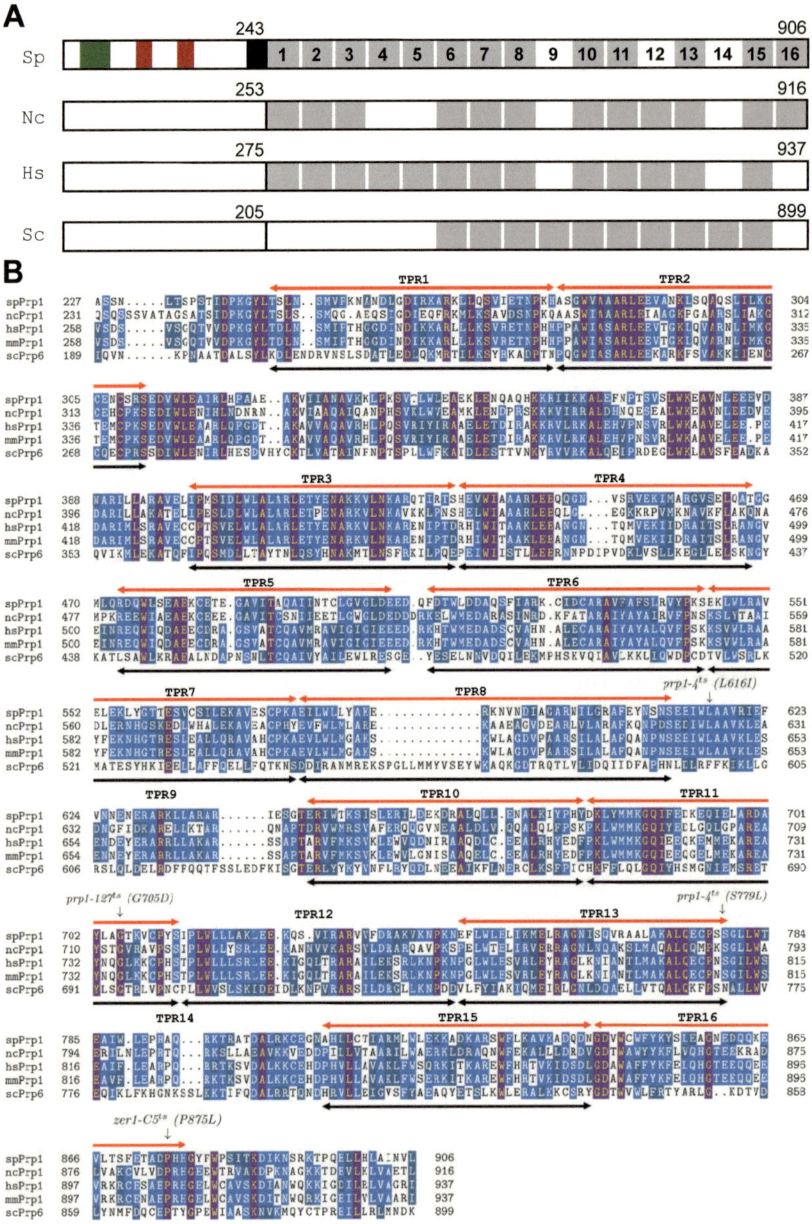

Figure 3. (A) Schematic representation of Prp1 from *S. pombe*, *N. crassa*, *H. sapiens* and *S. cerevisiae*. Conserved sequence elements (see Fig. 3) within the N-terminus are coloured in green, red and black. Tetratrico peptide repeats (TPRs) within the C-terminus are drawn as grey boxes. Positions of the TPR sequences were determined using the program TPRpred [28]. Only TPRs with a P-value lower than P = 0.01 are shown. **(B)** ClustalX alignment of the Prp1 C-terminal domain. Red arrows (↔) above the alignment mark TPR sequences within spPrp1, black arrows (↔) below indicate TPR positions of hsPrp1. Mutated amino acid residues of the spPrp1 temperature-sensitive alleles *prp1-127^{ts}*, *prp1-4^{ts}*, and *zer1-C5^{ts}* are indicated with arrows (↓).

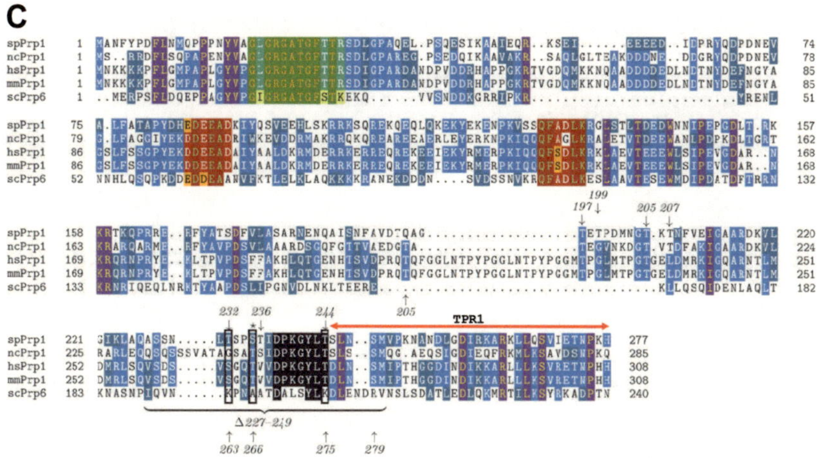

Figure 3. (C) ClustalX alignment of the Prp1 N-terminus. Conserved sequence elements are coloured in green, red and black. Positions of spPrp4 kinase *in vitro* phosphorylation sites are marked with arrows (↓) above the alignment. The *in vivo* phosphorylation site at pos. 235 of spPrp1, determined by phospho-proteome analysis [17] is marked with a star (⋆). Phosphorylation sites within hsPrp1 determined by [34] are indicated below the alignment (arrows, ↑). Amino acid residues which are phosphorylated in both spPrp1 and hsPrp1 are marked with a frame. The region containing most Prp1 phosphorylation sites, whose function was previously analysed by deletion mapping in [35], is marked with a brace (Δ227–249). GeneBank accession numbers of the sequences shown in the alignment are: spPrp1, CAA17050; ncPrp1, XP_958849; hsPrp1, NP_036601; mmPrp1, AAH23691; scPrp6, CAA84998.

including Prp6 of *S. cerevisiae* using TPRpred, a computer algorithm recently developed to find tetra-tricopeptide repeats [28]. Based on this analysis, Prp1 family members display 16 TPR positions in the C-terminus preceded by an N-terminal region of about 250 amino acids. Prp1 of fission yeast and the mammalian orthologs show 13 TPR repeats, of which 12 share the same positions. The sequences of *N. crassa* and *S. cerevisiae* display 12 and 10 TPR repeats, respectively (Figure 3A and 3B). A comparison of the N- termini revealed that there is only one highly conserved region comprising 32 amino acids with an identical core, GRGATGF, of seven amino acids proximately to the start codon. Two further conserved regions with the signatures, DEEAD and QFADLK at positions 85 and 129, respectively, were detected (Figure 3C). Most intriguingly, however, the fourth highly conserved signature sequence in the N-terminus, DPKGYLT, is directly next to the first TPR domain of fission yeast, *N. crassa* and the mammalian sequence, whereas the sequence in *S. cerevisiae* in this region is diverged and does not reveal a TPR repeat according to the algorithm used (Figure 3C). In addition, phosphoproteome analysis of fission yeast and human proteins revealed that the threonine in DPKGYLT is phosphorylated as documented in UniProtKB (PRP1_SCHPO, PRP6_HUMAN). Mapping the *in vitro* phosphorylation sites in Prp1 of fission yeast by recombinant Prp4 kinase using peptide fingerprinting revealed this site and additional sites close to this threonine [35]. Mass spectrometry analyses of *in vitro* assembled and purified pre-catalytic B complexes from HeLa cells treated with recombinant human Prp4K also show additional phosphorylation sites in this region [34]. The results of both analyses are shown in Figure 3C.

5. Participation of mammalian Prp4K in other cellular processes

Mammalian Prp4K has been shown to interact and colocalize with many diverse cellular structures and defined proteins, such as speckles, spliceosomal particles, chromatin organizing complexes and with proteins at the kinetocore organizing the spindle assembly checkpoint [12–14, 27, 36–39].

6. Role of Prp4 kinase in the activation process of pre-catalytic spliceosomes

The results discussed above, presenting the genetic, molecular and biochemical interactions of Prp4 kinase in fission yeast demonstrate genetic interactions with several major regulatory spliceosomal components, however, up to date a stable association with spliceosomal particles and any other cellular complexes was not detected. Prp4 kinase molecules in whole cell extract (WCE) sediment around 9S [30, 35, 40–42].

Particularly the lack of an *in vitro* splicing system in fission yeast, led us to use extensively the inducible and repressible expression systems available to switch-off and -on spliceosomal components and to express mutant versions for studying their molecular consequences *in vivo*. With this approach, we discovered that the expression of mutations in the N-terminus of Prp1 leads to the appearance of spliceosomal complexes containing the five snRNAs U1, U2, U5 and U4/U6 and pre-mRNAs. The mutations in the N-terminus, which prevent splicing to occur, include the identified phosphorylation sites of Prp4 kinase, as well as the other three highly conserved regions in the N-terminus (Figure 3C). This substantial mutational analysis revealed that the structural integrity of the N-terminus is required to mediate a splicing event, but that it is not necessary for the assembly of a pre-catalytic spliceosome. The purification of spliceosomal complexes by the tandem affinity purification (TAP) method, using the TAP-tagged spliceosomal component Prp31 of a strain expressing solely the N-terminal Prp1 mutant version in which the phosphorylation sites were deleted, yielded spliceosomal complexes containing pre-mRNA, the five snRNAs, Prp31-TAP, MycΔNPrp1 and HA-Cdc5, indicating that this complex is frozen or stalled in a pre-catalytic stage [35]. In fact, mass spectroscopy revealed a spliceosomal protein content clearly suggestive for a pre-catalytic complex containing all five snRNPs and the Prp19 complex (NTC) as shown for *in vitro* assembled mammalian B complexes (Lützelberger and Käufer, unpublished, [43]). Based on these observations, we hypothesized that phosphorylation of Prp1 by Prp4 kinase is involved in the activation of spliceosomes. However, it is not clear as of yet, whether this phosphorylation is involved directly, that is, inducing the rearrangements of the snRNPs for catalysis, or indirectly by recruiting other components necessary for the switch.

This in mind we employed again classical genetics to screen for suppressors and synthetic lethals of the three temperature sensitive alleles *prp1-127*^{ts}, *prp1-4*^{ts} and *zer1-C5*^{ts}, respectively (Figure 3B). For *prp1-127*^{ts}, displaying one point mutation, we found two extragenic suppressors, but none for the two other alleles [49]. In addition, we found a strong epistatic interaction between *prp1-4*^{ts}, displaying two point mutations, and a gene in fission yeast called *cdc28-P8*^{ts} [50]. This genetic interaction implicates that for proper processive action of Cdc28 a functional Prp1 is a prerequisite. The *cdc28* gene encodes the ortholog of Prp2 in *S.*

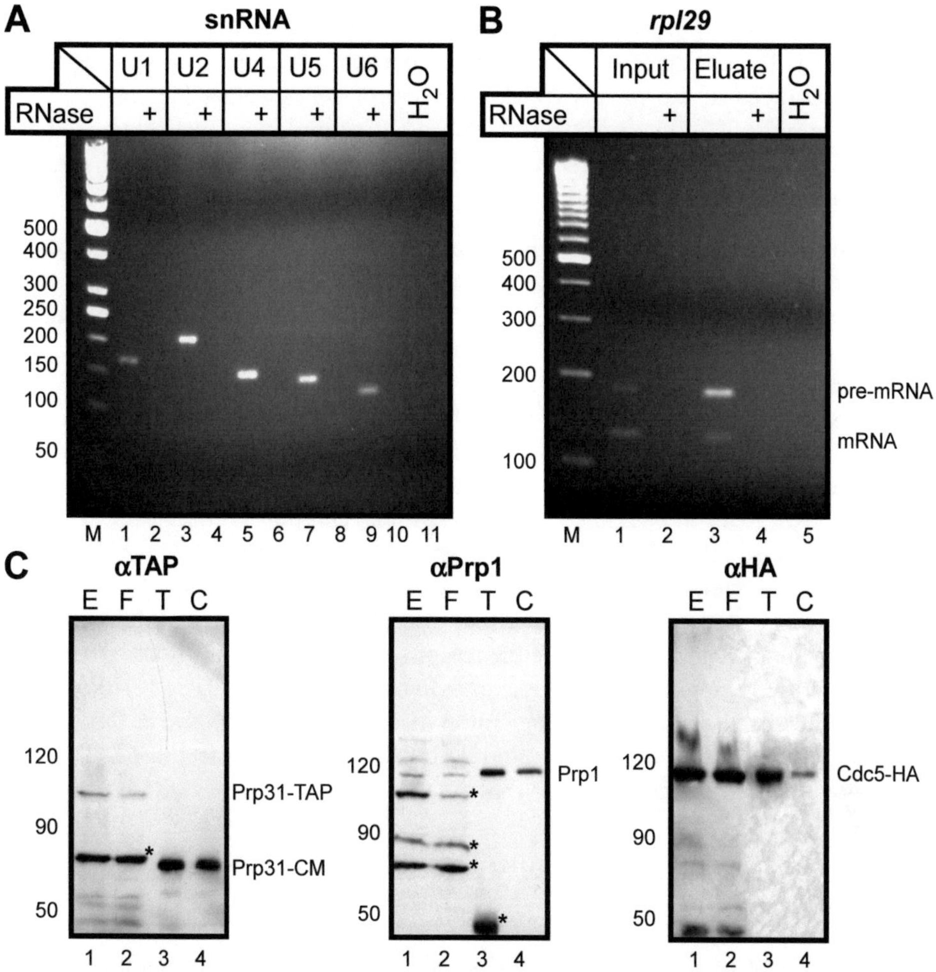

Figure 4. Tandem affinity purification (TAP) of pre-catalytic spliceosomal complexes. For this experiment a strain with the genotype h^{-s} *prp31 int::prp31-CTAP leu1-32 int::pMLtet*^{ON} *prp2*^{H539D} *cdc5 int::HA-cdc5* was used. In this strain, expression of a mutated Prp2 helicase is driven by a tet-inducible CaMV35S (tet^{ON}) promotor [44]. It has been shown that expression of Prp2^{H539D} leads to growth arrest by inhibition of pre-mRNA splicing [45–47] in yeast and human cells. TAP was performed as described in reference [48], after 3 hours of induction with 6 μM anhydro-tetracycline. RNA purified from the TAP eluate by phenol-extraction was analysed by RT-PCR in **(A)** using primer pairs amplifying the five snRNAs (U1–U6) and in **(B)** with a primer pair amplifying RNA expressed from the ribosomal protein gene *rpl29*, which contains a single intron of 53 nt. The PCR products of snRNA U1, U2, U4, U5 and U6 have a size of 166, 207, 149, 139 and 119 bp, respectively. The PCR products of *rpl29* pre-mRNA and mRNA migrate at 182 and 129 bp. Prior to reverse transcription, all samples were treated with DNase I. Samples were treated with RNase A as indicated (+), to verify that they were not contaminated with genomic DNA. **(C)** Whole cell extract, E, flow-through, F, eluate of the first-, T, and second TAP affinity column, C, were analysed for the presence of Prp31-CTAP (90.3 kDa; Prp31-CM after treatment with TEV protease, 62.6 kDa), Prp1 (103 kDa) and HA-Cdc5 (89.8 kDa) with a Western blot, using anti-TAP, anti-Prp1 and anti-HA antibodies as indicated on the top of each blot. Unspecifically recognized bands and degradation products of Prp31 and Prp1 are marked with asterisks ($\star$).

cerevisiae, DHX16 (hPrp2) in mammals and belongs to the DEAH subgroup of DExD/H-box ATPases/RNA helicases. Prp2 is required for the first catalytic step of the splicing pathway, and thus, is involved in the early activation process of spliceosomes [45, 46]. The stalled pre-catalytic complex found in fission yeast when ΔNPrp1 mutations were expressed did not contain Prp2, suggesting that, as observed for spliceosomes in mammals, the interaction of Prp2 with the spliceosome is transient.

Therefore, to study how this helicase affects pre-mRNA splicing in fission yeast, we made mutations in the conserved DEAH-box of Prp2 (spCdc28). In yeast and human, this mutation (Prp2^{H539D}) leads to a diminished helicase activity and inhibition of splicing, when overexpressed [45–47]. When we expressed the mutation with one of the inducible expression systems mentioned above, cells stopped mitotic growth within three hours. At this time point spliceosomes were purified using the TAP method [51, 52]. Spliceosomes purified under these conditions contained Prp31-TAP, Prp1, HA-Cdc5, all five snRNAs U1–U6 and pre-mRNA indicating the arrest of spliceosomes in a pre-catalytic stage (Figure 4). We have reason to believe that the protein composition of this spliceosomal complex is equivalent to the stalled spliceosomes purified after expressing the ΔNPrp1 mutations described above [35]. First, the results presented are consistent with the notion, that Prp1 operates in the activation center of a pre-catalytic spliceosome and emphasize that phosphorylation of Prp1 might be involved to recruit chaperones to induce the dynamic rearrangements of a spliceosome for activation. Second, and most intriguingly, the overexpression of mammalian DHX16/hPrp2 mutant versions in human cell lines led to the retention of unspliced pre-mRNA in the nucleus. It has been suggested that this nuclear retention is directly related to the fact that DHX16/hPrp2 functions after spliceosome formation [46, 53].

7. Inhibition of Prp4 kinase activity affects splicing of intron-containing genes differentially

Based on the observation that a relatively small number of intron-containing transcripts accumulated in cells expressing mutant versions, it was speculated that DHX16/hPrp2 might affect the splicing of different introns or different genes [46, 53]. These considerations prompted us to ask the question: Does the inhibition of Prp4 kinase in fission yeast affect splicing of intron-containing genes differentially?

Therefore we constructed a conditional analog sensitive (as) allele *prp4-as2* which allows to reversibly inhibit Prp4 kinase with ATP analogs [54]. Adding the inhibitor 1-NM-PP1 to a growing cell culture expressing Prp4-as2 leads to growth arrest [1]. We performed semi-quantitative RT-PCR analyses to detect mRNA and pre-mRNA of different intron containing genes, using RNA of a growing culture prepared 10, 20 and 30 minutes after adding the kinase inhibitor. Here we present selected data of the most interesting observations we made in these series of experiments.

We used, for example, *tbp1* encoding the TATA-binding protein. This gene contains three introns in the open reading frame (ORF). Within 30 min after adding the inhibitor, the ratio of *tbp1* mRNA and pre-mRNA is reversed, indicating that pre-mRNA is accumulating and mRNA degraded. In contrast, the ribosomal protein gene *rpl29* containing one intron of 53 bp is hardly affected, showing no significant change in mRNA concentration and a slight increase in pre-mRNA (Figure 5). We also used the genes *res1* and *res2* containing one intron in a similar 5′-position of the ORF with a size of 127 bp and 164 bp, respectively. Both genes, *res1* and *res2*, encode components of the Mlu1-binding factor (MBF). In fission yeast MBF is required together with the cyclin-dependent kinase Cdc2 for passage through Start in G1 phase by activating the transcription of genes for S phase. At this point the cell is in each cycle faced with a critical decision between vegetative proliferation by cell division or sexual conjugation followed by meiosis [55].

In case of *res1* only pre-mRNA is detected after 10 min exposure to the kinase inhibitor. Thus, splicing of this pre-mRNA is inhibited immediately and pre-mRNA accumulates, whereas the mRNA is rapidly degraded. On the contrary, *res2* is still efficiently spliced (Figure 5). These examples demonstrate that fission yeast contains genes with introns whose removal appears strictly dependent on Prp4 kinase activity, and also contains genes whose intron removal seems independent of kinase activity. The observed differences in mRNA and pre-mRNA concentrations detected indicate that there are major differences in pre-mRNA and mRNA stability of each gene (Figure 5).

It has been shown for several precursor pre-mRNA (*prp*) temperature sensitive mutants, that introns of different genes show a range of splicing defects in these strains. There are introns which are spliced independently of the large subunit of the U2 auxiliary factor ($U2AF^{59}$). Noteworthy here, $U2AF^{59}$ is essential for growth [56–58]. Moreover, there is some evidence that the recruitment of $U2AF^{59}$ to auxiliary factor dependent introns might be mediated by the SR protein Srp2, which has been shown above to be an *in vitro* substrate of Prp4 kinase [26]. However, we have no data, whether $U2AF^{59}$ dependent introns are also Prp4 kinase dependent introns.

This is the first report demonstrating Prp4 kinase dependent removal of introns from essential genes, such as *tbp1* and *res1*, respectively. Furthermore, inhibition of Prp4 kinase by the ATP-analog leads to growth arrest, and cells in this cell population are specifically arrested in G1 and G2 phase, respectively (Figure 5). These results are consistent with the notion that those cells in which the *res1* intron is not spliced out specifically arrest in G1 and, therefore, splicing control of *res1* might be involved in the regulatory switch between vegetative proliferation by cell division and sexual conjugation [59].

Apparently only few cases of pre-mRNA splicing regulation exist in fission yeast. A meiotic cyclin, Rem1, is only expressed when a 87-nt intron is spliced out of the *rem1* pre-mRNA. Splicing of *rem1* pre-mRNA is dependent on the meiosis specific transcription factor Mei4 regulating transcription of the *rem1* gene and recruiting the splicing machinery to the transcribed locus [60, 61]. About 45 % of the genes contain introns, whereas the genes contain from one to more than 10 introns. The introns are small with a mean size of 78 nt [62]. There is no known case of regulated alternative splicing in fission yeast producing different isoforms of a protein from the same open reading frame.

We have suggested that fission yeast represents the archetype of the pre-mRNA splicing machinery in eukaryotes [63]. And, we proposed that phosphorylation of Prp1 by Prp4 kinase is part of the process in which spliceosomes are activated: either the phosphorylation by Prp4

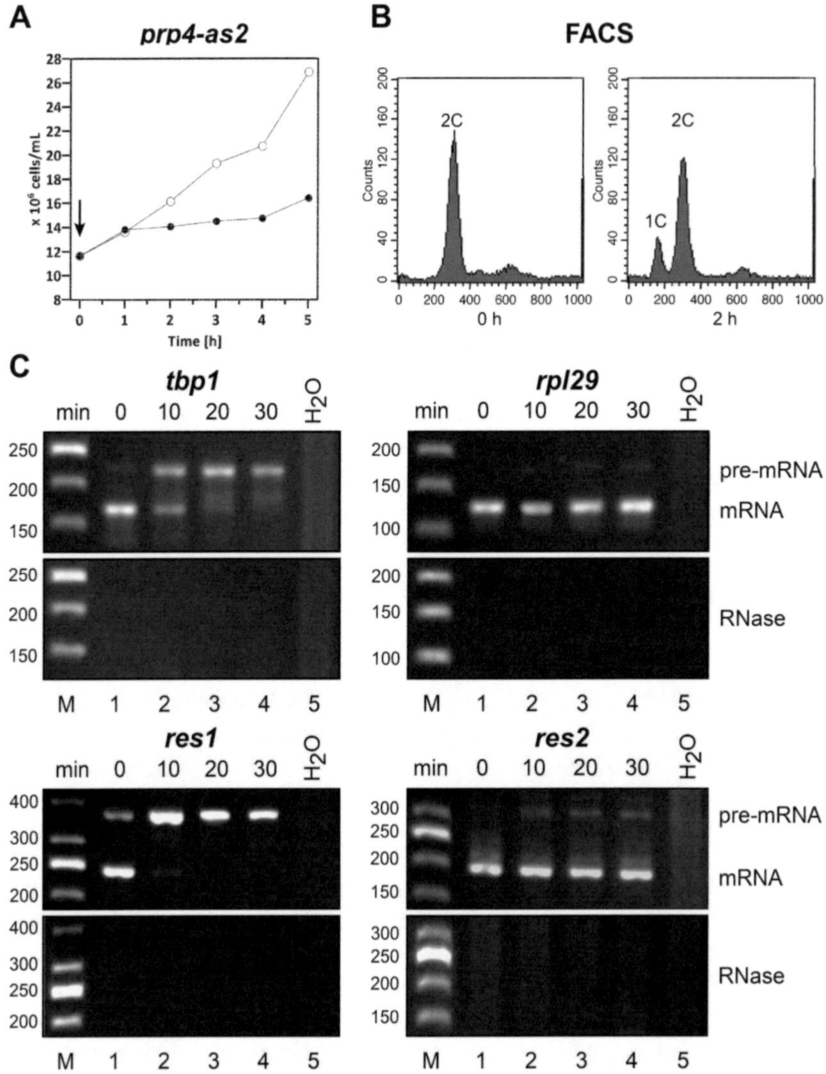

Figure 5. Inhibition of Prp4 kinase activity with 1-NM-PP1. **(A)** A strain with the genotype h^{-s} *prp4-as2* was grown to early log-phase. Then, 1-NM-PP1 was added to the culture medium (0 hours, arrow, ↓) at a final concentration of 10 μM. Growth of the culture was monitored by counting the number of cells/mL with a haemocytometer every hour (closed circles, •) and compared to a culture growing in absence of the inhibitor (open circles, ○). **(B)** Immediately before (0 hours) and 2 hours after addition of 1-NM-PP1, cells were analysed by FACS for their DNA content (1C, 2C). **(C)** RNA prepared after 0, 10, 20 and 30 min of inhibition with 1-NM-PP1 was analysed by RT-PCR, using primer pairs detecting *tbp1* (second intron), *rpl29*, *res1* and *res2* RNA, resulting in PCR products with a size of (pre-mRNA/mRNA) 225/173 bp for *tbp1*, 182/129 bp for *rpl29*, 374/247 bp for *res1* and 366/203 bp for *res2*. Prior to RT-PCR, all RNA samples were treated with DNase I. To verify that contaminating genomic DNA was completely removed, samples were treated with RNase as indicated. The analog-sensitive *prp4-as2* kinase allele was generated by introducing a point mutation within the kinase domain at position 238, changing the so-called "gate-keeper"amino acid [54] from phenylalanine to alanine.

kinase is part of a mechanism which signals that an intron is occupied by a splicing competent spliceosome in a sense of quality control and/or the phosphorylation is directly involved in inducing the rearrangements for catalysis [30, 35]. The results received since then, including those reported here, allow now a discussion which will help further to pinpoint the function of Prp4 kinase in pre-mRNA splicing.

8. Is Prp4 a pre-mRNA splicing checkpoint kinase?

The Prp4 kinase dependent genes we detected do not reveal any obvious sequence motifs indicating their Prp4 dependency. For example, the comparison of *res1* and *res2* exon and intron sequences did not offer anything clearly pointing into this direction. However, there is one tendency to observe: The removal of introns from transcripts which are encoded by genes that are essential for growth appears to be Prp4 kinase dependent.

In consideration of all the facts and thoughts presented above, we reason that in general, removal of introns in fission yeast during mitotic growth is constitutive by default. That means, the splicing machinery is recruited to the pre-mRNA and assembled on introns to form a splicing competent spliceosome. Spliceosomal ATPases/RNA helicases, including Prp2, have been identified as the candidates of a pre-mRNA splicing proofreading system in eukaryotes. They control stepwise induced conformational changes to turn a competent spliceosome into a catalytically active one [64–66]. Therefore, it is conceivable that phosphorylation of Prp1 by Prp4 kinase enhances the interaction of Prp1 with the ATPase/RNA helicase Prp2 to induce conformational changes in a pre-catalytic spliceosome. This suggestion does neither imply, nor exclude that the phosphorylation of Prp1 is the cause for the recruitment of Prp2 helicase. As a matter of fact, the Lührmann laboratory showed by using the mammalian HeLa cell splicing system that *in vitro* assembled pre-catalytic B-complexes are stabilized when Prp1 is phosphorylated by the Prp4K kinase *in vitro* [34]. This is consistent with our suggestion that stabilizing the pre-catalytic spliceosome *in vivo* by phosphorylation of Prp1 might increase time and chance for the ATPase(s) to operate as chaperone(s) at the pre-catalytic spliceosome.

In addition, while probing different transcripts containing multiple introns for their splicing defects, we discovered that pre-mRNAs containing introns larger than 250 nt never accumulate when splicing is inhibited *in vivo*. This occurred neither in cells where Prp4 kinase was inhibited by 1-NM-PP1 nor in cells containing the ts alleles *prp1-127*^{ts} or *prp1-4*^{ts} grown at the restrictive temperature, respectively (Eckert and Käufer, unpublished). It appears that transcripts containing introns of this size are rapidly degraded as a consequence of the splicing defect. This observation is consistent with the notion that this degradation of pre-mRNA most likely takes place in the nucleus. Noteworthy here, fission yeast contains only 9 % introns in the size range of 250–800 bp [62]. Preliminary results indicate that Rrp6, a subunit of the nuclear exosome, might be a candidate involved in this degradation process (Zock-Emmenthal and Käufer, unpublished).

Not much is known yet about the mechanisms of pre-mRNA degradation in the nucleus. However, distinct pathways of poly(A)-dependent mRNA degradation involving the nuclear poly(A)-binding protein (Pab2) and Rrp6 have been described in fission yeast [67–71].

Eukaryotic cells have developed several RNA surveillance pathways to prevent the expression of aberrant transcripts [72–74]. An early surveillance checkpoint acts at the transcription site and prevents the release of mRNAs that carry processing defects [75]. In mammals, the exosome including the Rrp6 subunit homolog PM/SCl-100, has been shown to be involved in many different RNA processing pathways. Based on these interactions of the exosome with multiple RNA processing machineries, it has been speculated that the production of a fully functional mRNA may be ensured through several different checkpoints [76].

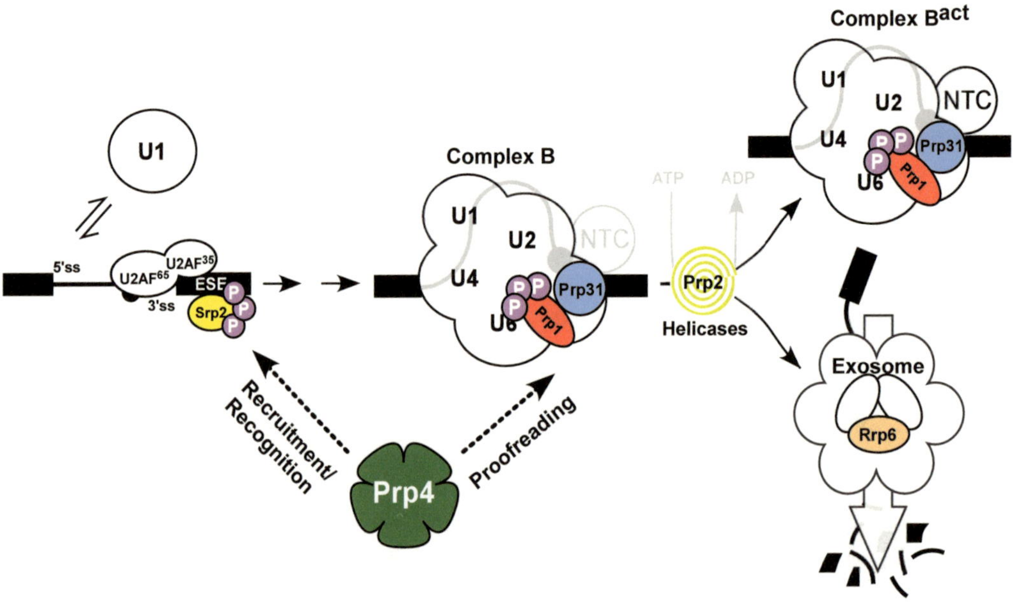

Figure 6. Checkpoints controlled by Prp4 kinase during splicing of a pre-mRNA. Phosphorylation of splicing factors, such as Srp2 may modulate their recruitment/binding to specific pre-mRNA substrates, thereby affecting the efficiency of intron recognition and removal. The phosphorylation of Prp1 acts as a "switch" to convert a fully assembled spliceosome into a catalytically active spliceosome. This is achieved, either directly or indirectly, by the recruitment of RNA helicases such as Prp2, which act as chaperones and aid in the proofreading of this process. Prp4 might also contribute in proofreading, i.e. by linking the splicing machinery to the nuclear exosome, which prevents that aberrant or unspliced pre-mRNA accumulates within the nucleus, if the transition from an inactive to an active spliceosome fails or the splicing reaction is unable to proceed. Exons of the pre-mRNA substrate are drawn as filled boxes, connected with a line (intron). Abbreviations: NTC, Nineteen Complex (containing Prp19, Cdc5 and other components, see reference [77]; ESE, Exonic Splicing Enhancer; U2AF, U2 auxiliary factor; ss, splice site.

We propose that Prp4 kinase is the pre-mRNA splicing checkpoint kinase, operating at the pre-catalytic spliceosome to provide splicing competent spliceosomes and to ensure that only properly spliced mRNA is transported out of the nucleus. Recruitment and/or enhancement of interactions between spliceosomal and exosomal components might be dependent on the phosphorylation of Prp1 by Prp4 kinase as suggested above for the ATPases (Figure 6). In the mammalian system Prp4K kinase appears also to phosphorylate hPrp31 *in vitro* which is a direct interaction partner of hPrp1 [34]. Interestingly, mutations in the hPrp31 phosphorylation sites seem to decrease the biochemical interaction capacity of pre-catalytic spliceosomes with the exosome [76]. Prp4 kinase of fission yeast does neither phosphorylate Prp31 *in vivo* nor *in vitro*. Two of the three mammalian phosphorylation sites are not conserved in the fission yeast homolog.

Collectively, we propose that phosphorylation of Prp1 determines the architecture of a platform for the proofreading and activation action of the ATPases at an assembled pre-catalytic spliceosome. At this level, the surveillance system is in close communication with the nuclear exosome and results in degradation of "aberrant" pre-mRNA at the transcriptional site (Fig. 6). All the questions which come up with our hypothesis can be experimentally approached and are currently under investigation. Further analysis will help to unravel in more detail the mechanism of this early surveillance checkpoint involved in controlling the expression of intron-containing genes.

Acknowledgements

We are grateful to Susanne Zock-Emmenthal, Daniela Eckert and Carolin Vogt for providing invaluable material and data for this chapter. Particularly, we want here to appreciate the input of Carolin Vogt who worked on the Srp2 project for her Masters Thesis (Technische Universität Braunschweig, 2011).

Author details

Martin Lützelberger and Norbert F. Käufer
Technische Universität Braunschweig, Institute of Genetics, Spielmannstr. 7, 38106 Braunschweig, Germany

9. References

[1] Cipak L, Zhang C, Kovacikova I, Rumpf C, Miadokova E, Shokat K M, Gregan J (2011) Generation of a set of conditional analog-sensitive alleles of essential protein kinases in the fission yeast *Schizosaccharomyces pombe*. Cell Cycle 10(20): 3527–3532.

[2] Käufer N F, Simanis V, Nurse P (1985) Fission yeast *Schizosaccharomyces pombe* correctly excises a mammalian RNA transcript intervening sequence. Nature 318(6041): 78–80.

[3] Gatermann K B, Hoffmann A, Rosenberg G H, Käufer N F (1989) Introduction of functional artificial introns into the naturally intronless ura4 gene of *Schizosaccharomyces pombe*. Mol Cell Biol 9(4): 1526–1535.

[4] Romfo C M, Alvarez C J, van Heeckeren W J, Webb C J, Wise J A (2000) Evidence for splice site pairing via intron definition in *Schizosaccharomyces pombe*. Mol Cell Biol 20(21): 7955–7970.

[5] Ram O, Ast G (2007) SR proteins: a foot on the exon before the transition from intron to exon definition. Trends Genet 23(1): 5–7.

[6] Potashkin J, Li R, Frendewey D (1989) Pre-mRNA splicing mutants of *Schizosaccharomyces pombe*. EMBO J 8(2): 551–559.

[7] Rosenberg G H, Alahari S K, Käufer N F (1991) *prp4* from *Schizosaccharomyces pombe*, a mutant deficient in pre-mRNA splicing isolated using genes containing artificial introns. Mol Gen Genet 226(1-2): 305–309.

[8] Alahari S K, Schmidt H, Käufer N F (1993) The fission yeast *prp4*$^{+}$ gene involved in pre-mRNA splicing codes for a predicted serine/threonine kinase and is essential for growth. Nucleic Acids Res 21(17): 4079–4083.

[9] Hanks S K, Quinn A M, Hunter T (1988) The protein kinase family: conserved features and deduced phylogeny of the catalytic domains. Science 241(4861): 42–52.

[10] Gross T, Lützelberger M, Wiegmann H, Klingenhoff A, Shenoy S, Käufer N F (1997) Functional analysis of the fission yeast Prp4 protein kinase involved in pre-mRNA splicing and isolation of a putative mammalian homologue. Nucleic Acids Res 25(5): 1028–1035.

[11] Beitz E (2000) TEXshade: shading and labeling of multiple sequence alignments using LATEX2 epsilon. Bioinformatics 16(2): 135–139.

[12] Tate P, Lee M, Tweedie S, Skarnes W C, Bickmore W A (1998) Capturing novel mouse genes encoding chromosomal and other nuclear proteins. J Cell Sci 111 (Pt 17): 2575–2585.

[13] Kojima T, Zama T, Wada K, Onogi H, Hagiwara M (2001) Cloning of human PRP4 reveals interaction with Clk1. J Biol Chem 276(34): 32247–32256.

[14] Dellaire G, Makarov E M, Cowger J J M, Longman D, Sutherland H G E, Lührmann R, Torchia J, Bickmore W A (2002) Mammalian PRP4 kinase copurifies and interacts with components of both the U5 snRNP and the N-CoR deacetylase complexes. Mol Cell Biol 22(14): 5141–5156.

[15] Kuhn A N, Käufer N F (2003) Pre-mRNA splicing in *Schizosaccharomyces pombe*: regulatory role of a kinase conserved from fission yeast to mammals. Curr Genet 42(5): 241–251.

[16] Aranda S, Laguna A, de la Luna S (2011) DYRK family of protein kinases: evolutionary relationships, biochemical properties, and functional roles. FASEB J 25(2): 449–462.

[17] Wilson-Grady J T, Villén J, Gygi S P (2008) Phosphoproteome analysis of fission yeast. J Proteome Res 7(3): 1088–1097.

[18] Zhong X Y, Wang P, Han J, Rosenfeld M G, Fu X D (2009) SR proteins in vertical integration of gene expression from transcription to RNA processing to translation. Mol Cell 35(1): 1–10.

[19] Gross T, Richert K, Mierke C, Lützelberger M, Käufer N F (1998) Identification and characterization of *srp1*, a gene of fission yeast encoding a RNA binding domain and a RS domain typical of SR splicing factors. Nucleic Acids Res 26(2): 505–511.

[20] Lützelberger M, Gross T, Käufer N F (1999) Srp2, an SR protein family member of fission yeast: *in vivo* characterization of its modular domains. Nucleic Acids Res 27(13): 2618–2626.

[21] Tang Z, Tsurumi A, Alaei S, Wilson C, Chiu C, Oya J, Ngo B (2007) Dsk1p kinase phosphorylates SR proteins and regulates their cellular localization in fission yeast. Biochem J 405(1): 21–30.

[22] Richert K (2003) Untersuchungen zur Aufklärung des Prä-mRNA Spleißvorgangs in der Spalthefe *Schizosaccharomyces pombe*: Genetische und biochemische Charakterisierung der Interaktionen des *prp4* Gens. Ph.D. thesis, Technische Universität Braunschweig. Available: `http://www.digibib.tu-bs.de/?docid=00001390`

[23] Tang Z, Kuo T, Shen J, Lin R J (2000) Biochemical and genetic conservation of fission yeast Dsk1 and human SR protein-specific kinase 1. Mol Cell Biol 20(3): 816–824.

[24] Tang Z, Käufer N F, Lin R J (2002) Interactions between two fission yeast serine/arginine-rich proteins and their modulation by phosphorylation. Biochem J 368(Pt 2): 527–534.

[25] Nilsen T W (2005) Spliceosome assembly in yeast: one ChIP at a time? Nat Struct Mol Biol 12(7): 571–573.

[26] Webb C J, Romfo C M, van Heeckeren W J, Wise J A (2005) Exonic splicing enhancers in fission yeast: functional conservation demonstrates an early evolutionary origin. Genes Dev 19(2): 242–254.

[27] Bennett E M, Lever A M L, Allen J F (2004) Human immunodeficiency virus type 2 Gag interacts specifically with PRP4, a serine-threonine kinase, and inhibits phosphorylation of splicing factor SF2. J Virol 78(20): 11303–11312.

[28] Karpenahalli M R, Lupas A N, Söding J (2007) TPRpred: a tool for prediction of TPR-, PPR- and SEL1-like repeats from protein sequences. BMC Bioinformatics 8: 2.

[29] Schmidt H, Richert K, Drakas R A, Käufer N F (1999) *spp42*, identified as a classical suppressor of *prp4-73*, which encodes a kinase involved in pre-mRNA splicing in fission yeast, is a homologue of the splicing factor Prp8p. Genetics 153(3): 1183–1191.

[30] Bottner C A, Schmidt H, Vogel S, Michele M, Käufer N F (2005) Multiple genetic and biochemical interactions of Brr2, Prp8, Prp31, Prp1 and Prp4 kinase suggest a function in the control of the activation of spliceosomes in *Schizosaccharomyces pombe*. Curr Genet 48(3): 151–161.

[31] Ritchie D B, Schellenberg M J, Gesner E M, Raithatha S A, Stuart D T, Macmillan A M (2008) Structural elucidation of a PRP8 core domain from the heart of the spliceosome. Nat Struct Mol Biol 15(11): 1199–1205.

[32] Maeder C, Kutach A K, Guthrie C (2009) ATP-dependent unwinding of U4/U6 snRNAs by the Brr2 helicase requires the C terminus of Prp8. Nat Struct Mol Biol 16(1): 42–48.

[33] Schwelnus W, Richert K, Opitz F, Gross T, Habara Y, Tani T, Käufer N F (2001) Fission yeast Prp4p kinase regulates pre-mRNA splicing by phosphorylating a non-SR-splicing factor. EMBO Rep 2(1): 35–41.

[34] Schneider M, Hsiao H H, Will C L, Giet R, Urlaub H, Lührmann R (2010) Human PRP4 kinase is required for stable tri-snRNP association during spliceosomal B complex formation. Nat Struct Mol Biol 17(2): 216–221.

[35] Lützelberger M, Bottner C A, Schwelnus W, Zock-Emmenthal S, Razanau A, Käufer N F (2010) The N-terminus of Prp1 (Prp6/U5-102 K) is essential for spliceosome activation *in vivo*. Nucleic Acids Res 38(5): 1610–1622.

[36] Huang Y, Deng T, Winston B W (2000) Characterization of hPRP4 kinase activation: potential role in signaling. Biochem Biophys Res Commun 271(2): 456–463.

[37] Huang B, Ahn Y T, McPherson L, Clayberger C, Krensky A M (2007) Interaction of PRP4 with Kruppel-like factor 13 regulates CCL5 transcription. J Immunol 178(11): 7081–7087.

[38] Montembault E, Dutertre S, Prigent C, Giet R (2007) PRP4 is a spindle assembly checkpoint protein required for MPS1, MAD1, and MAD2 localization to the kinetochores. J Cell Biol 179(4): 601–609.

[39] Duan Z, Weinstein E J, Ji D, Ames R Y, Choy E, Mankin H, Hornicek F J (2008) Lentiviral short hairpin RNA screen of genes associated with multidrug resistance identifies PRP-4 as a new regulator of chemoresistance in human ovarian cancer. Mol Cancer Ther 7(8): 2377–2385.

[40] Kuhn A N, Käufer N F (2004) The Molecular Biology of *Schizosaccharomyces pombe*, chapter Mechanism and Control of Pre-mRNA Splicing, 353–368. Springer, Heidelberg.

[41] Bottner C A (2006) Die Phosphorylierung von Prp1p durch Prp4p-Kinase ist notwendig zur Aktivierung von prä-katalytischen Spleißosomen. Ph.D. thesis, Technische Universität Braunschweig. Available: `http://www.digibib.tu-bs.de/?docid=00000030`

[42] Newo A N S, Lützelberger M, Bottner C A, Wehland J, Wissing J, Jänsch L, Käufer N F (2007) Proteomic analysis of the U1 snRNP of *Schizosaccharomyces pombe* reveals three essential organism-specific proteins. Nucleic Acids Res 35(5): 1391–1401.

[43] Fabrizio P, Dannenberg J, Dube P, Kastner B, Stark H, Urlaub H, Lührmann R (2009) The evolutionarily conserved core design of the catalytic activation step of the yeast spliceosome. Mol Cell 36(4): 593–608.

[44] Erler A, Maresca M, Fu J, Stewart A F (2006) Recombineering reagents for improved inducible expression and selection marker re-use in *Schizosaccharomyces pombe.* Yeast 23(11): 813–823.

[45] Kim S H, Lin R J (1996) Spliceosome activation by PRP2 ATPase prior to the first transesterification reaction of pre-mRNA splicing. Mol Cell Biol 16(12): 6810–6819.

[46] Gencheva M, Lin T Y, Wu X, Yang L, Richard C, Jones M, Lin S B, Lin R J (2010) Nuclear retention of unspliced pre-mRNAs by mutant DHX16/hPRP2, a spliceosomal DEAH-box protein. J Biol Chem 285(46): 35624–35632.

[47] Edwalds-Gilbert G, Kim D H, Kim S H, Tseng Y H, Yu Y, Lin R J (2000) Dominant negative mutants of the yeast splicing factor Prp2 map to a putative cleft region in the helicase domain of DExD/H-box proteins. RNA 6(8): 1106–1119.

[48] Gould K L, Ren L, Feoktistova A S, Jennings J L, Link A J (2004) Tandem affinity purification and identification of protein complex components. Methods 33(3): 239–244.

[49] Razanau A (2010) Isolation and characterization of suppressors of the *prp1* gene, encoding a regulatory component of the pre-catalytic spliceosome in fission yeast. Ph.D. thesis, Technische Universität Braunschweig. Available: `http://www.digibib.tu-bs.de/?docid=00036702`

[50] Lundgren K, Allan S, Urushiyama S, Tani T, Ohshima Y, Frendewey D, Beach D (1996) A connection between pre-mRNA splicing and the cell cycle in fission yeast: *cdc28*$^+$ is allelic with *prp8*$^+$ and encodes an RNA-dependent ATPase/helicase. Mol Biol Cell 7(7): 1083–1094.

[51] Rigaut G, Shevchenko A, Rutz B, Wilm M, Mann M, Séraphin B (1999) A generic protein purification method for protein complex characterization and proteome exploration. Nat Biotechnol 17(10): 1030–1032.

[52] Puig O, Caspary F, Rigaut G, Rutz B, Bouveret E, Bragado-Nilsson E, Wilm M, Séraphin B (2001) The tandem affinity purification (TAP) method: a general procedure of protein complex purification. Methods 24(3): 218–229.

[53] Gencheva M, Kato M, Newo A N S, Lin R J (2010) Contribution of DEAH-box protein DHX16 in human pre-mRNA splicing. Biochem J 429(1): 25–32.

[54] Gregan J, Zhang C, Rumpf C, Cipak L, Li Z, Uluocak P, Nasmyth K, Shokat K M (2007) Construction of conditional analog-sensitive kinase alleles in the fission yeast *Schizosaccharomyces pombe.* Nat Protoc 2(11): 2996–3000.

[55] Gómez-Escoda B, Ivanova T, Calvo I A, Alves-Rodrigues I, Hidalgo E, Ayté J (2011) Yox1 links MBF-dependent transcription to completion of DNA synthesis. EMBO Rep 12(1): 84–89.

[56] Potashkin J, Naik K, Wentz-Hunter K (1993) U2AF homolog required for splicing *in vivo.* Science 262(5133): 573–575.

[57] Habara Y, Urushiyama S, Shibuya T, Ohshima Y, Tani T (2001) Mutation in the *prp12*$^+$ gene encoding a homolog of SAP130/SF3b130 causes differential inhibition of pre-mRNA splicing and arrest of cell-cycle progression in *Schizosaccharomyces pombe.* RNA 7(5): 671–681.

[58] Sridharan V, Heimiller J, Singh R (2011) Genomic mRNA profiling reveals compensatory mechanisms for the requirement of the essential splicing factor U2AF. Mol Cell Biol 31(4): 652–661.
[59] Ayté J, Schweitzer C, Zarzov P, Nurse P, DeCaprio J A (2001) Feedback regulation of the MBF transcription factor by cyclin Cig2. Nat Cell Biol 3(12): 1043–1050.
[60] Malapeira J, Moldón A, Hidalgo E, Smith G R, Nurse P, Ayté J (2005) A meiosis-specific cyclin regulated by splicing is required for proper progression through meiosis. Mol Cell Biol 25(15): 6330–6337.
[61] Moldón A, Malapeira J, Gabrielli N, Gogol M, Gómez-Escoda B, Ivanova T, Seidel C, Ayté J (2008) Promoter-driven splicing regulation in fission yeast. Nature 455(7215): 997–1000.
[62] Kupfer D M, Drabenstot S D, Buchanan K L, Lai H, Zhu H, Dyer D W, Roe B A, Murphy J W (2004) Introns and splicing elements of five diverse fungi. Eukaryot Cell 3(5): 1088–1100.
[63] Käufer N F, Potashkin J (2000) Analysis of the splicing machinery in fission yeast: a comparison with budding yeast and mammals. Nucleic Acids Res 28(16): 3003–3010.
[64] Staley J P, Guthrie C (1998) Mechanical devices of the spliceosome: motors, clocks, springs, and things. Cell 92(3): 315–326.
[65] Tseng C K, Liu H L, Cheng S C (2011) DEAH-box ATPase Prp16 has dual roles in remodeling of the spliceosome in catalytic steps. RNA 17(1): 145–154.
[66] Horowitz D S (2011) The splice is right: guarantors of fidelity in pre-mRNA splicing. RNA 17(4): 551–554.
[67] Harigaya Y, Tanaka H, Yamanaka S, Tanaka K, Watanabe Y, Tsutsumi C, Chikashige Y, Hiraoka Y, Yamashita A, Yamamoto M (2006) Selective elimination of messenger RNA prevents an incidence of untimely meiosis. Nature 442(7098): 45–50.
[68] McPheeters D S, Cremona N, Sunder S, Chen H M, Averbeck N, Leatherwood J, Wise J A (2009) A complex gene regulatory mechanism that operates at the nexus of multiple RNA processing decisions. Nat Struct Mol Biol 16(3): 255–264.
[69] Yamanaka S, Yamashita A, Harigaya Y, Iwata R, Yamamoto M (2010) Importance of polyadenylation in the selective elimination of meiotic mRNAs in growing S. pombe cells. EMBO J 29(13): 2173–2181.
[70] Sugiyama T, Sugioka-Sugiyama R (2011) Red1 promotes the elimination of meiosis-specific mRNAs in vegetatively growing fission yeast. EMBO J 30(6): 1027–1039.
[71] Lemieux C, Marguerat S, Lafontaine J, Barbezier N, Bähler J, Bachand F (2011) A Pre-mRNA degradation pathway that selectively targets intron-containing genes requires the nuclear poly(A)-binding protein. Mol Cell 44(1): 108–119.
[72] Reznik B, Lykke-Andersen J (2010) Regulated and quality-control mRNA turnover pathways in eukaryotes. Biochem Soc Trans 38(6): 1506–1510.
[73] Houseley J, Tollervey D (2009) The many pathways of RNA degradation. Cell 136(4): 763–776.
[74] Doma M K, Parker R (2007) RNA quality control in eukaryotes. Cell 131(4): 660–668.
[75] Eberle A B, Hessle V, Helbig R, Dantoft W, Gimber N, Visa N (2010) Splice-site mutations cause Rrp6-mediated nuclear retention of the unspliced RNAs and transcriptional down-regulation of the splicing-defective genes. PLoS One 5(7): e11540.
[76] Nag A, Steitz J A (2012) Tri-snRNP-associated proteins interact with subunits of the TRAMP and nuclear exosome complexes, linking RNA decay and pre-mRNA splicing. RNA Biol 9(3).

[77] Grote M, Wolf E, Will C L, Lemm I, Agafonov D E, Schomburg A, Fischle W, Urlaub H, Lührmann R (2010) Molecular architecture of the human Prp19/CDC5L complex. Mol Cell Biol 30(9): 2105–2119.

Chapter 7

More Than Just an OFF-Switch: The Essential Role of Protein Dephosphorylation in the Modulation of BDNF Signaling Events

Katrin Deinhardt and Freddy Jeanneteau

Additional information is available at the end of the chapter

http://dx.doi.org/10.5772/50420

1. Introduction

Upon binding to their receptors, growth factors trigger intracellular signaling cascades. These cascades are propagated and modulated by many subsequent phosphorylation/ dephosphorylation events, which ultimately influence the cellular response. BDNF, a major growth factor of the central nervous system, is a member of the family of neurotrophins, which also comprises nerve growth factor (NGF) and neurotrophins (NT) 3 and 4. Neurotrophins bind to their cognate Trk receptor tyrosine kinases TrkA, B or C, to initiate downstream signaling events (Figure 1) (1, 2). During development, neurotrophins act as target-derived growth factors, which are essential for the survival of selective populations of neurons, especially within the peripheral nervous system (3). However, neurotrophin signaling extends well beyond effects on neuronal survival during development, and also plays important roles in higher order function in the adult, such as behavior, learning and memory. This is best characterized for BDNF- TrkB signaling. Mature BDNF facilitates long-term potentiation and dendritic spine formation in the hippocampus, a process that has been implicated in learning and memory (4). Animals with lower levels of BDNF or its receptor TrkB, as well as mice harboring a common polymorphism in the *bdnf* gene leading to decreased BDNF secretion, give rise to eating disorders and an increase in anxiety-related behaviour (5). Moreover, decreases in BDNF have been correlated with depression while increases in BDNF seem to have an antidepressant effect, and conversely, commonly prescribed anti-depressants raise BDNF levels (5, 6).

In this chapter, we will describe in detail examples of feedback and feed-forward loops downstream of BDNF-TrkB signaling, which transmit and adjust the signal, and therefore determine the ultimate physiological outcome. These cascades comprise multiple protein phosphorylation and dephosphorylation events to modulate both the duration and localization of the signal, as well as the downstream targets affected. These processes help shed light on how a single, well conserved ligand-receptor pair can have such diverse effects on cellular physiology as described above for BDNF-TrkB.

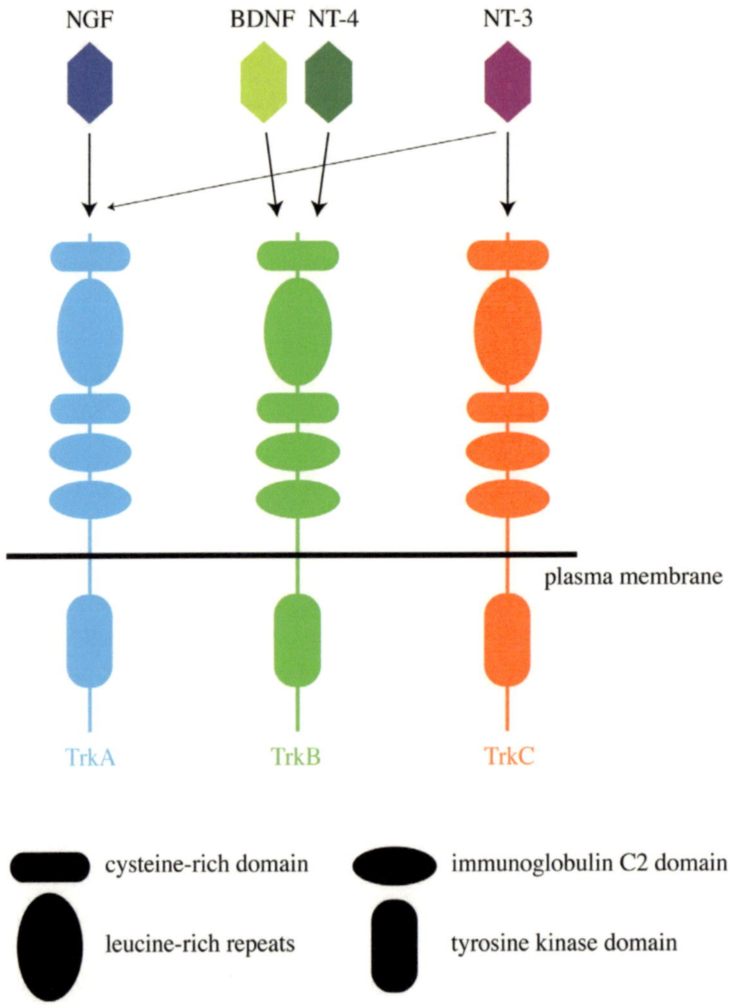

The neurotrophin family consists of four closely related proteins encoded by four different genes that include NGF (nerve growth factor), BDNF (brain-derived neurotrophic factor), NT-3 (neurotrophin-3) and NT-4 (neurotrophin-4). Neurotrophins act as homodimeric ligands for the Trk (tropomyosin-related kinase) receptors. Three Trk receptors encoded by independent genes afford selectivity among neurotrophins with NGF and NT-3 binding to TrkA, BDNF and NT-4 binding to TrkB and NT-3 binding to TrkC. All Trk receptors are composed of extracellular leucine-rich repeats, cysteine-rich domains and a single immunoglobulin C2 domain that ensure proper conformation of the ligand-binding pocket. Neurotrophin binding promotes homodimerization of Trk receptors, which in turn initiates intracellular phosphorylation cascades. The intracellular tyrosine kinase domain common to all Trk receptors is necessary for neurotrophin signaling as it allows transphosphorylation of several key tyrosine residues of the Trk receptor dimer at the origin of pleiotropic neurotrophic function. Several splice isoforms of the Trk receptors encode for a truncated protein that lack large portions of the intracellular domain. The TrkB.T1 and TrkB.T2 isoforms lack the prototypical tyrosine kinase domain. These isoforms are abundant in the adult brain and notably in glial cells. Nevertheless, glial cells respond to neurotrophin by eliciting distinct intracellular events. For instance, BDNF signaling mediated by the glial truncated TrkB.T1 isoform elevate intracellular calcium and associated phosphorylation waves mediated by calcium-sensing proteins kinases like CaMK2.

Figure 1. Neurotrophins and Trk neurotrophin receptor family of proteins.

2. Immediate changes in protein phosphorylation downstream of BDNF/ TrkB

Activation of TrkB upon BDNF binding leads to receptor dimerization and phosphorylation, thereby creating docking sites for effector proteins that initiate the activation of intracellular signaling pathways (7). The phosphorylated tyrosine residues Y516 and Y817 in human TrkB receptor serve as the main docking sites to initiate downstream signaling pathways, such as Src homology 2 containing protein (Shc), Akt, mitogen-activated protein kinase (MAPK)/ extracellular signal-regulated kinase (Erk) 1/2 and phospholipase C (PLC) γ (Figure 2) (1, 8). This in turn leads to the activation of various pathways involved in cellular functions that range from initiation of gene transcription and protein synthesis to decisions involved in cell growth and survival. The residues Y702, Y706 and Y707, located within the tyrosine kinase domain, can also recruit adaptor proteins when phosphorylated, including Grb2 and SH2B. At the same time as inducing multiple protein tyrosine, serine and threonine phosphorylation events in diverse proteins, BDNF stimulation may cause a reduction in the phosphorylation of other proteins, such as focal adhesion kinase (9), thereby reducing their activity. In the following paragraph, we will discuss in more detail multiple ways of neurotrophin-dependent activation of Erk1/2 signaling pathways.

3. Multiple cascades leading to BDNF-dependent Erk1/2 activation

Three major pathways mediate activation of Erk1/2 downstream of BDNF: PLCγ/ PKC signaling following phosphorylation of Y817 site, or Shc-Grb2 signaling through Ras or Rap1 (Figure 3) (1).

Phosphorylation of hTrkB (human TrkB) at the most C-terminal tyrosine, Y817, leads to the recruitment and activation of PLCγ, which hydrolyses phosphatidylinositol(4, 5)bisphosphate ($PI(4,5)P_2$) into diacylglycerol (DAG) and inositol tris-phosphate (IP_3). IP_3 subsequently leads to release of intracellular Ca^{2+}, which in turn activates Ca^{2+}-dependent enzymes such as Ca^{2+}-calmodulin-regulated protein kinases (CaM kinases), as well as the phosphatase calcineurin. Additionally, the release of Ca^{2+} and the production of DAG activate protein kinase C (PKC), which stimulates Erk1/2 signaling via activation of Raf and the mitogen activated protein kinase kinase MEK.

Along another pathway leading to active Erk, phosphorylation of hTrkB at the tyrosine residue closest to the plasma membrane, Y516, creates an Shc binding site to initiate downstream transient or prolonged Erk1/2 signaling. Transient activation follows the recruitment of a complex of growth factor receptor bound protein 2 (Grb2) and the Ras activator son of sevenless (SOS), which in turn stimulates activation of Ras and downstream, the activation of the c-Raf/ MEK/ Erk1/2 cascade. Erk in turn phosphorylates SOS, leading to the dissociation of the Grb2/ SOS complex, which then no longer activates the Ras/ c-Raf/ MEK cascade, thus only leading to transient activation of Erk.

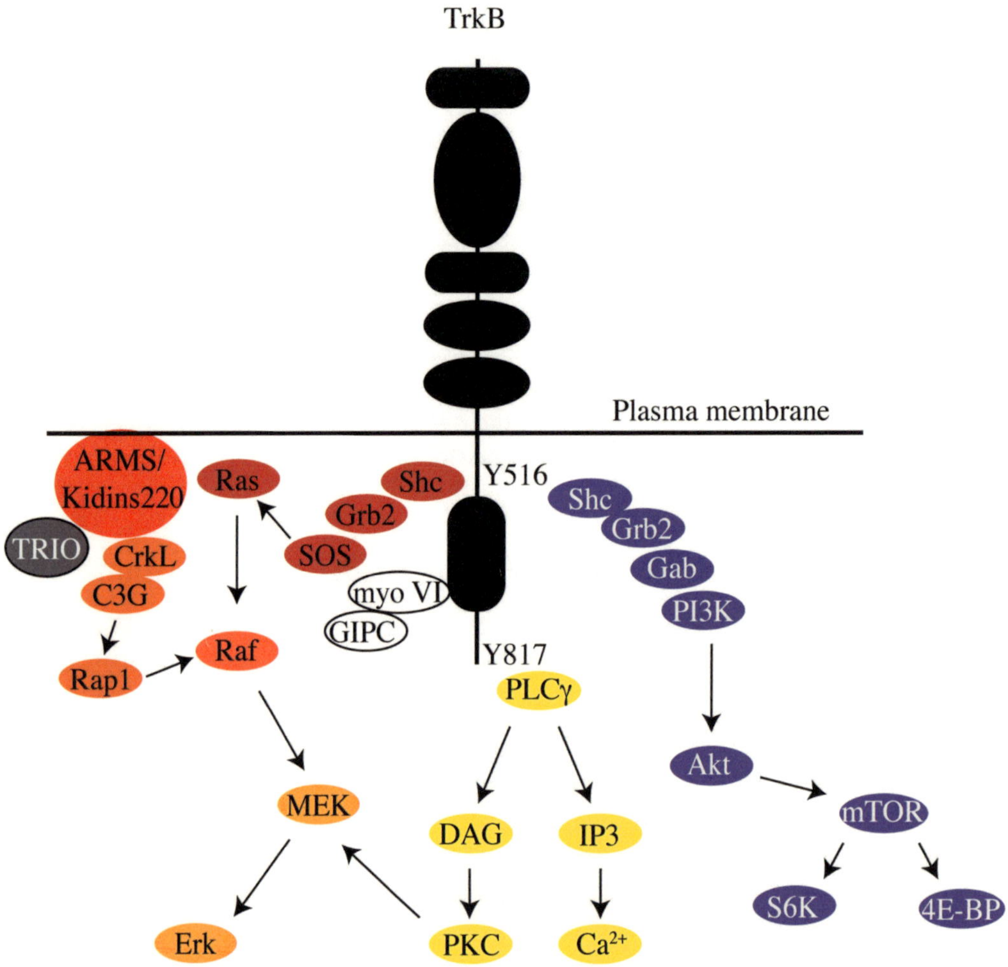

Upon binding to BDNF, a series of tyrosine phosphorylation events occur within TrkB cytoplasmic domain. These phospho-tyrosine residues form unique binding sites for intracellular adaptor proteins, Y516 and Y817 recruiting specifically Shc and PLCγ, respectively. The typical wave of second messengers involves, PLCγ, which raises intracellular calcium, the Ras-Erk and PI3-Kinase/Akt pathways. The elevation of intracellular calcium allows the activation of CAMK (calmodulin kinases), which converges with the Erk pathway to activate transcription factors like CREB within the nucleus by phosphorylation on S133. Trancription factors like CREB transform transient BDNF signaling into durable signaling by changing the expression of many selective target genes.

Figure 2. Proximal intracellular signaling of the TrkB receptor.

Prolonged Erk activation is also initiated at the Y516 site, but requires the adaptor protein ankyrin-rich membrane spanning protein (ARMS, also known as Kidins220), which recruits Grb2 and CrkL. This complex formation depends on tyrosine phosphorylation of ARMS at the residue Y1096. Binding to CrkL then activates the Rap exchange factor C3G and thus initiates prolonged Rap1/ Raf-dependent MEK/ Erk1/2 signaling. Accordingly, loss of ARMS impairs Rap1 activation and prolonged activation of Erk1/2, while early Erk1/2 activity is not affected (10).

Ultimately, Erk1/2 signaling not only promotes local axonal growth via cytosolic signaling events, but activated Erk1/2 can also translocate to the nucleus to phosphorylate and activate transcription factors, such as CREB (cAMP response element-binding), leading to the initiation of transcriptional events and the expression of immediate early genes (IEGs), which can further modulate the response (11).

4. The importance of signal duration

In the mid 1990s, it became widely recognized that the actual signal duration will critically influence the ultimate cellular outcome (12). Because the MAPK pathway (e.g. Erk1/2, JNK, P38) is central for the activation of transcription factors, the expression of a large array of genes is sensitive to extracellular trophic factors, such as BDNF (13). One classical example that highlights the importance of the temporal control of signaling is the activation of Erk1/2 downstream of NGF versus EGF in pheochromocytoma (PC12) cells (14). NGF leads to sustained activation of Erk1/2 by inducing a positive feedback loop on to the upstream activator Raf, whereas EGF activates a negative feedback loop to Raf and thus leads to transient activation of Erk1/2. As a consequence, EGF promotes cell division, while NGF initiates differentiation. This is not specific to PC12 cells, as sustained Erk1/2 activity also transforms fibroblasts and macrophages (15, 16). Indeed, under pathological conditions unrestricted activation of the Ras-Erk1/2 pathway through point mutations is one of the most frequently identified cellular defects leading to tumour formation and cancer (17).

One explanation for a differential duration of Erk1/2 activation downstream of different growth factors may be the expression levels of their cognate receptors. Indeed, PC12 clones with low amounts of the NGF receptor TrkA fail to differentiate in response to NGF, while PC12 cells overexpressing EGF receptor can undergo differentiation in response to EGF (18). In line with this, tumour cells frequently upregulate growth factor receptors, leading to aberrant activation and transformation (19).

In addition to activation through distinct cascades, both positive and negative feedback loops further influence the amplitude and duration of MAPK signals. For example, BDNF induces its own release, thus initiating further rounds of receptor-mediated signal activation (20). On the other hand, Erk1/2 phosphorylates SOS, which impairs SOS-Grb2 complex formation and thus decreases further activation of Erk1/2 (21). Moreover, multiple phosphatases (PP1, PP2a and MKPs) inactivate ERKs, implying that the duration and extent of ERK activation is controlled by the balanced activities of the upstream ERK kinases, MEKs, as well as MEK and ERK phosphatases (22-24). Modeling approaches showed that these multiple layers of feedback along the MAPK cascade can not only determine the strength and timing of the signal, but also induce robust and sustained signal oscillations, thereby ultimately allowing for a multitude of biological outcomes (25).

5. Localizing the signal: Signal transduction cascades versus trafficking and intracellular localization of the ligand-receptor complex

Receptor tyrosine kinases are activated by ligand binding at the cell surface. They are subsequently internalized into the endosomal pathway and either recycled back to the plasma membrane for further rounds of activation, or sorted to the lysosome for degradation. For a long time, the classical belief was that signal transduction terminates with receptor internalization. However, receptors are internalized very rapidly upon activation, thus leaving only a short time window to induce signal transduction. In the mid 1990s the view changed and it became accepted that receptors continue to signal following internalization, from so-called signaling endosomes (26-28). Much work has since focused on endosomes as signaling platforms, and it is now well established that cascades such as the Erk1/2 or Akt pathways can be initiated from endosomal membranes. For example, the MEK1 scaffold, MEK partner 1 (MP1), recruits MEK1 and Erk1/2 to endosomal membranes, and knockdown of MP1 leads to lack of recruitment and a concomitant reduction in Erk1/2 signaling (29).

The essential role of signaling from endosomes in physiological processes such as polarization and migration is widely accepted. In addition, a large body of work has highlighted the importance of signaling endosomes in neurons, where signals at times have to traverse large distances. For example, intracellular trafficking of the signal-receptor complex from the synapse along the axon and to the cell body is essential for health and survival of neurons of the peripheral nervous system, which depend on target-derived growth factors (30, 31). Consequently, mutations in genes involved in this retrograde axonal transport process are frequently associated with neuropathies (32).

Interestingly, two recent studies in cell lines questioned the view that intracellular trafficking of the activated ligand-receptor complex is critical for downstream cellular responses (33, 34). Following EGF stimulation, they demonstrated that the cascades eventually influencing transcriptional changes are already initiated at the plasma membrane, and within a short time after ligand binding. Consequently, interfering with subsequent ligand-receptor sorting had only minor effects on the overall transcriptional response. How these findings apply to different cell systems, for example in highly polarized cells such as neurons, remains to be seen. At least for peripheral neurons, it has been demonstrated that internalization of the NGF-TrkA complex at the distal axon is strictly required for activation of CREB, initiation of transcription, and survival (28).

6. Activation of an essential CREB co-activator through dephosphorylation

Phosphorylation of CREB is an activation mark that is required but not sufficient to induce the expression of responsive-genes (35). The CREB co-activator, transducer of regulated CREB (TORC or CRTC) must be actively transported to the nucleus to allow CREB-dependent transcription of target genes (35). There are three members of the CRTC family (CRTC1/2/3) that are encoded by independent genes. Each isoform presents specific expression profile and binding to CREB-occupied genes, but redundancy was highlighted by loss-of-function experiments (36). For instance, CRTC1 null mice decrease BDNF expression in the prefrontal cortex and hippocampus down to 40 % of wildtype levels, suggesting additional mechanisms of regulation and/ or compensatory mechanisms (37). Knockdown of CRTC1, the major isoform in the limbic brain is sufficient to prevent BDNF-induced structural plasticity such as dendritic and axonal arborization, as well as physiological features like long-term potentiation that also depends on BDNF/TrkB signaling (38, 39). Because the transcriptional activity of CREB downstream of BDNF depends on CRTC1 and perhaps other CRTC isoforms, it is now interesting to describe how CRTC1 function is regulated.

When phosphorylated, CRTC proteins reside in the cytoplasm of resting neurons via high affinity interactions with 14-3-3, a family of cytoplasmic scaffold proteins that help organize and sequester phosphorylated proteins in the cytoplasm. Upon neuronal activation, CRTC proteins become dephosphorylated notably at residues S171, S275 and S307, which unmask a nuclear localization sequence and permit the translocation of CRTC proteins into the nucleus (40). If at the same time CREB is phosphorylated, the formation a CREB-CRTC1-CBP protein complex can drive transcription at target genes (Figure 3). Such a mode of action raises questions about the coincidence detection mechanisms that allow the convergence of CREB phosphorylation and CRTC dephosphorylation. Calcineurin, a calcium sensing phosphatase, directly dephosphorylates CRTC proteins. BDNF signaling induces robust and sustained phosphorylation of CREB, but cannot elicit nuclear translocation of CRTC1 (38). In similar experiments conducted in hypothalamic neurons, where CRTC2 is the major isoform expressed, BDNF signaling did not elicit CRTC2 translocation to the nucleus, while cAMP-elevating drugs or drugs that elevate intracellular calcium did (41). Although BDNF/TrkB signaling has been previously shown to elevate cAMP and calcium levels in neurons (1, 42), it is believed to occur and remain local, such as neurite terminals (20). However, it is clear that elevation of intracellular cAMP or calcium facilitate the functional and morphological synaptic responses to BDNF signaling (43, 44). Elevation of intracellular calcium activates calcineurin whereas cAMP activates PKA, which in turn phosphorylates and deactivates the upstream CRTC kinase, salt-inducible kinase (SIK). Only such coordinated signaling guarantees efficient translocation of CRTC proteins to the nucleus (Figure 3). So, what neuronal mechanisms mediate calcineurin-dependent dephosphorylation of CRTC protein? Neuronal activity via calcium-permeable glutamate ion channels not only phosphorylates CREB, but also triggers the calcineurin-dependent dephosphorylation of CRTC1 in cortical neurons and of CRTC2 in hypothalamic neurons that is necessary to activate CREB-mediated transcription (38, 41).

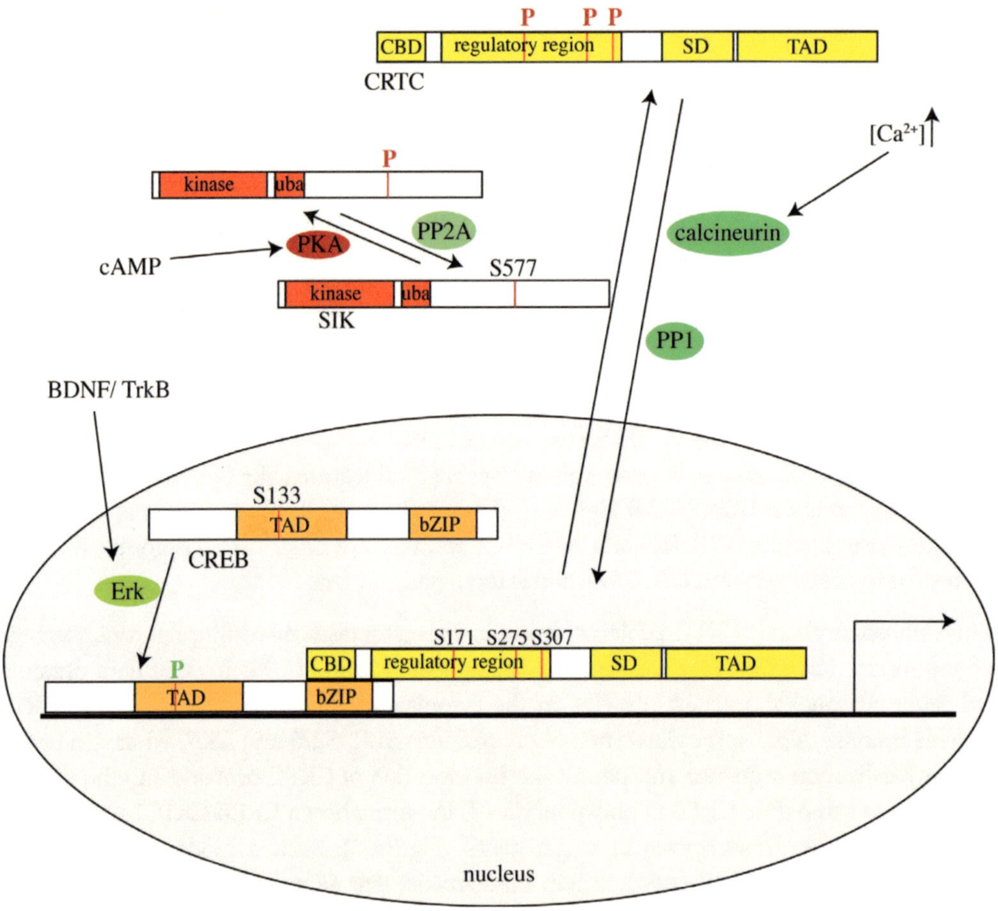

Figure 3. Subcellular compartmentalization of CRTC proteins regulates their function as necessary CREB-cofactors. CRTC proteins are constitutively phosphorylated in many cell types including neurons. Consequently, they reside in the cytoplasm via sequestration by the 14-3-3 family of proteins. When actively dephosphorylated by the calcium-sensing phosphatase calcineurin, a nuclear localization sequence is unmasked and CRTC translocates to the nucleus. Efficient translocation of CRTC protein to the nucleus is also governed by concomitant inactivation of the CRTC upstream kinases like SIK (Salt-inducible kinase) via its phoshorylation by the protein kinase A. Once in the nucleus, CRTC proteins form a multi-complex with the phosphorylated form of CREB, thus, acting as a permissive signal for robust and specific genomic signaling response.

7. Wait a minute: Immediate-early gene expression following BDNF stimulation

Following the immediate phosphorylation and dephosphorylation events, BDNF signaling eventually results in a nuclear response and immediate-early gene (IEG) expression. This process starts within minutes, and the first translated proteins are detectable within 30 min following the initial stimulation. Many IEGs are themselves transcription factors, such as fos, which will set off a series of transcription/ translation waves to adjust the cellular transcriptome and proteome. Other IEGs directly modulate cellular shape and responsiveness. The probably best-characterized BDNF-sensitive IEG is Arc (Arg3.1), a modulator of actin depolymerizing factor (ADF)/ cofilin activity and regulator of AMPA receptor trafficking (45). Local translation of Arc plays an essential role in the consolidation of long-term potentiation, which equates to an increase in synaptic transmission in response to neuronal activity. In addition, BDNF initiates its own synthesis and release, thereby strengthening and prolonging its own signal and starting a positive feedback loop. Other IEGs induced by Erk1/2 signaling are phosphatases, which provide a negative feedback loop. For example, we recently reported that BDNF-TrkB signaling induces the expression of the dual-specificity phosphatase MKP-1 (MAP kinase phosphatase 1, also known as DUSP1) (46). MKPs comprise a family if phosphatases that recognize and dephosphorylate both the threonine (T) and tyrosine (Y) within a TxY motif in the catalytic core that is conserved among the family of MAPKs (24). Below, the role of MKP-1 expression in modulating MAPK signaling, and its ultimate cellular consequences, will be discussed in greater detail.

8. MKP-1 molds the MAPK signal and neuronal morphology

Basal MKP-1 protein levels within the cell are very low, but its expression is induced following Erk1/2 activation by growth factors in a variety of cell types (47). Generally, MKPs have a preference for specific members of the MAPK family, and the favored substrates for MKP-1 are JNK, p38 and Erk1/2. Therefore, MKP-1 can terminate the signal that initially induced its expression (24). This form of feedback inhibition is a common theme in many signal transduction events, such as discussed above for Erk1/2 signaling. After induction, MKP-1 is rapidly degraded by the proteasome within one hour post stimulation. But BDNF signaling prolongs MKP-1 protein stability by several hours (46). Erk1/2-dependent phosphorylation of carboxy-terminal serine residues can modulate the half-life of MKP-1 protein. One study proposed that phosphorylation of serines 296 and 323 is required for recognition of MKP-1 by the ubiquitin ligase, thereby promoting degradation (48), while another study suggested that phosphorylation at serines 359 and 364 interferes with ubiquitination and thus prevents degradation (49). Serial mutagenesis of such signature motifs helped crack MKP-1 phosphorylation code (Figure 4). Only the mutations of all four phospho-sites alter significantly MKP-1 protein half-life whereas mutations of individual phospho-sites or motifs (S296/S323 and S359/S364) are mainly ineffective. Notably, alanine mutations in place of serines 359 and 364 as well as phospho-mimicking glutamate mutations in place of serines 296 and 323 in a single quadruple mutant diminish MKP-1 protein stability despite BDNF signaling. Therefore, BDNF signaling not only induces *mkp-1* expression but also prolongs MKP-1 protein half-life as a result of phosphorylation/ dephosphorylation of MKP-1 C-terminal signature motifs (Figure 4) (46). If the kinase involved in MKP-1 phosphorylation at serine 359 in neurons is Erk1/2, the identity of the phosphatases for serines 296 and 323 are presently unknown.

Within the immune system, MKP-1 is largely nuclear. One of its best-described functions is terminating cytokine production and therefore the immune response by inactivating p38 and p38-mediated transcription following an immune challenge. Indeed, mice lacking

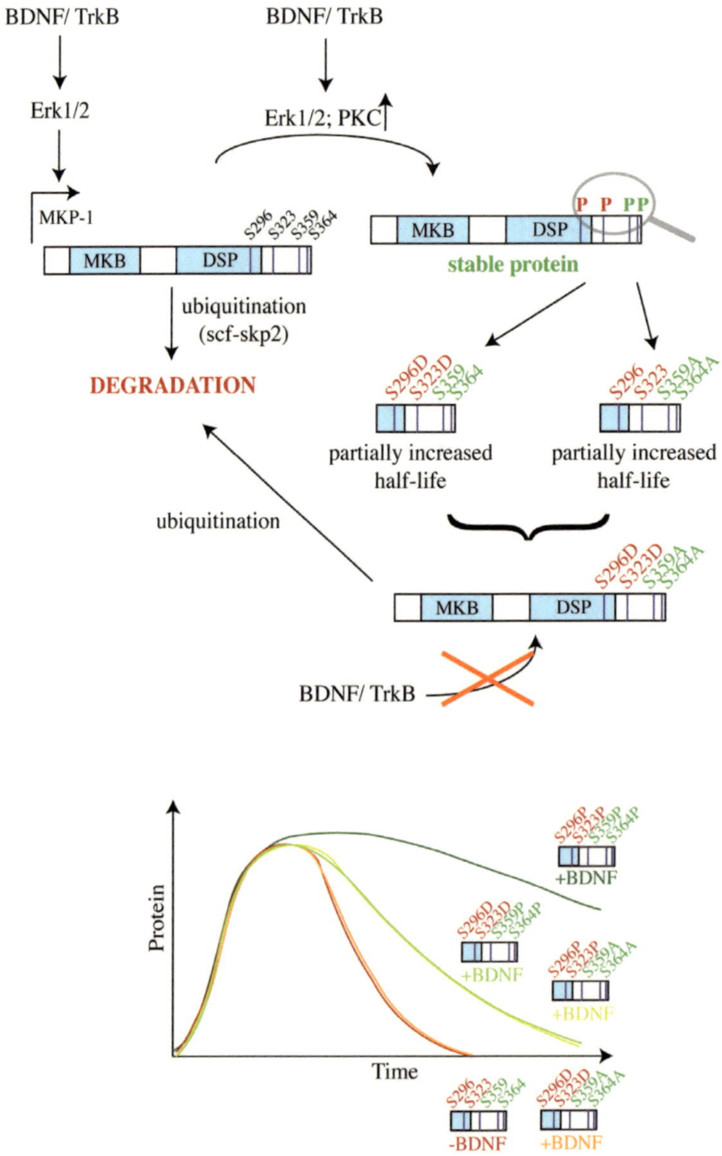

Figure 4. *Mkp-1* is a BDNF and CREB sensitive gene. Among the many genes regulated by CREB, *mkp-1* is an immediate early gene that can be expressed within minutes of BDNF stimulation. With low basal expression in resting neurons, the induction of the *mkp-1* gene product represents a mechanism of activation necessarily delayed in time from the initial BDNF signaling cascade. It is thought that MKP-1 protein serves to terminate the MAPK signaling via a negative feedback loop mechanism, since MKP-1 is a deactivating MAPK phosphatase. To support this view, the protein turnover of MKP-1 is extremely rapid (< 1 hour) allowing the rapid reinstatement of basal MAPK signaling homeostasis. Of note, phosphorylation of MKP-1 by Erk is sufficient to stabilize the protein. This serves to maintain MKP-1 function where needed in the cell whereas other signaling compartments lacking Erk signaling are preserved. So, MKP-1 induction and stabilization offers a sophisticated mode of regulation for MAPK signaling in time and space.

MKP-1 die due to cytokine overproduction after activation of the immune system (50). In neurons, MKP-1 localises to the cytosol. Here, it inactivates JNK, which is constitutively active within axons of neurons of the central nervous system (51). Prolonged MKP-1 expression thus leads to decreased phosphorylation of JNK substrates. Among the neuronal JNK substrates are many cytoskeleton-associated proteins, such as neurofilaments, tau and stathmins (46). The role of neurofilament phosphorylation is still debated, but has been suggested to influence its axonal transport rate and therefore subcellular localization. Tau has an exceptionally complex phosphorylation signature, and its over 30 phosphorylation sites are affected by many different kinases and phosphatases (52). Under physiological conditions, tau binds to and stabilizes existing microtubules and promotes microtubule growth, but pathological hyperphosphorylation leads to self-assembly of tau, which results both in tau tangles and also in microtubule detabilization. In contrast, the role of phosphorylation on stathmin activity is much better elucidated. Stathmins have four phosphorylation sites, all of them serine residues (53). When phosphorylated at these residues, stathmins are inactive, and dephosphorylation therefore equates to activation. Active stathmins sequester free tubulin dimers, the building blocks for microtubules, and therefore passively decrease microtubule growth (53). This results in an increase in microtubule dynamics or a decrease in microtubule stability.

Spatio-temporal control of MKP-1 expression is critical to increase dynamic microtubules, a prerequisite for the remodeling of the cytoskeleton that manifests in the forms of branching or pruning of axonal collateral arbors. For instance, transient expression of MKP-1 permits branching of axons (46). On the other hand, disruption of such spatio-temporal expression of MKP-1, in the forms of ectopic expression or sustained protein half-life over prolonged periods of time impedes axonal growth or prunes axons, depending on the developmental window.

9. From behavior to MKP-1 and back

Arborization of axons is critical to adjust neural network wiring to environmental needs. Behavioral experience evokes multiple signaling pathways that converge to cytoskeletal remodeling via both slow genomic and rapid non-genomic mechanisms. Protein phosphorylation is instrumental in the signaling toolbox that controls both of these programs. The balance of phosphorylation and dephosphorylation of the molecular components of the cytoskeletal machine dictates, in part, its continuous plasticity (54). By challenging this equilibrium at defined subcellular locations, timely, BDNF signaling instructs the position of branching points that mold the topographic maps of innervation. The manifold aspects of phosphorylation on BDNF signaling in this process can be illustrated by the molecular mechanisms that regulate the expression, localization and degradation of MKP-1, the dual specificity MAPK phosphatase. Induction of MKP-1 requires both a linear phosphorylation cascade through the MAPK-ERK1/2-CREB pathway and a feed-forward dephosphorylation switch via the calcineurin-CRTC1/2 pathway (Figure 5). Failure of either signaling branches prevents *mkp-1* expression, which impinge on activity-dependent remodeling of the cytoskeleton. Baseline *mkp-1* mRNA expression is limited in the brain of naturally behaving songbirds and rodents (55, 56). But hearing song, seeing visual stimuli, or performing motor behavior robustly increases *mkp-1* transcripts respectively, in auditory, visual, and somatosensory neurons (56-58). Therefore, expression of *mkp-1* is driven by neural activity in the primary sensory areas of the brain. What may result from the deregulation of MKP-1 expression during higher order behaviors? When ectopically expressed in humans and animal models, MKP-1 triggers depressive behavior (55). In contrast, genetic disruption of *mkp-1* protects from stress in an animal model (55). Therefore, too little MKP-1 may prevent activity-dependent remodeling of axons and dendrites that is necessary for behavioral adaptation, learning and memory. In contrast, too much MKP-1, as observed in depression and stress, may destabilize cytoskeletal architecture that impinges on the maintenance of functional neural networks. How titration of MKP-1 levels affects structural characteristics such as dendritic spines, physiological features like long-term potentiation and cognitive performance like learning and memory is unknown. Future investigations will shed light into these possibilities.

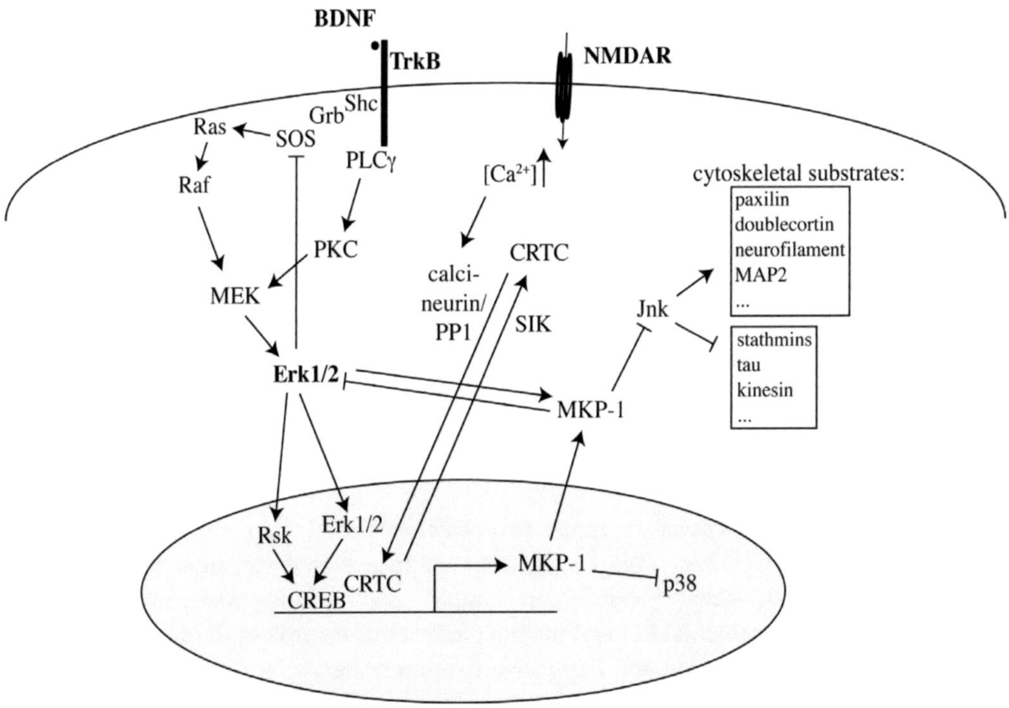

Figure 5. BDNF signaling from the plasma membrane to the nucleus. Activation of TrkB by BDNF rapidly elicits numerous waves of protein phosphorylation that converge to the nucleus to trigger a genomic response. Coincidence detectors like CRTC proteins may determine the nature of the genomic response based on the cellular context. In effect, phosphorylation of CREB by BDNF signaling is required but not sufficient to elicit a transcriptional response. Neuronal activity and excitatory neurotransmitter, glutamate signaling converge to CREB activation via the dephosphorylation and nuclear translocation of the CREB-coactivors, CRTC. Among the regulated genes, MKP-1 is a MAPK phosphatase that terminates upstream BDNF-induced signaling in a delayed fashion. But MKP-1 serves also to deactivate JNK, which is constitutively activated in the axon. In consequence, many of the JNK substrates that serve cytoskeletal attributes are dephosphorylated. Numerous cytoskeletal-binding proteins that are substrates of JNK are either activated or deactivated upon phosphorylation. Spatio-temporal phosphorylation and dephosphorylation of these proteins helps maintain the integrity of the cytoskeletal architecture of the axon, as much as its remodeling capacity.

10. Conclusion

We have described how multiple steps of phosphorylation and dephosphorylation along the signaling pathways initiated by the neurotrophin BDNF determine its function via its receptor TrkB. These phosphorylation and dephosphorylation loops serve to efficiently activate in time and space the downstream components of BDNF signaling either proximal to the plasma membrane or distal in the nucleus. Concurrent activation of a kinase and deactivation of the substrate's phosphatase is a common, but not exclusive mechanism to ensure both the robustness and fidelity of the output signal. Indeed, phosphorylated or dephosphorylated residues may serve to accelerate or delay the target protein's turnover as exemplified by MKP-1. Where BDNF signaling is not capable of initiating its entire signaling machinery such as the dephosphorylation of CRTC proteins, it relies on converging signaling pathways. Coincidence detectors, like CRTC proteins may serve to 'gate' neurotrophin signaling and filter the physiological output consequences as a function of the cellular context.

Author details

Katrin Deinhardt and Freddy Jeanneteau
Molecular Neurobiology Program; Skirball Institute of Biomolecular Medicine; New York University Langone School of Medicine; New York, NY, USA

Acknowledgement

Brain and Behavior foundation (FJ) and Human Frontiers (KD).

The authors declare no conflict of interest.

11. References

[1] Huang EJ, Reichardt LF. Trk receptors: roles in neuronal signal transduction. Annu Rev Biochem. 2003;72:609-42.
[2] Chao MV. Neurotrophins and their receptors: a convergence point for many signalling pathways. Nat Rev Neurosci. 2003 Apr;4(4):299-309.
[3] Woo N, Je H-s, Lu B. Role of neurotrophins in the formation and maintenance of synapses. Molecular mechanisms of synaptogenesis. [Book chapter]. 2006;Part II / Roles of cell adhesion and secreted molecules in synaptic differentiation:179-94.
[4] Poo MM. Neurotrophins as synaptic modulators. Nat Rev Neurosci. 2001 Jan;2(1):24-32.
[5] Autry AE, Monteggia LM. Brain-derived neurotrophic factor and neuropsychiatric disorders. Pharmacol Rev. 2012 Apr;64(2):238-58.
[6] Castren E, Rantamaki T. The role of BDNF and its receptors in depression and antidepressant drug action: Reactivation of developmental plasticity. Dev Neurobiol. 2010 Apr;70(5):289-97.
[7] Cunha C, Brambilla R, Thomas KL. A simple role for BDNF in learning and memory? Front Mol Neurosci. 2012;3:1.

[8] Arevalo JC, Wu SH. Neurotrophin signaling: many exciting surprises! Cell Mol Life Sci. 2006 Jul;63(13):1523-37.

[9] Spellman DS, Deinhardt K, Darie CC, Chao MV, Neubert TA. Stable isotopic labeling by amino acids in cultured primary neurons: application to brain-derived neurotrophic factor-dependent phosphotyrosine-associated signaling. Mol Cell Proteomics. 2008 Jun;7(6):1067-76.

[10] Arevalo JC, Yano H, Teng KK, Chao MV. A unique pathway for sustained neurotrophin signaling through an ankyrin-rich membrane-spanning protein. EMBO J. 2004 Jun 16;23(12):2358-68.

[11] Shaywitz AJ, Greenberg ME. CREB: a stimulus-induced transcription factor activated by a diverse array of extracellular signals. Annu Rev Biochem. 1999;68:821-61.

[12] Chao MV. Growth factor signaling: where is the specificity? Cell. 1992 Mar 20;68(6):995-7.

[13] Glorioso C, Sabatini M, Unger T, Hashimoto T, Monteggia LM, Lewis DA, et al. Specificity and timing of neocortical transcriptome changes in response to BDNF gene ablation during embryogenesis or adulthood. Mol Psychiatry. 2006 Jul;11(7):633-48.

[14] Marshall CJ. Specificity of receptor tyrosine kinase signaling: transient versus sustained extracellular signal-regulated kinase activation. Cell. 1995 Jan 27;80(2):179-85.

[15] Mansour SJ, Matten WT, Hermann AS, Candia JM, Rong S, Fukasawa K, et al. Transformation of mammalian cells by constitutively active MAP kinase kinase. Science. 1994 Aug 12;265(5174):966-70.

[16] Whalen AM, Galasinski SC, Shapiro PS, Nahreini TS, Ahn NG. Megakaryocytic differentiation induced by constitutive activation of mitogen-activated protein kinase kinase. Mol Cell Biol. 1997 Apr;17(4):1947-58.

[17] Dhillon AS, Hagan S, Rath O, Kolch W. MAP kinase signalling pathways in cancer. Oncogene. 2007 May 14;26(22):3279-90.

[18] Traverse S, Seedorf K, Paterson H, Marshall CJ, Cohen P, Ullrich A. EGF triggers neuronal differentiation of PC12 cells that overexpress the EGF receptor. Curr Biol. 1994 Aug 1;4(8):694-701.

[19] Brodeur GM, Minturn JE, Ho R, Simpson AM, Iyer R, Varela CR, et al. Trk receptor expression and inhibition in neuroblastomas. Clin Cancer Res. 2009 May 15;15(10):3244-50.

[20] Cheng PL, Song AH, Wong YH, Wang S, Zhang X, Poo MM. Self-amplifying autocrine actions of BDNF in axon development. Proc Natl Acad Sci U S A. 2011 Nov 8;108(45):18430-5.

[21] Langlois WJ, Sasaoka T, Saltiel AR, Olefsky JM. Negative feedback regulation and desensitization of insulin- and epidermal growth factor-stimulated p21ras activation. J Biol Chem. 1995 Oct 27;270(43):25320-3.

[22] Boutros T, Chevet E, Metrakos P. Mitogen-activated protein (MAP) kinase/MAP kinase phosphatase regulation: roles in cell growth, death, and cancer. Pharmacol Rev. 2008 Sep;60(3):261-310.

[23] Jaumot M, Hancock JF. Protein phosphatases 1 and 2A promote Raf-1 activation by regulating 14-3-3 interactions. Oncogene. 2001 Jul 5;20(30):3949-58.

[24] Owens DM, Keyse SM. Differential regulation of MAP kinase signalling by dual-specificity protein phosphatases. Oncogene. 2007 May 14;26(22):3203-13.

[25] Kholodenko BN. Cell-signalling dynamics in time and space. Nat Rev Mol Cell Biol. 2006 Mar;7(3):165-76.

[26] Baass PC, Di Guglielmo GM, Authier F, Posner BI, Bergeron JJ. Compartmentalized signal transduction by receptor tyrosine kinases. Trends Cell Biol. 1995 Dec;5(12):465-70.

[27] Miller FD, Kaplan DR. Neurobiology. TRK makes the retrograde. Science. 2002 Feb 22;295(5559):1471-3.

[28] Ye H, Kuruvilla R, Zweifel LS, Ginty DD. Evidence in support of signaling endosome-based retrograde survival of sympathetic neurons. Neuron. 2003 Jul 3;39(1):57-68.

[29] Teis D, Wunderlich W, Huber LA. Localization of the MP1-MAPK scaffold complex to endosomes is mediated by p14 and required for signal transduction. Dev Cell. 2002 Dec;3(6):803-14.

[30] Riccio A, Ahn S, Davenport CM, Blendy JA, Ginty DD. Mediation by a CREB family transcription factor of NGF-dependent survival of sympathetic neurons. Science. 1999 Dec 17;286(5448):2358-61.

[31] Riccio A, Pierchala BA, Ciarallo CL, Ginty DD. An NGF-TrkA-mediated retrograde signal to transcription factor CREB in sympathetic neurons. Science. 1997 Aug 22;277(5329):1097-100.

[32] Perlson E, Maday S, Fu MM, Moughamian AJ, Holzbaur EL. Retrograde axonal transport: pathways to cell death? Trends Neurosci. 2010 Jul;33(7):335-44.

[33] Brankatschk B, Wichert SP, Johnson SD, Schaad O, Rossner MJ, Gruenberg J. Regulation of the EGF transcriptional response by endocytic sorting. Sci Signal. 2012 Mar 13;5(215):ra21.

[34] Sousa LP, Lax I, Shen H, Ferguson SM, Camilli PD, Schlessinger J. Suppression of EGFR endocytosis by dynamin depletion reveals that EGFR signaling occurs primarily at the plasma membrane. Proc Natl Acad Sci U S A. 2012 Mar 20;109(12):4419-24.

[35] Conkright MD, Canettieri G, Screaton R, Guzman E, Miraglia L, Hogenesch JB, et al. TORCs: transducers of regulated CREB activity. Mol Cell. 2003 Aug;12(2):413-23.

[36] Altarejos JY, Montminy M. CREB and the CRTC co-activators: sensors for hormonal and metabolic signals. Nat Rev Mol Cell Biol. 2011 Mar;12(3):141-51.

[37] Breuillaud L, Rossetti C, Meylan EM, Merinat C, Halfon O, Magistretti PJ, et al. Deletion of CREB-Regulated Transcription Coactivator 1 Induces Pathological Aggression, Depression-Related Behaviors, and Neuroplasticity Genes Dysregulation in Mice. Biol Psychiatry. 2012 May 14.

[38] Finsterwald C, Fiumelli H, Cardinaux JR, Martin JL. Regulation of dendritic development by BDNF requires activation of CRTC1 by glutamate. J Biol Chem. 2011 Sep 10;285(37):28587-95.

[39] Kovacs KA, Steullet P, Steinmann M, Do KQ, Magistretti PJ, Halfon O, et al. TORC1 is a calcium- and cAMP-sensitive coincidence detector involved in hippocampal long-term synaptic plasticity. Proc Natl Acad Sci U S A. 2007 Mar 13;104(11):4700-5.

[40] Uebi T, Tamura M, Horike N, Hashimoto YK, Takemori H. Phosphorylation of the CREB-specific coactivator TORC2 at Ser(307) regulates its intracellular localization in COS-7 cells and in the mouse liver. Am J Physiol Endocrinol Metab. 2010 Sep;299(3):E413-25.

[41] Jeanneteau FD, Lambert WM, Ismaili N, Bath KG, Lee FS, Garabedian MJ, et al. BDNF and glucocorticoids regulate corticotrophin-releasing hormone (CRH) homeostasis in the hypothalamus. Proc Natl Acad Sci U S A. 2012 Jan 24;109(4):1305-10.

[42] Gao Y, Nikulina E, Mellado W, Filbin MT. Neurotrophins elevate cAMP to reach a threshold required to overcome inhibition by MAG through extracellular signal-regulated kinase-dependent inhibition of phosphodiesterase. J Neurosci. 2003 Dec 17;23(37):11770-7.

[43] Ji Y, Pang PT, Feng L, Lu B. Cyclic AMP controls BDNF-induced TrkB phosphorylation and dendritic spine formation in mature hippocampal neurons. Nat Neurosci. 2005 Feb;8(2):164-72.

[44] Mai J, Fok L, Gao H, Zhang X, Poo MM. Axon initiation and growth cone turning on bound protein gradients. J Neurosci. 2009 Jun 10;29(23):7450-8.

[45] Bramham CR, Worley PF, Moore MJ, Guzowski JF. The immediate early gene arc/arg3.1: regulation, mechanisms, and function. J Neurosci. 2008 Nov 12;28(46):11760-7.

[46] Jeanneteau F, Deinhardt K, Miyoshi G, Bennett AM, Chao MV. The MAP kinase phosphatase MKP-1 regulates BDNF-induced axon branching. Nat Neurosci. 2010 Nov;13(11):1373-9.

[47] Jeanneteau F, Deinhardt K. Fine-tuning MAPK signaling in the brain: The role of MKP-1. Commun Integr Biol. 2011 May;4(3):281-3.

[48] Lin YW, Yang JL. Cooperation of ERK and SCFSkp2 for MKP-1 destruction provides a positive feedback regulation of proliferating signaling. J Biol Chem. 2006 Jan 13;281(2):915-26.

[49] Brondello JM, Pouyssegur J, McKenzie FR. Reduced MAP kinase phosphatase-1 degradation after p42/p44MAPK-dependent phosphorylation. Science. 1999 Dec 24;286(5449):2514-7.

[50] Liu Y, Shepherd EG, Nelin LD. MAPK phosphatases--regulating the immune response. Nat Rev Immunol. 2007 Mar;7(3):202-12.

[51] Oliva AA, Jr., Atkins CM, Copenagle L, Banker GA. Activated c-Jun N-terminal kinase is required for axon formation. J Neurosci. 2006 Sep 13;26(37):9462-70.

[52] Stoothoff WH, Johnson GV. Tau phosphorylation: physiological and pathological consequences. Biochim Biophys Acta. 2005 Jan 3;1739(2-3):280-97.

[53] Curmi PA, Gavet O, Charbaut E, Ozon S, Lachkar-Colmerauer S, Manceau V, et al. Stathmin and its phosphoprotein family: general properties, biochemical and functional interaction with tubulin. Cell Struct Funct. 1999 Oct;24(5):345-57.

[54]Lin YC, Koleske AJ. Mechanisms of synapse and dendrite maintenance and their disruption in psychiatric and neurodegenerative disorders. Annu Rev Neurosci. 2010;33:349-78.

[55] Duric V, Banasr M, Licznerski P, Schmidt HD, Stockmeier CA, Simen AA, et al. A negative regulator of MAP kinase causes depressive behavior. Nat Med. 2010 Nov;16(11):1328-32.

[56] Horita H, Wada K, Rivas MV, Hara E, Jarvis ED. The dusp1 immediate early gene is regulated by natural stimuli predominantly in sensory input neurons. J Comp Neurol. 2010 Jul 15;518(14):2873-901.

[57] Chen MF, Chen HI, Jen CJ. Exercise training upregulates macrophage MKP-1 and affects immune responses in mice. Med Sci Sports Exerc. 2010 Dec;42(12):2173-9.

[58] Doi M, Cho S, Yujnovsky I, Hirayama J, Cermakian N, Cato AC, et al. Light-inducible and clock-controlled expression of MAP kinase phosphatase 1 in mouse central pacemaker neurons. J Biol Rhythms. 2007 Apr;22(2):127-39.

Chapter 8

Signalling DNA Damage

Andres Joaquin Lopez-Contreras and Oscar Fernandez-Capetillo

Additional information is available at the end of the chapter

http://dx.doi.org/10.5772/50863

1. Introduction

1.1. Types and sources of DNA damage

During our lifetime, the genome is constantly being exposed to different types of damage caused either by exogenous sources (radiations and/or genotoxic compound) but also as byproducts of endogenous processes (reactive oxigen species during respiration, stalled forks during replication, eroded telomeres, etc).

From a structural point of view, there are many types of DNA damage including single or double strand breaks, base modifications and losses or base-pair mismatches. The amount of lesions that we face is enormous with estimates suggesting that each of our 10^{13} cells has to deal with around 10.000 lesions per day [1]. While the majority of these events are properly resolved by specialized mechanisms, a deficient response to DNA damage, and particularly to DSB, harbors a serious threat to human health [2].

DSB can be formed [1] following an exposure to ionizing radiation (X- or γ-rays) or clastogenic drugs; [2] endogenously, during DNA replication, or [3], as a consequence of reactive oxygen species (ROS) generated during oxidative metabolism. In addition, programmed DSB are used as repair intermediates during V(D)J and Class-Switch recombination (CSR) in lymphocytes [3], or during meiotic recombination [4]. Because of this, immunodeficiency and/or sterility problems are frequently associated with DDR-related pathologies.

2. DNA repair of DSB. NHEJ and HR

Mammalian cells are equipped with two mechanisms that repair DSB and prevent dangerous chromosomal rearrangements; [1] *Non-homologous end joining (NHEJ)*, which links together the two ends of broken DNA by direct ligation, and [2] *Homologous Recombination (HR)*, which is only available S and G2 phases when a sister chromatid can be used as a template for the repair reaction (see Figure 1).

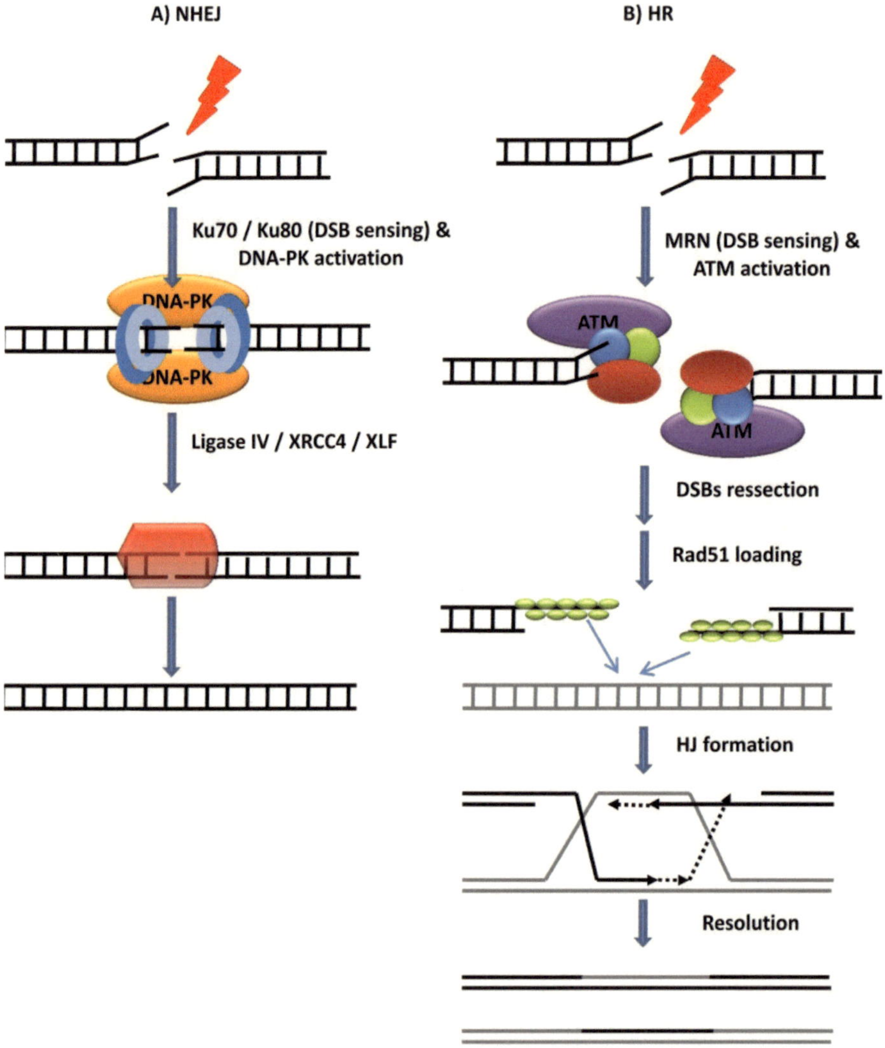

Figure 1. DSBs repair mechanisms. *A) NHEJ*. DSBs are sensed by the ring-shape heterodimer Ku70/Ku80 which then stabilizes the two DNA ends and recruits DNA-PK. Next, DNA-PK phosphorylates and activates the NHEJ effector complex (ligase IV/XRC44/XLF) that finally religates the broken DNA. *B) HR*. The ATM kinase is recruited to DSB via an interaction with the MRN (Mre11-Rad50-Nbs1) complex. Once at the break, ATM that becomes activated, phosphorylating multiple substrates. In a reaction that depends in multiple endo and exonuclease activities (including Mre11, Exo1 and CtIP) DSBs are resected forming ssDNA strands. These ssDNA regions attract Rad51 and other associated proteins. The Rad51-coated nucleoprotein filaments then invade the undamaged sister strands forming HJ structures. HR is completed by new DNA synthesis and still to be identified HJ "resolvase" enzymes.

2.1. Non Homologous End Joining (NHEJ)

NHEJ is simpler and faster than HR, and can take place in any cell cycle stage. However, NHEJ can process altered or improper ends is thus more error-prone that HR. Therefore, HR is the preferred repair mechanisms during S/G2 phases. However, due to the preponderance of the G0/G1 stage, NHEJ is key to safeguard genomic integrity in mammalian organisms. Moreover, and probably due to the larger genomes and abundant repetitive sequences which limit HR proficiency, mammalian genomes are also frequently healed by NHEJ in S/G2 [5].

The mechanism by which NHEJ rejoins a DSB is fairly understood. First, DSB are recognized by a heterodimer formed by **Ku70** and **Ku80** proteins [6]. Ku proteins display a ring-like structure and are able to bind and stabilize the ends of DSB, acting as sensors, and subsequently attracting the transducer kinase, **DNA-PK** (DNA dependent protein Kinase). DNA-PK is a large Ser/Thr kinase (about 470 Kda), which belongs to the PIKK family (PI3-kinase like family of protein kinases). Other members of this family, ATM (ataxia talangectasia mutated) and ATR (ATM and RAD3-related), are key kinases in the DDR and will be explained in futher detail below. Once DNA-PK is located to the DSB it becomes activated and phosphorylates several substrates involved in the processing and ligation of DNA ends. Significantly, DNA-PK can also auto-phosphorylate in several residues, which seems to be essential for its repair capacity [7].

Finally, the main effectors of NHEJ form a multimeric complex (**DNA Ligase IV-XRCC4-XLF**), which is recruited to DSB and activated by DNA-PK dependent phosphorylation. This complex is responsible for the actual rejoining of the ends [8]. Ligase IV provides the catalytic activity for the rejoining, while XRCC4 stabilizes and stimulates its activity [9].

Ku70 and Ku 80 (sensors), DNA-PK (transducer) and DNA ligase IV and XRCC4 (effectors) are the core component of NHEJ. But often other accessory components are required for the conversion of altered broken ends. For instance, DSB produced by IR usually requires an end-processing step prior to relegation, such as the one regulated by **Artemis**, a 5′- 3′ exonuclease, that acquires endonuclease activity when phosphorylated by DNA-PK [10]. This activity of Artemis is important to open closed hairpins in which the two strands of the DSB have linked together. Importantly, such hairpins are normally generated at the DSB generated by RAG nucleases during V(D)J recombination. Note that ATM can also induce the phosphorylation and activation of Artemis [11]. In fact, and in addition to be important for the repair of accidental DSB, NHEJ carries out several specialized functions in lymphocytes during V(D)J and CSR [12, 13]. Accordingly, patients with mutation in Artemis, ATM or DNA-PKcs, as well as in other NHEJ components, often suffer from immune deficiencies as well as from an increased predisposition to cancer [14].

Another context in which difficult-to repair DSB are formed relates to chromatin accessibility. For instance, it is estimated that around 10% of radiation induced DSB are repaired with slow kinetics, this population being enriched adjacent to compacted chromatin (heterochromatin). In this case, ATM and not DNAPK will play an important role in the NHEJ-mediated repair of these difficult-to-repair breaks. In this context, ATM activation is necessary to phosphorylate some substrates like H2AX or KAP1, which would relax chromatin compaction allowing the access of repair proteins to DSB at heterochromatin [11, 15]. Nevertheless, it should be noted that the main cell-type that suffers from ATM deficiency is Purkinje cells which are almost devoid of heterochromatin, so that ATM must play additional roles in euchromatin [16].

2.2. Homologous recombination

The other mechanism that cells use for DSB repair, and the most important for replicating cells, is Homologous Recombination. In contrast to NHEJ, during HR DSB need to be first extensively processed to allow for the search of the homologous undamaged template. First, ends undergo 5′-3′ resection producing two single stranded DNA regions. Rad51-coated ssDNA stretches invade the sister chromatid DNA duplex forming inter-strand structures. How these heteroduplexes are finally resolved is still not fully characterized.

Since HR repairs DSB using the sister chromatid as template, it is restricted to S and G2 phases. Restricting HR in G1 is in fact critical, since if HR takes place in G1 it could lead to loss of heterozigosity (LOH) or chromosomal translocations [17]. To avoid this problem the activity of several HR components is regulated by several S-G2 specific CDKs (cyclin dependent kinases) [18].

For teaching purposes, and trying to simplify the complex process that takes place during HR, we will artificially divide it in 4 independent stages. We acknowledge that many of the stepwise events described here are still to be fully validated, but just want to transmit a holistic view of how a DSB can be sensed, signaled and repaired by HR:

a. **Recruitment to the DSB: *Foci* forming factors**

The **Mre11-Rad50-Nbs1** (MRN) complex is one of the first in being recruited to DSB [19]. Next, through a direct interaction, MRN recruits **ATM** which, among other things, phophorylates H2AX (a variant of the canonical histone H2A) at serine 139, forming **γH2AX** [20]. Direct phospho-binding to γH2AX recruits the adaptor protein **MDC1** [21], which through interaction with ATM and Nbs1 forms a positive feedback loop that amplifies the γH2AX signal [22]. In addition, ATM-dependent phosphorylation of MDC1 is recognized by the E3 ubiquitin ligase **RNF8**, that ubiquitinates histones in the vicinity of the DSB [23, 24]. Another E3 ubiquitin ligase, **RNF168** (mutated in the human RIDDLE immunodeficiency syndrome), is also recruited and amplifies the ubqutylation signal, in both cases mediated by **UBC13** E2 ligase, eventually recruiting 53BP1 and BRCA1 to DSB-associated foci [25-27]. In the case of BRCA1, **RAP80** binds to ubiquinylated substrates at DSB through its UIM (Ubiquitin Interaction Motif) [23]. RAP80 then interacts with **Abraxas** [28], the deubiquitylating (DUB) enzyme **BRCC36** and **BRCA1** (breast cancer 1, early onset). BRCA1 is a well known human breast cancer susceptibility gene, responsible for the third part of familiar breast cancer [29]. BRCA1 is a large protein (over 200 kDa) that is constitutively bound to BARD1. Together, BRCA1/BARD1 present E3 ubiquitin ligase activity [30]. Although BRCA1 has been the subject of many studies and it is known to participate in HR, its exact role(s) and whether its ubiquitin ligase activity is critical for its activity is still not well understood. Whereas the road from DSB to BRCA1 is more understood, how 53BP1 is loaded to substrates modified by RNF8/RNF168 remains unknown.

Importantly, it should be noted that all of these events have been inferred from the formation or absence of *foci* at DSB and, to date, it is not clear to what extent capacity to recruit to foci represents an accurate measurement of the function of the protein [31].

b. Processing of the end: Resection

As mentioned before, the resection of the two 5′ ends of the DSB is an essential step for HR. Three exonucleases (Mre11, Exo1 and CtIP) and one helicase (BLM) have been involved in resection [32-34]. Importantly, ATM dependent phosphorylation seems to stimulate CtIP-mediated resection, linking DNA damage signaling with the processing of DNA ends [35]. In addition to ATM, ssDNA is quickly coated by RPA (replication protein A) and triggers a parallel pathway resulting in the activation of the kinase ATR [18, 36-38], that will be described below. It remains to be seen to what extent ATM, ATR, and perhaps DNA-PK collaborate in the processing of DSB for HR. One important recent development is the finding that, against all expectations, 53BP1 might limit resection [39]. This would explain how the absence of 53BP1 rescues the cancer and ageing phenotypes of a BRCA1 mutant mouse model, which could be explained by an improved HR through enhanced resection [40].

c. Sister chromatid invasion

The initiation of recombination requires the loading of the **recombinase Rad51,** which replaces RPA coating on the ssDNA. Rad51, a protein with DNA-dependent ATPase activity, together with other associated proteins (DSS1, RAD52,RAD51B, RAD51C, RAD51D, XRCC2, XRCC3, RAD54, etc.) form a nucleoprotein filament that mediates strand invasion of the sister chromatid [41]. In mammals, Rad51 loading is mediated by **BRAC2** [42]. Once again, BRCA2 is another important breast cancer susceptibility gene suggesting a critical role of HR in the prevention of breast cancer [43]. In contrast to BRCA1, BRCA2 recruitment to DSB is not fully understood, one possible scenario being that BRCA1 could mediate the recruitment of **FancD2** and BRCA2 to DSB [44].

The nucleoprotein filament (ssDNA, RAD51 and other HR proteins) searches for an homologous region within the duplex DNA in the sister chromatid and displaces a DNA strand forming a D-loop structure and the 3′ end of the invading strand. This invading end then is extended by un unknown DNA polymerase (*in vitro* data indicates that DNA pol eta may be implicated [45]). The "X" shaped structure formed as a consequence of this invading process is called a Holliday Junction (HJ) [46]. When the other 3′ end of broken DNA enters the D-loop a double Holliday junction structure is formed. Noteworthy, whereas this model was proposed almost half a century ago, it was only recently that evidence for the double Holliday junction intermediates of repair was found [47]

d. Resolution

If HJ formation was remained elusive, the resolution of Holliday junctions is even a bigger mistery, many proteins having been proposed as candidates to be the HJ "resolvase". Such a protein should have helicase and nuclease activities, like BLM (Bloom syndrome protein), MUS81-EME1 complex or GEN1 [48-51]. All of them have been proposed to be the missing HJ-resolvase at some point. Moreover, recent evidence suggests that another enzyme, SLX4, could be such missing link [52, 53]. Whereas it seems clear that many proteins can deal with HJ-resembling structures *in* vitro, only clean genetic data will finally resolve this "resolution" problem. We should mention that although the HR classical model consists in the formation of these two Holliday Junctions, there are other alternative models that explain the HR process.

In addition to its role at DSB, HR also has a key role in restarting stalled replication forks (RF). SSBs, interstrand crosslinks or other lesions in the DNA promote stalling of the RF which, if persistent, could lead to breakage that has to be resolved by HR [54]. ATR, another PIKK kinase that is essential for an appropriate progression of RF, may be regulating HR in this case. In fact, ATR and its target kinase Chk1 phosphorylate a number of HR-related proteins such as BRCA1, BLM and Rad51 [55-57].

HR also participates in the maintenance of **telomere length**, by promoting inter-telomeric HR in the absence of telomerase. This pathway is known as alternative lengthening of telomeres (ALT) [58]. Finally, HR is the repair pathway of the recombination reaction that occurs between homologous chromosomes in **meiosis**, where DSB are intentionally generated in order to increase genetic variability.

Whereas we here provided a simplified view of DSB repair, it should be noted that other still poorly understood pathways of repair such as micro-homology directed NHEJ, which joins partially resected DSB, are emerging as important genome caretakers.

3. Signaling DSB

We here present a general view of how cells signal DSB, with a particular emphasis on phosphorylation, which is the most known mechanism to date.

3.1. Phosphorylation. The so-called DNA Damage Response (DDR)

The so-called DDR stands for a coordinated signaling response which starts at the DSB and which promotes DNA Repair while it limits the expansion of the damaged cell by apoptotic or cytostatic mechanisms. The canonical DDR begins with the activation of two PIKK, ATM and ATR, upon detection of DSB. The role of DNA-PK, another member of the PIKK family, is mainly to stimulate repair activities locally at the break but without triggering a cellular response. Thus, ATM and ATR are considered the main upstream kinases in the signaling of DNA damage. Whereas they are activated by different types of damage and have some specific substrates and functions, their "response" is frequently interconnected. The activation of any of these kinases starts a phosphorylation cascade leading to cell cycle arrest (*Checkpoints)*. Among others, the tumor suppressor p53 plays a central role in coordinating the apoptotic and checkpoints initiated by DNA damage.

In the last decade the knowledge about the DDR has substantially increased, and besides the classical activation of the PIKK and phosphorylation cascades, other types of signaling such as ubiquitylation or sumoylation have burst [59]. A general overview of this complex pathway will be explained below.

3.1.1. Central players of the DDR: PIKK kinases: ATM, ATR and DNA-PK

The DDR has a well defined hierarchy. Their components have been classified into sensors, transducers, mediators and effectors. ATM and ATR kinases are considered the main DDR transducers.

As mentioned, ATM, ATR and DNA-PK belong to the PIKK (phosphatidylinositol-3-kinase related kinases) family [60]. They are large proteins (more than 300 kDa) with similar structure: a variable number of repeat domains in the N-terminus (HEAT domains), a FAT domain, a catalytic domain homologue to that in PI-3-Kinase (PI3K), a PIKK regulatory domain (PRD) and a FATC domain at the very C-terminus [61]. The PRD domain has been shown to mediate kinase activation, at least for ATR; and HEAT, FAT and FATC domains may be involved in the specific interactions of these proteins with their substrates and modulators [62].

ATM, ATR and DNA-PK specifically phosphorylate serine and threonine residues frequently followed by a glutamine. Upon activation, they are able to phosphorylate hundreds of common substrates regulating many cellular functions [63]. Noteworthy, some of them are preferred by one specific kinase, which is likely due to mediators. For instance, whereas all three can phosphorylate H2AX, Chk1 is only phosphorylated by ATR and this is explained by the need of **Claspin** in mediating the ATR/Chk1 interaction.

Despite their similarities, these kinases play different roles in the DDR. In brief, DNA-PK is activated in response to DSB and promotes their repair by NHEJ. However, if DSB are located in heterochromatin or they are too numerous, ATM activates additional repair mechanism (e.g. HR) and starts checkpoints signaling. In addition, ATR is activated by ssDNA, generated when DSB persist and are ressected into ssDNA, or when a replication fork is collapsed, promoting a strong checkpoint signaling. Besides, whereas ATM and DNA-PK are active through all the cell cycle, ATR activity is confined only to S and G2 phases [64]. One possible scenario is that the activity of the three kinases follows a stepwise activation if a DSB persist. This model is explained below.

a. DNA-PK. Stimulation of DNA Repair

The first step in this model will be the immediate activation of DNA-PK at a DSB. Previously in this chapter, we described how DNA-PK is activated and promotes NHEJ. In summary, the dimer Ku70/Ku80 binds and stabilizes the DSB ends, it recruits DNA-PK that activates the NHEJ effectors, LigaseIV-XRCC4-XLF. Thus, DNA-PK will provide a fast repair mechanism for easy-to-repair breaks, without the activation of checkpoint activities. It must be emphasized again, that DNA-PK has a very limited role in checkpoint signaling. However in the absence of ATM, DNA-PK may stay longer at the DSB and contribute to checkpoint functions [65].

b. ATM. DSB sensing and ATM Activation

If the DSB persist, one plausible scenario is that ATM could phosphorylate and displace DNA-PK from the DSB, so that repair and checkpoint activities are implemented. ATM is the most studied and likely best known DDR kinase. One reason for this is that its absence is responsible for the human **Ataxia-Telangiectasia (A-T)** hereditary disorder [66]. A-T is a severe autosomal recessive disease characterized by early onset progressive cerebellar ataxia, oculocutaneous telangectasia, immunodeficiency and lymphoid tumours [67]. Immunodeficiency and predisposition to lymphoid tumours is explained by the role of ATM during T and B lymphocyte development, where DSB are generated as by-products of immune rearrangements. Besides, cells of these patients present numerous breaks, what explains their increase predisposition also to other cancer types.

Whereas it seems clear that the main role of ATM is related to the DDR [68], the two symptoms that named the disease, ataxia and telangiectasia, are still not explained by the role of ATM in relation to DNA damage, suggesting that ATM may have other functions not related to DSB-signaling. Moreover, even though we have significant understanding of the effects of ATM activation, how this is accomplished is still a matter of debate.

As described above, ATM activation is triggered by the recruitment of the **MRN complex** (sensor) in response to DSB (Figure 2). MRN complex recruits ATM and collaborates for its activation [69]. However, the precise mechanism by which ATM becomes activated is still a matter of controversy [62]. Some authors claimed that, in basal conditions, ATM is an inactive homodimer which undergoes dissociation and activation in response to DSB, due to its autophosphorylation [70]. Importantly, it has later been shown that ATM autophosphorylation is not necessary for its activation *in vivo* [71, 72].

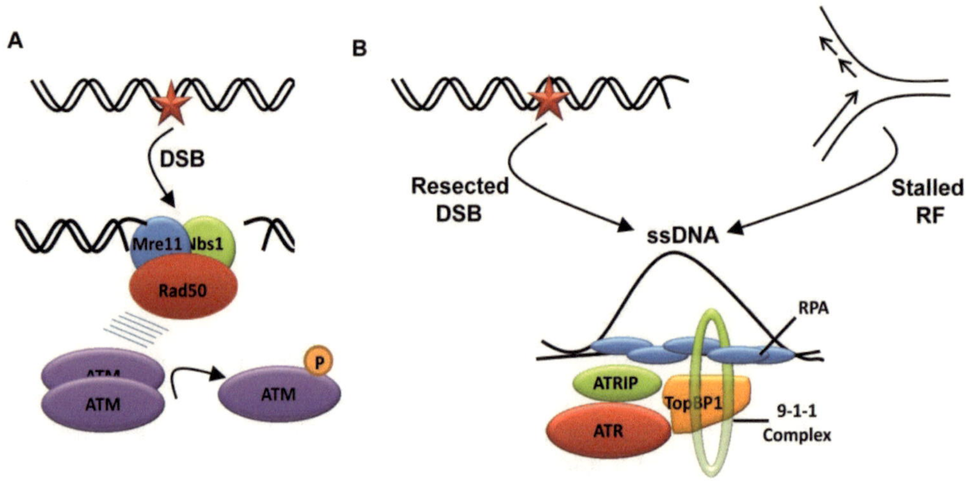

Figure 2. Mechanisms of ATM and ATR activation. *A) ATM activation.* DSBs (red asterisk) are sensed by the MRN (Mre11-Rad50-Nbs1) complex which attracts ATM and probably contributes to its activation. It is not well established how ATM is converted from its inactive to active status, one possibility being that it changes from an inactive dimer to an active monomeric form. *B) ATR activation.* The input for ATR activation is ssDNA, which can derive from resected DSB (left), or from stalled replication forks (right). RPA coated ssDNA loads the ATRIP-ATR complex and the 9-1-1 complex, which brings together ATR and its allosteric activator TopBP1.

Nbs1, part of the MRN complex, could contribute to ATM phosphorylation and activation [73], and several other proteins, such as the histone acetyl transferase Tip60 [74], have been reported to be involved in ATM activation. *In* vitro, ATM can be activated in the absence of MRN members. However, the MRN complex amplifies ATM activity and collaborates for an optimal ATM accumulation surrounding the DSB [75]. Noteworthy, defects in two members of the MRN complex cause A-T related syndromes: *Nijmegen breakage syndrome* (NBS1 mutants) and *A-T-like disorder* (MRE11 mutants) [76, 77].

ATM has been claimed to be activated by other stimuli rather than DNA damage, like chloroquine or osmotic shock [70]. However, whether those stimuli do not generate damage, particularly during replication, remains to be seen. There are some evidences of a cytoplasmic fraction of ATM that might be helpful to explain part of the symptoms of A-T disease not related to the DDR like the early neurodegeneration. Of note, ATM in neuronal cells has been found predominantly cytosolic [78].

c. ATR. Activation by ssDNA

The last (in fact, its activation occurs later than ATM) main PIKK kinase in the signaling of DSB is ATR. As noted before, despite their homology, ATR responds to different types of stresses than ATM does, and although these two kinases share several substrates, ATR regulates different processes. ATR has an essential role during replication, sensing alterations in fork progression and activating cellular checkpoints if necessary [79, 80].

In contrast to ATM, ATR is essential at the organism and the cellular level [81]. Consequently there is not any human disease lacking ATR. However, patients of a very rare ATR-related disease known as the Seckel syndrome are alive with very low amounts of ATR [82].

The input for ATR is not the DSB itself, but rather unusual large strands of ssDNA that can be generated in several circumstances [64]:

- RS (*replication stress*) is a not well defined concept that refers to a variety of alterations in the normal progression of the replication fork, caused by lesions encountered in the DNA (SSBs, crosslinks, base adducts), dNTPs deficiency or other problems at the RF. When RS is prolonged or, in the absence of ATR, RF collapse and DSB are generated. Notice that there is no such a thing as RS-free replication, and thus ATR is essential to complete replication even in the absence of exogenous DNA damage.
- *End resection of DSB*. Initially DSB lead to DNA-PK and ATM activation. However if DSB occurs in S or G2 phases and they persist enough, DSB are resected by ATM-stimulated exonucleases generating strands of ssDNA which then activate ATR.
- *Telomeres*. ssDNA can be also generated at uncapped telomeres that have lost its capping function, leading to ATR activation.
- *NER (nucleotide excision repair)*. The process of NER can generate patches of ssDNA as repair intermediates, which lead to the activation of ATR, perhaps even in G1 [83].

In contrast to ATM, the molecular mechanism of ATR activation by ssDNA is well established (Figure 2). **RPA-coated ssDNA** [84] recruits the **ATR-ATRIP** (ATR interacting protein) complex [85]. At the same time, **Rad17** and subsequently the **9-1-1** (Rad9-Rad1-Hus1] complex are also brought to the damage sites by RPA [86]. The 9-1-1 complex, with a PCNA-like clamp conformation, then brings the allosteric activator TopBP1 (topoisomerase-binding protein 1] into close proximity of ATR [87]. The interaction of ATR with **TopBP1** is then sufficient to unleash ATR activity [88]. Of note, activation of ATR by TopBP1 even in the absence of DNA breaks is sufficient to promote a robust cellular response including senescence, demonstrating the key role of the DDR in responding to DNA damage [89].

3.1.2. Mediators and DDR amplification. Foci forming factors

Downstream of the PIKK, DDR signaling is amplified by several mechanisms, allowing the response to achieve its final cellular outcomes. On one hand, the DDR, like any other phosphorylation cascade, amplifies its signal in subsequent (enzymatic) step. This involves the participation of *mediators*, which are proteins acting downstream of the transducer kinases ATM and ATR. Several substrates, regulators, recruiters and others proteins acting as scaffold are considered mediators (e.g. Mdc1, 53BP1, MRN complex, Claspin, BRCA1), and, they modulate the activation of the effectors. Another mean of amplifying the signal, is an intense accumulation of many of their components surrounding the DNA lesions in spots so-called *IRIF (Ionizing Radiation Induced Foci).*

Once ATM or DNA-PK are activated, the rapid phosphorylation of the histone H2AX (*γH2AX*) is key for subsequent events. The γH2AX mark is accumulated in such a large amount in the proximity of DSB that can be visualized in spots (IRIF) by standard immunofluorescence techniques. Many DDR proteins (MRN complex, ATM, 53BP1, BRCA1 and others) form IRIF that co-localize with γH2AX foci. Actually, γH2AX modulates the accumulation of repair and signaling proteins in chromatin regions distal to the DSB. However, this has nothing to do with the recruitment of the proteins to the DSB, and rather by altering chromatin conformation in the vicinity of the break [90]. But what are foci good for? One likely possibility is that the accumulation of DDR proteins surrounding DNA lesions is necessary to build a signaling threshold in conditions of limited damage [91].

Among the different factors, 53BP1 is probably one of the most studied examples of an IRIF forming protein. 53BP1 has a pan-nuclear location which, after exposure to genotoxic agents, is quickly repositioned to IRIF. 53BP1 localization into foci is dependent on several upstream events including H2AX phosphorylation [90], recruitment of MDC1, ubiquitinating activity of RNF8 and RNF168 [23, 25, 92, 93], and methylation of histones H3 and H4 [94, 95]. Regardless of their importance for our understanding of the DDR, the absence of foci does not seem to be essential for a proficient DDR. Thus, mouse models lacking H2AX or MDC1, that abolishes IRIF formation, as well as 53BP1 null mice, are viable, but they exhibit phenotypes related to DDR deficiency like genome instability, cancer predisposition or immunodeficiency [22, 96, 97]. In summary, while not essential, IRIF seem to modulate the amplitude of the signaling of DSB which might be important in conditions of low numbers of DSB.

In contrast to ATM, ATR does not undergo any post-translational modifications which would modify its activity, such as autophosphorylation. Nevertheless, a number of mediators of ATR signaling are indeed regulated through phosphorylation. For instance, the ATR activator TopBP1 is phosphorylated by ATM at resected DSB [98]; and probably also by ATR in response to RS. In addition, Claspin phosphorylation is also required for ATR-dependent phosphorylation of Chk1 in response to DSB [99].

In summary, ATM and ATR signaling are amplified and driven by these and many other mediators. The endpoint of the signaling cascade arrives with the activation of the effectors, which would finally be responsible for the cellular responses.

3.1.3. *Effectors and cellular outcomes of the DDR*

In addition to promote the repair of DNA lesions, the DDR can orchestrate multiple cellular responses orientated to safeguard genome integrity or, in some cases, to avoid transmission of harmful alterations by activating apoptosis or senescence. In this context, one of the main effectors of the DDR is the transcription factor p53 which provides a late sustained response to DNA damage. p53 up-regulation contributes to the activation of checkpoints, and, if the damage persists, may activate senescence, apoptosis or cell differentiation programmes.

Regardless of this p53-centric view, it is clear that many p53-independent pathways are also stimulated by the DDR. For instance, a single proteomic study identified more than 700 ATM/ATR phosphorylation substrates, pointing out the wide variety of effectors and pathways that are regulated by the DDR [63].

Given that there are multiple reviews elsewhere that focus on these cellular responses, we here only briefly describe the main cellular responses promoted by the DDR: cell cycle checkpoints, senescence, apoptosis and differentiation.

3.1.3.1. Transient cell cycle delay: Checkpoints

The transitions through the different stages of the cell cycle are tightly regulated by the activity of cyclin-dependent kinases (CDKs). CDKs are activated by cyclins and inhibited by CDK inhibitors (CKIs) or inhibitory tyrosine phosphorylations [100]. In brief, a simplified scheme depicts that four CDKs are involved in the regulation of cell cycle; CDK2, CDK4 and CDK6 during interphase, and CDK1 being considered the mitotic CDK. An activated DDR can limit the activity of CDKs and thus prevent cell cycle progression into the next stage (G1/S and the G2/M). In addition, the DDR can also slow down replication (intra-S checkpoint), but this is not a full stop and cells with damage in S-phase progress into G2 stop at the G2/M checkpoint [101]. The way that the DDR gets to the CDKs is through effectors that limit CDK activity which we now briefly summarize.

First, the main PIKK targets that regulate checkpoints are the so-called checkpoint kinases Chk1 and Chk2, direct substrates of ATR and ATM respectively [102, 103]. Checkpoint kinases act by regulating CDK inhibitory effectors such as Cdc25a, Wee1 or p53. *Cdc25*a is a phosphatase that controls CDK1 and CDK2 activities. In response to DNA damage, ATR-activated Chk1 phosphorylates Cdc25a inducing its degradation [104, 105], and thereby, inhibition of CDK activity [106]. An opposing force for Cdc25a is *Wee1*, the kinase that counteracts Cdc25a activity. Finally, a major mediator of cellular responses to DNA damage is p53. *p53* is rapidly stabilized upon DNA damage by a number of inter-dependent PTMs. ATM, ATR, Chk1 and Chk2 are all able to phosphorylate p53 contributing to its stabilization [107, 108]. Besides its apoptotic targets, p53 has a number of transcriptional targets that contribute to checkpoint function, perhaps the most notorious being the CKI $p21^{cip1}$ which is an important regulator of the G1/S checkpoint.

Specifically, the ***G1/S checkpoint*** avoids the replication of damaged DNA (see Figure 3 for a scheme of checkpoint responses). The transition from G1 to S is directed by an increase in CDK2 activity induced by cyclin E [109]. As such, the G1/S checkpoint is directed to limit this burst in CDK activity. An early and late component checkpoint can be separated. First, the G1/S checkpoint is initiated by degradation of Cdc25a, leading to the accumulation of inhibitory phosphorylations on CDK2 [110, 111]. This is an early response that does not require the synthesis of new proteins. If the damage persists, p53-dependent transcriptional upregulation of $p21^{cip1}$ would implement a stronger G1/S arrest [112].ATM and Chk2, but not ATR/Chk1 are the main DDR mediators of the G1/S transition.

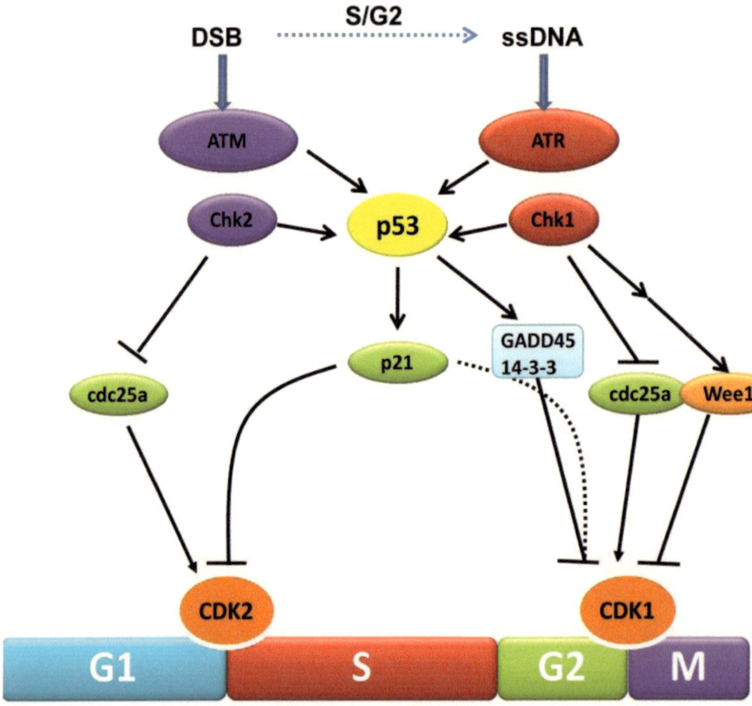

Figure 3. Chekpoint regulation by the DDR. ATM and ATR orchestrate a transitory delay of the cell cycle in response to DSBs and ssDNA, respectively. Wherease direct phosphorylation of of cdc25a and wee1 allow a rapid establishment of the G1/S and G2/M checkpoints, p53-dependent regulation contributes to checkpoint maintenance at later timepoints. During S and G2 phases DSBs can be resected leading to the generation of ssDNA, which also activates ATR-signaling.

If damage arises in S phase, the ***intra-S checkpoint*** is also mainly regulated by the phosphatase Cdc25a, but now under de control of ATR and Chk1 [102]. In addition, DDR-promoted replication inhibition is in part mediated by Cdt1, which participates in the loading of MCM helicases that facilitate DNA unwinding ahead of the RF [113]. How the DDR promotes Cdt1 degradation and thus replication control is yet uncharacterized.

The last key control point is the ***G2/M checkpoint***, that "checks" genome integrity before proceeding into chromosome segregation. Here, the transition from G2 into M is governed by an increase cyclinB-CDK1 activity. Once again, this checkpoint is also established by Cdc25a phosphorylation, in this case mediated by the ATR-dependent Chk1 kinase. In addition, the kinase Wee1 also contributes to the G2/M checkpoint. In a normal G2/M transition Plk1 (Polo kinase 1) phosphorylates Wee1 inducing its degradation and entry into mitosis. Upon damage ATM and ATR are able to phosphorylate and inhibit Plk1, contributing to an increase of Wee1 and therefore reduced CDK1 activity [100]. In addition to this early checkpoint, p53 also regulates the maintenance or sustained G2/M arrest. In this case, rather than mediated by p21, which has little CDK1 inhibitory capacity, other p53 targets such as GADD45 and 14-3-3 act as effectors [114].

3.1.3.2. Permanent cell cycle arrest: Senescence

By definition, checkpoints are a transitory state from which cells can escape if repair is accomplished and the signal is turned off. In contrast, cellular senescence is a persistent and irreversible cell cycle arrest. It was firstly observed in cell culture in 1965 [115]. Depending on the load of DNA damage or the cell type, a persistent activation of the DDR might direct cells into senescence [89].

Besides the presence of DSB, other cellular stresses can also promote senescence. These include telomere shortening [116], oxidative stress [117] and oncogenes [118-121]. Nevertheless, all of these stimuli can activate the DDR, so that DNA damage might be the ultimate cause of the senescent response. First, short or unprotected telomeres resemble and are actually sensed by cell as DSB [122, 123]. Second, reactive oxygen species generated by oxidative stress are an obvious source of DNA damage. Finally, several oncogenes have been shown to induce RS so that oncogene-induced senescence (OIS) would be linked to the DDR [124-126]. Importantly, and as it will be discussed below, OIS has been suggested as an early anti-cancer barrier in vivo, providing a link between the DDR and cancer development [127]. However, it must be pointed out that alternative, DDR-independent pathways of promoting OIS and which operate through the Ink4a/ARF locus have been described [128].

3.1.3.3. Apoptosis

Apoptosis, or programmed cell death, is other phenomenon activated by the DDR in order to eliminate cells with intolerable amounts of DNA damage. As such, apoptosis has an important role in eliminating damaged cells during aging [129] or in the acute responses genotoxic cancer therapies. In addition, apoptosis is a physiological process essential for normal development.

As in the case of senescence, apoptosis is also chiefly governed by p53. DDR-induced p53 promotes the expression of several pro-apoptotic factors, such as Puma, Noxa and Bax [130-132]. This pro-apoptotic p53 program leads to mitochondrial membrane permeabilzation [133], allowing the exit of cytochrome c to the cytosol, forming the apoptosome, which finally activates effector caspases [134].

Why some cells undergo apoptosis and other senescence in response to DNA damage is still a matter of study [135]. Although most cells are capable of both phenomenons, cell type is indeed determinant to undergo one or another. For instance, whereas DNA damage in fibroblasts and epithelial cells specially promotes senescence, low amounts of DNA breaks in lymphocytes are sufficient to trigger apoptosis. Of note, post-mitotic cells like neurons, have a limited capacity to become senescent or undergo apoptosis which might be due to their particular cell cycle status.

3.1.3.4. Other cellular pathways stimulated by the DDR

Given the large amount of PIKK phospho-targets and p53 transcriptional targets it is not surprising that the DDR exerts its function in many cellular processes by means that remain poorly understood. For instance, high doses of DNA damage can induce the *differentiation* of melanocyte stem cells (SC), resulting in their depletion and thereby promoting aging phenotypes on the skin [136]. Similar results linking the DDR and differentiation have been found in neurons [137]. Related to this, p53 has been shown to regulate the *polarity* of mammary cancer stem cell divisions [138]. p53 loss promotes symmetric and promiscuous cancer stem cell divisions, which contribute to the expansion of premalignant pools. It is therefore tempting to speculate that one of the means by which DNA damage leads to stem cell exhaustion is by promoting p53-dependent asymmetric cell divisions in SC.

Finally, another process that might be modulated by DNA damage is *autophagy*, which functions to promote cell survival through the degradation of damaged organelles and molecules. Interestingly, one of the key regulators of autophagy is mTOR (mammalian target of Rapamycin), another member of the PIKK family. Whereas the mechanism remains to be solved, recent studies suggest a connection between the DDR and mTOR that could be the responsible for DNA damage induced autophagy [139, 140]. To what extent these additional effects of the DDR impact on the physiological consequences of a deficient DDR, remains to be seen.

3.1.4. Physiological consequences of the DDR

DDR deficiencies cause important physiological consequences. As commented on this chapter, DSB are physiologically generated during B and T lymphocyte maturation and during meiotic recombination, and many DDR-related proteins are required for normal functioning of these processes. In addition, the DDR has an essential role in facing the stochastic DNA damage that our cells acquire through our lifetimes. In this context, it is not surprising that deficiencies in DDR components cause human diseases associated to immune deficiencies, sterility, premature aging and cancer predisposition. Alterations during embryonic development are also frequent, suggesting that the high division rates occurring at this stage might be prone to accumulate DNA damage, particularly RS.

DDR-mutant mouse models recapitulate many of the phenotypes found in DDR-associated human syndromes. Some of the most relevant DDR-related diseases are shown in **table 1**. Most of them are of recessive nature, with some exceptions such as variants of Li-Fraumeni, which can be caused by dominant mutations in just one allele of p53.

3.1.4.1. The DDR and cancer: Protector and target

The relationship between the DDR and cancer is of particular interest from multiple points of view. First, the DDR is critical **to prevent the accumulation of spontaneous pro-cancerous mutations** and overall genomic instability. This is why most DDR-related human diseases are prone to cancer development. In addition, the DDR is particularly relevant in preventing chromosome rearrangements during lymphoid maturation which makes lymphomas one of the most frequent cancer in Genomic Instability Syndromes. Note that in some cases mutations

Disease	Mutated gen	Clinical feature
Ataxia Telangiectasia	ATM	Cerebellar ataxia, telangiectasia, inmunodeficiency, lymphoid tumours.
Nijmegen breakage syndrome	Nbs1	Growth retardation, microcephaly, immunodeficiency, lymphoid tumours.
A-T like disorder	Mre11	Cerebellar ataxia, mild predisposition to tumours.
Seckel Syndrome	ATR	Progeria, microcephaly and other developmental defects.
Li-Fraumeni	p53	Early development of cancer (breast cancer, sarcomas, brain tumours, leukemias, etc.)
Riddle syndrome	RNF168	Inmunodeficiency, dysmorphic features, mental retardation.
Werner syndrome	RECQL2 (WRN)	Progeria and age-associated disorders
Fanconi Anemia	13 different FA genes	Bone marrow failure, predisposition to leukemias and solid tumours.

Table 1. Several human genetic syndromes related to DDR components.

in only one allele convey a dramatic increase in cancer predisposition. This is the case for BRCA1 and BRCA2 mutations carriers, whose life-time breast cancer risk raise up to 80%.

Second, **the DDR is activated by oncogenes** in early stages of tumorigenesis [124, 141]. These studies proposed a model where the activation of certain oncogenes could generate RS which, by activating the DDR, would limit cancer development by promoting cell senescence [142, 143]. In fact, convincing evidence exists to show that certain oncogenes indeed are able to generate DNA damage trough promoting abnormal replication [124, 125]. Note that this type of damage, known as RS, is sensed and signaled mainly by ATR rather than ATM [83], raising the relevance of ATR-signaling in the oncogene-activated DDR model of cancer progression.

Finally, many of the current **anti-cancer therapies** (including radiotherapy) operate by generating high loads of DNA damage that activate the DDR towards apoptosis. In this regard, there is increasing interest in the development of new anti-cancer strategies that take advantage of our knowledge of the DDR to specifically target tumor cells. The idea behind these new strategies is to exploit synthetic lethal interactions that will only occur in cancer cells. For instance, one of the most promising approaches in this regard is the use of *PARP inhibitors* for the treatment of BRCA1/2 deficient breast cancers. These inhibitors block a ssDNA repair pathway which is mostly dispensable for normal cells, but essential for cells deficient in HR, such as BRCA1/2 mutant cells [144]. Other examples of synthetic lethality could be the use of Chk1 inhibitors and ATR inhibitors, to treat p53 deficient tumors [145-148].

3.1.4.2. The role of the DDR in ageing

Ageing is intuitively associated with the natural degeneration of our tissues, which would derive from the accumulation of some "toxic" factor. Studies mostly performed in the last decade have identified DNA damage as this deleterious factor that is associated to the onset of ageing [149, 150]. For instance, aged tissues or stem cells show evidences of an activated DDR [151, 152]. Moreover, most DDR-related genetic diseases suffer from premature ageing, which is likely due to a faster accumulation of intolerable amounts of DNA damage.

The most accepted theory is that DNA damage, when accumulated in SC, activates a DDR that limits their regenerative capacity and thus promotes ageing [151, 153]. To what extent DNA damage is the natural cause of actual ageing in humans, and which types of DNA damage (RS, eroded telomeres, ROS…) are most important in this process, remains to be understood. In what regards to RS, the faster nature of embryonic cell divisions might make this stage particularly susceptible to this type of damage. In fact, recent studies in ATR hypomorphic mice revealed that an intra-uterine exposure to RS can accelerate the later onset ageing [146, 154]. Whereas the exact mechanism of this intrauterine programming of ageing is not fully understood, it raises the question about to what extent our adult well-being can be already conditioned by the stresses to which we were exposed *in utero*.

3.2. Other posttranslational modifications in the DDR

There is little doubt that PIKK-mediated phosphorylation is a major controller of the DDR. Nevertheless, to end this chapter we would want to describe the role that non-phosphorylation based signaling of DNA damage might play in genome protection. In the light of recent discoveries, DNA damage signaling through other PTMs such as acetylation, methylation, ubiquitination and, sumoylation might also play crucial roles for appropriate DNA damage signaling.

3.2.1. Ubiquitination

Ubiquitination is a highly regulated process that promotes covalent modification of specific proteins substrates with the 76-amino acid protein *ubiquitin*, catalyzed in three sequential steps by *E1* (*ubiquitin-activating enzyme*), *E2* (*ubiquitin-conjugating enzyme*) and E3 (*ubiquitin ligase*) enzymatic activities [155]. Classically, ubiquitination (UQ) was described as a mechanism to target proteins for proteasome mediated degradation. However, at present, other functions of UQ such as during protein localization or in mediating protein-protein interactions are known. In fact, phosphorylation signaling (not only by the DDR) is often coupled to substrate ubiquitination, which increases the potential network of protein-protein interaction [156, 157].

UQ presents seven lysines in its surface: K6, K11, K27, K29, K33, K48 and K63. Whereas poly-ubiquitination linked to K48 residues is usually related to proteasomal degradation [158], K63-linked polyubiquitin chains are more related to other regulatory functions [159]. In addition to the conjugating lysine, ubiquitin chains display an ample structural diversity, that has its counterpart in many different *ubiquitin interactif motifs (UIM)* in other proteins [160]. The role of UQ is counteracted by *deubiquitianting enzymes (DUB),* which are responsible for the elimination of UQ conjugates.

Several ubiquitination events have been assoctaied to DSB signaling. As previously discussed, PIKK activation is followed by ubiquitination of various substrates. Again, ATM-dependent phosphorylation of H2AX and MDC1 are sufficient to recruit the E3 ubiquitin ligase *RNF8*. Together with another E3 ligase known as RNF168, and with *Ubc13* as the E2 ligase, RNF8 promotes the accumulation of ubiquitinylated substrates in the vicinity of the DSB. Of note,

RNF168 loading to foci occurs trough direct recognition of RNF8-deposited UQ chains through its UIM domains [25, 26]. These poly-ubiquitinations are mainly K63-linked and contribute to attract specific UIM-containing proteins and/or to modulate chromatin architecture via histone ubiquitinylation [159]. Recent works have shown that HERC2 (Hect Domain and RLD2) is an important regulator of RNF8 and RNF168-dependent ubiquitinitalion which mediates through promoting the binding to the E2 ligase Ubc13 [161].

This coordinated cascade of UQ modifications generated at DSB is necessary for the formation of BRCA1 and 53BP1 foci. However, once again, the absence of RNF8 does not lead to major BRCA1 phenotypes, which challenges the relevance of IRIF as predictors of functionality. It should be noted also that there is no evidence of direct binding of 53BP1 to ubiquitin chains, and how UQ mediates 53BP1 foci remains a mistery. In addition, 53BP1 can bind methylated histones which may provide an independent way of loading to DSB [94, 95, 162].

In contrast to 53BP1, the relationship of BRCA1 foci with UQ is well characterized. *RAP80*, a protein containing several UIMs in tandem, binds to ubiquitinated substrates (perhaps histones) [23], and brings Abraxas [28] and BRCA1. Interestingly, RAP80 also interacts with *BRCC36*, a DUB, which activity is also required for proper DSB repair and signaling [163, 164]. Thus, ordered ubiquitinylation and deubuquitinylation may be needed during the signaling of DNA damage.

The UQ pathway does not end with 53BP1 or BRCA1. *BRCA1* itself is an E3 ubiquitin ligase activity resident in the N-terminal RING domain of this large protein. In fact, this is the only enzymatic activity found in BRCA1. While BRCA1 has E3 activity by itself, this activity increases in several orders of magnitude when bound to its constitutive partner BARD1 [30]. To date, the only well characterized BRCA1 substrates are BRCA1 itself and CtIP. CtIP ubiquitination by BRCA1 [165] has been proposed to promote the resection of DSB, leading to HR and a regulation of the G2/M checkpoint through ATR-activity. Hence, in this system UQ would be upstream of the phosphorylation DDR.

To complicate things further, BRCA1 auto-ubiquitination is linked to K6, which is mediated by the E2 enzyme Ubch5c [166]. Ubiquitinated BRCA1 is found at DSB and also in several endogenous spots during S phase. Interestingly, even though 20% of human BRCA1 mutations predisposing to breast and ovarian cancer are found in the RING domain [30], recent data emerging from mouse models suggest that the E3 ligase activity of BRCA1 might be unrelated to genome maintenance and its tumor suppression role [167, 168]. However, other studies [169, 170] indicate the importance of the RING domain in BRCA1 tumor suppressor function. Certainly, further work needs to be done to solve these divergent observations.

Finally, regardless of DSB there is solid evidence that UQ-mediated signaling pathways also contribute to other genome protective pathways. For instance, UQ plays a key role in the *Fanconi Anemia* pathway. Fanconi Anemia (FA) is a recessive disease characterized by developmental abnormalities, bone marrow failure and cancer predisposition [171]. The disease is caused by mutations in at least 13 genes which mutations compromise the repair of interstrand DNA cross-links. A key event on the activation of the FA pathway is the monoubiquitination of FancD2 and FancI proteins, with is thought to be essential for its localization at chromatin [44, 172, 173]. Again, there is evidence to suggest that FANCD2 ubiquitinylation is downstream of ATR signaling, providing a further example of the constant interaction between the different signaling pathways that are activated by DNA damage [55].

3.2.2. *SUMOylation*

SUMO stands for Small Ubiquitin-like modifier due to its similarities with UQ. In fact, SUMOylation is a similar process to ubiquitinylation involving E1, E2 and E3 enzymes. Importantly, very few SUMO E3 ligases exist in the mammalian proteome, which limits the search for potential ligases. In addition, SUMO E3 ligases are mostly dispensable and E2 ligases can complete the SUMOylation reaction largely by themselves. In contrast to UQ, three SUMO variants (SUMO1, SUMO2 and SUMO3 exist [174].

A number of SUMO roles with genome maintenance pathways have been discovered. In what regards to the DDR, two recent studies identified a SUMO-related signaling cascade that also coordinates the foci formation of BRCA1 and 53BP1 in response to DSB [175, 176]. At present, *PIAS1* (*Protein Inhibitor of Activated STAT-1*) and *PIAS4*, are the E3 SUMO ligase enzymes found to participate in the DDR, using *SAE1* (*SUMO activating enzyme subunit 1)* as E1 and *UBC9* (Ubiquitin Conjugating Enzyme 9) as E2 enzymes. All these proteins, as well as SUMO1 and SUMO2/3 conjugates are rapidly recruited to DSB, forming IRIF. Whereas the mechanism is still not totally clear, it seems that PIAS1 promotes SUMO2/3 modification of BRCA1, and PIAS4 is mainly involved in SUMO1 modifications of both 53BP1 and BRCA1. Together, these SUMOylations seem to be necessary for RNF8 and RNF168 function, providing another instance of inter-PTM signaling at DSB [175, 176]. A summary of key SUMO and UQ modifications in the DSB response is illustrated in **table 2**.

E3 Ligase	E2 Ligase	Main substrates	Function
		Ubiquitinations	
FancL	Unknown	FancD2	DNA Cross-link repair
BRCA1 / BARD1	Ubch5c	BRCA1	Unknown,
		CtIP	DSB resection
RNF8	Ubc13	H2A, H2AX	DSB signaling
RNF168	Ubc13	H2A, H2AX	DSB signaling
		SUMOylations	
PIAS1	Ubc9	BRCA1	DSB signaling
PIAS4	Ubc9	BRCA1, 53BP1	DSB signaling

Table 2. Relevant ubiquitinations and SUMOylations in genome maintenance.

Regardless of the DDR, other genome maintenance pathways are also controlled by SUMO. One example is the role of a SUMO ligase called Mms21, which is an essential component of a cohesin and condensin related complex formed by Smc5 and Smc6 [177]. Whereas the role of this complex is far from being understood, it seems it might be important to prevent the accumulation of hemicatenates at stalled replication forks [178].

3.2.3. *Interplay of PTMs in the DDR*

Other post-translational modifications, such as methylation and acetylation, are also involved in the regulatory network of the DDR. A paradigm of multiple and interconnected PTM is found in the **regulation of p53** levels, that involves a coordinated network of phosphorylation, acetylation, methylation and ubiquitination [179].

In the absence of DNA damage, p53 levels are kept low due to its *ubiquitination* by the E3 UQ ligase MDM2 and rapid degradation by the proteasome [180]. In fact, one of the ways by which DNA damage and other stress signals promote p53 stabilization is by PTMs which alters the MDM2/p53 interaction. p53 also suffers DDR-dependent *phosphorylations* [107] are thought to stabilize the protein and allow its association with the CBP/p300 acetyltransferase complex, promoting p53 *acetylation* and further stabilization [181]. Besides, p53 activity is limited by Set8/Pr-Set7 mediated methylations [182], which are also upon DNA damage [183].

Another relevant example of the interplay between different PTMs in the DDR is found in **histones.** Indeed, post-translational modifications of histones regulate many other processes related to chromatin compaction and structure, such as replication and transcription. The best known histone modification upon DNA damage is the already described *phosphorylation* of H2AX, that it is mediated by ATM, ATR or DNA-PK [20]. We also discussed how RNF8 and RNF168 can *ubiquitinate* histones in the proximity of DSB [26, 92]. Finally, *methylations* of histones H3 and H4 could modulates the recruitment of 53BP1 [94, 95, 162]; and several *acetylations* of histones have been described to play roles in genome maintenance which are still not completely understood [184-186]. How histone modifications enhance DSB repair is a very active area of research and discussion. One possibility is that histone modifications could increase chromatin accessibility, which would therefore facilitate the repair and signaling of the breaks [187].

4. Future perspectives

We have here provided a general overview of how cells signal the presence of DNA damage, and how a proper signaling is necessary to maintain a healthy genome. Still, whereas the amount of PTMs that coordinate the cellular response to DNA damage is already intimidating, it is likely that we are only seeing the tip of the iceberg. Many other targets and even PTM (ADP-rybosylation, Neddylation, N-terminal glycosylation, etc...) will probably be involved in mounting a proper DDR. Without a doubt, the fast development of massive proteomic technologies will soon provide a breathtaking picture of how cells detect, signal and repair DNA breaks; by promoting a myriad of PTMs in almost every molecule involved in the DDR.

Author details

Andres Joaquin Lopez-Contreras*
Genomic Instability Group, Spanish National Cancer Research Centre (CNIO), Madrid, Spain

* Corresponding Author

Oscar Fernandez-Capetillo
Genomic Instability Group, Spanish National Cancer Research Centre (CNIO), Madrid, Spain

5. References

[1] Lindahl T, Barnes DE. Repair of endogenous DNA damage. Cold Spring Harb Symp Quant Biol2000;65:127-33.
[2] Jackson SP, Bartek J. The DNA-damage response in human biology and disease. Nature2009 Oct 22;461(7267):1071-8.
[3] Dudley DD, Chaudhuri J, Bassing CH, Alt FW. Mechanism and control of V(D)J recombination versus class switch recombination: similarities and differences. Adv Immunol2005;86:43-112.
[4] Zickler D, Kleckner N. The leptotene-zygotene transition of meiosis. Annu Rev Genet1998;32:619-97.
[5] Mao Z, Bozzella M, Seluanov A, Gorbunova V. Comparison of nonhomologous end joining and homologous recombination in human cells. DNA Repair (Amst)2008 Oct 1;7(10):1765-71.
[6] Doherty AJ, Jackson SP. DNA repair: how Ku makes ends meet. Curr Biol2001 Nov 13;11(22):R920-4.
[7] Burma S, Chen DJ. Role of DNA-PK in the cellular response to DNA double-strand breaks. DNA Repair (Amst)2004 Aug-Sep;3(8-9):909-18.
[8] Martin IV, MacNeill SA. ATP-dependent DNA ligases. Genome Biol2002;3(4):REVIEWS3005.
[9] Calsou P, Delteil C, Frit P, Drouet J, Salles B. Coordinated assembly of Ku and p460 subunits of the DNA-dependent protein kinase on DNA ends is necessary for XRCC4-ligase IV recruitment. J Mol Biol2003 Feb 7;326(1):93-103.
[10] Ma Y, Pannicke U, Schwarz K, Lieber MR. Hairpin opening and overhang processing by an Artemis/DNA-dependent protein kinase complex in nonhomologous end joining and V(D)J recombination. Cell2002 Mar 22;108(6):781-94.
[11] Riballo E, Kuhne M, Rief N, Doherty A, Smith GC, Recio MJ, et al. A pathway of double-strand break rejoining dependent upon ATM, Artemis, and proteins locating to gamma-H2AX foci. Mol Cell2004 Dec 3;16(5):715-24.
[12] Gu Y, Jin S, Gao Y, Weaver DT, Alt FW. Ku70-deficient embryonic stem cells have increased ionizing radiosensitivity, defective DNA end-binding activity, and inability to support V(D)J recombination. Proc Natl Acad Sci U S A1997 Jul 22;94(15):8076-81.
[13] Chaudhuri J, Alt FW. Class-switch recombination: interplay of transcription, DNA deamination and DNA repair. Nat Rev Immunol2004 Jul;4(7):541-52.
[14] Moshous D, Pannetier C, Chasseval Rd R, Deist Fl F, Cavazzana-Calvo M, Romana S, et al. Partial T and B lymphocyte immunodeficiency and predisposition to lymphoma in patients with hypomorphic mutations in Artemis. J Clin Invest2003 Feb;111(3):381-7.
[15] Goodarzi AA, Noon AT, Deckbar D, Ziv Y, Shiloh Y, Lobrich M, et al. ATM signaling facilitates repair of DNA double-strand breaks associated with heterochromatin. Mol Cell2008 Jul 25;31(2):167-77.

[16] Fernandez-Capetillo O, Nussenzweig A. ATM breaks into heterochromatin. Mol Cell2008 Aug 8;31(3):303-4.
[17] Richardson C, Jasin M. Frequent chromosomal translocations induced by DNA double-strand breaks. Nature2000 Jun 8;405(6787):697-700.
[18] Jazayeri A, Falck J, Lukas C, Bartek J, Smith GC, Lukas J, et al. ATM- and cell cycle-dependent regulation of ATR in response to DNA double-strand breaks. Nat Cell Biol2006 Jan;8(1):37-45.
[19] de Jager M, van Noort J, van Gent DC, Dekker C, Kanaar R, Wyman C. Human Rad50/Mre11 is a flexible complex that can tether DNA ends. Mol Cell2001 Nov;8(5):1129-35.
[20] Fernandez-Capetillo O, Lee A, Nussenzweig M, Nussenzweig A. H2AX: the histone guardian of the genome. DNA Repair (Amst)2004 Aug-Sep;3(8-9):959-67.
[21] Stucki M, Clapperton JA, Mohammad D, Yaffe MB, Smerdon SJ, Jackson SP. MDC1 directly binds phosphorylated histone H2AX to regulate cellular responses to DNA double-strand breaks. Cell2005 Dec 29;123(7):1213-26.
[22] Lou Z, Minter-Dykhouse K, Franco S, Gostissa M, Rivera MA, Celeste A, et al. MDC1 maintains genomic stability by participating in the amplification of ATM-dependent DNA damage signals. Mol Cell2006 Jan 20;21(2):187-200.
[23] Mailand N, Bekker-Jensen S, Faustrup H, Melander F, Bartek J, Lukas C, et al. RNF8 ubiquitylates histones at DNA double-strand breaks and promotes assembly of repair proteins. Cell2007 Nov 30;131(5):887-900.
[24] Santos MA, Huen MS, Jankovic M, Chen HT, Lopez-Contreras AJ, Klein IA, et al. Class switching and meiotic defects in mice lacking the E3 ubiquitin ligase RNF8. J Exp Med May 10;207(5):973-81.
[25] Doil C, Mailand N, Bekker-Jensen S, Menard P, Larsen DH, Pepperkok R, et al. RNF168 binds and amplifies ubiquitin conjugates on damaged chromosomes to allow accumulation of repair proteins. Cell2009 Feb 6;136(3):435-46.
[26] Stewart GS, Panier S, Townsend K, Al-Hakim AK, Kolas NK, Miller ES, et al. The RIDDLE syndrome protein mediates a ubiquitin-dependent signaling cascade at sites of DNA damage. Cell2009 Feb 6;136(3):420-34.
[27] Bohgaki T, Bohgaki M, Cardoso R, Panier S, Zeegers D, Li L, et al. Genomic instability, defective spermatogenesis, immunodeficiency, and cancer in a mouse model of the RIDDLE syndrome. PLoS Genet Apr;7(4):e1001381.
[28] Wang B, Elledge SJ. Ubc13/Rnf8 ubiquitin ligases control foci formation of the Rap80/Abraxas/Brca1/Brcc36 complex in response to DNA damage. Proc Natl Acad Sci U S A2007 Dec 26;104(52):20759-63.
[29] Fackenthal JD, Olopade OI. Breast cancer risk associated with BRCA1 and BRCA2 in diverse populations. Nat Rev Cancer2007 Dec;7(12):937-48.
[30] Hashizume R, Fukuda M, Maeda I, Nishikawa H, Oyake D, Yabuki Y, et al. The RING heterodimer BRCA1-BARD1 is a ubiquitin ligase inactivated by a breast cancer-derived mutation. J Biol Chem2001 May 4;276(18):14537-40.
[31] Fernandez-Capetillo O, Celeste A, Nussenzweig A. Focusing on foci: H2AX and the recruitment of DNA-damage response factors. Cell Cycle2003 Sep-Oct;2(5):426-7.
[32] Paull TT, Gellert M. The 3' to 5' exonuclease activity of Mre 11 facilitates repair of DNA double-strand breaks. Mol Cell1998 Jun;1(7):969-79.

[33] Nimonkar AV, Ozsoy AZ, Genschel J, Modrich P, Kowalczykowski SC. Human exonuclease 1 and BLM helicase interact to resect DNA and initiate DNA repair. Proc Natl Acad Sci U S A2008 Nov 4;105(44):16906-11.

[34] Sartori AA, Lukas C, Coates J, Mistrik M, Fu S, Bartek J, et al. Human CtIP promotes DNA end resection. Nature2007 Nov 22;450(7169):509-14.

[35] You Z, Shi LZ, Zhu Q, Wu P, Zhang YW, Basilio A, et al. CtIP links DNA double-strand break sensing to resection. Mol Cell2009 Dec 25;36(6):954-69.

[36] Cuadrado M, Martinez-Pastor B, Murga M, Toledo LI, Gutierrez-Martinez P, Lopez E, et al. ATM regulates ATR chromatin loading in response to DNA double-strand breaks. J Exp Med2006 Feb 20;203(2):297-303.

[37] Adams KE, Medhurst AL, Dart DA, Lakin ND. Recruitment of ATR to sites of ionising radiation-induced DNA damage requires ATM and components of the MRN protein complex. Oncogene2006 Jun 29;25(28):3894-904.

[38] Myers JS, Cortez D. Rapid activation of ATR by ionizing radiation requires ATM and Mre11. J Biol Chem2006 Apr 7;281(14):9346-50.

[39] Bunting SF, Callen E, Wong N, Chen HT, Polato F, Gunn A, et al. 53BP1 inhibits homologous recombination in Brca1-deficient cells by blocking resection of DNA breaks. Cell Apr 16;141(2):243-54.

[40] Cao L, Xu X, Bunting SF, Liu J, Wang RH, Cao LL, et al. A selective requirement for 53BP1 in the biological response to genomic instability induced by Brca1 deficiency. Mol Cell2009 Aug 28;35(4):534-41.

[41] Baumann P, Benson FE, West SC. Human Rad51 protein promotes ATP-dependent homologous pairing and strand transfer reactions in vitro. Cell1996 Nov 15;87(4):757-66.

[42] Tarsounas M, Davies D, West SC. BRCA2-dependent and independent formation of RAD51 nuclear foci. Oncogene2003 Feb 27;22(8):1115-23.

[43] Wagner JE, Tolar J, Levran O, Scholl T, Deffenbaugh A, Satagopan J, et al. Germline mutations in BRCA2: shared genetic susceptibility to breast cancer, early onset leukemia, and Fanconi anemia. Blood2004 Apr 15;103(8):3226-9.

[44] Garcia-Higuera I, Taniguchi T, Ganesan S, Meyn MS, Timmers C, Hejna J, et al. Interaction of the Fanconi anemia proteins and BRCA1 in a common pathway. Mol Cell2001 Feb;7(2):249-62.

[45] McIlwraith MJ, Vaisman A, Liu Y, Fanning E, Woodgate R, West SC. Human DNA polymerase eta promotes DNA synthesis from strand invasion intermediates of homologous recombination. Mol Cell2005 Dec 9;20(5):783-92.

[46] Holliday R. The Induction of Mitotic Recombination by Mitomycin C in Ustilago and Saccharomyces. Genetics1964 Sep;50:323-35.

[47] Bzymek M, Thayer NH, Oh SD, Kleckner N, Hunter N. Double Holliday junctions are intermediates of DNA break repair. Nature Apr 8;464(7290):937-41.

[48] Wu L, Hickson ID. The Bloom's syndrome helicase suppresses crossing over during homologous recombination. Nature2003 Dec 18;426(6968):870-4.

[49] Chen XB, Melchionna R, Denis CM, Gaillard PH, Blasina A, Van de Weyer I, et al. Human Mus81-associated endonuclease cleaves Holliday junctions in vitro. Mol Cell2001 Nov;8(5):1117-27.

[50] Constantinou A, Chen XB, McGowan CH, West SC. Holliday junction resolution in human cells: two junction endonucleases with distinct substrate specificities. EMBO J2002 Oct 15;21(20):5577-85.
[51] Svendsen JM, Harper JW. GEN1/Yen1 and the SLX4 complex: Solutions to the problem of Holliday junction resolution. Genes Dev Mar 15;24(6):521-36.
[52] Fekairi S, Scaglione S, Chahwan C, Taylor ER, Tissier A, Coulon S, et al. Human SLX4 is a Holliday junction resolvase subunit that binds multiple DNA repair/recombination endonucleases. Cell2009 Jul 10;138(1):78-89.
[53] Svendsen JM, Smogorzewska A, Sowa ME, O'Connell BC, Gygi SP, Elledge SJ, et al. Mammalian BTBD12/SLX4 assembles a Holliday junction resolvase and is required for DNA repair. Cell2009 Jul 10;138(1):63-77.
[54] Helleday T. Homologous recombination in cancer development, treatment and development of drug resistance. Carcinogenesis Mar 29.
[55] Andreassen PR, D'Andrea AD, Taniguchi T. ATR couples FANCD2 monoubiquitination to the DNA-damage response. Genes Dev2004 Aug 15;18(16):1958-63.
[56] Tibbetts RS, Cortez D, Brumbaugh KM, Scully R, Livingston D, Elledge SJ, et al. Functional interactions between BRCA1 and the checkpoint kinase ATR during genotoxic stress. Genes Dev2000 Dec 1;14(23):2989-3002.
[57] Davies SL, North PS, Dart A, Lakin ND, Hickson ID. Phosphorylation of the Bloom's syndrome helicase and its role in recovery from S-phase arrest. Mol Cell Biol2004 Feb;24(3):1279-91.
[58] Henson JD, Neumann AA, Yeager TR, Reddel RR. Alternative lengthening of telomeres in mammalian cells. Oncogene2002 Jan 21;21(4):598-610.
[59] Harper JW, Elledge SJ. The DNA damage response: ten years after. Mol Cell2007 Dec 14;28(5):739-45.
[60] Shiloh Y. ATM and related protein kinases: safeguarding genome integrity. Nat Rev Cancer2003 Mar;3(3):155-68.
[61] Lovejoy CA, Cortez D. Common mechanisms of PIKK regulation. DNA Repair (Amst)2009 Sep 2;8(9):1004-8.
[62] Lavin MF. Ataxia-telangiectasia: from a rare disorder to a paradigm for cell signalling and cancer. Nat Rev Mol Cell Biol2008 Oct;9(10):759-69.
[63] Matsuoka S, Ballif BA, Smogorzewska A, McDonald ER, 3rd, Hurov KE, Luo J, et al. ATM and ATR substrate analysis reveals extensive protein networks responsive to DNA damage. Science2007 May 25;316(5828):1160-6.
[64] Zou L, Elledge SJ. Sensing DNA damage through ATRIP recognition of RPA-ssDNA complexes. Science2003 Jun 6;300(5625):1542-8.
[65] Callen E, Jankovic M, Wong N, Zha S, Chen HT, Difilippantonio S, et al. Essential role for DNA-PKcs in DNA double-strand break repair and apoptosis in ATM-deficient lymphocytes. Mol Cell2009 May 15;34(3):285-97.
[66] Savitsky K, Bar-Shira A, Gilad S, Rotman G, Ziv Y, Vanagaite L, et al. A single ataxia telangiectasia gene with a product similar to PI-3 kinase. Science1995 Jun 23;268(5218):1749-53.
[67] Boder E. Ataxia-telangiectasia: an overview. Kroc Found Ser1985;19:1-63.

[68] Shiloh Y. The ATM-mediated DNA-damage response: taking shape. Trends Biochem Sci2006 Jul;31(7):402-10.
[69] Uziel T, Lerenthal Y, Moyal L, Andegeko Y, Mittelman L, Shiloh Y. Requirement of the MRN complex for ATM activation by DNA damage. EMBO J2003 Oct 15;22(20):5612-21.
[70] Bakkenist CJ, Kastan MB. DNA damage activates ATM through intermolecular autophosphorylation and dimer dissociation. Nature2003 Jan 30;421(6922):499-506.
[71] Daniel JA, Pellegrini M, Lee JH, Paull TT, Feigenbaum L, Nussenzweig A. Multiple autophosphorylation sites are dispensable for murine ATM activation in vivo. J Cell Biol2008 Dec 1;183(5):777-83.
[72] Pellegrini M, Celeste A, Difilippantonio S, Guo R, Wang W, Feigenbaum L, et al. Autophosphorylation at serine 1987 is dispensable for murine Atm activation in vivo. Nature2006 Sep 14;443(7108):222-5.
[73] Difilippantonio S, Celeste A, Fernandez-Capetillo O, Chen HT, Reina San Martin B, Van Laethem F, et al. Role of Nbs1 in the activation of the Atm kinase revealed in humanized mouse models. Nat Cell Biol2005 Jul;7(7):675-85.
[74] Sun Y, Xu Y, Roy K, Price BD. DNA damage-induced acetylation of lysine 3016 of ATM activates ATM kinase activity. Mol Cell Biol2007 Dec;27(24):8502-9.
[75] Lavin MF. ATM and the Mre11 complex combine to recognize and signal DNA double-strand breaks. Oncogene2007 Dec 10;26(56):7749-58.
[76] Matsuura S, Tauchi H, Nakamura A, Kondo N, Sakamoto S, Endo S, et al. Positional cloning of the gene for Nijmegen breakage syndrome. Nat Genet1998 Jun;19(2):179-81.
[77] Stewart GS, Maser RS, Stankovic T, Bressan DA, Kaplan MI, Jaspers NG, et al. The DNA double-strand break repair gene hMRE11 is mutated in individuals with an ataxia-telangiectasia-like disorder. Cell1999 Dec 10;99(6):577-87.
[78] Barlow C, Ribaut-Barassin C, Zwingman TA, Pope AJ, Brown KD, Owens JW, et al. ATM is a cytoplasmic protein in mouse brain required to prevent lysosomal accumulation. Proc Natl Acad Sci U S A2000 Jan 18;97(2):871-6.
[79] Shechter D, Costanzo V, Gautier J. Regulation of DNA replication by ATR: signaling in response to DNA intermediates. DNA Repair (Amst)2004 Aug-Sep;3(8-9):901-8.
[80] Lopez-Contreras AJ, Fernandez-Capetillo O. The ATR barrier to replication-born DNA damage. DNA Repair (Amst) Dec 10;9(12):1249-55.
[81] Brown EJ, Baltimore D. ATR disruption leads to chromosomal fragmentation and early embryonic lethality. Genes Dev2000 Feb 15;14(4):397-402.
[82] O'Driscoll M, Ruiz-Perez VL, Woods CG, Jeggo PA, Goodship JA. A splicing mutation affecting expression of ataxia-telangiectasia and Rad3-related protein (ATR) results in Seckel syndrome. Nat Genet2003 Apr;33(4):497-501.
[83] Cimprich KA, Cortez D. ATR: an essential regulator of genome integrity. Nat Rev Mol Cell Biol2008 Aug;9(8):616-27.
[84] Fanning E, Klimovich V, Nager AR. A dynamic model for replication protein A (RPA) function in DNA processing pathways. Nucleic Acids Res2006;34(15):4126-37.
[85] Cortez D, Guntuku S, Qin J, Elledge SJ. ATR and ATRIP: partners in checkpoint signaling. Science2001 Nov 23;294(5547):1713-6.
[86] Yang XH, Zou L. Recruitment of ATR-ATRIP, Rad17, and 9-1-1 complexes to DNA damage. Methods Enzymol2006;409:118-31.

[87] Lee J, Kumagai A, Dunphy WG. The Rad9-Hus1-Rad1 checkpoint clamp regulates interaction of TopBP1 with ATR. J Biol Chem2007 Sep 21;282(38):28036-44.
[88] Kumagai A, Lee J, Yoo HY, Dunphy WG. TopBP1 activates the ATR-ATRIP complex. Cell2006 Mar 10;124(5):943-55.
[89] Toledo LI, Murga M, Gutierrez-Martinez P, Soria R, Fernandez-Capetillo O. ATR signaling can drive cells into senescence in the absence of DNA breaks. Genes Dev2008 Feb 1;22(3):297-302.
[90] Celeste A, Fernandez-Capetillo O, Kruhlak MJ, Pilch DR, Staudt DW, Lee A, et al. Histone H2AX phosphorylation is dispensable for the initial recognition of DNA breaks. Nat Cell Biol2003 Jul;5(7):675-9.
[91] Fernandez-Capetillo O, Chen HT, Celeste A, Ward I, Romanienko PJ, Morales JC, et al. DNA damage-induced G2-M checkpoint activation by histone H2AX and 53BP1. Nat Cell Biol2002 Dec;4(12):993-7.
[92] Huen MS, Grant R, Manke I, Minn K, Yu X, Yaffe MB, et al. RNF8 transduces the DNA-damage signal via histone ubiquitylation and checkpoint protein assembly. Cell2007 Nov 30;131(5):901-14.
[93] Kolas NK, Chapman JR, Nakada S, Ylanko J, Chahwan R, Sweeney FD, et al. Orchestration of the DNA-damage response by the RNF8 ubiquitin ligase. Science2007 Dec 7;318(5856):1637-40.
[94] Huyen Y, Zgheib O, Ditullio RA, Jr., Gorgoulis VG, Zacharatos P, Petty TJ, et al. Methylated lysine 79 of histone H3 targets 53BP1 to DNA double-strand breaks. Nature2004 Nov 18;432(7015):406-11.
[95] Botuyan MV, Lee J, Ward IM, Kim JE, Thompson JR, Chen J, et al. Structural basis for the methylation state-specific recognition of histone H4-K20 by 53BP1 and Crb2 in DNA repair. Cell2006 Dec 29;127(7):1361-73.
[96] Celeste A, Petersen S, Romanienko PJ, Fernandez-Capetillo O, Chen HT, Sedelnikova OA, et al. Genomic instability in mice lacking histone H2AX. Science2002 May 3;296(5569):922-7.
[97] Ward IM, Difilippantonio S, Minn K, Mueller MD, Molina JR, Yu X, et al. 53BP1 cooperates with p53 and functions as a haploinsufficient tumor suppressor in mice. Mol Cell Biol2005 Nov;25(22):10079-86.
[98] Yoo HY, Kumagai A, Shevchenko A, Dunphy WG. Ataxia-telangiectasia mutated (ATM)-dependent activation of ATR occurs through phosphorylation of TopBP1 by ATM. J Biol Chem2007 Jun 15;282(24):17501-6.
[99] Kumagai A, Dunphy WG. Claspin, a novel protein required for the activation of Chk1 during a DNA replication checkpoint response in Xenopus egg extracts. Mol Cell2000 Oct;6(4):839-49.
[100] Guardavaccaro D, Pagano M. Stabilizers and destabilizers controlling cell cycle oscillators. Mol Cell2006 Apr 7;22(1):1-4.
[101] Abraham RT. Cell cycle checkpoint signaling through the ATM and ATR kinases. Genes Dev2001 Sep 1;15(17):2177-96.
[102] Bartek J, Lukas J. Chk1 and Chk2 kinases in checkpoint control and cancer. Cancer Cell2003 May;3(5):421-9.

[103] Smits VA, Reaper PM, Jackson SP. Rapid PIKK-dependent release of Chk1 from chromatin promotes the DNA-damage checkpoint response. Curr Biol2006 Jan 24;16(2):150-9.
[104] Jin J, Shirogane T, Xu L, Nalepa G, Qin J, Elledge SJ, et al. SCFbeta-TRCP links Chk1 signaling to degradation of the Cdc25A protein phosphatase. Genes Dev2003 Dec 15;17(24):3062-74.
[105] Xiao Z, Chen Z, Gunasekera AH, Sowin TJ, Rosenberg SH, Fesik S, et al. Chk1 mediates S and G2 arrests through Cdc25A degradation in response to DNA-damaging agents. J Biol Chem2003 Jun 13;278(24):21767-73.
[106] Boutros R, Dozier C, Ducommun B. The when and wheres of CDC25 phosphatases. Curr Opin Cell Biol2006 Apr;18(2):185-91.
[107] Canman CE, Lim DS, Cimprich KA, Taya Y, Tamai K, Sakaguchi K, et al. Activation of the ATM kinase by ionizing radiation and phosphorylation of p53. Science1998 Sep 11;281(5383):1677-9.
[108] Shieh SY, Ahn J, Tamai K, Taya Y, Prives C. The human homologs of checkpoint kinases Chk1 and Cds1 (Chk2) phosphorylate p53 at multiple DNA damage-inducible sites. Genes Dev2000 Feb 1;14(3):289-300.
[109] Geng Y, Eaton EN, Picon M, Roberts JM, Lundberg AS, Gifford A, et al. Regulation of cyclin E transcription by E2Fs and retinoblastoma protein. Oncogene1996 Mar 21;12(6):1173-80.
[110] Falck J, Mailand N, Syljuasen RG, Bartek J, Lukas J. The ATM-Chk2-Cdc25A checkpoint pathway guards against radioresistant DNA synthesis. Nature2001 Apr 12;410(6830):842-7.
[111] Mailand N, Falck J, Lukas C, Syljuasen RG, Welcker M, Bartek J, et al. Rapid destruction of human Cdc25A in response to DNA damage. Science2000 May 26;288(5470):1425-9.
[112] Bartek J, Lukas J. Pathways governing G1/S transition and their response to DNA damage. FEBS Lett2001 Feb 16;490(3):117-22.
[113] Arias EE, Walter JC. Strength in numbers: preventing rereplication via multiple mechanisms in eukaryotic cells. Genes Dev2007 Mar 1;21(5):497-518.
[114] Taylor WR, Stark GR. Regulation of the G2/M transition by p53. Oncogene2001 Apr 5;20(15):1803-15.
[115] Hayflick L. The Limited in Vitro Lifetime of Human Diploid Cell Strains. Exp Cell Res1965 Mar;37:614-36.
[116] Harley CB, Futcher AB, Greider CW. Telomeres shorten during ageing of human fibroblasts. Nature1990 May 31;345(6274):458-60.
[117] Parrinello S, Samper E, Krtolica A, Goldstein J, Melov S, Campisi J. Oxygen sensitivity severely limits the replicative lifespan of murine fibroblasts. Nat Cell Biol2003 Aug;5(8):741-7.
[118] Serrano M, Lin AW, McCurrach ME, Beach D, Lowe SW. Oncogenic ras provokes premature cell senescence associated with accumulation of p53 and p16INK4a. Cell1997 Mar 7;88(5):593-602.

[119] Lin AW, Barradas M, Stone JC, van Aelst L, Serrano M, Lowe SW. Premature senescence involving p53 and p16 is activated in response to constitutive MEK/MAPK mitogenic signaling. Genes Dev1998 Oct 1;12(19):3008-19.

[120] Michaloglou C, Vredeveld LC, Soengas MS, Denoyelle C, Kuilman T, van der Horst CM, et al. BRAFE600-associated senescence-like cell cycle arrest of human naevi. Nature2005 Aug 4;436(7051):720-4.

[121] Zhu J, Woods D, McMahon M, Bishop JM. Senescence of human fibroblasts induced by oncogenic Raf. Genes Dev1998 Oct 1;12(19):2997-3007.

[122] d'Adda di Fagagna F, Reaper PM, Clay-Farrace L, Fiegler H, Carr P, Von Zglinicki T, et al. A DNA damage checkpoint response in telomere-initiated senescence. Nature2003 Nov 13;426(6963):194-8.

[123] Martens UM, Chavez EA, Poon SS, Schmoor C, Lansdorp PM. Accumulation of short telomeres in human fibroblasts prior to replicative senescence. Exp Cell Res2000 Apr 10;256(1):291-9.

[124] Bartkova J, Rezaei N, Liontos M, Karakaidos P, Kletsas D, Issaeva N, et al. Oncogene-induced senescence is part of the tumorigenesis barrier imposed by DNA damage checkpoints. Nature2006 Nov 30;444(7119):633-7.

[125] Di Micco R, Fumagalli M, Cicalese A, Piccinin S, Gasparini P, Luise C, et al. Oncogene-induced senescence is a DNA damage response triggered by DNA hyper-replication. Nature2006 Nov 30;444(7119):638-42.

[126] Mallette FA, Gaumont-Leclerc MF, Ferbeyre G. The DNA damage signaling pathway is a critical mediator of oncogene-induced senescence. Genes Dev2007 Jan 1;21(1):43-8.

[127] Halazonetis TD, Gorgoulis VG, Bartek J. An oncogene-induced DNA damage model for cancer development. Science2008 Mar 7;319(5868):1352-5.

[128] Serrano M. The INK4a/ARF locus in murine tumorigenesis. Carcinogenesis2000 May;21(5):865-9.

[129] Pollack M, Phaneuf S, Dirks A, Leeuwenburgh C. The role of apoptosis in the normal aging brain, skeletal muscle, and heart. Ann N Y Acad Sci2002 Apr;959:93-107.

[130] Miyashita T, Reed JC. Tumor suppressor p53 is a direct transcriptional activator of the human bax gene. Cell1995 Jan 27;80(2):293-9.

[131] Nakano K, Vousden KH. PUMA, a novel proapoptotic gene, is induced by p53. Mol Cell2001 Mar;7(3):683-94.

[132] Oda E, Ohki R, Murasawa H, Nemoto J, Shibue T, Yamashita T, et al. Noxa, a BH3-only member of the Bcl-2 family and candidate mediator of p53-induced apoptosis. Science2000 May 12;288(5468):1053-8.

[133] Martinou JC, Green DR. Breaking the mitochondrial barrier. Nat Rev Mol Cell Biol2001 Jan;2(1):63-7.

[134] Ferri KF, Kroemer G. Organelle-specific initiation of cell death pathways. Nat Cell Biol2001 Nov;3(11):E255-63.

[135] Campisi J. Aging and cancer cell biology, 2007. Aging Cell2007 Jun;6(3):261-3.

[136] Inomata K, Aoto T, Binh NT, Okamoto N, Tanimura S, Wakayama T, et al. Genotoxic stress abrogates renewal of melanocyte stem cells by triggering their differentiation. Cell2009 Jun 12;137(6):1088-99.

[137] Tedeschi A, Di Giovanni S. The non-apoptotic role of p53 in neuronal biology: enlightening the dark side of the moon. EMBO Rep2009 Jun;10(6):576-83.

[138] Cicalese A, Bonizzi G, Pasi CE, Faretta M, Ronzoni S, Giulini B, et al. The tumor suppressor p53 regulates polarity of self-renewing divisions in mammary stem cells. Cell2009 Sep 18;138(6):1083-95.

[139] Budanov AV, Karin M. p53 target genes sestrin1 and sestrin2 connect genotoxic stress and mTOR signaling. Cell2008 Aug 8;134(3):451-60.

[140] Alexander A, Cai SL, Kim J, Nanez A, Sahin M, MacLean KH, et al. ATM signals to TSC2 in the cytoplasm to regulate mTORC1 in response to ROS. Proc Natl Acad Sci U S A Mar 2;107(9):4153-8.

[141] Gorgoulis VG, Vassiliou LV, Karakaidos P, Zacharatos P, Kotsinas A, Liloglou T, et al. Activation of the DNA damage checkpoint and genomic instability in human precancerous lesions. Nature2005 Apr 14;434(7035):907-13.

[142] Braig M, Lee S, Loddenkemper C, Rudolph C, Peters AH, Schlegelberger B, et al. Oncogene-induced senescence as an initial barrier in lymphoma development. Nature2005 Aug 4;436(7051):660-5.

[143] Collado M, Gil J, Efeyan A, Guerra C, Schuhmacher AJ, Barradas M, et al. Tumour biology: senescence in premalignant tumours. Nature2005 Aug 4;436(7051):642.

[144] Lord CJ, Ashworth A. Targeted therapy for cancer using PARP inhibitors. Curr Opin Pharmacol2008 Aug;8(4):363-9.

[145] Chen Z, Xiao Z, Gu WZ, Xue J, Bui MH, Kovar P, et al. Selective Chk1 inhibitors differentially sensitize p53-deficient cancer cells to cancer therapeutics. Int J Cancer2006 Dec 15;119(12):2784-94.

[146] Murga M, Bunting S, Montana MF, Soria R, Mulero F, Canamero M, et al. A mouse model of ATR-Seckel shows embryonic replicative stress and accelerated aging. Nat Genet2009 Aug;41(8):891-8.

[147] Toledo LI, Murga M, Zur R, Soria R, Rodriguez A, Martinez S, et al. A cell-based screen identifies ATR inhibitors with synthetic lethal properties for cancer-associated mutations. Nat Struct Mol Biol Jun;18(6):721-7.

[148] Murga M, Campaner S, Lopez-Contreras AJ, Toledo LI, Soria R, Montana MF, et al. Exploiting oncogene-induced replicative stress for the selective killing of Myc-driven tumors. Nat Struct Mol Biol Dec;18(12):1331-5.

[149] Garinis GA, van der Horst GT, Vijg J, Hoeijmakers JH. DNA damage and ageing: new-age ideas for an age-old problem. Nat Cell Biol2008 Nov;10(11):1241-7.

[150] Lombard DB, Chua KF, Mostoslavsky R, Franco S, Gostissa M, Alt FW. DNA repair, genome stability, and aging. Cell2005 Feb 25;120(4):497-512.

[151] Rossi DJ, Bryder D, Seita J, Nussenzweig A, Hoeijmakers J, Weissman IL. Deficiencies in DNA damage repair limit the function of haematopoietic stem cells with age. Nature2007 Jun 7;447(7145):725-9.

[152] Sedelnikova OA, Horikawa I, Zimonjic DB, Popescu NC, Bonner WM, Barrett JC. Senescing human cells and ageing mice accumulate DNA lesions with unrepairable double-strand breaks. Nat Cell Biol2004 Feb;6(2):168-70.

[153] Rossi DJ, Jamieson CH, Weissman IL. Stems cells and the pathways to aging and cancer. Cell2008 Feb 22;132(4):681-96.

[154] Fernandez-Capetillo O. Intrauterine programming of ageing. EMBO Rep Jan;11(1):32-6.

[155] Pickart CM. Ubiquitin enters the new millennium. Mol Cell2001 Sep;8(3):499-504.

[156] Haglund K, Dikic I. Ubiquitylation and cell signaling. EMBO J2005 Oct 5;24(19):3353-9.

[157] Schwartz AL, Ciechanover A. Targeting proteins for destruction by the ubiquitin system: implications for human pathobiology. Annu Rev Pharmacol Toxicol2009;49:73-96.

[158] Pickart CM, Cohen RE. Proteasomes and their kin: proteases in the machine age. Nat Rev Mol Cell Biol2004 Mar;5(3):177-87.

[159] Messick TE, Greenberg RA. The ubiquitin landscape at DNA double-strand breaks. J Cell Biol2009 Nov 2;187(3):319-26.

[160] Grabbe C, Dikic I. Functional roles of ubiquitin-like domain (ULD) and ubiquitin-binding domain (UBD) containing proteins. Chem Rev2009 Apr;109(4):1481-94.

[161] Bekker-Jensen S, Rendtlew Danielsen J, Fugger K, Gromova I, Nerstedt A, Lukas C, et al. HERC2 coordinates ubiquitin-dependent assembly of DNA repair factors on damaged chromosomes. Nat Cell Biol Jan;12(1):80-6; sup pp 1-12.

[162] Sanders SL, Portoso M, Mata J, Bahler J, Allshire RC, Kouzarides T. Methylation of histone H4 lysine 20 controls recruitment of Crb2 to sites of DNA damage. Cell2004 Nov 24;119(5):603-14.

[163] Shao G, Lilli DR, Patterson-Fortin J, Coleman KA, Morrissey DE, Greenberg RA. The Rap80-BRCC36 de-ubiquitinating enzyme complex antagonizes RNF8-Ubc13-dependent ubiquitination events at DNA double strand breaks. Proc Natl Acad Sci U S A2009 Mar 3;106(9):3166-71.

[164] Shao G, Patterson-Fortin J, Messick TE, Feng D, Shanbhag N, Wang Y, et al. MERIT40 controls BRCA1-Rap80 complex integrity and recruitment to DNA double-strand breaks. Genes Dev2009 Mar 15;23(6):740-54.

[165] Yu X, Fu S, Lai M, Baer R, Chen J. BRCA1 ubiquitinates its phosphorylation-dependent binding partner CtIP. Genes Dev2006 Jul 1;20(13):1721-6.

[166] Brzovic PS, Lissounov A, Christensen DE, Hoyt DW, Klevit RE. A UbcH5/ubiquitin noncovalent complex is required for processive BRCA1-directed ubiquitination. Mol Cell2006 Mar 17;21(6):873-80.

[167] Reid LJ, Shakya R, Modi AP, Lokshin M, Cheng JT, Jasin M, et al. E3 ligase activity of BRCA1 is not essential for mammalian cell viability or homology-directed repair of double-strand DNA breaks. Proc Natl Acad Sci U S A2008 Dec 30;105(52):20876-81.

[168] Shakya R, Reid LJ, Reczek CR, Cole F, Egli D, Lin CS, et al. BRCA1 tumor suppression depends on BRCT phosphoprotein binding, but not its E3 ligase activity. Science Oct 28;334(6055):525-8.

[169] Drost R, Bouwman P, Rottenberg S, Boon U, Schut E, Klarenbeek S, et al. BRCA1 RING function is essential for tumor suppression but dispensable for therapy resistance. Cancer Cell Dec 13;20(6):797-809.

[170] Zhu Q, Pao GM, Huynh AM, Suh H, Tonnu N, Nederlof PM, et al. BRCA1 tumour suppression occurs via heterochromatin-mediated silencing. Nature Sep 8;477(7363):179-84.

[171] Moldovan GL, D'Andrea AD. How the fanconi anemia pathway guards the genome. Annu Rev Genet2009;43:223-49.

[172] Wang W. Emergence of a DNA-damage response network consisting of Fanconi anaemia and BRCA proteins. Nat Rev Genet2007 Oct;8(10):735-48.
[173] Matsushita N, Kitao H, Ishiai M, Nagashima N, Hirano S, Okawa K, et al. A FancD2-monoubiquitin fusion reveals hidden functions of Fanconi anemia core complex in DNA repair. Mol Cell2005 Sep 16;19(6):841-7.
[174] Yeh ET. SUMOylation and De-SUMOylation: wrestling with life's processes. J Biol Chem2009 Mar 27;284(13):8223-7.
[175] Galanty Y, Belotserkovskaya R, Coates J, Polo S, Miller KM, Jackson SP. Mammalian SUMO E3-ligases PIAS1 and PIAS4 promote responses to DNA double-strand breaks. Nature2009 Dec 17;462(7275):935-9.
[176] Morris JR, Boutell C, Keppler M, Densham R, Weekes D, Alamshah A, et al. The SUMO modification pathway is involved in the BRCA1 response to genotoxic stress. Nature2009 Dec 17;462(7275):886-90.
[177] Potts PR. The Yin and Yang of the MMS21-SMC5/6 SUMO ligase complex in homologous recombination. DNA Repair (Amst)2009 Apr 5;8(4):499-506.
[178] Branzei D, Sollier J, Liberi G, Zhao X, Maeda D, Seki M, et al. Ubc9- and mms21-mediated sumoylation counteracts recombinogenic events at damaged replication forks. Cell2006 Nov 3;127(3):509-22.
[179] Benkirane M, Sardet C, Coux O. Lessons from interconnected ubiquitylation and acetylation of p53: think metastable networks. Biochem Soc Trans Feb;38(Pt 1):98-103.
[180] Momand J, Zambetti GP, Olson DC, George D, Levine AJ. The mdm-2 oncogene product forms a complex with the p53 protein and inhibits p53-mediated transactivation. Cell1992 Jun 26;69(7):1237-45.
[181] Ito A, Lai CH, Zhao X, Saito S, Hamilton MH, Appella E, et al. p300/CBP-mediated p53 acetylation is commonly induced by p53-activating agents and inhibited by MDM2. EMBO J2001 Mar 15;20(6):1331-40.
[182] Shi X, Kachirskaia I, Yamaguchi H, West LE, Wen H, Wang EW, et al. Modulation of p53 function by SET8-mediated methylation at lysine 382. Mol Cell2007 Aug 17;27(4):636-46.
[183] Ivanov GS, Ivanova T, Kurash J, Ivanov A, Chuikov S, Gizatullin F, et al. Methylation-acetylation interplay activates p53 in response to DNA damage. Mol Cell Biol2007 Oct;27(19):6756-69.
[184] Tjeertes JV, Miller KM, Jackson SP. Screen for DNA-damage-responsive histone modifications identifies H3K9Ac and H3K56Ac in human cells. EMBO J2009 Jul 8;28(13):1878-89.
[185] van Attikum H, Gasser SM. Crosstalk between histone modifications during the DNA damage response. Trends Cell Biol2009 May;19(5):207-17.
[186] Yuan J, Pu M, Zhang Z, Lou Z. Histone H3-K56 acetylation is important for genomic stability in mammals. Cell Cycle2009 Jun 1;8(11):1747-53.
[187] Fernandez-Capetillo O, Murga M. Why cells respond differently to DNA damage: a chromatin perspective. Cell Cycle2008 Apr 15;7(8):980-3.

Section 3

Tyrosine Protein Kinases in Receptor Signaling and Diseases

Chapter 9

Tyrosine Phosphorylation of the NMDA Receptor Following Cerebral Ischaemia

Dmytro Pavlov and John G. Mielke

Additional information is available at the end of the chapter

http://dx.doi.org/10.5772/52316

1. Introduction

Cerebral ischaemia (stroke) describes a condition wherein blood flow to the brain is reduced such that neurological function is disrupted, and neural cell death becomes possible. For several decades, stroke has remained a leading international cause of death and disability, which is the reason considerable effort has been applied to improve understanding of its pathogenesis; however, only a modest comprehension of the complex cellular processes underlying ischaemia-mediated cell death can currently be claimed. Our limited knowledge regarding how the brain is changed by an ischaemic event is part of the explanation for the absence of a successful clinical intervention, despite the examination of more than a thousand potential pharmacotherapies during the past fifty years [61, 69, 169].

Phosphorylation is the most broadly examined post-translational modification within the central nervous system [125, 222, 244]. Physiological shifts in neuronal activity, such as those that occur during memory formation, can lead to changes in protein phosphorylation; in a similar fashion, pathological changes in brain activity, such as those that occur during cerebral ischaemia, can also affect phosphorylation status. One principal means whereby the pattern of phosphorylation, especially at tyrosine residues [45, 80], can affect brain function is by regulating the activity of ionotropic receptors, which mediate the vast majority of rapid signal transmission. While the phosphoregulation of many ionotropic receptors has been examined, the NMDA sub-type of receptors that respond to the excitatory neurotransmitter glutamate has been the subject of a disproportionate level of attention due to its key role in neuronal communication.

To contribute to ongoing efforts directed at developing improved pharmacotherapies for stroke, the present review will provide a reflection on the manner in which ischaemic injury may alter neuronal physiology through changes in the tyrosine phosphorylation of the NMDA receptor; in particular, three goals will aim to be accomplished: (a) providing a general review of the primary upstream changes initiated by cerebral ischaemia, and, in so doing, highlighting the importance of the NMDA receptor (b) offering a summary of the structure and function of the NMDA receptor, and the evidence that establishes how the receptor's function and cellular distribution are altered by tyrosine phosphorylation (c) outlining what is known about how ischaemia may set in motion cellular changes leading to the aberrant, potentially harmful, and possibly self-amplifying over-activation of the NMDA receptor.

2. Cerebral ischaemia

2.1. Definition, prevalence, and risk factors

Insufficient cerebral blood supply may result from either the collapse of systemic circulation (leading to global ischaemia), or from the occlusion of a vessel that supplies a discrete region of the brain (leading to focal ischaemia). Although there are several possible causes of focal occlusions, they are predominantly the result of a foreign substance travelling within the cerebral circulation until the lumen becomes too narrow to permit further movement (embolism) [240]; the principal source of emboli is believed to be atherosclerotic plaques [187]. While uncontrolled bleeding from a vessel (haemorrhage) can also cause ischaemia of a focal nature, occlusion is thought to account for approximately 80% of focal events [198, 230].

For several decades, stroke has consistently been recognised as one of the leading causes of death worldwide, and one of the major causes of severe disability. Globally, over 15 million people per year are diagnosed with stroke, and a third of those afflicted die from complications relating to the injury [255]. In addition to significant medical consequences for affected individuals, cerebral ischaemia also presents enormous socioeconomic costs; for example, recent estimates place the direct and indirect annual costs associated with stroke in the United States at approximately 65 billion USD [47], while similarly constructed European estimates place the annual costs at approximately 77 billion USD [172]. Given that those who survive an ischaemic attack must cope with a variety of significant cognitive deficits (including aphasia, hemiparesis, and memory problems) that often lack treatment, the social costs of stroke are as enduring as they are significant.

Understanding the underlying causes of cerebral ischaemia requires an appreciation for the numerous genetic and environmental factors that contribute to its development, and that its determinants may be divided into non-modifiable and modifiable categories. The primary, and most significant, non-modifiable risk factor is age. The incidence of stroke rises exponentially with age, and the majority of strokes are seen within individuals who are older than 65 years of age [83, 203]. Gender is also an important consideration, for stroke incidence among men has consistently been shown to be approximately one-third greater than among women [203]. In addition, numerous American studies have indicated that the occurrence of stroke among multiple non-white demographic groups is greater than among white individuals, even when socioeconomic factors are considered [95, 202]. The principal modifiable risk factor for cerebral ischaemia is hypertension, and a large body of work has illustrated that the likelihood of stroke rises proportionately with increasing blood pressure [210, 256]. As well, cardiac disease, notably atrial fibrillation and coronary artery disease [203, 257], and metabolic disease, particularly type II diabetes and dyslipidaemia [189, 256], are also associated with elevated stroke risk. Finally, several lifestyle factors, including physical activity levels, cigarette smoking, alcohol consumption, and diet, have been shown to independently affect the potential for stroke development [13, 92, 93, 251].

2.2. Pathogenesis

Despite comprising only about 2% of total body weight, the brain receives 15% of cardiac output and consumes about 20% of the oxygen utilised by the body [28]. The brain's disproportionate circulatory demands are attributable to a high metabolic rate based almost exclusively upon cellular respiration; in addition, unlike most other organs, glucose stores in the brain are sufficient to cover energy requirements for only about one minute [83]. In a relatively quick manner, reduction of blood flow beyond a critical threshold results in the inability of neurones to fire action potentials, and, if sufficiently extensive, may lead to the failure of oxidative phosphorylation, which is the principal method of cellular energy production [5]. To avert the cellular energy crisis that rapidly follows reduced blood supply, cells in an affected area rely increasingly upon glycolysis; consequently, tissue concentrations of lactate and hydrogen ions increase dramatically, causing acidosis [214]. However, the comparatively meagre amount of energy provided by anaerobic metabolism provides limited compensation, and, in a short period of time, the lack of high-energy phosphate, combined with decreased pH, precipitates a multifactorial increase of membrane permeability.

A number of ionic gradients exist across the neuronal membrane (high intracellular [K^+] and low intracellular [Na^+], [Cl^-], and [Ca^{2+}]), and these are quickly disrupted by the collapse of various energy-dependent pumps and transporters. Of particular note is Na^+/K^+-ATPase pump failure, which allows Na^+ to move into the cell causing neuronal depolarisation accompanied by the passive diffusion of Cl^- and water [126, 230]. In combination, the normalisation of ions across the cellular membrane and the concomitant movement of water lead to intracellular swelling that causes osmolysis (cytotoxic oedema), which significantly contributes to acute neuronal cell death [60].

Disrupted ionic homeostasis also leads to a dramatic and unregulated increase in the fusion of neurotransmitter storage vesicles with pre-synaptic membranes, which causes a massive release of vesicular content. Of the transmitters that flood the synapse following ischaemia, the most intensely studied has been the amino acid glutamate, which is the principal mediator of excitatory neurotransmission within the mammalian brain. The harm that might result from excessive glutamate was first observed in studies that found its systemic administration caused pronounced retinal degeneration [142, 173], a phenomenon described as "excitotoxicity". A substantial body of subsequent work has established that glutamate is a key element of neurodegeneration in general, and of ischaemic cell death in particular [119, 133, 199]. For example, glutamate efflux precedes widespread injury to cellular membranes and enzyme systems [2], the extracellular concentration of glutamate rises dramatically during ischaemia [63, 84], glutamate release is correlated with insult severity [29, 224], and glutamate receptor antagonists provide significant protection against ischaemic brain damage [119, 155, 215].

The widespread release of glutamate and the excessive stimulation of its high-affinity post-synaptic receptors are thought to act as critical elements that permit a profound rise of the intracellular calcium ion concentration. Calcium ions are involved in an array of neuronal functions, and their intracellular concentration is rigourously maintained at a level approximately 10^4 times lower than their extracellular concentration [143] by a combination of specialised binding proteins [8], sequestration within organelles [77], and extrusion [232]. One of the first studies to recognise the importance of calcium ions in cell death found that degeneration following axonal amputation occurred only when calcium ions were present in the bathing medium [208]. Subsequently, the essential role played by Ca^{2+} in glutamate-mediated cell death became established by studies that used mouse neocortical cultures [36, 88], rat hippocampal cultures [115, 190], and rat brain slices [57, 137]. Furthermore, work with culture [37, 67, 207], slice [276], and *in vivo* [15] models of ischaemia went on to reveal that a specific sub-type of glutamate receptor - the ionotropic NMDA receptor (section 3) - accounts for the majority of Ca^{2+} entry during and immediately after an ischaemic insult.

The dysregulation of intracellular Ca^{2+} has become recognised as a central branch point within the ischaemic cascade [11, 133, 213, 223], and serves as an important link between upstream activation of glutamate receptors and downstream stimulation of cell death mediators; for example, catalytic enzymes and free radicals. Several cytodestructive enzymes appear to be activated by cerebral ischaemia [119, 133, 185, 192], including proteases, phospholipases, and endonucleases. One set of enzymes that has received significant attention is the calpains, which are cytosolic cysteine proteases with variable Ca^{2+}-binding domains [217]. Calpains are ubiquitously expressed in the CNS, and a clear rise in their levels has been observed in models of both transient focal and global ischaemia [272, 280]. As well, activated calpains have been associated with damage to a variety of proteins [10, 241, 254], and calpain inhibitors have been found to provide a measure of protection in both culture [10] and *in vivo* models of ischaemia [12].

Free radicals have emerged as important players in the development of ischaemia-induced neuronal damage [3, 111, 133, 139]. The detection of free radical production following excitotoxicity caused by NMDA receptor stimulation has been clearly demonstrated in a variety of cultured rodent neurones [50, 76, 117, 194], and various groups have shown neuroprotection against excitotoxicity using antioxidant compounds [119]. As well, the mechanism of excitotoxicity-induced free radical production has been linked to Ca^{2+} by a report that demonstrated exposing isolated mitochondria to increasing calcium and sodium concentrations elevated free radical production [52], and another that showed removing extracellular calcium attenuated free radical production following NMDA application [50]. In addition to mitochondrial impairment, increased levels of reactive oxygen and nitrogen species are likely due to a combination of suppressed free radical scavengers and the elevation of formative enzymes, such as xanthine oxidase, cyclooxygenase, and nitrogen oxide synthases. Collectively, the cellular changes caused by increased free radical activity are extensive, and include lipid peroxidation, protein denaturation, and nucleic acid modification.

Slight changes in cerebral blood supply can be effectively managed by autoregulatory mechanisms that govern blood flow and oxygen extraction; however, decreases beyond this primary threshold initiate numerous cellular changes that become more severe in direct relation to the extent of the disturbance. The critical stages of stroke pathogenesis (figure 1) develop following a rapid and sustained drop of neuronal energy supply, and are generally thought to include a loss of ionic homeostasis, the unregulated release of the excitatory transmitter glutamate, the profound over-activation of glutamate receptors (particularly, the NMDA receptor), the dysregulation of intracellular Ca^{2+} levels, and the activation of a number of calcium-mediated internal changes that broadly affect cellular structure and function. While the exact manner and time course of ischaemia-mediated changes can be varied, and is influenced by factors such as insult severity, neuronal maturation, phenotype, and connectivity, the one thing held in common is the ultimate development of extensive neuronal cell death.

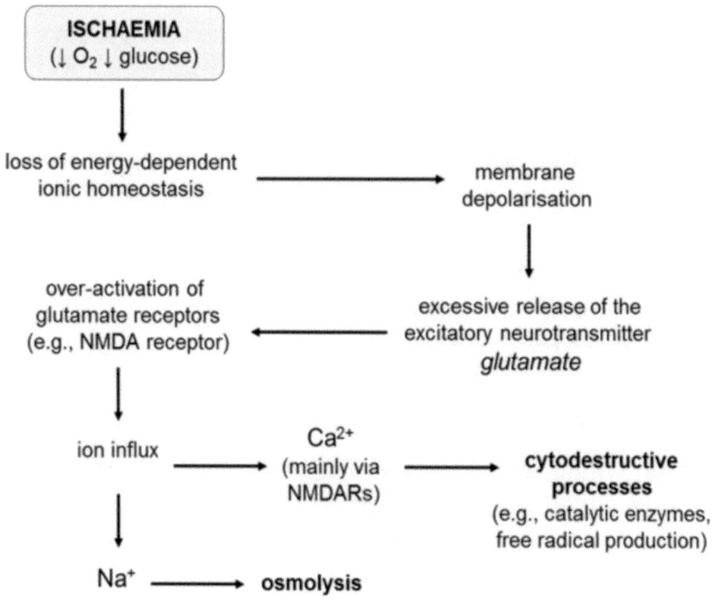

Figure 1. Summary of major elements in the early stages of ischaemic pathogenesis.

3. The NMDA receptor

3.1. Historical overview

Glutamate receptors (GluRs) mediate the majority of excitatory transmission in the vertebrate CNS, and participate in a number of physiological processes, including the formation of neuronal networks during development [43, 110], the pattern of ongoing synaptic communication [236], and the cellular plasticity believed to underlie learning and memory [21, 146]. In addition to an intimate involvement with the brain's physiology, glutamate responsive receptors are also of central importance in several neuropsychiatric conditions. For example, the GluRs have been implicated in neurodevelopmental disorders (e.g., schizophrenia) [59], mood disorders (e.g., depression) [149], chronic neurodegeneration (e.g., Alzheimer's disease, Parkinson's disease, and amyotrophic lateral sclerosis) [1, 22, 100], and pain transmission [20], in addition to brain injury (e.g., head trauma and stroke).

The broad influence of glutamate-mediated signalling upon synaptic function and dysfunction is attributable to the broad anatomical and cellular distribution of GluRs, and that they exist in two functionally and pharmacologically distinct varieties: metabotropic (mGluRs) and ionotropic (iGluRs). The metabotropic receptors are coupled to G-proteins, and, while structurally related to one another, do vary appreciably in their distribution and signal transduction mechanisms [175, 193]. The ionotropic receptors are non-specific cation channels that possess a common general structure, but vary considerably in both distribution and function [153, 175, 236]. As well, the iGluRs have been divided into three sub-types based upon relative selectivity to three exogenous agonists: N-methyl-D-aspartate (NMDA), α-amino-3-hydroxy-5-methyl-4-isoxazolepropionic acid (AMPA), and kainate.

Important preliminary evidence for diversity within excitatory neurotransmission was found in the early 1960s when the synthetic GluR agonist NMDA was shown to potently excite neurones [44]. Subsequent work in the 1970s, using radioligand binding and specific antagonists, established the existence of a specific NMDA subtype of iGluR (NMDAR) [154]. Following the advent of molecular cloning technology in the 1980s, a receptor complex possessing the functional characteristics ascribed to the NMDAR was characterised [158], which confirmed the existence of this particular iGluR sub-type, and helped to foment investigation into its physiopathological roles.

3.2. Subunit structure and assembly

The NMDA receptor is thought to be a heteromeric complex formed from a combination of four subunits: GluN1, GluN2 (with four known sub-types, labelled A-D), and GluN3 (with two identified sub-types, labelled A and B); notably, the nomenclature for GluR subunits has recently changed [42]. The GluN1 subunit has been shown to be essential to the formation of functional receptors [55], while the GluN2 and GluN3 subunits are believed to impart distinct gating and ion conductance properties [236]. Although the stoichiometry of subunits remains to be definitively resolved, endogenous NMDA receptors are thought to require the assembly of two GluN1 subunits with either two GluN2 subunits, or a combination of GluN2 and GluN3 subunits [19, 236]. Regardless of their ultimate arrangement, similar to other iGluRs, NMDARs are thought to be held within the endoplasmic reticulum until they assemble in a manner sufficient to permit counteraction of a retention signal [183].

One important limitation to improved understanding of NMDAR composition is the significant degree of developmental and anatomical heterogeneity that exists within subunit expression. The GluN1 subunit displays a peak degree of expression late in embryonic life before slightly declining to a relatively stable level of post-natal expression, while the GluN2 subunits vary considerably in their expression across the lifespan [53, 252]. For example, the GluN2A and GluN2C subunits are found post-natally, the GluN2B is expressed both before and after birth, although expression levels decline considerably between the early post-natal period and adulthood, and the GluN2D subunit is overwhelmingly restricted to embryonic development. As well, the GluN1 subunit is found in all central neurones, but a significant degree of anatomical heterogeneity exists among GluN2 subunits; in particular, the GluN2A and GluN2B subunits are found throughout the forebrain, the GluN2C subunit is limited to the cerebellum, and the GluN2D subunit is found predominantly within the midbrain [53, 156, 252, 253].

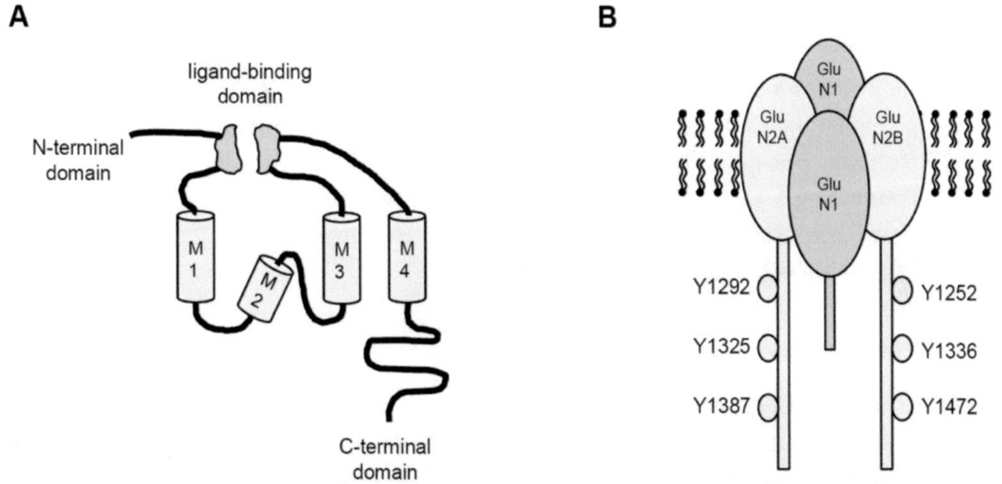

Figure 2. (A) Diagram of the structure for a typical NMDA receptor subunit. (B) Schematic illustrating one possible heterotetrameric combination of GluN subunits, along with identification of those GluN2 C-terminal tyrosine residues believed most relevant to phosphorylation-mediated changes in receptor gating and surface expression.

Despite being variably expressed, each NMDA receptor subunit shares a similar general architecture: a large extracellular region that consists of the amino-terminal and ligand binding domains, a pore-forming transmembrane region, and an intracellular region containing the carboxy-terminal domain [19, 56, 236] (figure 2). The N-terminal domain, at least in certain GluN2 subunits, is believed to allow receptor activity to be non-competitively inhibited by ligands such as zinc [177], although this may be an artifact of heterologous expression [261]. The adjacent ligand-binding domain is elegantly formed by two, non-contiguous segments that are separated by a portion of the polypeptide sequence thought to weave its way through most of the transmembrane region; as a result, conformational changes within the ligand-binding domain are thought to influence opening of the channel pore [56]. Four hydrophobic domains are believed to form the transmembrane region: the M1, M3, and M4 are predicted to cross the membrane as helices, while the M2, which lines the lumen of the pore, is expected to be a re-entrant loop that connects M1 and M3 [14, 19].

Among the NMDAR subunits, the C-terminal domain (CTD) is regarded as the most divergent region of the protein sequence [201], and can vary between 80-600 amino acids [56]. In addition to accounting for almost half the length of certain subunits (e.g., GluN2A and GluN2B), the CTD appears to be particularly important for intracellular signalling, trafficking, and localisation of the receptors due to the presence of multiple protein motifs that permit interaction with a variety of enzymes and scaffolding molecules. In particular, the intracellular region contains multiple locations for post-translational modifications, such as tyrosine phosphorylation [31, 125, 205, 236].

While the comparatively short CTD of the GluN1 does possess a tyrosine residue (Y837) [204], the subunit does not appear to experience tyrosine phosphorylation [121]; in contrast, each CTD of the GluN2 subunit contains 25 tyrosine residues, although not all of these residues will accept a phosphate group. On the GluN2A subunit, Y1292, Y1325, and Y1387 are thought to be the primary tyrosine residues subject to phosphoregulation [114]. On the GluN2B subunit, phosphorylation of Y1252, Y1336, and Y1472 has been reported [163]. Despite comprising a relatively small number of sites within the extensive CTD, tyrosine residues have become regarded as crucial points of convergence for signalling pathways that modulate NMDAR activity [170, 204, 205, 237].

3.3. Receptor function and cellular distribution

The basic pattern of excitatory signal transmission between the overwhelming majority of central neurones in the mammalian brain involves the pre-synaptic release of glutamate, its passage across the synaptic cleft, and its interaction with post-synaptically positioned GluRs. While basal synaptic transmission tends to be mediated by the AMPA sub-type of iGluR, periods of higher frequency synaptic activation (such as those that would tend to be present during an ischaemic event) recruit the NMDAR; the primary reason for the distinct activation profiles rests with a unique characteristic of the receptor. During basal transmission, the NMDAR's endogenous agonist (i.e., glutamate, which binds to an extracellular segment of GluN2 or GluN3 subunits) and its co-agonist (i.e., glycine, which binds to an extracellular segment of the GluN1 subunit) are present, yet the receptor remains functionally silent (i.e., ion conductance does not occur). The lack of basal NMDAR activity is attributable to a voltage-dependent blockade of the channel pore. At resting membrane potentials, external magnesium ions (which experience a significant inward driving force due to their high external concentration) enter the NMDAR pore, and bind in a manner that prevents further ion passage; however, membrane depolarisation of a sufficient magnitude and duration leads to the expulsion of Mg^{2+} from the pore, which permits the subsequent movement of cations [168].

Upon activation, glutamate receptors become permeable to both monovalent and, in some cases, divalent cations; however, the nature and degree of ion flux is not equivalent across iGluRs, and the NMDA sub-type has become acknowledged as the primary mediator of Ca^{2+} passage [57, 152, 236]. The ability to permit the entry of calcium ions is a primary reason that NMDARs make substantial contributions to both physiological and pathological phenomena [223, 236], although their pattern of cellular distribution also plays a role in their wide functional reach. Similar to many other ion channels, NMDARs are recognised as being widely dispersed across the cellular surface, however, information regarding the manner in which membrane bound receptors are distributed has only recently begun to be gathered. The available evidence indicates that NMDARs are not uniformly distributed at the plasma membrane, but can be divided into three spatially defined categories: synaptic, peri-synaptic and extra-synaptic [70].

The post-synaptic population exhibits the greatest density, relative to the other sub-regions, and responds directly to pre-synaptically released glutamate [70]. Peri-synaptic NMDARs have been operationally defined as those located within a 300 nm range of the post-synaptic terminal [70, 184, 275], and are believed to be activated by glutamate released from the pre-synaptic terminal following strong stimulation. Approximately half of all surface NMDARs, depending upon the developmental stage, are located extra-synaptically; however, relative to synaptic receptors, this compartment has a low density given the much broader area [72, 233]. Under physiological conditions, extra-synaptic NMDARs are unlikely to be activated by pre-synaptically released glutamate; however, they could be stimulated by glutamate released either from other sources [104, 128], or following the spillover of synaptic glutamate caused by ischaemia.

4. Regulation of NMDA receptors by tyrosine phosphorylation

4.1. Phosphorylation as a key determinant of ligand-gated ion channel function

Proteins exist as part of a complex system of elements that interact with one another to allow a cell to respond, directly or indirectly, to changes in its environment. Over several decades, the cellular distribution and molecular interactions of many proteins have been shown to be fundamentally regulated by post-translational modification in the form of phosphorylation [178, 238]. In essence, phosphorylation involves the protein kinase-mediated transfer of the γ-phosphate from adenosine triphosphate to a serine, threonine, or tyrosine residue of a substrate (although other amino acids may also be modified [40]), and is a process counteracted by protein phosphatases, which catalyse dephosphorylation.

Near the end of the 1980s, phosphorylation began to emerge as an important determinant in the function of a class of proteins essential for most neuronal communication – ligand-gated ion channels (LGICs). The first study to illustrate that LGICs could be regulated by phosphorylation revealed that NMDA currents recorded from cultured hippocampal neurones gradually declined during dialysis with an intracellular solution, but that the loss of receptor activity could be prevented by the addition of an ATP regenerating solution to the dialysate [148]. In the mid-1990s, further work not only confirmed that the NMDA receptor was indeed regulated by phosphorylation, but also that a critical site for the modification was at tyrosine residues [249]. Subsequent reports established that a variety of other LGICs, such as the inhibitory GABA-A receptor [159] and the nicotinic acetylcholine receptor [246], were also regulated by the activities of tyrosine kinases and phosphatases, and helped to establish the importance of phosphorylation in the control of synaptic function.

4.2. Regulation of NMDA receptors by tyrosine phosphorylation

Electrophysiological studies have established that NMDAR function is regulated by a balance between phosphorylation and dephosphorylation of tyrosine residues [31, 204, 205]. Within mammalian neurones, introducing an exogenous protein tyrosine kinase (PTK), or inhibiting endogenous protein tyrosine phosphatase (PTP) activity enhances NMDAR currents [249]; in contrast, inhibiting PTK activity [249, 250], or introducing an exogenous PTP [250] suppresses NMDAR currents. In addition, exogenous PTKs have been shown to potentiate currents mediated by recombinant NMDARs [32, 108]. During the past twenty years, members of the Src family of PTKs have emerged as the predominant tyrosine kinases responsible for mediating activity of the NMDA receptor.

4.2.1. Src Family Kinases (SFKs) and the brain: An introduction

The Src family of non-receptor, protein tyrosine kinases (SFKs) consists of several lower molecular weight proteins (52 to 62 kDa) that share a common domain organisation, which includes a catalytic region (the Src homology 1 or SH1 domain) and two regions that guide protein-protein interactions (the SH2 and SH3 domains) [170, 204]. Given that Src, the prototypical SFK, was initially identified as a proto-oncogene [218], SFKs in the brain were originally believed to influence only those processes related to the regulation of neuronal proliferation and differentiation [102, 116]. However, SFKs were subsequently shown to be expressed in differentiated, post-mitotic neurones, which suggested that these kinases might participate in neural activity past the point of early development [86, 220]. Notably, significant changes in neuronal plasticity and behaviour have been observed in adult mice lacking certain SFKs [68, 239], while the expression and activity of Src was shown to increase during spatial learning [278].

Within the mammalian nervous system, the expression of five members of the SFKs has been established; of these, Src [101], Fyn [221], and Yes [105] have been found within the post-synaptic density (PSD), which is a specialised region of the post-synaptic terminal thought to provide a molecular scaffold that helps regulate proper protein placement. In addition, Src [270], Fyn [267], and Yes [105] have been shown to be components of a large complex in the PSD that includes the NMDA receptor. Considered together, the biochemical analyses reveal that several SFKs have a spatial distribution appropriate to permit regulation of NMDAR function.

4.2.2. *Evidence to support SFKs as modulators of NMDAR channel gating*

When activated, ion channels, such as the NMDAR, passively conduct charged particles (i.e., they permit current flow) across the plasma membrane in a direction influenced by electrostatic forces and the ionic concentration gradient. The transition of a channel between closed and open states (i.e., from non-conducting to conducting) is referred to as gating, and requires a dramatic, albeit temporary, change in the channel's structure. The first evidence that SFKs might affect NMDAR function through alterations in channel gating was provided by a study that recorded channel currents from dissociated neurones [270]. A specific, high-affinity activator of SFKs [134] increased synaptic NMDAR-mediated currents, while an antibody that inhibited SFKs (anti-cst1; [195]), but not other protein tyrosine kinases, depressed NMDAR channel gating. A subsequent report, which recorded activity within neurones from acutely prepared brain slices, confirmed that the phosphopeptide SFK activator was able to significantly enhance NMDAR gating [141].

Additional support for the ability of SFKs to mediate NMDAR function was provided by a study that found protein tyrosine phosphatase alpha (PTPα) enhanced NMDAR-mediated synaptic currents in both cultured neurones and brain slices, while reducing PTPα activity with an inhibitory peptide reduced NMDAR currents [127]. Although the findings appear superficially paradoxical, PTPα is thought to activate SFKs by selectively dephosphorylating a residue in their regulatory domain, and thereby interfering with an intramolecular interaction that maintains the kinases in an inactive state [176]. In support of the proposed mechanism of action, PTPα has been shown to activate several different SFK members within cell lines [17, 87, 279], and SFK activity is substantially reduced in PTPα deficient mice [186]. As well, in cells lacking SFKs, or in which SFK activity is inhibited, PTPα has no effect on NMDAR currents [127].

While little doubt can exist that SFKs are involved in regulating NMDAR activity, the identities of the family members that might contribute to the process are not definitively known; however, considerable evidence has drawn attention to at least two kinases. The first candidate to be examined was Src, which was implicated by experiments illustrating that application of Src-specific inhibitors (the antibody anti-src1, and the peptide Src(40-58), which was the immunogen used to create the antibody) significantly decreased synaptic NMDAR-mediated currents and NMDAR channel gating [270]. As well, the Src-specific inhibitors were found to prevent the increased channel activity produced by application of a high-affinity SFK-activating peptide, which suggested that endogenous Src is required for SFK-mediated upregulation of NMDAR activity. To provide a structural complement to the functional studies, recent work with GluN2A subunits expressed in a heterologous expression system has found that Src directly interacts with segments in the C-terminus [75].

The second SFK member considered to have a role in NMDAR activity is Fyn, which was initially implicated by experiments wherein exogenous Fyn was shown to modulate glutamate-evoked currents mediated by recombinant NMDARs expressed in HEK293 cells [108]. Subsequently, co-expression of a constitutively active form of Fyn with GluN1 and GluN2B subunits in cerebellar granule cells was found to cause a significant increase in the amplitude of NMDA miniature excitatory post-synaptic currents [188]. In addition, several groups have reported that Fyn is able to phosphorylate both GluN2A and GluN2B within post-synaptic densities of the rodent forebrain [237].

Along with a direct effect upon NMDARs, SFKs may influence channel activity by phosphorylating proteins that associate with the receptor. For example, the post-synaptic density contains several proteins that are both tyrosine phosphorylated and potentially connected with NMDAR function, such as the scaffold protein PSD-93 [161, 206]. As well, phosphorylation of GluN2B may recruit signalling proteins, such as phosphatidylinositol 3-kinase, which has been shown to associate with the subunit [94, 182]. In addition, tyrosine phosphorylation of GluN2 subunits may prevent the loss of signalling molecules from the NMDA receptor by limiting degradation caused by calpain [18, 197], one of the principal proteases activated following ischaemia (section 2.2). Taken together, the variety of evidence suggests that SFKs may indirectly influence NMDAR function by altering the manner in which scaffolding and signalling proteins interact with GluN subunits.

4.2.3. Evidence to support SFKs as modulators of NMDAR trafficking

Rapid synaptic communication was traditionally believed to be altered by structural changes in ligand-gated ion channels that affected gating properties, such as mean open time and open probability. However, during the past fifteen years, cellular trafficking events, which modify the surface density of ion channels, have attracted considerable attention as an additional means whereby synaptic transmission can be regulated [41]. Although the inhibitory GABA-A receptor was the first LGIC found to undergo changes in cell surface expression in response to extracellular signals [245], the trafficking of other receptors, notably the NMDAR, has been the subject of growing interest over the past decade [70, 120, 183]. In particular, a number of studies have revealed that NMDARs are quite mobile, and undergo regulated trafficking between intracellular organelles and the plasma membrane [51, 64, 74, 124, 188, 191] and between extra-synaptic and synaptic sites [65, 71, 234].

The earliest evidence that NMDAR trafficking could be influenced through tyrosine phosphorylation was provided by a study wherein the repeated application of glutamate to heterologously expressed GluN1 and GluN2A subunits lead to an increase in receptor internalisation that could be prevented by application of Src [242]; using site-directed mutagenesis, the authors found that agonist-mediated dephosphorylation of a single tyrosine residue in the C-terminus of the GluN2A subunit was responsible for the reduced surface expression of functional channels. Subsequent studies wherein tyrosine phosphatase activity was reduced have demonstrated that phosphorylation of the NMDAR is positively associated with its surface expression. For example, brief treatment of cultured striatal neurones with a general inhibitor of tyrosine phosphatases increased the level of GluN2 subunit tyrosine phosphorylation and their surface expression [85]. As well, treatment of cultured cortical cells with a short interfering RNA to reduce the expression of a tyrosine phosphatase known to interact with the NMDAR lead to both an increase in its surface expression and the level of Ca^{2+} influx after agonist stimulation [24].

While enhanced surface expression of a receptor would reasonably be expected to increase its activity, the possibility that such a change will have a functional outcome is greater if the insertion occurs at synaptic membranes. In acutely prepared striatal slices from adult animals, a tyrosine phosphatase inhibitor was observed to increase the phosphorylation state of GluN2 subunits and increase their association with synaptosomal membranes; notably, treatment with a tyrosine kinase inhibitor had effects in the opposite direction [51]. An ensuing study that used tissue slices from the adult hippocampus and a separate set of tyrosine kinase and phosphatase inhibitors found the same general pattern tying together changes in GluN2 subunit phosphorylation status with synaptosomal membrane density [64]. Intriguingly, a further report revealed that the surface location to which GluN2 subunits are trafficked may be differentially affected by changes in tyrosine phosphorylation [65]. In particular, increasing the phosphorylation level of GluN2B subunits through the application of a tyrosine phosphatase inhibitor tended to increase the extra-synaptic expression of the NMDAR more greatly than its synaptic expression.

4.2.4. Balancing of SFK activity by tyrosine dephosphorylation

The level of NMDAR tyrosine phosphorylation is currently understood to be regulated by a balance between the activity of SFKs and protein tyrosine phosphatases [170, 204, 205] (figure 3). The PTPs are a large, structurally diverse family of enzymes [247] that play a number of important roles in the CNS, including contributing to the regulation of neural development [162, 219]. The striatal enriched phosphatase (STEP) is a brain-specific, non-receptor PTP that was originally found to be highly expressed within the adult rodent striatum [66, 138], and has subsequently been identified in other regions, such as the hippocampus [23]. While STEP immunoreactivity can be observed throughout the soma and processes of neurons [23], its presence at the post-synaptic density [174], a prominent structure at excitatory synapses, and its direct interaction with NMDARs [181], strongly suggest that the phosphatase contributes to signal transduction.

The ability of broad PTP inhibition to increase, and broad PTP activation to decrease, NMDAR gating in spinal cord neurones provided the initial evidence that the receptor was modulated by a phosphatase [250]. However, the identification of STEP as the putative candidate was not proposed until a report using the same experimental preparation showed that recombinant STEP reduced NMDAR activity, while the intracellular application of a function-blocking STEP antibody increased synaptic NMDAR-mediated currents [181]. Furthermore, within hippocampal slices, inhibition of STEP was shown to increase NMDAR activity, while recombinant STEP was able to occlude the development of a form of NMDAR-dependent synaptic plasticity.

The modulation of NMDA receptor function by STEP has become associated with its ability to affect the level of phosphorylation at a single tyrosine residue (Y1472) located in the distal portion of the GluN2B C-terminus [123, 196]. When dephosphorylated, the unique residue, which is part of a short motif (YXXϕ, where X is any amino acid and ϕ = a bulky hydrophobic amino acid), promotes endocytosis by allowing the development of hydrophobic interactions between cargo molecules and clathrin adaptor proteins, such as AP-2 [235]. Notably, the phosphorylation of Y1472 and the association of GluN2B with adaptor proteins are inversely associated [164], and the overexpression of a Y1472 mutant unable to interact with AP-2 leads to a significant increase in the number of NMDA receptors at the synapse [188]. As well, STEP co-immunoprecipitates with the GluN1 subunit [181], directly dephosphorylates Y1472 [216], and, when deleted from the mouse genome, causes hyperphosphorylation of Y1472 in synaptosomal membranes prepared from the hippocampus [277]. Along with a direct effect upon Y1472, STEP may also act indirectly by dephosphorylating regulatory residues in the catalytic domains of Fyn, which is the principal SFK acting at Y1472 [165], and proline-rich tyrosine kinase 2 (Pyk2), which is an upstream activator of SFKs [262].

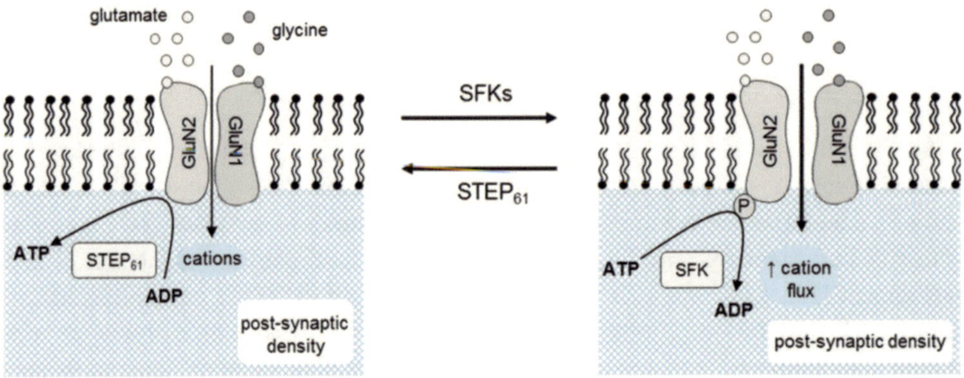

Figure 3. A simplified illustration of the key elements that regulate tyrosine phosphorylation of the NMDA receptor at the post-synaptic terminal.

5. Ischaemia-related changes in tyrosine phosphorylation of the NMDA receptor

5.1. Effects of ischaemia upon NMDA receptor subunit expression

Ischaemia causes a dramatic change in gene expression, which is largely attributable to a broad reduction in gene transcription and/or the inhibition of protein translation [109, 112]. While the general pattern of change suggests the level of most genes (and their protein products) will be reduced after ischaemia, several genes do show an increased level of expression; for example, certain ones associated with neuronal survival, such as members of the heat shock family of proteins. The first study to examine the effect of transient global ischaemia upon GluN2 subunits found that mRNA of both the GluN2A and GluN2B subunit declined in a progressive manner over 24 h of reperfusion, and that the transcriptional change was reflected in a pronounced loss of the proteins over the same time period [274]; notably, the study employed an antibody that detected an epitope shared between the subunits, so the relative nature of the protein loss was not apparent. A subsequent study that used subunit specific antibodies revealed that the pattern of reduced protein expression may not be equal, for the loss of the GluN2A subunit was greater [228]. In agreement with the possibility that GluN2 subunits may be differentially affected by ischaemic insult, hypoxia-ischaemia applied to rats at post-natal day seven caused a reduction of GluN2A protein levels within one hour of reperfusion, while a reduction in the GluN2B subunit was not observed; in contrast, similar experiments performed with animals at post-natal day 21 showed a significant reduction of only the GluN2B subunit [82].

While evidence does exist that the expression of GluN2 subunit proteins may be decreased by ischaemia, a comparatively greater amount of work suggests that the level of the subunits is not altered. For example, no change in GluN2B immunolabelling was detected in hippocampal synaptosomes prepared six hours after a period of transient global ischaemia in gerbils [179]. As well, the level of GluN2A and GluN2B subunit proteins in either hippocampal homogenates [227], or forebrain post-synaptic densities [226] prepared six hours following global ischaemia in rats did not appear to differ from the levels seen in control samples [227]; in agreement, a large group of studies that employed the same experimental approach failed to find an effect of the insult upon hippocampal protein expression of the GluN2A subunit (the GluN2B subunit was not examined) [33, 98, 136, 144, 248]. When the period of reperfusion was extended to 24 h, one study continued to find no change [97], while another found a slight, albeit significant, decline in GluN2A protein levels in whole hippocampal homogenates (again, the GluN2B subunit was not assessed) [135]. Collectively, the data strongly suggest that GluN2 subunit protein expression, particularly of the GluN2A variant, is not likely to be altered within the first 24 h after a brief period of global ischaemia in adult animals.

5.2. Ischaemia and the general cellular pattern of tyrosine phosphorylation

In the early 1990s, a brief stimulation of cultured hippocampal neurones with either glutamate, or NMDA was shown to cause a significant increase in tyrosine phosphorylation of mitogen activated protein kinase (MAPK, a class of kinases that respond to extracellular signals and mediate proliferation, differentiation, and cell survival) in a manner sensitive to blockade of the NMDA receptor [7]. Given the establishment of a connection between NMDA receptor activation and downstream tyrosine phosphorylation, subsequent reports sought to determine whether the excessive stimulation of the receptor that occurs during ischaemia would cause a similar pattern of change. Indeed, a brief period of bilateral carotid artery occlusion in gerbils (which would cause global ischaemia) was found to very quickly evoke a significant and transient increase in hippocampal MAPK phosphorylation that could be prevented through NMDAR antagonism [30, 107].

Once the association between ischaemia-mediated activation of the NMDA receptor and MAPK phosphorylation had been confirmed, a search for other proteins that might experience an induced change in tyrosine phosphorylation began in earnest. Within gerbils, global ischaemia was clearly shown to cause a rapid and significant increase in the level of tyrosine phosphorylation of a number of hippocampal proteins, particularly those with a higher molecular weight [171, 179, 269]. Within rats, both transient forebrain [99, 209] and global [34, 225, 228] ischaemia were found to induce a sustained increase in tyrosine phosphorylation of higher molecular weight proteins in the hippocampus. In addition, acutely prepared hippocampal slices subjected to *in vitro* models of ischaemia (i.e., oxygen-glucose deprivation) also displayed changes in the general level of tyrosine phosphorylation; however, while the magnitude of the effect was similar to that observed with the *in vivo* models, the direction of the effect was the opposite [6, 26].

Intriguingly, the post-ischaemic increase in tyrosine phosphorylation observed with *in vivo* injury did not appear uniformly throughout the hippocampus, which is composed of three major sub-fields: *cornu ammonis* (or CA) sector 1, CA3, and the dentate gyrus [54, 131]. Immunohistochemical labelling of hippocampal slices prepared at several time points following global ischaemia indicated that the CA3 and dentate gyrus appear to have the most intense initial increases in phosphorylation, but that, over several days, the CA1 region becomes more strongly labelled [269]. Immunoblotting revealed that the CA3 and dentate gyrus regions displayed greater tyrosine phosphorylation, particularly of higher molecular weight proteins, during the first two days after insult [228]. A disproportionate increase of tyrosine phosphorylation in the CA3-dentate gyrus was also observed in synaptosomes (sub-cellular fractions of pre-synaptic terminals that also include remnants of many post-synaptic sites) during the first day after ischaemia [99].

The elevated level of tyrosine phosphorylation routinely observed in various models of ischaemic brain injury would intuitively be attributable to increases in the activity of tyrosine kinases, decreases in the activity of tyrosine phosphatases, or a combination of the two. Within whole hippocampal homogenates, the level of Src was not found to change during a six hour period of reperfusion following either global ischaemia in adult animals [273], or hypoxia-ischaemia in pre-weanling animals [103]. In contrast, during the same length of time after global ischaemia the level of both Src and Fyn proteins were observed to experience about a twofold increase within the post-synaptic density [16, 34, 226].

Autophosphorylation of Y416 in the catalytic domain of SFKs is necessary to permit enzyme activity [204, 211, 266]. Within several hours of reperfusion following global ischaemia, a general increase in the level of tyrosine phosphorylation at hippocampal Src was observed [135, 136]; as well, a specific increase in Y416 phosphorylation was found within the whole hippocampus [38, 79, 248, 258, 273], and the CA1 [130, 264, 273] and CA3-dentate gyrus [79] regions. The level of phosphorylated Y416 was also found to be increased in both synaptosomes [160] and post-synaptic densities [16, 35, 160] prepared from the rodent forebrain region after the return of blood supply to the insulted area. In agreement with the immunoblotting data, *in vitro* enzyme activity assays confirmed that Src function in either whole hippocampal homogenates [78], or hippocampal synaptosomes [180] was clearly greater several hours after a brief period of global ischaemia.

While understanding how ischaemia may alter tyrosine kinase activity has been the principal focus of many studies, a developing body of work has chosen to examine changes at the level of tyrosine phosphatases; in particular, attention has been drawn to STEP. Glutamate-mediated excitotoxicity within cultured cortical neurones lead to the cleavage of STEP (i.e., $STEP_{61}$, a membrane-associated isoform localised to the endoplasmic reticulum and post-synaptic density) into a lower molecular weight isoform [66, 166, 263]. In agreement with the cell culture work, transient hypoxia-ischaemia in younger rats [81], brief focal ischaemia in adult rats [25], and global ischaemia in gerbils [89] caused the loss of $STEP_{61}$, and a concomitant rise of lower molecular weight STEP in the affected brain areas. Quite likely, STEP degradation is mediated by Ca^{2+}-activated proteases, such as calpain; for example, the *in vitro* incubation of isolated PSDs with calpain causes $STEP_{61}$ breakdown [81, 166], while treatment with a calpain inhibitor (calpeptin) prevents glutamate-activated $STEP_{61}$ cleavage [263]. Ischaemia also appears to reduce STEP levels at the transcriptional level by causing a rapid and significant reduction in its mRNA expression [25]. In addition, the exposure of cultured neurones to oxidative stress, using a free radical that undergoes increased production after ischaemia [4], results in greater oligomerisation of $STEP_{61}$, which causes a reduction in its activity level [46]. Considered together, the data indicate that ischaemia initiates a series of different processes that reduce STEP activity, and thereby contributes to enhanced levels of tyrosine phosphorylation.

5.3. The NMDAR as a specific substrate of ischaemia-mediated tyrosine phosphorylation

5.3.1. Evidence to illustrate ischaemic alteration of GluN2 phosphotyrosine status

The knowledge that ischaemia can bring about changes in the broad pattern of tyrosine phosphorylation, particularly of a glycoprotein with a molecular weight of 180 kDa, began to acquire additional significance after the identification of the GluN2B subunit as the major tyrosine phosphorylated, higher molecular weight glycoprotein associated with the post-synaptic density [157]. Shortly thereafter, came the first direct demonstration that ischaemia could specifically alter the tyrosine phosphorylation of NMDA receptor subunits; in particular, for several hours after a brief period of global ischaemia in adult rats, Takagi et al. [225] observed a rapid and dramatic rise in tyrosine phosphorylation of hippocampal GluN2A and GluN2B subunits. Although the modified phosphorylation pattern of the subunits was still clear 24 h after the insult, the GluN2A subunit consistently displayed a degree of change several times greater than that observed for the GluN2B subunit. As well, the magnitude of the effect was substantially greater in the hippocampus than either the cerebral cortex, or the striatum. The seminal report showed that ischaemia can cause a sharp and sustained rise in NMDAR tyrosine phosphorylation that differentially affects the receptor's constituent subunits and develops in an anatomically heterogeneous manner; in addition, the findings helped to influence a number of studies that confirmed ischaemia initiates cellular changes that ultimately modify the degree of tyrosine phosphorylation at GluN2 subunits (Table 1).

As noted, one of the first details to emerge regarding the pathological modification of NMDAR phosphorylation was the swift manner in which the change developed. Subsequent work revealed that within twenty minutes of reperfusion following a brief period of global ischaemia, a substantial rise in tyrosine phosphorylation of the GluN2A subunit could be detected [33, 34, 135]. As well, the magnitude of the GluN2A subunit modification was shown to increase during at least the first six hours of reperfusion, and was seen to slowly return to basal levels over 2-3 days [135, 228]. Using a similar *in vivo* model of ischaemia coupled with immunoprecipitation-based experiments, several groups confirmed a significant rise in the tyrosine phosphorylation of GluN2A subunits in either whole hippocampal homogenates [98, 136, 144, 226, 248], or CA1 homogenates [264] prepared within six hours of reperfusion.

While an increase in tyrosine phosphorylation of the GluN2B subunit was also detected after ischaemia, those studies that examined both subunits tended to find that the effect upon the GluN2A subunit was more pronounced [16, 160, 225, 226, 228]. One exception, was a study that applied global ischaemia to gerbils; however, the variation may have been, in part, attributable to a species difference [271]. In contrast to adult animals, ischaemic injury in weanling rats (post-natal day 21) was found to affect tyrosine levels of the GluN2A and GluN2B subunits in a similar fashion, and was shown to have a significantly greater effect upon the GluN2B subunit in pre-weanling rats (post-natal day 7); as well, the change in phosphorylation appeared to be more transient, for the levels had returned to baseline within a day of reperfusion [82, 103]. While the effect of oxygen-glucose deprivation (OGD) upon cultured neurones tended to match well with the effect of *in vivo* ischaemia upon the GluN2A subunit [248], the application of OGD to acutely prepared hippocampal slices caused an apparent decrease in the level of tyrosine phosphorylation at both subunits [6, 26]; notably, Src protein levels have been shown to rise in hippocampal slices after OGD [9], which suggests that the unexpectedly reduced level of phosphorylation might be attributable to a comparatively greater elevation in the expression and/or activity of tyrosine phosphatases.

In addition to an obvious effect upon GluN2 subunit phosphorylation at the cellular level (i.e., within whole homogenates of a brain region), several reports observed that ischaemia also clearly modified subunits located within synaptic compartments. For example, the immunoprecipitation of GluN2A and GluN2B subunits from post-synaptic densities after global ischaemia in the rat revealed a clear rise in tyrosine phosphorylation during the first six hours of reperfusion [34], while immunoblotting with antibodies directed against phosphotyrosine residues in the GluN2A (Y1387) and GluN2B (Y1472) subunits displayed a similar effect [16]. In agreement, several hours after transient restriction in blood supply to the rat cerebral cortex, tyrosine phosphorylation of both the GluN2A and GluN2B subunits was found to be increased in both post-synaptic densities and synaptosomes [160]. As well, the phosphotyrosine level of the GluN2B subunit in synaptosomes enriched from gerbil hippocampus was markedly increased within six hours of reperfusion after global ischaemia [179].

Reference	Species	Age or Weight	Ischaemia Model	GluN2A pY Change Relative to Control	GluN2B pY Change Relative to Control	Sample Size
16	rat	200-250 g	4VO & 6 h REP	pY1387: ~3.5 fold increase	pY1472: ~2.8 fold increase	5
26	rat	150-200 g	OGD	↓ in sample blot, no measurement	↓ in sample blot, no measurement	-
33	rat	250-300 g	4VO & 15 min REP	~4 fold increase	not examined	3
34	rat	200-250 g	4VO & 6 h REP	↑ in sample blot, no measurement	~4.0 fold increase	3
35	rat	200-250 g	4VO & 45 min REP	not examined	↑ pY1472 in sample blot, no measurement	1
82	rat	PND 7, PND 21	permanent right CCAO + hypoxia & 1 h REP	PND 7: similar PND 21: ~3.2 fold increase	PND 7: ~3.5 fold increase pY1472 (PND 7): ~2 fold increase PND 21: ~3.2 fold increase pY1472 (PND 21): ~8 fold increase	3-4
98	rat	250-300 g	4VO & 6 h REP	~6.2 fold increase	not examined	3
103	mouse	PND 7	permanent right CCAO + hypoxia	~2 fold increase (15 min REP)	~3 fold increase (15 min REP)	7
135	rat	200-250 g	4VO & 0-72 h REP	~6.8 fold increase (6 h REP)	not examined	3
136	rat	220-270 g	4VO & 6 h REP	~2.8 fold increase	not examined	4
144	rat	250-300 g	4VO & 6 h REP	~4.8 fold increase	not examined	3
160	rat	7-8 wks; 240-360 g	right MCAO & 4 h REP	~4.7 fold increase	pY1336: ~3.9 fold increase pY1472: ~3.3 fold increase	5
179	gerbil	60-75 g	BCAO & 6 h REP	not examined	~1.9 fold increase	3
225	rat	200-250 g	4VO & 6 h REP	~30 fold increase	~2.2 fold increase	5
226	rat	200-250 g	4VO & 1 h REP	~6.6 fold increase	~3.1 fold increase	4
228	rat	200-250 g	4VO & 1 h REP	CA1: ~13.5 fold increase CA3/DG: ~14.0 fold increase	CA1: ~3.0 fold increase CA3/DG: ~5.4 fold increase	5 5
248	rat	220-250 g	4VO & 6 h REP	~2.6 fold increase	not examined	4
264	rat	250-300 g	4VO & 6 h REP	~2 fold increase	pY1472: ~1.5 fold increase	5
268	rat	16 DIV	OGD	~5 fold increase	not examined	5
271	gerbil	50-70 g	BCAO & 3 h REP	~1.6 fold increase	~2.2 fold increase	6
273	rat	250-300 g	4VO & 6 h REP	~1.9 fold increase	not examined	4

Table 1. Studies examining GluN2 tyrosine phosphorylation following experimental ischaemia. 4VO, four vessel occlusion; BCAO, bilateral carotid artery occlusion; CCAO, common carotid artery occlusion; DIV, days *in vitro*; OGD, oxygen-glucose deprivation; PND, post-natal day; pY, phosphotyrosine; REP, reperfusion

5.3.2. Interaction of GluN2 with synaptic elements may influence its phosphorylation

Along with changes in the synaptic concentration and/or activity of those tyrosine kinases and phosphatases that act upon the NMDA receptor, the increased degree of tyrosine phosphorylation observed at GluN2 subunits after an ischaemic insult may also be attributable to changes in how the receptor directly interacts with SFKs. In particular, there may be greater association between phosphotyrosine sequences within GluN2 subunits and the segment of SFKs containing SH2 domains, which are relatively short amino acid modules believed to be necessary to permit the interactions that underlie many tyrosine based signalling cascades [150, 243]. Notably, ischaemia-mediated tyrosine phosphorylation was found to increase, by approximately twofold, the association of Src and Fyn with both GluN2A and GluN2B during reperfusion [226]. In agreement, a number of subsequent studies also observed greater association of SFKs with GluN2A during the first six hours following global ischaemia in adult rats [97, 98, 135, 248, 273]. As well, hypoxia-ischaemia applied to neonatal rats [103] and OGD of cultured neurones prepared from late-stage embryonic animals [268] also lead to greater co-immunoprecipitation of SFKs and the GluN2A subunit. Despite being examined to a lesser degree, the interaction between GluN2B and SFKs has also been clearly demonstrated after neonatal hypoxia-ischaemia [103], following global ischaemia in adult rats [179], and in response to global ischaemia within adult gerbils [271].

An additional component that may facilitate ischaemia-mediated changes in GluN2 phosphorylation is its enhanced interaction with a prominent post-synaptic scaffolding protein. The post-synaptic density 95 kDa (PSD-95) protein is a member of the membrane-associated guanylate kinase (MAGUK) family, and functions as an integral scaffolding protein in excitatory post-synaptic terminals [106, 265]. Like other MAGUK relatives, PSD-95 displays a modular structure that consists of three N-terminal PDZ domains (PDZ 1-3), an SH3 domain, and C-terminal guanylate-kinase domain. Through the PDZ1/2 domains, in particular, PSD-95 has been shown to bind with a conserved ES(E/D)V amino acid sequence located in the distal portion of GluN2 C-termini [113, 167], which permits PSD-95 to influence gating and surface expression of the receptor [39, 132]. A series of studies that employed multiple co-immunoprecipitation experiments helped to establish that an enhanced association of PSD-95 with the GluN2A subunit develops during the first few hours of post-insult reperfusion [33, 97, 144, 248, 273]. As well, an increased degree of binding with PSD-95 has been displayed by GluN2A subunits after OGD with cultured neurones [268] and by hippocampal GluN2B subunits within a few hours after global ischaemia in the gerbil [271].

Ischaemia clearly enhanced the interaction of GluN2 subunits with both SFKs and PSD-95, and increased the level of interaction between SFKs and PSD-95 [33, 49, 97, 144], presumably at its SH3 domain. As well, SFK-mediated tyrosine phosphorylation of GluN2 fusion proteins augmented their binding to PSD-95 [197], and co-expressing PSD-95 with the GluN2A subunit improved its ability to be phosphorylated by SFKs [231]. Considered together, these data suggest that the post-ischaemic increase of GluN2 tyrosine phosphorylation (section 5.3.1) is attributable to a pathologically heightened and, potentially, self-amplifying degree of interaction among GluN2 subunits, PSD-95, and SFKs. Our understanding of how the tripartite complex operates following ischaemia has been greatly aided by a set of elegant studies that used molecular level approaches to alter its assembly. Reducing by approximately one-third the hippocampal expression of PSD-95 protein, through the repeated intracerebroventricular injection of antisense oligonucleotides, sharply attenuated both the post-ischaemic rise in GluN2A tyrosine phosphorylation and the elevated binding of SFKs with the GluN2A subunit [98]. In addition, adenoviral-mediated overexpression of the PSD-95 PDZ1 domain was able to nearly eliminate ischaemia-mediated changes in GluN2A phosphorylation, and prevented the expected increased interactions between the GluN2A subunit, PSD-95, and Src [248].

5.4. Ischaemic changes that may contribute to increased SFK activation

The elevation of tyrosine phosphorylation within neurones, in general, and at GluN2 subunits, in particular, would seem to be a consistent feature in the array of changes that follows cerebral ischaemia. Proximally, the ischaemia-mediated interactions of a complex formed between GluN2 subunits, synaptic scaffolding proteins, and members of the SFKs provide at least one working explanation for the increased pattern of phosphorylation; however, the fashion in which these components begin to assemble is still unclear. A starting point in understanding, from a slightly more distal perspective, the reason for heightened GluN2 phosphotyrosine levels may be to focus on SFKs; specifically, to ask why might SFK activity rise after ischaemia? Fortunately, the answer to the question is beginning to take shape, and appears to involve the activity of two other, putatively interconnected, kinases. The first one is protein kinase C (PKC), which acts upon serine-threonine residues and exists in at least ten different isoforms, most of which are heterogeneously distributed within the brain [229]. While the various members of the PKC family have different mechanisms underlying their activation, many of them are stimulated by changes in Ca^{2+} dynamics and the generation of free radicals [27], which are key consequences following from the over-activation of NMDARs that characterises ischaemic injury (section 1). Also, the translocation of PKC to the post-synaptic density after ischaemia has been well established [35, 151].

The signalling cascade initiated by the stimulation of PKC is quite diverse, however, the ability of the activated enzyme to enhance NMDA receptor function [147, 260] and surface expression [118], is, to a large extent, attributable to its engagement of SFK activity. For example, the ability of PKC activators to potentiate NMDA-evoked currents in dissociated neurones was blocked by both tyrosine kinase inhibitors and Src-specific blocking peptides; as well, the PKC-dependent upregulation of the receptor was absent in neurones isolated from mice with a targeted deletion of the Src gene [140]. In addition, the stimulation of PKC activity in hippocampal slices was able to dramatically increase the level of phosphotyrosine detected within immunoprecipitated GluN2A and GluN2B subunits [73]. Direct support for the possibility that a PKC-dependent tyrosine kinase signalling cascade contributes to ischaemic changes in GluN2 tyrosine phosphorylation was provided by a study wherein a PKC inhibitor administered immediately after an ischaemic challenge was able to reduce, by approximately half, Src Y416 phosphorylation, general GluN2A tyrosine phosphorylation, and GluN2B Y1472 phosphorylation [35].

The second kinase that may serve to regulate post-ischaemic SFK activity is the proline-rich tyrosine kinase 2, which is a member of the focal adhesion kinase family and highly expressed within the brain [62, 259]. Through mechanisms that are still being uncovered, Pyk2 stimulation (permitted by phosphorylation of its Y402 residue) can be initiated through either depolarisation-induced Ca^{2+} influx, or PKC activation [101, 129, 212]; notably, the level of total and phosphorylated Pyk2 in the post-synaptic density increases sharply less than an hour after post-ischaemic reperfusion has begun [34, 35]. Upon phosphorylation, Pyk2 has been observed to interact with the Src SH2 domain to form a complex that enhances Src function [48, 101, 122]. In addition, the degree of interaction between Pyk2 and GluN2A is quickly amplified in the hippocampus during reperfusion after global ischaemia in either rat [135, 145], or gerbil [271]. Together, the data strongly suggest that ischaemia actuates Pyk2 and enhances its interaction with GluN2 subunits, which, in turn, likely allows Pyk2 to bind and activate the SFKs that would also have been drawn into a complex with NMDA receptors (figure 4).

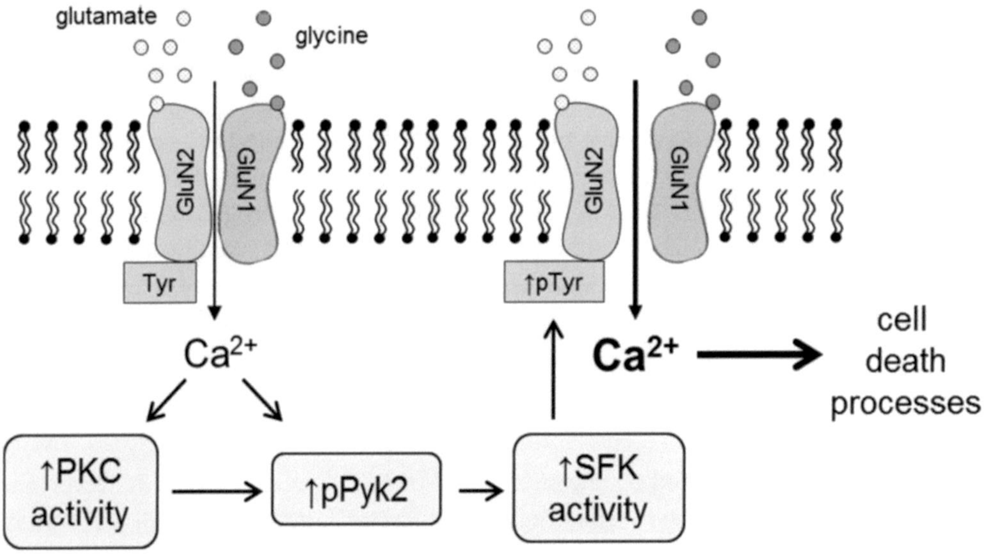

Figure 4. Model summarising the proximal steps leading to the ischemia-mediated increase in tyrosine phosphorylation of the NMDA receptor, and the possible association of its post-translational modification with upstream processes leading to cell death.

Direct support for Pyk2 as a critical component in the pathologic increase of GluN2 phosphorylation has been provided by a set of elegant studies that used either pharmacologic, or genetic approaches to downregulate the kinase's activity. The first study used lithium chloride (LiCl), which has been shown to protect neurones from ischaemic injury [200]. The application of LiCl for several days to cultured cortical neurones was able to dramatically reduce the basal level of both activated Src and phosphorylation at Y1472 of GluN2B [90, 91]; more importantly, administration of LiCl to animals for several days prior to global ischaemia was able to reduce insult-mediated increases in tyrosine phosphorylation of GluN2A [144]. As well, pre-ischaemic LiCl was observed to reduce both the phosphorylation of Y402 of Pyk2 and Y416 of Src, and to diminish the association of both Pyk2 and Src with GluN2A that generally accompanies ischaemic reperfusion [145]. The second study involved the intracerebroventricular injection of Pyk2 antisense oligonucleotides, which lead to a reduction of nearly one-quarter in the enzyme's protein expression within the hippocampus [136]. Animals in which Pyk2 levels had been downregulated displayed not only very little post-ischaemic change in the level of GluN2A tyrosine phosphorylation, but also very little change in the activity of Pyk2 and Src and their ability to be co-immunoprecipitated with GluN2A.

6. Conclusions

A short period of time after the circulation of blood to a region of the brain is substantially reduced, a series of escalating changes is initiated that can very quickly place neurones on a path leading to cell death. One of the principal elements in the pathologic cascade is the excessive stimulation of the excitatory NMDA receptor, which initiates a broad array of potentially cytodestructive changes; most germanely, a disruption in the usually strict regulation of the intracellular calcium ion concentration. One consequence of the elevated level of internal Ca^{2+} is the initiation of an enzyme cascade that involves either the direct, or indirect (through the serine-threonine PKC) stimulation of the tyrosine kinase Pyk2, followed by the subsequent activation of SFK members that go on to increase the tyrosine phosphorylation of GluN2 subunits. Notably, the post-translational modification of the GluN2 subunits is likely both a consequence, and, potentially, a cause of the post-ischaemic enhancement of the degree of interaction between the subunits and Pyk2, SFKs, and PSD-95. One important outcome of the ischaemia-mediated increase of GluN2 tyrosine phosphorylation that is quite likely concerns the enhancement of NMDA receptor gating properties and surface expression, which would serve as a form of signal amplification with the undesirable effect of contributing to increased cell death.

Preliminary support for the possibility that elevated NMDA receptor phosphorylation may contribute to post-ischaemic neuronal loss is found in a collection of studies that have sought to manipulate the cellular level of tyrosine phosphorylation for a neuroprotective effect. The first report in the area revealed that the intracerebral injection of specific inhibitors of protein tyrosine kinases minutes prior to a brief period of global ischaemia was able to prevent the significant degree of neuronal loss that would normally have been seen within the CA1 sub-field of the gerbil hippocampus a week after the insult [107]. Subsequently, the intraperitoneal injection of a selective inhibitor of Src shortly after forebrain ischaemia was found to significantly reduce not only the usual increases in Src activity and general tyrosine phosphorylation, but also the level of cell death observed in the hippocampus four days after the insult [171]. A group of successive studies observed that pretreatment of rats with PP2 (4-amino-5-(4-chlorophenyl)-7-(*t*-butyl)pyrazolo[3,4-*d*]pyrimidine), a selective SFK inhibitor, 0.5 h prior to global ischaemia was able to reduce by greater than half the usual increase in phosphorylated Src [130, 273] and GluN2A tyrosine phosphorylation [96, 273] seen after six hours of reperfusion; as well, cell density of the hippocampal CA1 sub-field five days after the insult was approximately 7-8 fold greater in the treated animals [96, 130, 273]. In addition, the injection of PP2 into neonatal mice shortly after hypoxia-ischaemia was able to reduce by about a third the degree of hippocampal cell loss observed several days after the insult [103].

By using tyrosine kinase inhibitors to control the level of GluN2 tyrosine phosphorylation after an ischaemic challenge, the excessive NMDA receptor activation that plays a critical upstream role in the resulting cell death may be, at least partially, addressed. As a result, a foundation may begin to be constructed that will serve as inspiration for the careful development of new approaches to address the discouraging absence of treatments for brain injury. Regardless of the outcome displayed by future studies that explore how understanding the causes and consequences of NMDA receptor tyrosine phosphorylation may be applied therapeutically, the activity will undoubtedly continue to add important details to our understanding of how the phosphorylation of brain proteins influences neuronal communication and synaptic dysfunction

Author details

Dmytro Pavlov and John G. Mielke*
School of Public Health and Health Systems, University of Waterloo, Waterloo, Canada

Acknowledgement

The preparation of this chapter was supported by a Discovery Grant from the Natural Sciences and Engineering Council of Canada (NSERC) awarded to J.G. Mielke.

7. References

[1] Ahmed I, Bose SK, Pavese N, Ramlackhansingh A, Turkheimer F, Hotton G, Hammers A, Brooks DJ. (2011) Glutamate NMDA receptor dysregulation in Parkinson's disease with dyskinesias. Brain 134(4):979-986.

[2] Ahmed SH, Hu CJ, Paczynski R, Hsu CY. (2001) Pathophysiology of ischemic injury. In Stroke Therapy, 2nd Edition, Butterworth-Heinemann, Boston, pp. 25-57.

[3] Allen CL, Bayraktutan U. (2009) Oxidative stress and its role in the pathogenesis of ischaemic stroke. Int J Stroke 4(6):461-470.

* Corresponding Author

[4] Armogida M, Nisticò R, Mercuri NB. (2012) Therapeutic potential of targeting hydrogen peroxide metabolism in the treatment of brain ischaemia. Br J Pharmacol 166(4):1211-1224.

[5] Astrup J, Skovsted P, Gjerris F, Sørensen HR. (1981) Increase in extracellular potassium in the brain during circulatory arrest: effects of hypothermia, lidocaine, and thiopental. Anesthesiology (3):256-262.

[6] Au KN, Gurd JW. (1995) Tyrosine phosphorylation in a model of ischemia using the rat hippocampal slice: specific, long-term decrease in the tyrosine phosphorylation of the postsynaptic glycoprotein PSD-GP180. J Neurochem 65(4):1834-1841.

[7] Bading H, Greenberg ME. (1991) Stimulation of protein tyrosine phosphorylation by NMDA receptor activation. Science 253(5022):912-914.

[8] Baimbridge KG, Celio MR, Rogers JH. (1992) Calcium-binding proteins in the nervous system. Trends Neurosci 15:303-308.

[9] Barr CS, Dokas LA. (2001) Regulation of pp60(c-src) synthesis in rat hippocampal slices by in vitro ischemia and glucocorticoid administration. J Neurosci Res 65(4):340-345.

[10] Bano D, Young KW, Guerin CJ, Lefeuvre R, Rothwell NJ, Naldini L, Rizzuto R, Carafoli E, Nicotera P. (2005) Cleavage of the plasma membrane Na+/Ca2+ exchanger in excitotoxicity. Cell 120(2):275-285.

[11] Bano D, Nicotera P. (2007) Ca^{2+} signals and neuronal death in brain ischemia. Stroke 38(Suppl 2):674-676.

[12] Bartus RT, Baker KL, Heiser AD. (1994) Postischemic administration of AK275, a calpain inhibitor, provides substantial protection against focal ischemic brain damage. J Cereb Blood Flow Metab 14:537-544.

[13] Batty GD, Lee IM. (2002) Physical activity for preventing strokes. BMJ 325:350-351.

[14] Bennett JA, Dingledine R. (1995) Topology profile for a glutamate receptor: three transmembrane domains and a channel-lining reentrant membrane loop. Neuron 14(2):373-384.

[15] Benveniste H, Jorgensen MB, Diemer NH, Hansen AJ. (1988) Calcium accumulation by glutamate receptor activation is involved in hippocampal cell damage after ischemia. Acta Neurol Scand 78(6):529-536.

[16] Besshoh S, Bawa D, Teves L, Wallace MC, Gurd JW. (2005) Increased phosphorylation and redistribution of NMDA receptors between synaptic lipid rafts and post-synaptic densities following transient global ischemia in the rat brain. J Neurochem 93(1):186-194.

[17] Bhandari V, Lim KL, Pallen CJ. (1998) Physical and functional interactions between receptor-like protein-tyrosine phosphatase alpha and p59fyn. J Biol Chem 273(15):8691-8698.

[18] Bi R, Rong Y, Bernard A, Khrestchatisky M, Baudry M. (2000) Src-mediated tyrosine phosphorylation of NR2 subunits of N-methyl-D-aspartate receptors protects from calpain-mediated truncation of their C-terminal domains. J Biol Chem 275(34):26477-26483.

[19] Blanke ML, VanDongen A. (2009) Activation mechanisms of the NMDA receptor. In Biology of the NMDA Receptor, CRC Press, New York, pp. 283-312.

[20] Bleakman D, Alt A, Nisenbaum ES. (2006) Glutamate receptors and pain. Semin Cell Dev Biol 17(5):592-604.

[21] Bliss TV, Collingridge GL. (1993) A synaptic model of memory: long-term potentiation in the hippocampus. Nature 361(6407):31-39.

[22] Bogaert E, d'Ydewalle C, Van Den Bosch L. (2010) Amyotrophic lateral sclerosis and excitotoxicity: from pathological mechanism to therapeutic target. CNS Neurol Disord Drug Targets 9(3):297-304.

[23] Boulanger LM, Lombroso PJ, Raghunathan A, During MJ, Wahle P, Naegele JR. (1995) Cellular and molecular characterization of a brain-enriched protein tyrosine phosphatase. J Neurosci 15(2):1532-1544.

[24] Braithwaite SP, Adkisson M, Leung J, Nava A, Masterson B, Urfer R, Oksenberg D, Nikolich K. (2006) Regulation of NMDA receptor trafficking and function by striatal-enriched tyrosine phosphatase (STEP). Eur J Neurosci 23(11):2847-2856.

[25] Braithwaite SP, Xu J, Leung J, Urfer R, Nikolich K, Oksenberg D, Lombroso PJ, Shamloo M. (2008) Expression and function of striatal enriched protein tyrosine phosphatase is profoundly altered in cerebral ischemia. Eur J Neurosci 27(9):2444-2452.

[26] Braunton JL, Wong V, Wang W, Salter MW, Roder J, Liu M, Wang YT. (1998) Reduction of tyrosine kinase activity and protein tyrosine dephosphorylation by anoxic stimulation in vitro. Neuroscience 82(1):161-170.

[27] Bright R, Mochly-Rosen D. (2005) The role of protein kinase C in cerebral ischemic and reperfusion injury. Stroke 36(12):2781-2790.

[28] Brust JC. (2000) Circulation of the brain. In Principles of Neural Science, 4th Edition, McGraw-Hill, New York, pp. 1302-1316.

[29] Butcher SP, Bullock R, Graham DI, McCulloch J. (1990) Correlation between amino acid release and neuropathologic outcome in rat brain following middle cerebral artery occlusion. Stroke 21:1727-1733.

[30] Campos-González R, Kindy MS. (1992) Tyrosine phosphorylation of microtubule-associated protein kinase after transient ischemia in the gerbil brain. J Neurochem 59(5):1955-1958.

[31] Chen BS, Roche KW. (2007) Regulation of NMDA receptors by phosphorylation. Neuropharmacology 53(3):362-368.

[32] Chen C, Leonard J. (1996) Protein tyrosine kinase-mediated potentiation of currents from cloned NMDA receptors. J Neurochem 67:194-200.

[33] Chen M, Hou X, Zhang G. (2003) Tyrosine kinase and tyrosine phosphatase participate in regulation of interactions of NMDA receptor subunit 2A with Src and Fyn mediated by PSD-95 after transient brain ischemia. Neurosci Lett 339(1):29-32.

[34] Cheung HH, Takagi N, Teves L, Logan R, Wallace MC, Gurd JW. (2000) Altered association of protein tyrosine kinases with postsynaptic densities after transient cerebral ischemia in the rat brain. J Cereb Blood Flow Metab 20(3):505-512.

[35] Cheung HH, Teves L, Wallace MC, Gurd JW. (2003) Inhibition of protein kinase C reduces ischemia-induced tyrosine phosphorylation of the N-methyl-d-aspartate receptor. J Neurochem 86(6):1441-1449.

[36] Choi DW. (1985) Glutamate neurotoxicity in cortical cell culture is calcium dependent. Neurosci Lett 58(3):293-297.

[37] Choi DW. (1987) Ionic dependence of glutamate neurotoxicity. J Neurosci 7:369-379.

[38] Choi JS, Kim HY, Chung JW, Chun MH, Kim SY, Yoon SH, Lee MY. (2005) Activation of Src tyrosine kinase in microglia in the rat hippocampus following transient forebrain ischemia. Neurosci Lett 380(1-2):1-5.

[39] Chung HJ, Huang YH, Lau LF, Huganir RL. (2004) Regulation of the NMDA receptor complex and trafficking by activity-dependent phosphorylation of the NR2B subunit PDZ ligand. J Neurosci 24(45):10248-10259.

[40] Ciesla J, Fraczyk T, Rode W. (2011) Phosphorylation of basic amino acid residues in proteins: important but easily missed. Acta Biochim Pol 58(2):137-147.

[41] Collingridge G, Isaac J, Wang YT. (2004) Receptor trafficking and synaptic plasticity. Nat Rev Neurosci 5(12):952-962.

[42] Collingridge GL, Olsen RW, Peters J, Spedding M. (2009) A nomenclature for ligand-gated ion channels. Neuropharmacology 56(1):2-5.

[43] Constantine-Paton M. (1990) NMDA receptor as a mediator of activity-dependent synaptogenesis in the developing brain. Cold Spring Harbour Symp Quant Biol 55:431-443.

[44] Curtis D, Watkins J. (1961) Analogues of glutamic and gamma-amino-n-butyric acids having potent actions on mammalian neurones. Nature 191:1010-1011.

[45] Dabrowski A, Umemori H. (2011) Orchestrating the synaptic network by tyrosine phosphorylation signalling. J Biochem 149(6):641-653.

[46] Deb I, Poddar R, Paul S. (2011) Oxidative stress-induced oligomerization inhibits the activity of the non-receptor tyrosine phosphatase STEP61. J Neurochem 116(6):1097-1111.

[47] Demaerschalk BM, Hwang HM, Leung G. (2010) US cost burden of ischemic stroke: a systematic literature review. Am J Manag Care 16(7):525-533.

[48] Dikic I, Tokiwa G, Lev S, Courtneidge SA, Schlessinger J. (1996) A role for Pyk2 and Src in linking G-protein-coupled receptors with MAP kinase activation. Nature 383(6600):547-550.

[49] Du CP, Gao J, Tai JM, Liu Y, Qi J, Wang W, Hou XY. (2009) Increased tyrosine phosphorylation of PSD-95 by Src family kinases after brain ischaemia. Biochem J 417(1):277-285.

[50] Dugan LL, Sensi SL, Canzoniero LM, Handran SD, Rothman SM, Lin TS, Goldberg MP, Choi DW. (1995) Mitochondrial production of reactive oxygen species in cortical neurons following exposure to N-methyl-D-aspartate. J Neurosci 15(10):6377-6388.

[51] Dunah AW, Standaert DG. (2001) Dopamine D1 receptor-dependent trafficking of striatal NMDA glutamate receptors to the postsynaptic membrane. J Neurosci 21(15):5546-5558.

[52] Dykens JA. (1994) Isolated cerebral and cerebellar mitochondria produce free radicals when exposed to elevated CA^{2+} and Na^{+}: implications for neurodegeneration. J Neurochem 63:584-591.

[53] Ewald RC, Cline HT. (2009) NMDA receptors and brain development. In Biology of the NMDA Receptor, CRC Press, New York, pp. 1-15.
[54] Fanselow MS, Dong HW. (2010) Are the dorsal and ventral hippocampus functionally distinct structures? Neuron 65(1):7-19.
[55] Forrest D, Yuzaki M, Soares HD, Ng L, Luk DC, Sheng M, Stewart CL, Morgan JI, Connor JA, Curran T. (1994) Targeted disruption of NMDA receptor 1 gene abolishes NMDA response and results in neonatal death. Neuron 13(2):325-338.
[56] Frank R. (2011) Endogenous ion channel complexes: the NMDA receptor. Biochem Soc Trans 39:707-718.
[57] Garaschuk O, Schneggenburger R, Schirra C, Tempia F, Konnerth A. (1996) Fractional Ca2+ currents through somatic and dendritic glutamate receptor channels of rat hippocampal CA1 pyramidal neurones. J Physiol 491(3):757-772.
[58] Garthwaite G, Hojos F, Garthwaite J. (1986) Ionic requirements for neurotoxic effects of excitatory amino acid analogues in rat cerebellar slices. Neuroscience 18:437-447.
[59] Gilmour G, Dix S, Fellini L, Gastambide F, Plath N, Steckler T, Talpos J, Tricklebank M. (2012) NMDA receptors, cognition and schizophrenia - testing the validity of the NMDA receptor hypofunction hypothesis. Neuropharmacology 62(3):1401-1412.
[60] Ginsberg MD. (1996) Pathophysiology and mechanisms of ischemic brain injury. In New Approaches to the Treatment of Ischemic Stroke: Part I. Ischemic Stroke: A Disease Update. Excerpta Medica, New Jersey, pp. 11-17.
[61] Ginsberg MD. (2009) Current status of neuroprotection for cerebral ischemia: synoptic overview. Stroke 40(3 Suppl):S111-S114.
[62] Girault JA, Costa A, Derkinderen P, Studler JM, Toutant M. (1999) FAK and PYK2/CAKbeta in the nervous system: a link between neuronal activity, plasticity and survival? Trends Neurosci 22(6):257-263.
[63] Globus MY, Busto R, Martinez E, Valdes I, Dietrich WD, Ginsberg MD. (1991) Comparative effect of transient global ischemia on extracellular levels of glutamate, glycine, and gamma-aminobutyric acid in vulnerable and nonvulnerable brain regions in the rat. J Neurochem 57(2):470-478.
[64] Goebel SM, Alvestad RM, Coultrap SJ, Browning MD. (2005) Tyrosine phosphorylation of the N-methyl-D-aspartate receptor is enhanced in synaptic membrane fractions of the adult rat hippocampus. Brain Res Mol Brain Res 142(1):65-79.
[65] Goebel-Goody SM, Davies KD, Alvestad Linger RM, Freund RK, Browning MD. (2009) Phospho-regulation of synaptic and extrasynaptic N-methyl-d-aspartate receptors in adult hippocampal slices. Neuroscience 158(4):1446-1459.
[66] Goebel-Goody SM, Baum M, Paspalas CD, Fernandez SM, Carty NC, Kurup P, Lombroso PJ. (2012) Therapeutic implications for striatal-enriched protein tyrosine phosphatase (STEP) in neuropsychiatric disorders. Pharmacol Rev 64(1):65-87.
[67] Goldberg MP, Choi DW. (1993) Combined oxygen and glucose deprivation in cortical cell culture: calcium-dependent and calcium-independent mechanisms of neuronal injury. J Neurosci 13(8):3510-3524.

[68] Grant SG, O'Dell TJ, Karl KA, Stein PL, Soriano P, Kandel ER. (1992) Impaired long-term potentiation, spatial learning, and hippocampal development in fyn mutant mice. Science 258(5090):1903-1910.

[69] Green AR, Odergren T, Ashwood T. (2003) Animal models of stroke: do they have value for discovering neuroprotective agents? *Trends Pharmacol Sci* 24(8):402-408.

[70] Groc L, Bard L, Choquet D. (2009) Surface trafficking of N-Methyl-D-Aspartate receptors: physiological and pathological perspectives. Neuroscience 158:4-18.

[71] Groc L, Heine M, Cognet L, Brickley K, Stephenson FA, Lounis B, Choquet D. (2004) Differential activity-dependent regulation of the lateral mobilities of AMPA and NMDA receptors. Nat Neurosci 7(7):695-696.

[72] Groc L, Heine M, Cousins SL, Stephenson FA, Lounis B, Cognet L, Choquet D. (2006) NMDA receptor surface mobility depends on NR2A-2B subunits. Proc Natl Acad Sci USA 103:18769-18774.

[73] Grosshans DR, Browning MD. (2001) Protein kinase C activation induces tyrosine phosphorylation of the NR2A and NR2B subunits of the NMDA receptor. J Neurochem 76(3):737-744.

[74] Grosshans D, Clayton D, Coultrap S, Browning M. (2002) LTP leads to rapid surface expression of NMDA, but not AMPA, receptors. Nature Neurosci 5:27-33.

[75] Groveman BR, Xue S, Marin V, Xu J, Ali MK, Bienkiewicz EA, Yu XM. (2011) Roles of the SH2 and SH3 domains in the regulation of neuronal Src kinase functions. *FEBS J* 278:643-653.

[76] Gunasekar PG, Kanthasamy AG, Borowitz JL, Isom GE. (1995) NMDA receptor activation produces concurrent generation of nitric oxide and reactive oxygen species: implication for cell death. J Neurochem 65(5):2016-2021.

[77] Gunter TE, Pfeiffer D. (1990) Mechanisms by which mitochondria transport calcium. Am J Physiol 258:C755-C786.

[78] Guo J, Meng F, Zhang G, Zhang Q. (2003) Free radicals are involved in continuous activation of nonreceptor tyrosine protein kinase c-Src after ischemia/reperfusion in rat hippocampus. Neurosci Lett 345(2):101-104.

[79] Guo J, Wu HW, Hu G, Han X, De W, Sun YJ. (2006) Sustained activation of Src-family tyrosine kinases by ischemia: a potential mechanism mediating extracellular signal-regulated kinase cascades in hippocampal dentate gyrus. Neuroscience 143(3):827-836.

[80] Gurd JW. (1997) Protein tyrosine phosphorylation: implications for synaptic function. Neurochem Int 31(5):635-649.

[81] Gurd JW, Bissoon N, Nguyen TH, Lombroso PJ, Rider CC, Beesley PW, Vannucci SJ. (1999) Hypoxia-ischemia in perinatal rat brain induces the formation of a low molecular weight isoform of striatal enriched tyrosine phosphatase (STEP). J Neurochem 73(5):1990-1994.

[82] Gurd JW, Bissoon N, Beesley PW, Nakazawa T, Yamamoto T, Vannucci SJ. (2002) Differential effects of hypoxia-ischemia on subunit expression and tyrosine phosphorylation of the NMDA receptor in 7- and 21-day-old rats. J Neurochem 82(4):848-856.

[83] Hacke W, Hennerici M, Gelmers HJ, Kramer G. (1991) Epidemiology and classification of strokes. In Cerebral Ischaemia, Springer-Verlag, New York, pp. 31-52.

[84] Hagberg H, Lehmann A, Sandberg M, Nystrom B, Jacobson I, Hamberger A. (1985) Ischemia-induced shift of inhibitory and excitatory amino acids from intra to extracellular compartments. J Cereb Blood Flow Metab 5:925-929.

[85] Hallett PJ, Spoelgen R, Hyman BT, Standaert DG, Dunah AW. (2006) Dopamine D1 activation potentiates striatal NMDA receptors by tyrosine phosphorylation-dependent subunit trafficking. J Neurosci 26(17):4690-4700.

[86] Hanley MR. (1988) Proto-oncogenes in the nervous system. Neuron 1(3):175-182.

[87] Harder KW, Moller NP, Peacock JW, Jirik FR. (1998) Protein-tyrosine phosphatase alpha regulates Src family kinases and alters cell-substratum adhesion. J Biol Chem 273(48):31890-31900.

[88] Hartley DM, Kurth MC, Bjerkness L, Weiss JH, Choi DW. (1993) Glutamate receptor-induced Ca^{2+} accumulation in cortical cell culture correlates with subsequent neuronal degeneration. J Neurosci 13(5):1993-2000.

[89] Hasegawa S, Morioka M, Goto S, Korematsu K, Okamura A, Yano S, Kai Y, Hamada JI, Ushio Y. (2000) Expression of neuron specific phosphatase, striatal enriched phosphatase (STEP) in reactive astrocytes after transient forebrain ischemia. Glia 29(4):316-329.

[90] Hashimoto R, Fujimaki K, Jeong MR, Christ L, Chuang DM. (2003) Lithium-induced inhibition of Src tyrosine kinase in rat cerebral cortical neurons: a role in neuroprotection against N-methyl-D-aspartate receptor-mediated excitotoxicity. FEBS Lett 538(1-3):145-148.

[91] Hashimoto R, Hough C, Nakazawa T, Yamamoto T, Chuang DM. (2002) Lithium protection against glutamate excitotoxicity in rat cerebral cortical neurons: involvement of NMDA receptor inhibition possibly by decreasing NR2B tyrosine phosphorylation. J Neurochem 80(4):589-597.

[92] He J, Ogden LG, Vupputuri S, Bazzano LA, Loria C, Whelton PK. (1999) Dietary sodium intake and subsequent risk of cardiovascular disease in overweight adults. JAMA 282(21):2027-2034.

[93] He K, Rimm EB, Merchant A, Rosner BA, Stampfer MJ, Willett WC, Ascherio A. (2002) Fish consumption and risk of stroke in men. JAMA 288(24):3130-3136.

[94] Hisatsune C, Umemori H, Mishina M, Yamamoto T. (1999) Phosphorylation-dependent interaction of the N-methyl-D-aspartate receptor epsilon 2 subunit with phosphatidylinositol 3-kinase. Genes Cells 4(11):657-666.

[95] Horner RD, Matchar DB, Divine GW, Feussner JR. (1991) Racial variations in ischemic stroke-related physical and functional impairments. Stroke 22:1497-1501.

[96] Hou XY, Liu Y, Zhang GY. (2007) PP2, a potent inhibitor of Src family kinases, protects against hippocampal CA1 pyramidal cell death after transient global brain ischemia. Neurosci Lett 420(3):235-239.

[97] Hou XY, Zhang GY, Yan JZ, Chen M, Liu Y. (2002) Activation of NMDA receptors and L-type voltage-gated calcium channels mediates enhanced formation of Fyn-PSD95-NR2A complex after transient brain ischemia. Brain Res 955(1-2):123-132.

[98] Hou XY, Zhang GY, Zong YY. (2003) Suppression of postsynaptic density protein 95 expression attenuates increased tyrosine phosphorylation of NR2A subunits of N-methyl-D-aspartate receptors and interactions of Src and Fyn with NR2A after transient brain ischemia in rat hippocampus. Neurosci Lett 343(2):125-128.

[99] Hu BR, Wieloch T. (1994) Tyrosine phosphorylation and activation of mitogen-activated protein kinase in the rat brain following transient cerebral ischemia. J Neurochem 62(4):1357-1367.

[100] Hu NW, Ondrejcak T, Rowan MJ. (2012) Glutamate receptors in preclinical research on Alzheimer's disease: update on recent advances. Pharmacol Biochem Behav 100(4):855-862.

[101] Huang Y, Lu W, Ali DW, Pelkey KA, Pitcher GM, Lu YM, Aoto H, Roder JC, Sasaki T, Salter MW, MacDonald JF. (2001) CAKbeta/Pyk2 kinase is a signaling link for induction of long-term potentiation in CA1 hippocampus. Neuron 29(2):485-96.

[102] Ingraham CA, Cox ME, Ward DC, Fults DW, Maness PF. (1989) c-src and other proto-oncogenes implicated in neuronal differentiation. Mol Chem Neuropathol 10(1):1-14.

[103] Jiang X, Mu D, Biran V, Faustino J, Chang S, Rincón CM, Sheldon RA, Ferriero DM. (2008) Activated Src kinases interact with the N-methyl-D-aspartate receptor after neonatal brain ischemia. Ann Neurol 63(5):632-641.

[104] Jourdain P, Bergersen LH, Bhaukaurally K, Bezzi P, Santello M, Domercq M, Matute C, Tonello F, Gundersen V, Volterra A. (2007) Glutamate exocytosis from astrocytes controls synaptic strength. Nat Neurosci. 10(3):331-9.

[105] Kalia LV, Salter MW. (2003) Interactions between Src family protein tyrosine kinases and PSD-95. Neuropharmacology. 45(6):720-728.

[106] Kennedy MB. (1997) The postsynaptic density at glutamatergic synapses. Trends Neurosci 20(6):264-268.

[107] Kindy MS. (1993) Inhibition of tyrosine phosphorylation prevents delayed neuronal death following cerebral ischemia. J Cereb Blood Flow Metab 13(3):372-377.

[108] Kohr G, Seeburg P. (1996) Subtype-specific regulation of recombinant NMDA receptor channels by protein tyrosine kinases of the src family. J Physiol 492:445-452.

[109] Koistinaho J, Hökfelt T. (1997) Altered gene expression in brain ischemia. Neuroreport 8(2):i-viii.

[110] Komuro H, Rakic P. (1993) Modulation of neuronal migration by NMDA receptors. Science 260(5104):95-97.

[111] Kontos HA. (2001) Oxygen radicals in cerebral ischemia. The 2001 Willis Lecture. Stroke 32(11):2712-2715.

[112] Koritzinsky M, Wouters BG. (2007) Hypoxia and regulation of messenger RNA translation. Methods Enzymol 435:247-273.

[113] Kornau HC, Schenker LT, Kennedy MB, Seeburg PH. (1995) Domain interaction between NMDA receptor subunits and the postsynaptic density protein PSD-95. Science 269(5231):1737-1740.

[114] Krupp JJ, Vissel B, Thomas CG, Heinemann SF, Westbrook GL. (2002) Calcineurin acts via the C-terminus of NR2A to modulate desensitization of NMDARs. Neuropharmacology 42:593-602.

[115] Kudo Y, Ogura A. (1986) Glutamate-induced increase in intracellular Ca^{2+} concentration in isolated hippocampal neurones. Br J Pharmacol 89(1):191-198.

[116] Kuo WL, Chung KC, Rosner MR. (1997) Differentiation of central nervous system neuronal cells by fibroblast-derived growth factor requires at least two signaling pathways: roles for Ras and Src. Mol Cell Biol 17(8):4633-4643.

[117] Lafon-Cazal M, Pietri S, Culcasi M, Bockaert J. (1993) NMDA-dependent superoxide production and neurotoxicity. Nature 364(6437):535-537.

[118] Lan JY, Skeberdis VA, Jover T, Grooms SY, Lin Y, Araneda RC, Zheng X, Bennett MV, Zukin RS. (2001) Protein kinase C modulates NMDA receptor trafficking and gating. Nat Neurosci. 4(4):382-390.

[119] Lau A, Tymianski M. (2010) Glutamate receptors, neurotoxicity and neurodegeneration. Pflugers Arch 460(2):525-542.

[120] Lau C, Zukin R. (2007) NMDA receptor trafficking in synaptic plasticity and neuropsychiatric disorders. Nat Rev Neurosci 8(6):413-426.

[121] Lau L, Huganir R. (1995) Differential tyrosine phosphorylation of N-methyl-D-aspartate receptor subunits. J Biol Chem 270(34):20036-20041.

[122] Lauri SE, Taira T, Rauvala H. (2000) High-frequency synaptic stimulation induces association of fyn and c- src to distinct phosphorylated components. NeuroReport 11:997-1000.

[123] Lavezzari G, McCallum J, Lee R, Roche KW. (2003) Differential binding of the AP-2 adaptor complex and PSD-95 to the C-terminus of the NMDA receptor subunit NR2B regulates surface expression. Neuropharmacology 45(6):729-737.

[124] Lavezzari G, McCallum J, Dewey CM, Roche KW. (2004) Subunit-specific regulation of NMDA receptor endocytosis. J Neurosci 24(28):6383-6391.

[125] Lee HK. (2006) Synaptic plasticity and phosphorylation. Pharmacol Therapeutics 112:810-832.

[126] Lees GJ. (1991) Inhibition of sodium-potassium-ATPase: a potentially ubiquitous mechanism contributing to central nervous system pathology. Brain Res Rev 16(3):283-300.

[127] Lei G, Xue S, Chéry N, Liu Q, Xu J, Kwan CL, Fu YP, Lu YM, Liu M, Harder KW, Yu XM. (2002) Gain control of N-methyl-D-aspartate receptor activity by receptor-like protein tyrosine phosphatase alpha. EMBO J 21(12):2977-2989.

[128] Le Meur K, Galante M, Angulo MC, Audinat E. (2007) Tonic activation of NMDA receptors by ambient glutamate of non-synaptic origin in the rat hippocampus. J Physiol. 580(Pt. 2):373-83.

[129] Lev S, Moreno H, Martinez R, Canoll P, Peles E, Musacchio JM, Plowman GD, Rudy B, Schlessinger J. (1995) Protein tyrosine kinase PYK2 involved in Ca(2+)-induced regulation of ion channel and MAP kinase functions. Nature 376(6543):737-745.

[130] Li T, Yu XJ, Zhang GY. (2008) Tyrosine phosphorylation of HPK1 by activated Src promotes ischemic brain injury in rat hippocampal CA1 region. FEBS Lett 582(13):1894-1900.

[131] Li Y, Mu Y, Gage FH. (2009) Development of neural circuits in the adult hippocampus. Curr Top Dev Biol 87:149-174.

[132] Lin Y, Skeberdis VA, Francesconi A, Bennett MV, Zukin RS. (2004) Postsynaptic density protein-95 regulates NMDA channel gating and surface expression. J Neurosci 24(45):10138-10148.

[133] Lipton P (1999) Ischemic cell death in brain neurons. Physiol Rev 79(4):1431-1568.

[134] Liu X, Brodeur SR, Gish G, Songyang Z, Cantley LC, Laudano AP, Pawson T. (1993) Regulation of c-Src tyrosine kinase activity by the Src SH2 domain. Oncogene 8(5):1119-1126.

[135] Liu Y, Zhang G, Gao C, Hou X. (2001) NMDA receptor activation results in tyrosine phosphorylation of NMDA receptor subunit 2A(NR2A) and interaction of Pyk2 and Src with NR2A after transient cerebral ischemia and reperfusion. Brain Res 909(1-2):51-58.

[136] Liu Y, Zhang GY, Yan JZ, Xu TL. (2005) Suppression of Pyk2 attenuated the increased tyrosine phosphorylation of NMDA receptor subunit 2A after brain ischemia in rat hippocampus. Neurosci Lett 379(1):55-58.

[137] Lobner D, Lipton P. (1993) Intracellular calcium levels and calcium fluxes in the CA1 region of the rat hippocampal slice during in vitro ischemia: relationship to electrophysiological cell damage. J Neurosci 13:4861-4871.

[138] Lombroso PJ, Murdoch G, Lerner M. (1991) Molecular characterization of a protein-tyrosine-phosphatase enriched in striatum. Proc Natl Acad Sci USA 88(16):7242-7246.

[139] Love S. (1999) Oxidative stress in brain ischemia. Brain Pathol 9(1):119-131.

[140] Lu WY, Xiong ZG, Lei S, Orser BA, Dudek E, Browning MD, MacDonald JF. (1999) G-protein-coupled receptors act via protein kinase C and Src to regulate NMDA receptors. Nat Neurosci 2(4):331-338.

[141] Lu YM, Roder JC, Davidow J, Salter MW. (1998) Src activation in the induction of long-term potentiation in CA1 hippocampal neurons. Science 279(5355):1363-1367.

[142] Lucas DR, Newhouse JP. (1957) The toxic effects of sodium L-glutamate on the inner layer of the retina. Arch Ophthalm 58:193-201.

[143] Luiten PG, Stuiver B, de Jong GI, Nyakas C, De Keyser JH. (1997) Calcium homeostasis, nimodipine, and stroke. In Clinical Pharmacology of Cerebral Ischemia, Humana Press, New Jersey, pp. 67-99.

[144] Ma J, Zhang GY. (2003) Lithium reduced N-methyl-D-aspartate receptor subunit 2A tyrosine phosphorylation and its interactions with Src and Fyn mediated by PSD-95 in rat hippocampus following cerebral ischemia. Neurosci Lett 348(3):185-189.

[145] Ma J, Zhang GY, Liu Y, Yan JZ, Hao ZB. (2004) Lithium suppressed Tyr-402 phosphorylation of proline-rich tyrosine kinase (Pyk2) and interactions of Pyk2 and PSD-95 with NR2A in rat hippocampus following cerebral ischemia. Neurosci Res 49(4):357-362.

[146] MacDonald JF, Jackson MF, Beazely MA. (2006) Hippocampal long-term synaptic plasticity and signal amplification of NMDA receptors. Crit Rev Neurobiol 18(1-2):71-84.

[147] MacDonald JF, Kotecha SA, Lu WY, Jackson MF. (2001) Convergence of PKC-dependent kinase signal cascades on NMDA receptors. Curr Drug Targets 2(3):299-312.

[148] MacDonald JF, Mody I, Salter MW. (1989) Regulation of N-methyl-D-aspartate receptors revealed by intracellular dialysis of murine neurones in culture. J Physiol 414:17-34.

[149] Machado-Vieira R, Manji HK, Zarate CA. (2009) The role of the tripartite glutamatergic synapse in the pathophysiology and therapeutics of mood disorders. Neuroscientist 15(5):525-39.

[150] Machida K, Mayer BJ. (2005) The SH2 domain: versatile signaling module and pharmaceutical target. Biochim Biophys Acta 1747(1):1-25.

[151] Martone ME, Hu BR, Ellisman MH. (2000) Alterations of hippocampal postsynaptic densities following transient ischemia. Hippocampus 10(5):610-616.

[152] Mayer ML, Westbrook GL. (1987) Permeation and block of N-methyl-D-aspartic acid receptor channels by divalent cations in mouse cultured central neurones. J Physiol 394:501-527.

[153] Mayer M, Armstrong N. (2004) Structure and function of glutamate receptor ion channels. Annu Rev Physiol 66:161-181.

[154] McLennan H. (1983) Receptors for the excitatory amino acids in the mammalian central nervous system. Prog Neurobiol 20(3-4):251-271.

[155] Meldrum BS. (1990) Protection against ischemic neuronal damage by drugs acting on excitatory neurotransmission. Cerebrovasc Brain Metab Rev 2:27-57.

[156] Monyer H, Burnashev N, Laurie DJ, Sakmann B, Seeburg PH. (1994) Developmental and regional expression in the rat brain and functional properties of four NMDA receptors. Neuron 12:529–540.

[157] Moon IS, Apperson ML, Kennedy MB. (1994) The major tyrosine-phosphorylated protein in the postsynaptic density fraction is N-methyl-D-aspartate receptor subunit 2B. Proc Natl Acad Sci USA 91(9):3954-3958.

[158] Moriyoshi K, Masu M, Ishii T, Shigemotto R, Mizuno N, Nakanishi S. (1991) Molecular cloning and characterization of the rat NMDA receptor. Nature 354:31-37.

[159] Moss SJ, Gorrie GH, Amato A, Smart TG. (1995) Modulation of GABAA receptors by tyrosine phosphorylation. Nature 377(6547):344-348.

[160] Murotomi K, Takagi N, Takayanagi G, Ono M, Takeo S, Tanonaka K. (2008) mGluR1 antagonist decreases tyrosine phosphorylation of NMDA receptor and attenuates infarct size after transient focal cerebral ischemia. J Neurochem 105(5):1625-1634.

[161] Nada S, Shima T, Yanai H, Husi H, Grant SG, Okada M, Akiyama T. (2003) Identification of PSD-93 as a substrate for the Src family tyrosine kinase Fyn. J Biol Chem 278(48):47610-47621.

[162] Naegele JR, Lombroso PJ. (1994) Protein tyrosine phosphatases in the nervous system. Crit Rev Neurobiol 9(1):105-114.

[163] Nakazawa, T, Komai S, Tezuka T, Hisatsune C, Umemori H, Semba K, Mishina M, Manabe T, Yamamoto T. (2001) Characterization of Fyn-mediated tyrosine phosphorylation sites on GluR 2 (NR2B) subunit of the N-methyl-D-aspartate receptor. J Biol Chem 276: 693-699.

[164] Nakazawa T, Komai S, Watabe AM, Kiyama Y, Fukaya M, Arima-Yoshida F, Horai R, Sudo K, Ebine K, Delawary M, Goto J, Umemori H, Tezuka T, Iwakura Y, Watanabe M,

Yamamoto T, Manabe T. (2006) NR2B tyrosine phosphorylation modulates fear learning as well as amygdaloid synaptic plasticity. EMBO J 25(12):2867-2877.

[165] Nguyen TH, Liu J, Lombroso PJ. (2002) Striatal enriched phosphatase 61 dephosphorylates Fyn at phosphotyrosine 420. J Biol Chem 277(27):24274-24279.

[166] Nguyen TH, Paul S, Xu Y, Gurd JW, Lombroso PJ. (1999) Calcium-dependent cleavage of striatal enriched tyrosine phosphatase (STEP). J Neurochem 73(5):1995-2001.

[167] Niethammer M, Kim E, Sheng M. (1996) Interaction between the C terminus of NMDA receptor subunits and multiple members of the PSD-95 family of membrane-associated guanylate kinases. J Neurosci 16(7):2157-2163.

[168] Nowak L, Bregestovski P, Ascher P, Herbet A, Prochiantz A. (1984) Magnesium gates glutamate-activated channels in mouse central neurones. Nature 307(5950):462-465.

[169] O'Collins VE, Macleod MR, Donnan GA, Horky LL, van der Worp BH, Howells DW. (2006) 1,026 experimental treatments in acute stroke. Ann Neurol 59(3):467-477.

[170] Ohnishi H, Murata Y, Okazawa H, Matozaki T. (2011) Src family kinases: modulators of neurotransmitter function and behaviour. Trends Neurosci 34(12):629-637.

[171] Ohtsuki T, Matsumoto M, Kitagawa K, Mabuchi T, Mandai K, Matsushita K, Kuwabara K, Tagaya M, Ogawa S, Ueda H, Kamada T, Yanagihara T. (1996) Delayed neuronal death in ischemic hippocampus involves stimulation of protein tyrosine phosphorylation. Am J Physiol 271(4 Pt 1):C1085-1097.

[172] Olesen J, Gustavsson A, Svensson M, Wittchen HU, Jönsson B. (2012) The economic cost of brain disorders in Europe. Eur J Neurol 19(1):155-162.

[173] Olney JW. (1969) Glutamate-induced retinal degeneration in neonatal mice. Electron microscopy of the acutely evolving lesion. J Neuropathol Exp Neurol 28(3):455-474.

[174] Oyama T, Goto S, Nishi T, Sato K, Yamada K, Yoshikawa M, Ushio Y. (1995) Immunocytochemical localization of the striatal enriched protein tyrosine phosphatase in the rat striatum: a light and electron microscopic study with a complementary DNA-generated polyclonal antibody. Neuroscience 69(3):869-880.

[175] Ozawa S, Kamiya H, Tsuzuki K. (1998) Glutamate receptors in the mammalian central nervous system. Prog Neurobiol 54:581-618.

[176] Pallen CJ. (2003) Protein tyrosine phosphatase alpha (PTPalpha): a Src family kinase activator and mediator of multiple biological effects. Curr Top Med Chem 3(7):821-835.

[177] Paoletti P, Ascher P, Neyton J. (1997) High-affinity zinc inhibition of NMDA NR1-NR2A receptors. J Neurosci 17(15):5711-25.

[178] Pawson T, Scott JD. (2005) Protein phosphorylation in signaling - 50 years and counting. Trends Biochem Sci (6):286-290.

[179] Pei L, Li Y, Zhang GY, Cui ZC, Zhu ZM. (2000) Mechanisms of regulation of tyrosine phosphorylation of NMDA receptor subunit 2B after cerebral ischemia/reperfusion. Acta Pharmacol Sin 21(8):695-700.

[180] Pei L, Li Y, Yan JZ, Zhang GY, Cui ZC, Zhu ZM. (2000) Changes and mechanisms of protein-tyrosine kinase and protein-tyrosine phosphatase activities after brain ischemia/reperfusion. Acta Pharmacol Sin 21(8):715-720.

[181] Pelkey K, Askalan R, Paul S, Kalia L, Nguyen T, Pitcher G, Salter M, Lombroso P. (2002) Tyrosine phosphatase STEP is a tonic brake on induction of long-term potentiation. Neuron 34: 127-138.
[182] Perkinton MS, Ip JK, Wood GL, Crossthwaite AJ, Williams RJ. (2002) Phosphatidylinositol 3-kinase is a central mediator of NMDA receptor signalling to MAP kinase (Erk1/2), Akt/PKB and CREB in striatal neurones. J Neurochem 80(2):239-254.
[183] Petralia RS, Al-Hallaq R, Wenthold RJ. (2009) Trafficking and Targeting of NMDA receptors. In Biology of the NMDA Receptor, CRC Press, New York, pp. 149-200.
[184] Petralia RS, Sans N, Wang YX, Wenthold RJ. (2005) Ontogeny of postsynaptic density proteins at glutamatergic synapses. Mol Cell Neurosci 29:436-452.
[185] Phillis JW, O'Regan MH. (2004) A potentially critical role of phospholipases in central nervous system ischemic, traumatic, and neurodegenerative disorders. Brain Res Brain Res Rev 44(1):13-47.
[186] Ponniah S, Wang DZ, Lim KL, Pallen CJ. (1999) Targeted disruption of the tyrosine phosphatase PTPalpha leads to constitutive downregulation of the kinases Src and Fyn. Curr Biol 9(10):535-538.
[187] Powers WJ. (1990) Stroke. In Neurobiology of Disease, Oxford University Press, Toronto, pp. 339-355.
[188] Prybylowski K, Chang K, Sans N, Kan L, Vicini S, Wenthold RJ. (2005) The synaptic localization of NR2B-containing NMDA receptors is controlled by interactions with PDZ proteins and AP-2. Neuron 47(6):845-857.
[189] Qizilbash N, Duffy SW, Warlow C, Mann, J. (1992) Lipids are risk factors for ischemic stroke – review and overview. Cerebrovascular Disease 2:127-136.
[190] Randall RD, Thayer SA. (1992) Glutamate-induced calcium transient triggers delayed calcium overload and neurotoxicity in rat hippocampal neurons. J Neurosci 12:1882-1895.
[191] Rao A, Craig AM. (1997) Activity regulates the synaptic localization of the NMDA receptor in hippocampal neurons. Neuron 19(4):801-812.
[192] Ray SK. (2006) Currently evaluated calpain and caspase inhibitors for neuroprotection in experimental brain ischemia. Curr Med Chem 13(28):3425-3440.
[193] Récasens M, Guiramand J, Aimar R, Abdulkarim A, Barbanel G. (2007) Metabotropic glutamate receptors as drug targets. Curr Drug Targets 8(5):651-681.
[194] Reynolds IJ, Hastings TG. (1995) Glutamate induces the production of reactive oxygen species in cultured forebrain neurons following NMDA receptor activation. J Neurosci 15:3318-3327.
[195] Roche S, Koegl M, Barone MV, Roussel MF, Courtneidge SA. (1995) DNA synthesis induced by some but not all growth factors requires Src family protein tyrosine kinases. Mol Cell Biol 15(2):1102-1109.
[196] Roche KW, Standley S, McCallum J, Dune Ly C, Ehlers MD, Wenthold RJ. (2001) Molecular determinants of NMDA receptor internalization. Nat Neurosci 4(8):794-802.
[197] Rong Y, Lu X, Bernard A, Khrestchatisky M, Baudry M. (2001) Tyrosine phosphorylation of ionotropic glutamate receptors by Fyn or Src differentially

modulates their susceptibility to calpain and enhances their binding to spectrin and PSD-95. J Neurochem 79(2):382-390.

[198] Rosamond W, Flegal K, Friday G, et al. (2007) Heart disease and stroke statistics – 2007 update: a report from the American heart association statistics committee and stroke statistics subcommittee. Circulation 115, e69–e110.

[199] Rothman SM Olney JW. (1986) Glutamate and the pathophysiology of hypoxic-ischemic brain damage. Ann Neurol 19:105-111.

[200] Rowe MK, Chuang DM. (2004) Lithium neuroprotection: molecular mechanisms and clinical implications. Expert Rev Mol Med 6(21):1-18.

[201] Ryan TJ, Emes RD, Grant SG, Komiyama NH. (2008) Evolution of NMDA receptor cytoplasmic interaction domains: implications for organisation of synaptic signalling complexes. BMC Neurosci 9:6.

[202] Sacco RL, Boden-Albala B, Gan R, Chen X, Kargman DE, Shea S, Paik MC, Hauser WA. (1998) Stroke incidence among white, black, and Hispanic residents of an urban community. The Northern Manhattan Stroke Study. Am J Epidemiology 147:259-268.

[203] Sacco RL, Boden-Albala B. (2001) Stroke risk factors: identifiction and modification. In Stroke Therapy, 2nd Edition, Butterworth-Heinemann, U.S.A., pp. 1-24.

[204] Salter M, Kalia L. (2004) Src kinases: a hub for NMDA receptor regulation. Nat Rev Neurosci 5:317-328.

[205] Salter MW, Dong Y, Kalia LV, Liu XJ, Pitcher G. (2009) Regulation of NMDA receptors by kinases and phosphatases. In Biology of the NMDA Receptor, CRC Press, New York, pp. 123-148.

[206] Sato Y, Tao YX, Su Q, Johns RA. (2008) Post-synaptic density-93 mediates tyrosine phosphorylation of the N-methyl-D-aspartate receptors. Neuroscience 153(3):700-708.

[207] Sattler R, Charlton MP, Hafner M, Tymianski M. (1998) Distinct influx pathways, not calcium load, determine neuronal vulnerability to calcium neurotoxicity. J Neurochem 71(6):2349-2364.

[208] Schlaepfer WW, Bunge RP. (1973) Effects of calcium ion concentration on the degeneration of amputated axons in tissue culture. J Cell Biol 59:456-470.

[209] Shamloo M, Wieloch T. (1999) Changes in protein tyrosine phosphorylation in the rat brain after cerebral ischemia in a model of ischemic tolerance. J Cereb Blood Flow Metab 19(2):173-183.

[210] Shaper AG, Phillips AN, Pocock SJ, Walker M, Macfarlane PW. (1991) Risk factors for stroke in middle aged British men. BMJ 302(6785):1111-5.

[211] Sicheri F, Kuriyan J. (1997) Structures of Src-family tyrosine kinases. Curr Opin Struct Biol 7(6):777-785.

[212] Siciliano JC, Toutant M, Derkinderen P, Sasaki T, Girault JA. (1996) Differential regulation of proline-rich tyrosine kinase 2/cell adhesion kinase beta (PYK2/CAKbeta) and pp125(FAK) by glutamate and depolarization in rat hippocampus. J Biol Chem 271(46):28942-28946.

[213] Siesjo BK. (1986) Calcium and ischemic brain damage. Exp Neurol 25(Suppl 1):45-56.

[214] Siesjo BK, Katsura K, Mellergard P, Ekholm A, Lundgren J, Smith ML. (1993) Acidosis-related brain damage. Prog Brain Res 96:23-48.

[215] Simon RP, Swan JH, Griffiths T, Meldrum BS. (1984) Blockade of NMDA receptors may protect against ischemic damage in the brain. Science 226:850-852.

[216] Snyder EM, Nong Y, Almeida CG, Paul S, Moran T, Choi EY, Nairn AC, Salter MW, Lombroso PJ, Gouras GK, Greengard P. (2005) Regulation of NMDA receptor trafficking by amyloid-beta. Nat Neurosci 8(8):1051-1058.

[217] Sorimachi H, Ishiura S, Suzuki K. (1997) Structure and physiological function of calpains. Biochem J 328:721-732.

[218] Stehelin D, Varmus HE, Bishop JM, Vogt PK. (1976) DNA related to the transforming gene(s) of avian sarcoma viruses is present in normal avian DNA. Nature 260(5547):170-173.

[219] Stoker A, Dutta R. (1998) Protein tyrosine phosphatases and neural development. Bioessays 20(6):463-472.

[220] Sudol M, Grant SG, Maisonpierre PC. (1993) Proto-oncogenes and signaling processes in neural tissues. Neurochem Int 4:369-384.

[221] Suzuki T, Okumura-Noji K. (1995) NMDA receptor subunits epsilon 1 (NR2A) and epsilon 2 (NR2B) are substrates for Fyn in the postsynaptic density fraction isolated from the rat brain. Biochem Biophys Res Commun 216(2):582-588.

[222] Swope SL, Moss SJ, Raymond LA, Huganir RL. (1999) Regulation of ligand-gated ion channels by protein phosphorylation. Adv Second Messenger Phosphoprotein Res 33:49-78.

[223] Szydlowska K, Tymianski M. (2010) Calcium, ischemia and excitotoxicity. Cell Calcium 47(2):122-129.

[224] Takagi K, Ginsberg MD, Globus MY, Dietrich WD, Martinez E, Kraydieh S, Busto R. (1993) Changes in amino acid neurotransmitters and cerebral blood flow in the ischemic penumbral region following middle cerebral artery occlusion in the rat: correlation with histopathology. J Cereb Blood Flow Metab 13(4):575-585.

[225] Takagi N, Shinno K, Teves L, Bissoon N, Wallace MC, Gurd JW. (1997) Transient ischemia differentially increases tyrosine phosphorylation of NMDA receptor subunits 2A and 2B. J Neurochem 69(3):1060-1065.

[226] Takagi N, Cheung HH, Bissoon N, Teves L, Wallace MC, Gurd JW. (1999) The effect of transient global ischemia on the interaction of Src and Fyn with the N-methyl-D-aspartate receptor and postsynaptic densities: possible involvement of Src homology 2 domains. J Cereb Blood Flow Metab 19(8):880-888.

[227] Takagi N, Logan R, Teves L, Wallace MC, Gurd JW. (2000) Altered interaction between PSD-95 and the NMDA receptor following transient global ischemia. J Neurochem 74(1):169-178.

[228] Takagi N, Sasakawa K, Besshoh S, Miyake-Takagi K, Takeo S. (2003) Transient ischemia enhances tyrosine phosphorylation and binding of the NMDA receptor to the Src homology 2 domain of phosphatidylinositol 3-kinase in the rat hippocampus. J Neurochem 84(1):67-76.

[229] Tanaka C, Nishizuka Y. (1994) The protein kinase C family for neuronal signaling. Annu Rev Neurosci 17:551-567.

[230] Ter Horst G, Postigo A. (1997) Stroke: prevalence and mechanisms of cell death. In Clinical Pharmacology of Cerebral Ischaemia, Humana, New Jersey, pp. 1-30.

[231] Tezuka T, Umemori H, Akiyama T, Nakanishi S, Yamamoto T. (1999) PSD-95 promotes Fyn-mediated tyrosine phosphorylation of the N-methyl-D-aspartate receptor subunit NR2A. Proc Natl Acad Sci USA 96(2):435-440.

[232] Thayer SA, Usachev YM, Pottorf WJ. (2002) Modulating Ca^{2+} clearance from neurons. Frontiers Biosci 7:d1255-1279.

[233] Tovar KR, Westbrook GL (1999) The incorporation of NMDA receptors with a distinct subunit composition at nascent hippocampal synapses in vitro. J Neurosci 19:4180-4188.

[234] Tovar KR, Westbrook GL. (2002) Mobile NMDA receptors at hippocampal synapses. Neuron 34(2):255-264.

[235] Traub LM. (2009) Tickets to ride: selecting cargo for clathrin-regulated internalization. Nat Rev Mol Cell Biol 10(9):583-596.

[236] Traynelis SF, Wollmuth LP, McBain CJ, Menniti FS, Vance KM, Ogden KK, Hansen KB, Yuan H, Myers SJ, Dingledine R. (2010) Glutamate receptor ion channels: structure, regulation, and function. Pharmacol Rev 62(3):405-496.

[237] Trepanier CH, Jackson MF, MacDonald JF. (2012) Regulation of NMDA receptors by the tyrosine kinase Fyn. FEBS Journal 279:12-19.

[238] Ubersax JA, Ferrell JE Jr. (2007) Mechanisms of specificity in protein phosphorylation. Nat Rev Mol Cell Biol 8(7):530-541.

[239] Umemori H, Ogura H, Tozawa N, Mikoshiba K, Nishizumi H, Yamamoto T. (2003) Impairment of N-methyl-D-aspartate receptor-controlled motor activity in LYN-deficient mice. Neuroscience 118(3):709-713.

[240] Vaughan J & Bullock R. (1999) Cellular and vascular pathophysiology of stroke. In Stroke Therapy: Basic, Preclinical, and Clinical Directions, Wiley-Liss, Toronto, pp. 3-38.

[241] Vinade L, Petersen JD, Do K, Dosemeci A, Reese TS. (2001) Activation of calpain may alter the postsynaptic density structure and modulate anchoring of NMDA receptors. Synapse 40(4):302-309.

[242] Vissel B, Krupp JJ, Heinemann SF, Westbrook GL. (2001) A use-dependent tyrosine dephosphorylation of NMDA receptors is independent of ion flux. Nat Neurosci 4(6):587-596.

[243] Waksman G, Kumaran S, Lubman O. (2004) SH2 domains: role, structure and implications for molecular medicine. Expert Rev Mol Med 6(3):1-18.

[244] Walaas SI, Greengard P. (1991) Protein phosphorylation and neuronal function. Pharmacol Rev 43(3):299-349.

[245] Wan Q, Xiong ZG, Man HY, Ackerley CA, Braunton J, Lu WY, Becker LE, MacDonald JF, Wang YT. (1997) Recruitment of functional GABA(A) receptors to postsynaptic domains by insulin. Nature 388(6643):686-690.

[246] Wang K, Hackett JT, Cox ME, Van Hoek M, Lindstrom JM, Parsons SJ. (2004) Regulation of the neuronal nicotinic acetylcholine receptor by SRC family tyrosine kinases. J Biol Chem. 279(10):8779-8786.

[247] Wang WQ, Sun JP, Zhang ZY. (2003) An overview of the protein tyrosine phosphatase superfamily. Curr Top Med Chem 3(7):739-748.

[248] Wang WW, Hu SQ, Li C, Zhou C, Qi SH, Zhang GY. (2010) Transduced PDZ1 domain of PSD-95 decreases Src phosphorylation and increases nNOS (Ser847) phosphorylation contributing to neuroprotection after cerebral ischemia. Brain Res 1328:162-170.

[249] Wang Y, Salter M. (1994) Regulation of NMDA receptors by tyrosine kinases and phosphatases. Nature 369:233-235.

[250] Wang Y, Yu X, Salter M. (1996) Ca^{2+}-independent reduction of N-methyl-D-aspartate channel activity by protein tyrosine phosphatase. Proc Natl Acad Sci USA 93:1721-1725.

[251] Wannamethee G, Shaper AG. (1992) Physical activity and stroke in British middle aged men. BMJ 304:597-601.

[252] Watanabe M, Inoue Y, Sakimura K, Mishina M. (1992) Developmental changes in distribution of NMDA receptor channel subunit mRNAs. NeuroReport 3:1138-1140.

[253] Watanabe M, Inoue Y, Sakimura K, Mishina M. (1993) Distinct distributions of five N-methyl-D-aspartate receptor channel subunit mRNAs in the forebrain. J Comp Neurol 338(3):377-390.

[254] Wei G, Yin Y, Li W, Bito H, She H, Mao Z. (2012) Calpain-mediated degradation of myocyte enhancer factor 2D contributes to excitotoxicity by activation of extrasynaptic N-methyl-D-aspartate receptors. J Biol Chem 287(8):5797-5805.

[255] World Health Organization. Global Burden of Stroke. (2004) The atlas of heart disease and stroke. http://www.who.int/cardiovascular_diseases/en/cvd_atlas_15_burden_stroke.pdf.

[256] Wolf PA, D'Agostino RB, Belanger AJ, Kannel WB. (1991a) Probability of stroke: a risk profile from the Framingham study. Stroke 22:312-318.

[257] Wolf PA, Abbott RD, Kannel WB. (1991b) Atrial fibrillation as an independent risk factor for stroke: the Framingham study. Stroke 22:983-988.

[258] Wu HW, Li HF, Guo J. (2007) N-methyl-D-aspartate receptors mediate diphosphorylation of extracellular signal-regulated kinases through Src family tyrosine kinases and Ca2+/calmodulin-dependent protein kinase II in rat hippocampus after cerebral ischemia. Neurosci Bull 23(2):107-112.

[259] Xiong WC, Mei L. (2003) Roles of FAK family kinases in nervous system. Front Biosci 8:s676-s682.

[260] Xiong Z, Raouf R, Lu WY, Wang LY, Orser BA, Dudek EM, Browning MD, MacDonald JF. (1998) Regulation of N-methyl-D-aspartate receptor function by constitutively active protein kinase C. Mol Pharmacol 54(6):1055-1063.

[261] Xiong Z, Pelkey K, Lu W, Lu Y, Roder J, MacDonald J, Salter M. (1999) Src potentiation of NMDA receptors in hippocampal and spinal neurons is not mediated by reducing zinc inhibition. J Neurosci 19:RC37(1-6).

[262] Xu J, Kurup P, Bartos JA, Patriarchi T, Hell JW, Lombroso PJ. (2012) Striatal-enriched Protein-tyrosine Phosphatase (STEP) Regulates Pyk2 Kinase Activity. J Biol Chem 287(25):20942-20956.

[263] Xu J, Kurup P, Zhang Y, Goebel-Goody SM, Wu PH, Hawasli AH, Baum ML, Bibb JA, Lombroso PJ. (2009) Extrasynaptic NMDA receptors couple preferentially to excitotoxicity via calpain-mediated cleavage of STEP. J Neurosci 29(29):9330-9343.

[264] Xu J, Liu Y, Zhang GY. (2008) Neuroprotection of GluR5-containing kainate receptor activation against ischemic brain injury through decreasing tyrosine phosphorylation of N-methyl-D aspartate receptors mediated by Src kinase. J Biol Chem 283(43):29355-29366.

[265] Xu W. (2011) PSD-95-like membrane associated guanylate kinases (PSD-MAGUKs) and synaptic plasticity. Curr Opin Neurobiol 21(2):306-312.

[266] Xu W, Doshi A, Lei M, Eck MJ, Harrison SC. (1999) Crystal structures of c-Src reveal features of its autoinhibitory mechanism. Mol Cell 3(5):629-638.

[267] Yaka R, Thornton C, Vagts AJ, Phamluong K, Bonci A, Ron D. (2002) NMDA receptor function is regulated by the inhibitory scaffolding protein, RACK1. Proc Natl Acad Sci USA 99(8):5710-57155.

[268] Yan JZ, Liu Y, Zong YY, Zhang GY. (2012) Knock-down of postsynaptic density protein 95 expression by antisense oligonucleotides protects against apoptosis-like cell death induced by oxygen-glucose deprivation in vitro. Neurosci Bull 28(1):69-76.

[269] Yokota M, Saido TC, Miyaji K, Tani E, Kawashima S, Suzuki K. (1994) Stimulation of protein-tyrosine phosphorylation in gerbil hippocampus after global forebrain ischemia. Neurosci Lett 168(1-2):69-72.

[270] Yu XM, Askalan R, Keil GJ, Salter MW. (1997) NMDA channel regulation by channel associated protein tyrosine kinase Src. Science 275(5300):674-678.

[271] Zalewska T, Ziemka-Nałecz M, Domańska-Janik K. (2005) Transient forebrain ischemia effects interaction of Src, FAK, and PYK2 with the NR2B subunit of N-methyl-D-aspartate receptor in gerbil hippocampus. Brain Res 1042(2):214-223.

[272] Zhang C, Siman R, Xu YA, Mills AM, Frederick JR, Neumar RW. (2002) Comparison of calpain and caspase activities in the adult rat brain after transient forebrain ischemia. Neurobiol Dis 10(3):289-305.

[273] Zhang F, Li C, Wang R, Han D, Zhang QG, Zhou C, Yu HM, Zhang GY. (2007) Activation of GABA receptors attenuates neuronal apoptosis through inhibiting the tyrosine phosphorylation of NR2A by Src after cerebral ischemia and reperfusion. Neuroscience 150(4):938-949.

[274] Zhang L, Hsu JC, Takagi N, Gurd JW, Wallace MC, Eubanks JH. (1997) Transient global ischemia alters NMDA receptor expression in rat hippocampus: correlation with decreased immunoreactive protein levels of the NR2A/2B subunits, and an altered NMDA receptor functionality. J Neurochem 69(5):1983-1994.

[275] Zhang J, Diamond JS. (2006) Distinct perisynaptic and synaptic localization of NMDA and AMPA receptors on ganglion cells in rat retina. J Comp Neurol 498:810-820.

[276] Zhang Y, Lipton P. (1999) Cytosolic Ca^{2+} changes during in vitro ischemia in rat hippocampal slices: major roles for glutamate and Na^{+} dependent Ca^{2+} release from mitochondria. J Neurosci 19(9):3307-3315.

[277] Zhang Y, Kurup P, Xu J, Carty N, Fernandez SM, Nygaard HB, Pittenger C, Greengard P, Strittmatter SM, Nairn AC, Lombroso PJ. (2010) Genetic reduction of striatal-enriched tyrosine phosphatase (STEP) reverses cognitive and cellular deficits in an Alzheimer's disease mouse model. Proc Natl Acad Sci USA 107(44):19014-19019.

[278] Zhao W, Cavallaro S, Gusev P, Alkon DL. (2000) Nonreceptor tyrosine protein kinase pp60c-src in spatial learning: synapse-specific changes in its gene expression, tyrosine phosphorylation, and protein-protein interactions. Proc Natl Acad Sci USA 97(14):8098-8103.

[279] Zheng XM, Wang Y, Pallen CJ. (1992) Cell transformation and activation of pp60c-src by overexpression of a protein tyrosine phosphatase. Nature 359(6393):336-339.

[280] Ziemka-Nalecz M, Zalewska T, Zajac H, Domansk-Janik K. (2003) Decrease of PKC precedes other cellular signs of calpain activation in area CA1 of the hippocampus after transient cerebral ischemia. Neurochem Int 42(3):205-214.

Chapter 10

Function of Flotillins in Receptor Tyrosine Kinase Signaling and Endocytosis: Role of Tyrosine Phosphorylation and Oligomerization

Nina Kurrle, Bincy John, Melanie Meister and Ritva Tikkanen

Additional information is available at the end of the chapter

http://dx.doi.org/10.5772/48598

1. Introduction

There are two homologous members of the flotillin family which have been designated as flotillin-1/reggie-2 and flotillin-2/reggie-1, owing to their almost simultaneous discovery by two separate research groups (1, 2). In 1997, these proteins were described under the name "reggies", since they were found to be upregulated during the regeneration of retinal ganglion cells of the goldfish, following an optic nerve lesion (2). In the same year, Bickel *et al.* independently discovered them as components of detergent resistant fractions, and due to their ability to float in density gradients ascribed them as flotillins (1).

Biological membranes are complex structures composed of numerous proteins and lipids. As shown in Figure 1A, flotillin-1 and flotillin-2 are both constitutively associated with sphingolipid and cholesterol enriched membrane microdomains, known as lipid rafts (1, 3-5). Especially flotillin-1 is often considered as a *bona fide* marker protein for lipid rafts. The lipid raft concept was first postulated in 1997 by Kai Simons and Elina Ikonen (6), and has since then been refined and reshaped throughout the years. Nowadays, lipid rafts can be described as fluctuating nanoscale membrane assemblies composed of proteins, sphingolipids and cholesterol, which can coalesce to form platforms that are important for cell signaling, viral infection and membrane trafficking (7). It has been proposed that proteins with a high affinity for an ordered lipid environment, often achieved by post-translational modifications, will preferentially associate with lipid rafts (8). We have shown that flotillin proteins are linked to the plasma membrane by means of fatty acid modifications, especially myristoylation and palmitoylation (4), and both modifications facilitate the interaction with membrane cholesterol (our unpublished results). Earlier studies proposed that flotillins are localized in caveolae-type of lipid rafts, but later findings demonstrated that flotillins rather reside outside of caveolae and are thought to define their own subtype of lipid rafts (9).

The first description of flotillin-2 actually took place in 1994, when the group of Madeleine Duvic cloned an N-terminally truncated version of flotillin-2 from human epidermal keratinocytes and named it epidermal surface antigen (ESA) (10). However, in later studies by the same group, it turned out that the true ESA (ECS-1 antigen) is actually distinct from flotillin-2 (11). The flotillin-2 cDNA originally cloned by Schroeder *et al.* represents a truncated protein with a lower molecular mass that has not been detected *in vivo* and most likely came about due to a missing 5′ end of the cloned cDNA and false assignment of the ATG start codon. A monoclonal antibody ECS-1 raised against human keratinocytes was used for the identification of ESA. Curiously, a very similar approach with a monoclonal antibody against cell surface proteins was used by the Stuermer group to identify reggie-1/flotillin-2 and reggie-2/flotillin-1 as regeneration proteins of goldfish retinal ganglion cells (2). In this case, the true antigen of the M802 antibody was later shown to be identical with Thy-1, a glycophosphatidyl-inositol (GPI)-linked neuronal protein (12). Since flotillins have been shown not to traverse the membrane, it is unlikely that they were directly recognized by the antibodies used for the screenings. A more likely explanation is that flotillins were associated with the true antigens as molecular complexes and thus accidentally discovered. This is also supported by the data showing that flotillins are generally strongly associated with GPI-linked proteins (13-15). However, the details of their interaction have mechanistically not been clarified, since neither flotillins nor GPI-anchored proteins completely traverse the membrane. Thus, their interaction may be mediated by a yet to be identified transmembrane protein. Accordingly, we were able to show that both flotillins are coprecipitated after immunoprecipitation of surface biotinylated membrane proteins in confluent human epithelial MCF10A cells (our unpublished results).

Both flotillin-1 and flotillin-2 show a constitutive expression in almost all mammalian cell types and are highly conserved from fly to man (reviewed in 16). Furthermore, flotillin-like proteins are also present in bacteria (17), plants (18), fungi and metazoans but are absent in yeast and *Caenorhabditis elegans* (19). In humans, a 15 kb single-copy flotillin-1 gene with 13 exons is located on chromosome 6 (6p21.3), giving rise to a 1.9 kb mRNA transcript. The ORF encodes a 427 residue protein with a molecular mass of 47 kDa (20). A single copy of flotillin-2 gene is located on chromosome 17 (17q11-12) which encodes for a 48 kDa protein (10). Human flotillin-1 shares 98% identity with the murine protein and 47% identity with human flotillin-2. Flotillins are classified as part of the SPFH (Stomatin/ Prohibitin/ Flotillin/HflK/C) superfamily of proteins, also called prohibitin homology (PHB) proteins (21, 22). Different from other members of the SPFH superfamily, flotillins exhibit a conserved domain termed the flotillin domain C-terminally to the SPFH domain (Fig. 1B). This domain is characterized by several repeats of glutamic acid and alanine (EA repeats) and is predicted to form coiled coil structures (23, 24). A few years ago, the crystal structure of the core SPFH domain of mouse flotillin-2 was solved, and it shows partial similarity to the respective segment of *Pyrococcus horikoshii* stomatin (25). This structural region includes amino acids 43 to 173 of the SPFH domain of flotillin-2 and depicts that flotillin-2 SPFH domain has a compact, ellipsoid-globular structure, comprising four alpha helices and six beta strands. Although the structure of the flotillin domain has not yet been solved, it is predicted to show a high propensity for alpha helices. This could explain why flotillin domains are engaged in coiled coil structures that are important for the oligomerization of flotillins.

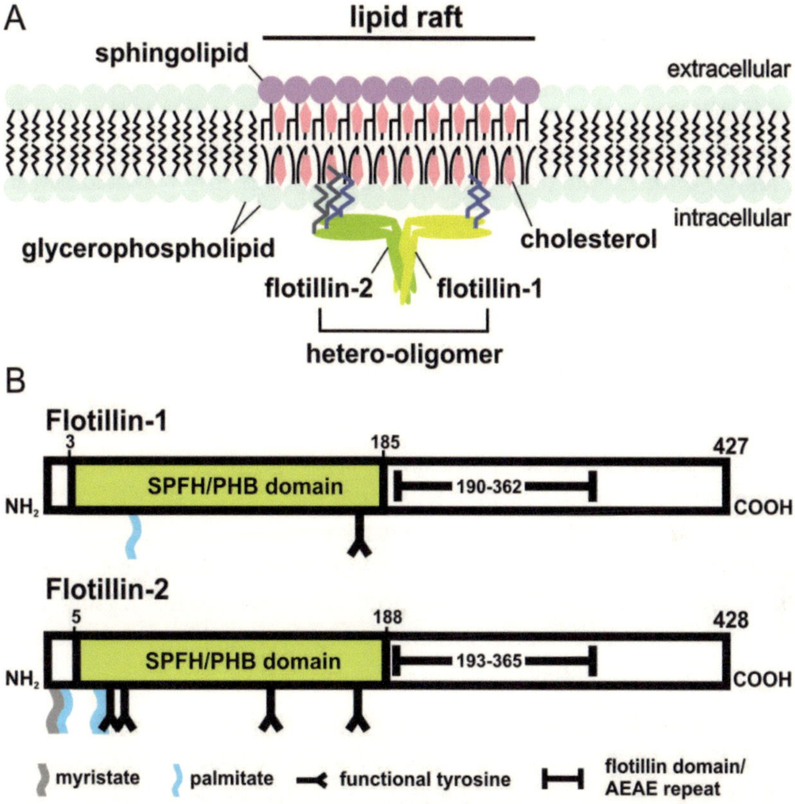

Figure 1. Flotillin-1 and flotillin-2 form oligomers in lipid rafts. A: Flotillin-1 and flotillin-2 are associated with specialized membrane microdomains, known as lipid rafts. Lipid rafts are defined as fluctuating nanoscale assemblies in membranes, composed of certain proteins and enriched in sphingolipids and cholesterol. They can coalesce to form platforms that are important for cell signaling, viral infection and membrane trafficking. Flotillin-1 and flotillin-2 are linked to the membrane by acylation, namely palmitoylation (both flotillins) and myristoylation (only flotillin-2). An important feature of flotillin function is the formation of homo- and hetero-oligomers. B: Flotillins contain in their N-terminal region a domain homologous with the prohibitin family of proteins, whereas their C-terminus is characterized by the unique flotillin domain with AEAE repeats.

2. Modifications, oligomerization and trafficking of flotillins

Flotillin-1 and flotillin-2 are ubiquitously expressed proteins and exhibit a relatively complementary tissue distribution. Northern blot analysis showed a high tissue-specific expression of flotillin-1 in murine brain, fat and heart tissue (1). High protein levels of flotillin-1 and flotillin-2 were found, e.g. in murine lung, thymus, bladder, cerebrum and hypothalamus tissue lysates (24, our unpublished results). Additionally, it has been shown that the expression of flotillin-2 increases during differentiation and myogenesis of C2C12 cells, whereas flotillin-1 increases during 3T3-L1 cell adipogenesis (1) and osteoclastogenesis (26). In contrast, during differentiation of rat pheochromocytoma PC12 cells, no change in the expression of flotillin-1 or flotillin-2 was observed (24).

The subcellular localization of flotillin-1 and flotillin-2 is as diverse as their tissue expression pattern and seems to be cell type specific. In glandular cervical cancer HeLa cells, PC12 cells, human hepatocellular carcinoma HepG2 cells, Chinese hamster ovary (CHO) cells and human breast cancer MCF-7 cells, flotillins mainly reside at the inner leaflet of the plasma membrane and to a minor extent in vesicular structures. A major localization in vesicular structures is found in astrocytes, the human HaCaT keratinocyte cell line and mouse embryonic fibroblast (MEF) cells. Colabeling experiments and immunogold electron microscopy studies identified the vesicular structures as endosomes and lysosomes in astrocytes, Jurkat, PC12 and HeLa cells (13, 14, 27-30). In line with the previous results, endogenous labeling of flotillin-2 in MCF10A cells shows a more prominent localization at the plasma membrane, whereas flotillin-1 is found in vesicular structures in non-confluent cells. However, with increasing confluency and advanced differentiation, flotillin-1 translocates to the plasma membrane (our unpublished results), a feature already observed in differentiating mouse 3T3-L1 cells (31). Rajendran *et al.* (32, 33) showed that flotillin-1 and flotillin-2 reside in preassembled structures under resting conditions in immature and mature hematopoietic cells, but they can move into uropods during cell migration and in immunological synapses during T-cell activation. These two studies highlight the fact that the subcellular localization of flotillin proteins is highly versatile and depends on the cell type and the differentiation status.

Total internal reflection fluorescence (TIRF) microscopy revealed that flotillin-1 and flotillin-2 exhibit a vesicular cycling at the plasma membrane (28), which seems to be independent of clathrin and caveolin (9, 13, 34, 35). Microtubule disruption in HeLa cells results in the accumulation of flotillin-1/flotillin-2 positive vesicles in the cytosol (28), while the same treatment in murine neuroblastoma N2a cells did not affect flotillin-2 localization (36). Manipulation of the actin cytoskeleton might also have a cell type dependent influence on the mobility of flotillins. In FRAP (fluorescence recovery after photobleaching) experiments, an increased lateral mobility of flotillin-2 after disruption of the actin cytoskeleton with cytochalasin D in N2a cells was observed, while treatment with the actin stabilizing compound jasplakinolide reduced the lateral mobility. On the contrary, the use of cytochalasin D in HeLa cells had no significant effect on flotillin-2 mobility (36). Recently, Affentrager *et al.* (37) showed that a dynamic actin turnover is required for capping of flotillin-1 and flotillin-2 in primary human peripheral blood T-lymphocytes, which underscores the importance of the actin cytoskeleton for flotillin localization and trafficking. The lateral motility is also dependent on the localization itself, since at least in Jurkat T cells, flotillin-2 is selectively immobilized in the region of the preformed cap and only shows a high lateral mobility at the plasma membrane outside the cap (29). In other studies, flotillin-

1 was found in exosomes of rat and human reticulocytes, human erythroleukemia K562 cells, lymphoid-B Daudi cells, human breast carcinoma MCF-7 cells and in exosomes of the cerebrospinal fluid (38-40). Flotillin-2 was detected in exosomes derived from MCF-7 cells and oligodendroglial Oli-neu cells (40, 41). Flotillin-1 was additionally found in mature phagosomes of murine J774 macrophages (42) and in the nucleus of human prostate cancer PC-3 cells (43).

Localization and trafficking of flotillins in the Golgi apparatus is still controversial. Nevertheless, evidence suggests that the involvement of Golgi in flotillin trafficking is also a cell type-specific process. In non-differentiated PC12, normal rat kidney (NRK), CHO and HeLa cells, flotillin-1 localizes to the Golgi complex (44-46). Also in rat brain tissue sections, flotillin-1 was found in the Golgi (47). In contrast, Morrow *et al.* (3) reported that flotillin-1 reaches the plasma membrane via a brefeldin A-resistant pathway in baby hamster kidney (BHK) cells. However, they did not rule out the possibility of Golgi involvement in flotillin-1 trafficking, as a GFP-tagged construct of the flotillin-1 SPFH domain colocalized with the cis-medial Golgi marker GM130 during early times of expression. Less is known about flotillin-2 and Golgi complex association. Only the study of Langhorst *et al.* (28) showed by immunogold EM microscopy that flotillin-2 was localized in vesicles in the Golgi field in Jurkat cells, but not in Golgi stacks.

Chemokines, growth factors and certain proteins can affect the localization and the trafficking of flotillin proteins. In Satb2-negative neuronal cells, flotillin-1 becomes more clustered in response to semaphorin 3a treatment, which acts as a potent guidance cue presented to cortical axons *in vivo* (48). In primary human peripheral blood T-lymphocytes, flotillin-1 and flotillin-2 are randomly distributed along the inner leaflet of the plasma membrane, and upon stimulation with stromal cell derived factor 1 (SDF-1), flotillins form stable caps in the uropod (32, 37). The best studied growth factor that has an effect on flotillin trafficking is the epidermal growth factor (EGF), as originally shown by us (30). Recently, we showed that flotillin-1 is indeed involved in the activation and downstream signaling of the EGF receptor (EGFR) (27). Upon stimulation with EGF, flotillin-2 becomes tyrosine phosphorylated at several tyrosine residues by Src kinases (30). This phosphorylation event is dependent on the activation of the EGFR, since the EGFR autophosphorylation inhibitor AG1478 prevents flotillin-2 phosphorylation. In regard to its localization, EGF stimulation results in a Tyr163-dependent translocation of flotillin-2 into the late endosomal compartment (30). Experiments in the group of B. Nichols confirmed our findings stating that Y163 is important for flotillin-2 internalization. In addition, it was shown that the corresponding tyrosine in flotillin-1, Y160, is crucial for flotillin-1 internalization (49). Other growth factors, such as hepatocyte growth factor (HGF) or insulin also affect the localization of flotillin proteins (Figure 2, and our unpublished results). Figure 2 shows that ten minutes after HGF stimulation, flotillin-1 is translocated from the plasma membrane to late endosomes/lysosomes where it colocalizes with LAMP3.

Posttranslational modifications of eukaryotic proteins are often important cues for localization, trafficking and membrane association of proteins (50). Two important modifications are N-myristoylation and S-palmitoylation. N-myristoylation is an irreversible

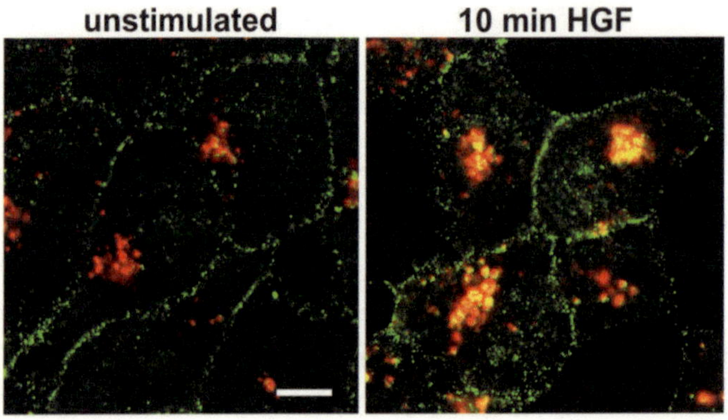

Figure 2. Flotillin-1 translocates to late endosomes upon 10 min of hepatocyte growth factor (HGF) stimulation. Staining of endogenous flotillin-1 (green) and endogenous lysosome-associated membrane glycoprotein 3 (LAMP-3; red) in HeLa cells stimulated for 10 minutes with HGF. Scale bar: 15 μm

acylation reaction at an N-terminal glycine residue, which is catalyzed by the enzyme N-myristoyl transferase (51). S-palmitoylation is a reversible reaction, in which the acyl group is transferred to cysteine residues by palmitoyl acyltransferases, referred to as the DHHC family (52, 53). In some proteins, e.g. Src-related protein tyrosine kinases, which are both myristoylated and palmitoylated, the myristoylation reaction is a prerequisite for the palmitoylation to occur (54). Our experiments with overexpressed flotillin-2 constructs in HeLa cells showed that flotillin-2 is myristoylated at Gly2 and palmitoylated at Cys4, Cys19 and Cys20, and Cys4 seems to be the major palmitoylation site (4). The myristoylation at Gly2 is essential for membrane targeting of flotillin-2, as the mutant flotillin-2 Gly2Ala remains fully soluble upon overexpression. Furthermore, the mutation of the cysteine residues to alanine and the concomitant loss of palmitoylation sites resulted in more soluble flotillin-2 mutants (4). In the study by Li *et al.* (53), the palmitoyl acyltransferase DHHC5 was identified as the enzyme to palmitoylate flotillin-2. In neuronal stem cells of DHHC5 gene-trapped mice, flotillin-2 palmitoylation was abolished. For flotillin-1, which is not myristoylated, it was shown that plasma membrane localization is dependent on palmitoylation of a conserved cysteine residue (Cys34) within its SPFH domain (3). This finding is supported by the study of Affentrager *et al.* (37), in which overexpressed flotillin-1 Cys34Ala exhibited a diffuse cytosolic localization in human T-lymphoblasts. In contrast, palmitoylation of this cysteine seems not to play a crucial role for plasma membrane targeting in adipocytes. Instead, deletion of the second hydrophobic stretch (residues 134 – 151) results in a similar cytoplasmic localization (31). This finding suggests that the effect of Cys34 palmitoylation in flotillin-1 function might be cell type specific.

Oligomeric proteins are prevalent in nature and comprise approximately one third of all known proteins. From the perspective of protein evolution, oligomerization may be of advantage for a functional control such as allosteric regulation (55). In the case of flotillin proteins, oligomerization is an essential feature for membrane raft association, endocytosis and EGF signaling (30, 56). Flotillin-1 and flotillin-2 form both homo- and hetero-oligomers (4, 5, 23, 34), and Solis *et al.* (23) suggested that flotillin oligomers exist in a monomer-tetramer equilibrium. The homo-oligomerization of flotillin-2 is mediated by the C-terminal half of the protein (amino acid residues 208-428), which seems to enhance the association of flotillin-2 with the plasma membrane and its membrane raft localization (4, 29). The C-terminal half of flotillin-1 and flotillin-2 contains the so called flotillin-domain, which contains several EAEA repeats and is predicted to form three adjacent coiled-coil structures. The formation of flotillin oligomers was shown to be dependent on the second and partially on the first coiled-coil structure (23). Using the flotillin-2 Y163A mutant, we showed that not the phosphorylation as such but hetero-oligomerization with flotillin-1 is indispensable for flotillin-2 endocytosis. In addition, our experimental data implicate that after EGF stimulation, preexisting flotillin oligomers form larger oligomeric complexes in which the stoichiometry of 1:1, also shown by Frick *et al.* (34), is preserved (56). In summary, these data show that not only the coiled coil structures within the C-terminal half of flotillins are important for the oligomerization, but also the tyrosine residue 163 in flotillin-2 plays a role in the hetero-oligomerization with flotillin-1.

Results of the Stuermer group have shown that ectopic expression of the presumed oligomerization domain of flotillin-2 comprising the amino acids 184 to 390 in Jurkat T cells interferes with function of flotillins in these cells and prevents the formation of macrodomains upon crosslinking of GM1 by cholera toxin (29). Hence, this fragment, termed R1EA, most likely prevents the proper oligomerisation of flotillins, thus functioning in a trans-negative manner. Upon overexpression of R1EA, insulin-like growth factor induced neurite outgrowth was abrogated in N2a neuroblastoma cells, and axon differentiation was impaired in hippocampal neurons (57). In addition, in R1EA expressing cells, recruitment of CAP/ponsin, which interacts with flotillin-1, to focal contacts was affected, resulting in imbalanced activation of Rho family GTPases Rac1 and Cdc42. Interestingly, focal adhesion kinase (FAK) activity was increased by R1EA expression. However, other signaling pathways such as ERK1/2, PKC, and PKB signals were unaltered (57). In line with this, previous studies have shown that upon growth factor stimulation of PC12 cells, protein kinase Pyk2, ubiquitin ligase Cbl and the CAP homolog ArgBP-2 are recruited to lipid rafts (58). Moreover, cholesterol depletion resulted in a diminished neurite outgrowth, suggesting involvement of membrane rafts (58). It has been proposed that ArgBP-2 associates with Cbl and Pyk2 via its SH3 domain and recruits them to lipid rafts by interacting with flotillin-1 through its SoHo domain (58). These findings point towards a vital role of flotillins in cytoskeletal remodeling and neurite growth at least in cultured cells. However, neither the flotillin-1 knockout mouse model (59) nor flotillin-2 deficient mice (our unpublished data) show a major neuronal phenotype. It thus remains to be clarified if flotillins are only required under conditions of neuronal regeneration or if they are generally important for the physiology of neurons in mammals.

3. In search of the molecular function of flotillins

As can be expected from such highly conserved and ubiquitous proteins, flotillins have been shown to play a role in a large number of vital cellular processes. Their original discovery as "reggies" suggested a function in neuronal regeneration in the goldfish (2, 45), which has been later verified by further studies from the same group (57, 60, 61). However, the regenerative capacity of the optic nerve is poorly conserved in mammals, making a generalization of the regenerative function of flotillins in the nervous system of mammals difficult. Recent studies have confirmed the relevance of flotillins for axon regeneration in zebrafish as well as in mammalian cell cultures. Apparently, downregulation of flotillins by flotillin specific morpholinos in the zebrafish resulted in a massive reduction in the number of regenerating axons (60). Since the role of flotillins in neuronal regeneration has recently been directly reviewed, we here omit a long discussion of the topic. Instead, the reader is referred to the recent review of C. Stuermer (62).

Flotillins also appear to be involved in membrane trafficking processes such as endocytosis and phagocytosis (13, 34, 42), and they have been suggested to be involved in the regulation the actin cytoskeleton (4, 11, 57). One emerging important function of flotillins, especially of flotillin-1, is the regulation of membrane receptor signaling, e.g. through mitogen activated protein kinases (MAPK) (27, 30, 43, 56, 63-67). Below, we have summarized the data on the function of flotillins in some of these processes.

Flotillins in endocytosis

During their discovery, flotillins were described to be associated with membrane rafts (1, 24). First findings suggested that flotillins would be integral membrane proteins of the cave-like invaginations called caveolae (1, 24), but these findings have later been disputed by several other studies (3, 9, 13, 34). However, the raft association of flotillins appears to be important for their function, and flotillin-1 has even been suggested to define a novel non-clathrin, non-caveolin endocytosis pathway that would operate via membrane rafts (13, 34). In eukaryotic cells, uptake of membrane bound molecules such as receptors can take place by means of several different pathways. The best characterized and the most common pathway for endocytosis is mediated by clathrin coated vesicles which are formed at the plasma membrane by the assembly of a coated pit which then forms a clathrin coated vesicle. However, recent research from several groups has revealed that endocytosis can be divided into numerous pathways, many of which do not require clathrin, and are thus designated as clathrin-independent. For a general introduction on endocytosis, the reader is referred to these excellent reviews (68-70). Some factors that regulate the clathrin independent pathways have been identified in the recent years, and it is clear that small GTPases such as Cdc42, Rho A or Arf (ADP ribosylation factor) family are involved, each determining their own endocytic pathway. The role of flotillins in endocytosis has recently been reviewed in detail (71), and we thus here only present a brief overview and a summary of the very recent studies not included in the review of Otto and Nichols.

Early after their discovery, flotillins were shown to associate and colocalize with GPI-anchored proteins. A role in the internalization of GPI-anchored proteins such as CD59 and of the glycosphingolipid GM1 has been demonstrated (13, 34, 72). Flotillins have also been suggested to be involved in the endocytosis of the GPI-linked Nodal coreceptor cripto (73). Although flotillins are affirmed regulators of cholera toxin subunit B endocytosis (13, 72), which is mediated by the binding of the toxin to GM1, no evidence for a direct role of flotillins in the endocytosis of the Shiga toxin or the plant toxin ricin was found (46). However, flotillins were shown to control other trafficking steps of these toxins, most likely a retrograde transport step towards Golgi/ER. Intriguingly, depletion of flotillins resulted in a higher degree of mannosylation of ricin, and the toxicity of both ricin and Shiga toxin was increased (46). Thus, flotillins are important factors in controlling not only the endocytosis but also other steps of the cellular trafficking of various molecules.

In addition to GPI-anchored proteins, flotillins have recently been shown to participate in the protein kinase C (PKC) induced endocytosis of neurotransmitter receptors such as the dopamine transporter DAT (also designed as solute carrier family 6, member 3 or SLC6A3) and glial glutamate transporter, GLT1 (74). PKC was shown to phosphorylate flotillin-1 at a Ser residue, and this phosphorylation was required for the endocytosis of DAT (74). Recent publications have revealed a role for flotillins in the endocytosis of the Alzheimer amyloid precursor protein (APP), the amyloidogenic processing of which requires its endocytosis (75). In addition, Niemann-Pick C1-like 1 (NPC1L1), an important mediator of the uptake of dietary cholesterol, relies on flotillins for its endocytosis, and depletion of flotillins drastically reduces cholesterol uptake in cultured cells (76). Curiously, APP, NPC1L1 and DAT are all endocytosed by means of clathrin mediated endocytosis, whereas flotillins as raft associated proteins have been rather suggested to define a non-clathrin endocytosis pathway, and there is very little colocalization between clathrin and flotillins (13). Thus, it is possible that rather than directly mediating raft dependent endocytosis through flotillin microdomains, flotillins might exert their function by first facilitating the uptake of some cargo molecules into rafts and their efficient clustering, but the act of endocytosis may only take place after transfer of the cargo into clathrin coated pits. Hence, it will be important in the future to study the exact relationship of flotillins and clathrin dependent endocytosis.

We have recently shown that flotillins are involved in EGFR/MAP kinase signaling, and siRNA mediated downregulation of flotillin-1 results in severe impairment of both EGFR phosphorylation and MAPK signaling (27). Since flotillins also become phosphorylated upon EGFR signaling (30), it would not be surprising if they were involved in EGFR endocytosis, which has been shown to take place by means of both clathrin dependent and raft mediated endocytosis (77, 78). However, according to our recent findings, flotillin-1 depletion does not significantly affect the EGF-induced endocytosis of EGFR (27). Furthermore, EGFR is efficiently endocytosed even in cells depleted of both clathrin and flotillin-1 (our unpublished data). Interestingly, recent findings from the Stuermer group have implicated that depletion of flotillin-2/reggie-1 may affect the endocytosis of EGFR (79). This finding is somewhat counter intuitive as flotillin-2 depletion induces a significant depletion of flotillin-1 as well, and flotillin-2 knockdown cells express only minor amounts of both flotillins. Flotillin-1 knockdown cells in turn still exhibit substantial flotillin-2 expression. Thus, these results imply that the flotillin-2 homo-oligomers that are still present in flotillin-1 knockdown cells may be capable of supporting normal EGFR endocytosis, whereas in the absence of flotillins, EGFR uptake from the plasma membrane is impaired. However, one also has to keep in mind some important methodological differences between our study (27) and that of Solis *et al.* (79). Our EGF uptake assays were performed with surface-bound iodinated EGF using short endocytosis times (up to 6 min), which allows the calculation of endocytosis rate constants for the receptor, providing a reliable and truly quantitative measurement of the early endocytosis and uptake of the receptor from the plasma membrane (80). We observed no difference between flotillin-1 knockdown and control cells even after very short endocytosis times (2, 4 or 6 min). However, Solis *et al.* used methods such as continuous uptake of fluorescent EGF for 5-10 min, or endocytosis of biotinylated EGFR for 120 min. In the latter assay, they observed an increased amount of EGFR remaining at the cell surface of flotillin-2 knockdown cells. However, also the total EGFR was increased in flotillin-2 depleted cells after 120 min EGF stimulation. Since substantial degradation of EGFR (and EGF) will evidently take place over such a long time, these results might indicate that the degradation and not endocytosis of EGFR is impaired, resulting in generally higher amount of remaining EGFR in flotillin-2 knockdown cells. Furthermore, when longer time points are used (10 - 120 min), some of the receptor will also be recycled back to the plasma membrane, thus biasing these results. In fact, considerable recycling of EGFR has been shown to take place in A431 cells (81). Hence, an increased amount of EGFR on the surface of flotillin-2 knockdown cells could also be a result of increased recycling combined with a reduced degradation. In addition to this, the A431 cells used by Solis *et al.* massively overexpress EGFR and are thus widely considered as a poor model system for EGFR trafficking, since the high amounts of EGFR may result in saturation of the endocytosis pathways normally used by the receptor and redirection of the receptor to pathways that otherwise play a negligible role. Therefore, the role of each flotillin in EGFR endocytosis should be reevaluated and directly compared in the same cell system with methods that are suitable for unbiased measurement of endocytosis, such as iodinated EGF uptake.

One important open question on the role of flotillins in endocytosis is if the flotillin-mediated endocytosis of various cargo molecules is dependent on the GTPase dynamin or not, since the studies have resulted in contradictory results, depending on the cell system used and cargo molecules studied. Since flotillins are endocytosed from the plasma membrane as a result of EGF stimulation (30) but appear not to directly affect EGFR endocytosis (27), they may in some cases also themselves represent cargo molecules whose cellular localization needs to be regulated during signaling. It is possible that depending on the endocytic process, cargo and stimulus, mechanistically different pathways are used. For a further discussion of this idea, please refer to the recent review of Otto and Nichols (71). Another important question is how the modifications (such as phosphorylation) and oligomerization of flotillins affect the trafficking of their putative cargo molecules. This topic is discussed more in detail below in the chapter "*Functional significance of phosphorylation and oligomerization of flotillins*".

Functions of flotillins in cell migration and adhesion

Already the discovery of flotillins by using antibodies directed against cell surface proteins led to the assumption of a functional role of flotillin proteins in cell adhesion (2, 82). Up to date, much has been speculated about this attribute, but only a few studies actually showed an involvement of flotillins in the establishment and maintenance of cell-cell and cell-matrix adhesion structures. One of the first functional hints was obtained in the study by Hoehne *et al.* (83), in which they investigated the functional role of flotillins in the model organism *Drosophila melanogaster*. The null mutant of flotillin-2 in *Drosophila* is viable and showed no visible phenotype, whereas Mz1369-Gal4 regulated overexpression of flotillin-2 alone or together with flotillin-1 resulted in a severe disturbance of the ommatidial pattern in regard to the number of primary pigment cells and cone cells. Furthermore, staining with antibodies against the cell adhesion molecules Roughest, Kin-of-irre and Sticks-and-Stones of the IgCAM protein family showed a strong labeling of an abnormal accumulation of multivesicular bodies in interommatidial cells. These observations led to the conclusion that flotillins interfere with the distribution of cell adhesion and signaling molecules in imaginal discs of *Drosophila*. In 2009, Málaga-Trillo *et al.* (15) published that the loss of the prion protein (PrP) in zebrafish embryos is characterized by the loss of embryonic cell adhesion. They presented confocal images of drosophila S2 cells, in which overexpressed mouse PrP-EGFP colocalized with overexpressed rat flotillin-2-dsRed at cell-cell contact sites. Similar results were obtained with overexpressed zebrafish PrP-2-EGFP with rat flotillin-1-dsRed and flotillin-2-dsRed as well as zebrafish flotillin-1a-dsRed. (15)

One major type of cell-cell contact in multicellular organisms is the adherens junction. The core of adherens junctions is composed of proteins of the cadherin and catenin family (84). Insights into a functional association of flotillins with this cell-cell contact type were obtained in the study of Bodrikov *et al.* (85), who showed that a transient knockdown of flotillin-2 in primary hippocampal neurons perturbed axon growth and differentiation. This phenotype was rescued in 62% of the neurons by overexpression of the constitutive active mutant of the GTPase TC10 which participates in the exocyst dependent polarized delivery of cargo to the growth cone (86). Interestingly, the amount of coprecipitated of N-Cadherin, which is a core protein of adherens junctions in adult neuronal cells, increased in flotillin-2 immunoprecipitates from mouse hippocampal HPL3-4 cells after application of PrP-Fc. Overexpression of a dominant negative TC10 blocked this effect, which indicates that the PrP together with flotillin-2 is important for the recruitment of N-Cadherin, which in turn takes place in a TC10-dependent manner (85). Very recently, the Stuermer group could show that flotillins together with the PrP play a role in E-Cadherin recruitment to adherens junctions (79). They showed that both proteins colocalized with E-cadherin at the plasma membrane in human epidermoid carcinoma A431 cells. Knockdown of flotillin-2 or PrP resulted in an abnormal shape of adherens junctions, causing overlapping of neighboring cells (79). In addition, electron microscopy revealed that the length of adherens junctions was shorter in flotillin-2 and PrP knockdown cells (79).

The complexing of the junctional proteins p120-catenin (p120ctn) and N-Cadherin at cell-cell contact sites was shown to occur in cholesterol rich membrane domains in mouse C2C12 cells (87). A similar observation was made in differentiated human colon adenocarcinoma HT-29 cells, in which the interaction of E-Cadherin with p120ctn preferentially takes place in lipid rafts. A stable knockdown of flotillin-1 resulted in a diffuse localization of p120ctn and an impaired recruitment of p120ctn and E-Cadherin in lipid rafts. In addition, flotillin-1 depletion decreased the enzymatic activity of ALP and DPPIV during the enterocytic differentiation process (88). This study revealed a novel function of flotillin-1 in a lipid raft mediated maturation of adherens junctions and in intestinal cell differentiation.

Other studies implicated that flotillins seem to be of functional relevance for cell-matrix adhesion processes. We showed that the transient knockdown of flotillin-2 in HeLa cells impaired cell spreading on fibronectin, as compared to cells transfected with control siRNA (30). Overexpression of flotillin-2-EGFP enhanced cell spreading and induced filopodia-like protrusions in an expression-level dependent manner in several epithelial cells lines, e.g. HaCaT cells (4, 30). The observed enrichment of flotillin-2 fusion proteins at cell-cell contact sites and the induction of filopodia suggest an active link to the cytoskeleton. Indeed, use of *in vivo* colocalization assays, *in vitro* binding assays and actin polymerization assays suggested that flotillin-2 interacts with F-actin via its SPFH domain, and that this binding mediates the anchoring of the actin cytoskeleton to the plasma membrane (36).

Role of flotillins in EGF receptor and mitogen activated protein kinase signaling

In the last 12 years, various studies have shown that flotillin-1 and flotillin-2 are physically and functionally linked to signal transduction pathways of several membrane receptors, especially receptor tyrosine kinases such as the insulin receptor (IR), the nerve growth factor (NGF) receptor, tropomyosin-related kinase A (TrkA), the polymeric Immunoglobulin E (IgE) receptor, fibroblast growth factor receptor (FGFR) and the epidermal growth factor receptor (EGFR) (27, 30, 63, 65, 89, 90). However, the mechanisms how flotillins may regulate the signaling process have not been dissected in detail. Only recently, we have shed light on the molecular mechanisms of flotillin-1 function in EGFR/MAPK signaling (27, 89). We showed that flotillin-1 actually plays a dual role by first regulating the clustering of EGFR in the plasma membrane after EGF stimulation and, later on during signaling, by functioning as a MAPK scaffolder protein (27). We also demonstrated that flotillin-1, but not flotillin-2, interacts with Fibroblast Growth Factor Receptor Substrates 2 and 3 (FRS2 and FRS3) (89) which have previously been shown to be involved in MAPK signaling (91-93). (See Figure 3).

Depletion of flotillin-1 in HeLa cells results in a decreased tyrosine phosphorylation of the EGFR especially at Tyr1173 already after a short EGF stimulation, and the reduced phosphorylation persists up to a time point where no phosphorylation of EGFR can be detected (27). By means of TIRF microscopy, we showed that the formation of EGFR clusters at the cell surface upon EGF stimulation is impaired after flotillin-1 knockdown. This fits well with the findings of Schneider *et al.* (75) who showed that flotillins might be important for the clustering of APP on the cell surface before its endocytosis. In addition to EGFR clustering, flotillin-1 depletion also prevents the association of EGFR and some of its downstream signaling partners with membrane rafts (27). Although the fraction of total cellular EGFR that is found in rafts is very low, this might be the population of the receptors that is capable of fast signaling upon stimulation. Earlier findings from Hofman *et al.* have suggested that the raft associated EGFR actually resides in two separate populations of rafts which then coalesce after stimulation, bringing the required signaling molecules in close

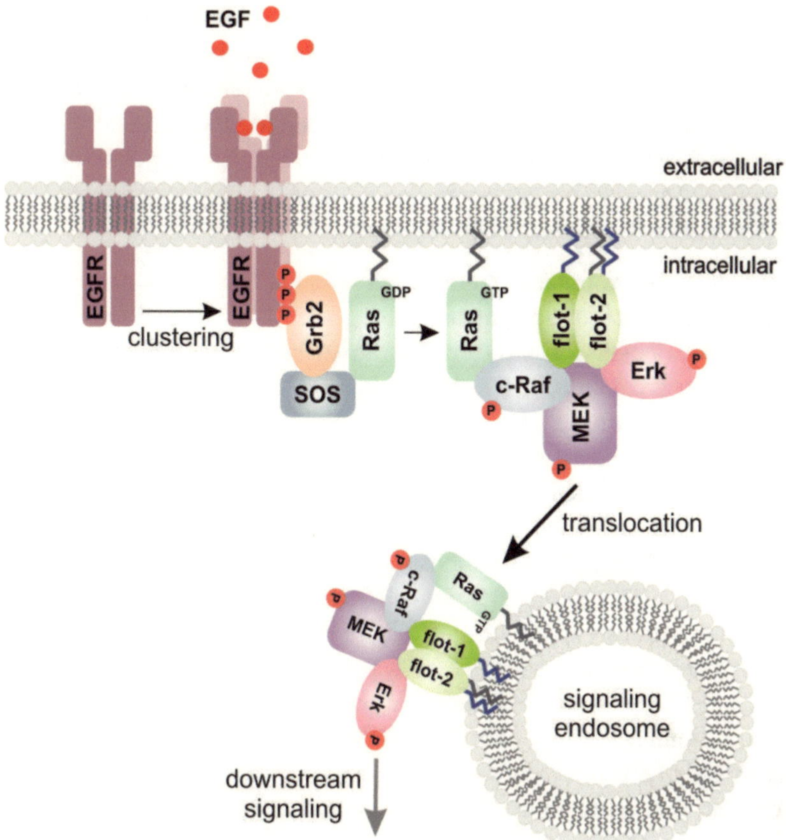

Figure 3. Flotillin-1 is a MAPK scaffolder - the role of flotillins in EGFR/MAPK signaling. Binding of the ligand EGF results in dimerization and activation of the EGFR. Thereby, several Tyr residues in its kinase domain become either autophosphorylated or phosphorylated by other kinases. These phosphorylation events lead to the recruitment of further signaling components, especially those of the MAPK signaling pathway. Grb2 binds to the phosphorylated EGFR kinase domain and transmits the downstream signal via Ras, c-Raf and MEK to the MAPK ERK1/2. The EGF-induced signaling through MAPK is initiated at the plasma membrane but later on translocates to specialized endosomes, i.e. signaling endosomes. Flotillins are able to associate with the EGFR itself and regulate the clustering of the receptor at the plasma membrane. Flotillin-1 directly interacts with the components of the MAPK signaling pathway, e.g. c-Raf, MEK, KSR1 and ERK and can thus be classified as a novel MAPK scaffolder.

contact (94). This model is well in line with our earlier findings showing that upon EGF stimulation, the molecular mass of flotillin oligomers increases, most likely due to their coalescence into larger complexes (56).

We also observed a reduced downstream signaling towards the canonical MAPK pathway and Protein Kinase B/Akt after stimulation with EGF or basic fibroblast growth factor (bFGF) upon flotillin-1 knockdown (27), implicating that flotillin-1 is not only involved in EGFR but also in FGFR signaling. Similar results with EGF have later on been obtained by

Solis *et al.* (79) in A431 cells, which overexpress EGFR to a very high degree, after flotillin-2 depletion. This is somewhat in contrast to our unpublished results in HeLa cells, which express physiological amounts of EGFR. In these cells, depletion of flotillin-2, resulting in nonexpression of flotillin-1, actually causes an increased MAPK phosphorylation upon EGF stimulation (A. Banning & R.T., unpublished findings). This again stresses the importance of using analogous cell systems for studies in signaling, as the degree of downstream signaling is highly dependent on the amount of EGFR expressed.

Flotillin-1 depletion also resulted in reduced activation of the MAPK pathway, especially of ERK kinases, which are required for transmitting the MAPK signal into the nucleus (27). Although flotillin-1 depletion clearly impairs an early step, EGFR clustering, during the signaling, which alone would be sufficient to inhibit MAPK signaling, this appears not to be the only reason for the reduced ERK activity. Incubation of the cells with phorbol myristate acetate (PMA) results in the activation of PKC, which in turn can active the cRAF kinase in the absence of an upstream EGFR signal (95, 96). Our attempt to overcome the downstream ERK inhibition by PKC-mediated activation of cRAF resulted in normal activation of cRAF and MEK kinases, whereas the ERK phosphorylation could not be rescued in flotillin-1 knockdown cells (27). This demonstrates that flotillin-1 must play a role not only at the plasma membrane but also at the level of ERK activation. Accordingly, we showed that flotillin-1 directly interacts with several MAPK pathway proteins, namely cRAF, MEK1 and ERK2. This interaction was not dependent on the MAPK scaffolder Kinase Suppressor of Ras (KSR), since flotillin-1 was found to coprecipitate with the MAPK component also in KSR1 depleted cells (27). Thus, these results suggest that flotillin-1 is indeed a *bona fide* MAPK scaffolder that is capable of directly interacting with several MAPK pathway proteins. Interestingly, the flotillin-1 interactor FRS2 has also been suggested to function as a scaffolding protein for the MAPK proteins (92, 97). Furthermore, our yeast two-hybrid studies have revealed another MAPK scaffolding protein, Mitogen-activated Protein Kinase Organizer 1 (MORG1) as an interaction partner of flotillins (our unpublished data). In future studies, it will be interesting to dissect the details of the regulation of MAPK signaling by flotillin-1, e.g. how these complexes are regulated during signaling in terms of their molecular composition and cellular localization.

The role of flotillins in EGFR signaling is supported by our recent findings in stable flotillin-1 and flotillin-2 knockdown human breast cancer MCF-7 cells (Figure 4). Comparable to HeLa cells, in MCF7 cells the stability of flotillin-1 is strongly dependent on flotillin-2, since the knockdown of flotillin-2 resulted also in a loss of flotillin-1. However, knockdown of flotillin-1 had no effect on flotillin-2 expression. Immunoblot analysis showed that the amount of EGFR is increased in flotillin-1 and flotillin-2 knockdown cells (Figure 4A). This effect is only visible in stable knockdown cells and not in transient knockdown cells, most likely due to an adaption of the EGFR amount to overcome the decreased EGFR-MAPK signaling in flotillin knockdown cells. We have previously observed this effect also in HeLa cells and other cell lines (our unpublished results). The EGFR, also known as ErbB1/Her1, is one of the four known members of the ErbB/Her protein-tyrosine kinase family (reviewed in (98)). Analysis of the protein amount of ErbB2/Her2 and ErbB3/Her3 showed no detectable

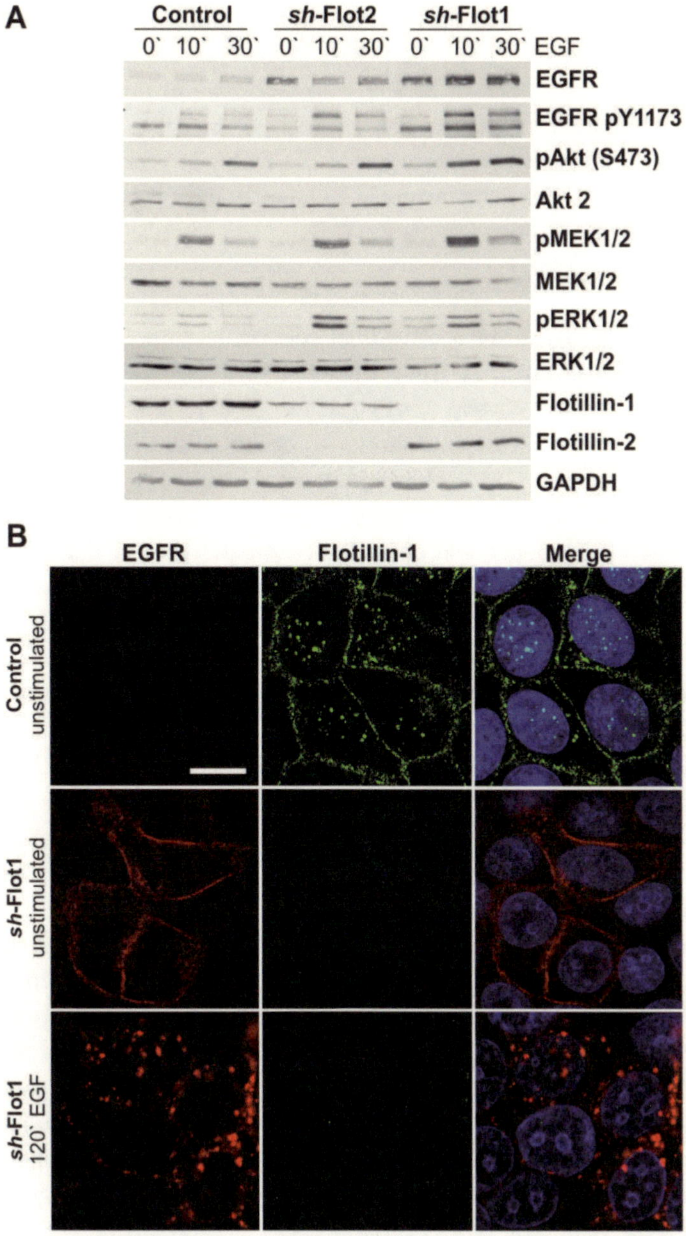

Figure 4. The reduced activation of the MAPK signaling pathway due to fiotillin depletion is compensated by an increased protein expression level of the epidermal growth factor receptor (EGFR) in MCF-7 cells. (A) Stimulation of stable flotillin-1 and flotillin-2 MCF-7 knockdown cells with EGF for 10 minutes and 30 minutes. The reduced activation of the MAPK signaling in flotillin knockdown cells is compensated by an upregulation of the EGFR protein level. (B) Immunofluorescence of endogenous EGFR (red) and endogenous flotillin-1 (green) in unstimulated and EGF-stimulated (120 min) flotillin-1 knockdown cells (sh-Flot1). Control cells are shown only in unstimulated state, due to undetectable EGFR level by immunofluorescence. Scale bar: 20 μm

change in the protein level (data not shown), which indicates that flotillin depletion specifically affects the protein level of the EGFR. In general, the endogenous EGFR is not detectable by immunofluorescence in MCF-7 cells, whereas in flotillin-1 depleted MCF-7 cells, a prominent staining at the plasma membrane is visible (Figure 4B). Stimulation with EGF for 120 minutes results in a translocation of the EGFR in vesicular structures in these cells. This is in line with our previous results in HeLa cells, indicating that the endocytosis of the EGFR is not affected by flotillin-1 depletion (27).

Flotillins and other receptor tyrosine kinases

The first experimental evidence for a functional role of flotillins in insulin signaling was presented by the Saltiel group (63). They demonstrated that flotillin-1 forms a ternary complex with c-Cbl-associated protein (CAP) and the E3 ubiquitin protein ligase Cbl upon insulin stimulation (Figure 5). This was shown to be important for lipid raft association, downstream signaling of the CAP-Cbl complex and finally for glucose uptake by the glucose transporter GLUT4 in 3T3-L1 adipocytes (63). Previously, the interaction of CAP with Cbl was shown to be independent of insulin stimulation *in vivo* and *in vitro* and to be mediated by SH3 domains (99, 100). In line with this, expression of CAPΔSH3 inhibited the translocation of GLUT4 from storage vesicle to the plasma membrane upon insulin stimulation (63). Further analysis of the flotillin-1 interaction mode with murine CAP isoforms showed that flotillin-1 only interacts with the isoform CAP-4 via its first hydrophobic domain, but not with the isoforms CAP-1, -2, and -3 (31). In CAP, the sorbin homology domain (SoHo) seems to be important for flotillin-1 binding, as the expression of CAPΔSoHo prevented the translocation of Cbl to lipid rafts in 3T3-L1 adipocytes (101). Since the murine CAP isoforms 1-4 all contain the SoHo domain, a predicted 70 amino acids long proline-rich region N-terminal to the SoHo domain in CAP-4 might also be of importance for flotillin-1 binding (102). While flotillin-1 was found in perinuclear regions in differentiated skeletal muscle cells (103), it was located at the plasma membrane in adipocytes (31) under basal conditions, suggesting that the role of flotillin-1 in targeting GLUT4 to the plasma membrane after insulin stimulation may differ between muscle and adipose tissue. Indeed, Fecchi *et al.* (103) showed that flotillin-1 colocalized with GLUT4 in the perinuclear region of myotubes, and both proteins translocated to the sarcolemma in a PI3K/ PKCζ- and caveolin-3 dependent manner upon stimulation with insulin. In addition, it was demonstrated that caveolin-3 is involved in the PI3K-dependent insulin signaling pathway, whereas flotillin-1 is crucial for the PI3K-independent insulin signaling pathway by interacting with the main scaffolding protein CAP. The interaction with CAP was also shown for flotillin-1 and flotillin-2 in mouse neuroblastoma N2a cells, in which overexpressed flotillin-1 and flotillin-2 colocalized with endogenous CAP at focal adhesion sites (57). This result indicates that by means of their interaction with CAP, flotillins might play an additional role in focal adhesion dynamics and integrin signaling.

Receptor tyrosine kinases of the Trk receptor family regulate various cellular processes, such as proliferation and differentiation, through several cellular signal cascades. Three types of Trk receptors exist in humans, including TrkA, TrkB and TrkC, which have varying affinities to neutrotrophins such as NGF. TrkA is specifically activated by NGF (reviewed in (104, 105). Downstream signaling by TrkA seems to be dependent on the lipid raft association of TrkA. Upon NGF stimulation, TrkA is recruited to lipid rafts in PC12 cells, a process dependent on its association with CAP, which in turn binds to flotillin-1 (65). The deletion of the CAP SoHo domain abolishes the lipid raft association of TrkA and further downstream signaling events such as ERK1/2 phosphorylation (65). (See Figure 5)

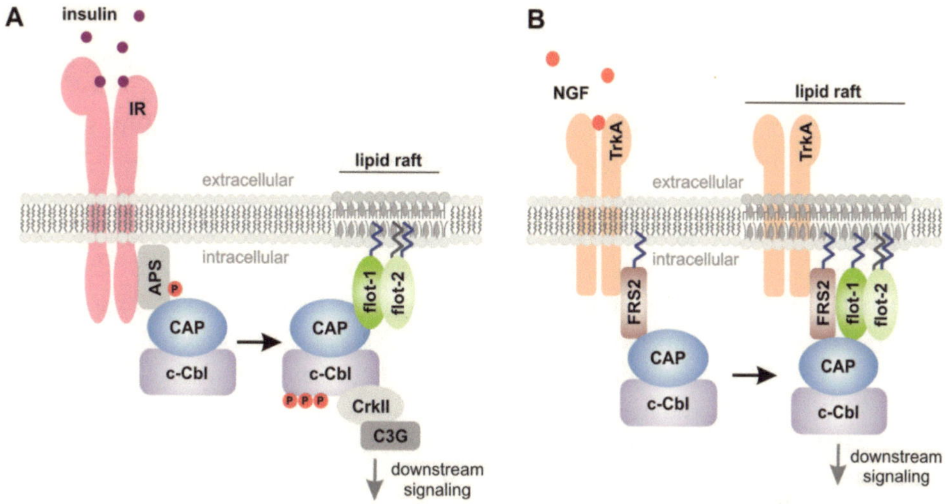

Figure 5. Proposed functional role of flotillin proteins in insulin and NGF signaling cascades. (A) Insulin is the major hormone controlling essential metabolic processes such as glucose and lipid turnover. Insulin binding to the extracellular subunits of the insulin receptor tyrosine kinase (IR) induces a conformational change and results in the autophosphorylation of several tyrosine residues in the cytoplasmic part of the IR. In adipocytes, the constitutive complex of the E3 ubiquitin ligase c-Cbl with the c-Cbl associated protein (CAP) is recruited to the active receptor. The interaction of CAP/c-Cbl complex with the IR was found to be indirect and mediated via the Adapter protein with Pleckstrin homology and Src homology 2 domains (APS). To initiate downstream signaling events, the CAP/c-Cbl complex then dissociates from the IR and is recruited to lipid rafts by forming a ternary complex with flotillin-1. (B) Receptor tyrosine kinases of the Trk receptor family regulate various cellular processes in the mammalian neuronal system, such as proliferation and differentiation by activation through neutrophins. The receptor TrkA is activated by the neutrophin nerve growth factor (NGF), which leads to the recruitment of the CAP/c-Cbl complex to TrkA. Since the fibroblast growth factor substrate 2 (FRS2) is also capable of binding to TrkA and CAP, it might be possible that the CAP/c-Cbl complex is recruited to TrkA by its interaction with FRS2. Most likely by the scaffolding activity of flotillin-1, the complex including the TrkA receptor is translocated to lipid rafts for a proper initiation and amplification of the downstream signal.

Recently, we have demonstrated that flotillin-1 directly interacts *in vitro* and *in vivo* with FRS2, a protein suggested to function in insulin signaling (106), by means of its N-terminal phosphotyrosine binding (PTB) domain and competes for the binding with FGFR (89). Interestingly, FRS2 was shown to interact directly through its PTB domain with TrkA in a phosphotyrosine-dependent manner after NGF stimulation (107, 108). Furthermore, we showed that in addition to flotillin-1, FRS2 also binds CAP by means of both its PTB domain and the C-terminal domain. In CAP, the SoHo domain in cooperation with the third SH3 domain mediate FRS2 binding (89). Both flotillin-1 and CAP bind to the PTB domain of FRS2, which suggests that CAP and flotillin-1 may compete for FRS2 binding to regulate the formation of signaling complexes.

Animal models for the function of flotillins

Flotillins are highly conserved proteins which are assumed, mainly on the basis of cell culture studies, to play multifaceted roles in developmental regulation. Hoehne *et al.* carried out initial studies of loss- and gain-of function of flotillins in wild type and mutant *Drosophila melanogaster* to investigate their role during morphogenesis and organogenesis (83). According to this study, flotillin proteins are highly expressed in embryonic neuronal tissues, and during later developmental stages flotillins showed an enhanced expression pattern in axon fascicles (83). Additionally, flotillin specific antibodies labeled in particular the *Drosophila* mushroom body, which is a paired structure of insect central brain responsible for higher-order sensory integration and learning. Flotillins showed a categorical neuronal expression, as antibody staining was restricted to optic lobes and central brain but was not observed in glial cells. A P-element-induced null mutant for flotillin-2 was viable, fertile and with no apparent deficits in behavior or overall activity. In this flotillin-2 null mutant, the expression of flotillin-1 was undetectable even though the mRNA transcript was present (83). Conversely, overexpression of flotillin-1 and flotillin-2 proteins either alone or together in the eye imaginal discs lead to mislocalization of adhesion molecules of the immunoglobulin superfamily (IgCAMs; please also refer to the chapter *"Functions of flotillins in cell migration and adhesion"*). Additionally, the adult flies showed a variable phenotype affecting bristles, ocelli, eyes, wings, abdominal segments and thoracic structures. A severe wing phenotype, including blistering and melanotic cells, was caused by flotillin overexpression in wing imaginal discs. Moreover, a later study showed that flotillin-2 deficiency resulted in reduced spreading of the morphogens Wnt and hedgehog, whereas flotillin-2 overexpression resulted in increased morphogen secretion and expanded diffusion. These findings qualify flotillin-2 as a novel component of the Wnt and hedgehog secretion pathway in D*rosophila* (64).

Flotillins are also implicated to regulate axon regeneration in a zebrafish model. As a consequence of gene duplication in fish, there are two copies of each flotillin gene. To understand the essential role of flotillins in axon regeneration, specific morpholino (Mo) antisense nucleotides were used to transiently downregulate flotillin-1a, flotillin-1b and flotillin-2a in zebrafish (60). Interestingly, the number of retinal ganglion cells (RGC) undergoing axon regeneration was reduced by 69% in flotillin-Mo treated eyes after 7 days (60). Recently, a zebrafish model was employed to study the role of flotillins in cholera intoxication. Consequently, flotillin-1 and flotillin-2 knockdown prevented cholera intoxication in zebrafish embryos. Moreover, cholera toxin subunit B (CTxB) colocalized with flotillins at the plasma membrane and in endosomes in COS1 cells (109). Thus, these results suggest flotillins as essential elements for axon regeneration and indicate a novel cholera intoxication *in vivo* model dependent on flotillins for trafficking between plasma membrane/endosomes to the ER in the zebrafish.

Cell migration is an essential mechanism during the development and maintenance of multicellular organisms. It requires the constant turnover of cell-matrix adhesion structures, e.g., integrin-based focal contacts. Results presented by Ludwig *et al.* (110) strongly suggest a functional role of flotillin microdomains during neutrophil migration, in uropod formation, and in the regulation of myosin IIa activity. They generated and characterized C57BL6/J mice lacking exon 3-8 of the gene for flotillin-1. In line with the observations in *Drosophila*, these flotillin-1$^{-/-}$ mice are viable, fertile, and have no readily apparent phenotype. On the cellular level, absence of flotillin-1 resulted in a greatly reduced flotillin-2 expression, and the residual flotillin-2 was not found in detergent-resistant fractions of flot-1 $^{-/-}$ MEF cells. These data suggest that deletion of flotillin-1 leads to the abrogation of flotillin microdomain function. Furthermore, isolated flotillin-1$^{-/-}$ neutrophils exhibited a defect in chemotaxis when exposed to the chemoattractant N-formyl-Met-Leu-Phe (fMLP). Previous reports have already shown that, upon stimulation with chemoattractants, flotillin microdomains rapidly distribute to the uropod, a contractile structure at the back of leukocytes (32, 111). This suggested that these microdomains could participate in polarization and/or chemotaxis. Ludwig *et al.* were also able to show by mass spectrometry of isolated flotillin microdomains and immunoprecipitation of flotillin-2-EGFP an association of flotillin microdomains with myosin IIa, α-spectrin and β-spectrin. Flotillin overexpression led to an increase of myosin IIa activity, whereas the loss of flotillins caused a reduction as measured by using phosphospecific antibodies (110). The regulatory effect of flotillins on myosin IIa activity strengthens the assumption that both proteins exhibit a functional role during cell migration, as myosin IIa was shown to act as a negative regulator of epithelial cell migration, and its ablation results in severe defects in focal adhesion formation and actin stress fiber organization (112, 113).

4. Functional significance of phosphorylation and oligomerization of flotillins

Recent data from several groups have revealed flotillins as important regulators of vital cellular processes such as signaling and endocytosis. One major challenge in the future will be to dissect how the oligomerization and the covalent modifications of flotillins affect their function during these processes. Endocytosis of flotillins appears to be influenced by upstream signaling (30, 49, 56) and requires clustering of flotillin-1 and flotillin-2 molecules (34, 56). We have shown that EGF stimulation results in uptake of flotillins hetero-oligomers from the plasma membrane, and that hetero-oligomerization appears to be required for the endocytosis (30, 56). Mutation of a single Tyr residue, Tyr163, in flotillin-2 is sufficient to prevent the EGF-induced endocytosis of flotillins (30), and this mutation impairs the hetero-oligomerization of flotillin-2 with flotillin-1 (56). Flotillins are phosphorylated by the Src family kinases cSrc and Fyn (4, 49), but the direct role of Tyr phosphorylation in the endocytosis is still under debate. Our data show that inhibition of cSrc kinase, the activity of which is necessary for flotillin-2 phosphorylation (30), does not impair the endocytosis of flotillin-2 (16), whereas the mutation of the single Tyr residue Y163 does (30). Thus, it is more likely that this mutation affects the oligomerization of flotillins and thereby also endocytosis. However, phosphorylation of flotillins by the Fyn kinase appears to be sufficient to induce endocytosis of flotillins (49), suggesting that the Src family kinases might play different roles in terms of flotillin function. It is also important to keep in mind that PKC has recently been shown to phosphorylate flotillin-1 in Ser315, and that this phosphorylation is required for the endocytosis of the dopamin transporter DAT (74). Thus, phosphorylation seems to be an important direct or indirect regulator of flotillin trafficking.

Not only phosphorylation but also covalent modifications with fatty acids myristate and palmitate take place in the case of flotillins (3, 4, 53). Mutation of Gly2 prevents the myristoylation and the subsequent palmitoylation of flotillin-2, thus also inhibiting its membrane association and rendering the protein soluble (4). Recently, the palmitoyl transferase DHHC5 was shown to palmitoylate flotillin-2 (53). Interestingly, growth factor withdrawal, which induces neuronal differentiation, resulted in rapid degradation of DHHC5 (53), implicating that palmitoylation might be important for the well established function of flotillins in neurite outgrowth in cultured neuronal cells. Since the soluble, non-modified flotillin-2 with Gly2Ala mutation seems to function as a dominant negative protein during cell-matrix adhesion (30), and successive removal of the three palmitoylation sites affect the membrane association of flotillin-2 (4), the fatty acid modifications, especially the reversible palmitoylation, are most likely important for the regulation of flotillin function. Accordingly, we have observed that flotillin-2 expression is necessary for the membrane association of flotillin-1, which is not myristoylated and only palmitoylated in a single residue. Thus, ectopic expression of flotillin-1 in flotillin-2 depleted cells results in a soluble protein that is not capable of exerting its function (our unpublished data).

Our recent findings revealed flotillin-1 as a MAPK regulator (27). However, no data are so far available on the role of flotillin modifications such as phosphorylation in the regulation of MAPK signaling. Intriguingly, another SPFH/PHB family protein, prohibitin-1, has been shown to regulate an earlier step during MAPK signaling, namely signaling by the small GTPase Ras and RAF kinase (114, 115). Although the most evident cellular localization of prohibitin is the inner mitochondrial membrane, various studies have now shown that prohibitin is a substrate of several cytoplasmic kinases such as Akt, and it becomes Tyr phosphorylated upon insulin stimulation of cells (116, 117). Thus, at least a fraction of prohibitin must be found in another cellular localization such as the plasma membrane. Importantly, prohibitin has been shown to be essential for cell migration that is induced by the Ras-Raf-MAPK pathway (115), and very recent findings show that phosphorylation of prohibitin, which takes place in a raft domain, is necessary for the Ras-dependent enhancement of cellular metastasis (118), verifying the results of Rajalingam *et al.* (115). Thus, there are several parallels in prohibitin and flotillin function, including MAPK signaling and cell migration, although they appear to be involved in different steps of the signaling. Since some evidence for a hetero-oligomerization of different SPFH-PHB family members, namely prohibitin and stomatin family protein SLP-2 (119) has been presented, it would be important to study if flotillins and prohibitins are capable of hetero-oligomerizing with each other and how this affects their function, especially with respect to the MAPK signaling. In the future, it will also be of interest to study if the phosphorylation-incompatible forms of flotillins cause aberrant signaling and if this effect is linked on phosphorylation at specific sites. Our previous data show that the function of flotillin-2 in cell-matrix association is indeed dependent on specific Tyr residues, the mutations of which affect cell spreading (30). Similarly, mutations of phosphorylated residues in flotillin-1 might affect its role in MAPK signaling and its interaction with the MAPK proteins.

5. Flotillins in human diseases

Role of flotillins in cancers

Early findings already indicated that flotillins may be involved in the regulation of the actin cytoskeleton. Overexpression of flotillin-2 was found to result in induction of filopodia-like protrusions and changes in the cytoskeleton (4, 11). Furthermore, flotillins have been shown to be important for the polarization of various immune cells such as T cells and neutrophils (29, 32, 33, 37, 110, 111), and to be involved in the regulation of the activity of various small GTPases that control e.g. the remodeling of the actin cytoskeleton (36, 57). In fact, flotillin-2 has even been suggested to directly interact with actin (36), although this has not been verified in further studies. Thus, there are very strong implications that flotillins are required for a proper regulation of the actin cytoskeleton, which is necessary for e.g. the control of cell migration. Consequently, taking also into account the numerous reports on the involvement of flotillins in signaling, it is evident that flotillins are critical factors that regulate the cell physiology and cell growth. Thus, the findings showing that flotillins are involved in some types of cancer are well in accordance with this function.

The strongest evidence for the role of flotillins in cancer to date comes from studies on human malignant melanoma. The direct association of flotillins with human cancers was shown in 2004 when the group of M. Duvic demonstrated that flotillin-2 is highly expressed in various melanoma cell lines, and that flotillin-2 expression correlated with the progression of human melanoma (120). Furthermore, the thickness of primary melanoma lesions, so-called Breslow depth, which is a prognostic marker for the malignancy of a melanoma lesion, showed a correlation with the increased flotillin-2 expression (121). Importantly, benign, non-malignant cells could be converted into tumorigenic, metastatic ones upon overexpression of flotillin-2 (120). Furthermore, flotillin-2 was shown to be associated with the thrombin receptor PAR1, the expression of which was dependent on the level of flotillin-2 protein (120).

Lin *et al.* detected a high expression of flotillin-1 in the majority of the breast cancer specimens they studied (66). Furthermore, they revealed a significant correlation between the expression level of flotillin-1 and poor survival of the patients, suggesting that flotillins might prove useful as novel diagnostic markers for cancer. Knockdown of flotillin-1 was shown to result in inhibition of Akt activity and increased transcriptional activity of the transcription factor FOXO3a. Knockdown of flotillin-1 also inhibited the proliferation of breast cancer cell lines by inducing a G1-S phase arrest of the cell cycle. In line with this, the expression of the cyclin dependent kinase (CDK) regulator cyclin D1 was reduced after flotillin-1 silencing, whereas that of the CDK inhibitors $p21^{Cip1}$ and $p27^{Kip1}$ was considerably increased (66), suggesting that flotillin-1 is an important regulator of the cell cycle. This result is strongly supported by our findings showing that in flotillin-1 knockdown cells, cyclin D1 expression after EGF stimulation is severely impaired (27).

Although flotillins evidently play a role in cancer and their overexpression is associated with malignancy, very little is known about their transcriptional regulation. Flotillin-2 was shown to be a transcriptional target of the p53 family transcription factors p63 and p73 but not of p53 (122). We have recently addressed this question more in detail and shown that flotillins are transcriptionally regulated by the Extracellularly Regulated Kinase signaling and by the Retinoid X Receptor (Banning *et al.*, in revision). Due to their important role in cancer, a deeper knowledge on the transcriptional regulation of flotillins is essential for understanding the mechanisms of malignancy that results from flotillin upregulation.

Implications of flotillins in Alzheimer's Disease and other neurodegenerative disorders

Alzheimer's disease (AD) is the most common age-related neurodegenerative disorder whose most prominent pathological hallmarks include neuronal loss, neurofibrillary tangle formation and senile plaques throughout the brain cortex. The major component of the senile plaques is the amyloid β peptide (Aβ) comprising of 40-42 residues, which is generated by a proteolytic cleavage of a large transmembrane precursor protein named amyloid β precursor protein (APP). APP is subjected to proteolytic processing at several sites by a group of proteases called secretases. Sequential cleavage of APP by β-secretase (β–site APP cleaving enzyme or BACE) and γ-secretases generates Aβ and is hence termed the amyloidogenic pathway (reviewed in (123-126)). APP can also be processed through a non-amyloidogenic pathway, in which the α-secretase cleaves within the Aβ sequence, thereby precluding the formation of Aβ. It has been strongly implicated that the amyloidogenic processing of APP takes place in lipid rafts, which is supported by the findings showing that APP can be detected in rafts isolated from cortical neurons (124). Besides APP, other AD associated raft resident proteins include BACE-1 (127), endoproteolytic fragments of presenilin-1 (PS-1) and the presenilins (128, 129). Compelling evidence from various research groups shows that the flotillin family of proteins is partially associated with AD pathology and trafficking (47, 130, 131). Flotillins are considered as classic raft markers in neuronal tissue since they show an abundant expression in the brain, typically in pyramidal neurons and astrocytes. Kokubo *et al.* detected flotillin-1-positive rafts in the plasma membrane and membranes of intracellular organelles in rat brain tissue by using immunoelectron microscopy (47). Consequently, they showed that in APP transgenic mice, flotillin-1 and Aβ42 colocalized in approximately 10% of flotillin-1 positive rafts, and that flotillin-1 expression increased with the accumulation of Aβ (132).

Parallel studies in brain sections from AD, Down syndrome and non-demented subjects with plaques showed enhanced flotillin-1 expression with the progression of AD (130). Further insight was provided by Rajendran *et al.* who demonstrated that in AD patients, Aβ accumulates and is located in flotillin-1 positive endosomes. They also showed that flotillin-1 was not only linked with intracellular Aβ in transgenic mice but was also present in extracellular plaques of AD patient brain sections (131). Furthermore, comparison of flotillin-1 immunoreactivity in the hippocampus, the amygdala and the isocortex of AD and control patients implicated that flotillin-1 principally accumulates in lysosomes of tangle bearing neurons during the advanced stages of AD (133). To date, the precise functional significance of APP and flotillin association is enigmatic. Schneider *et al.* proposed that flotillins could function as scaffolding proteins, forming a platform for clustering of APP and consequent endocytosis. Accordingly, flotillin-2 knockdown in mouse neuroblastoma cells impaired APP endocytosis and processing, resulting in reduced Aβ production (75). It has previously been shown that the intracellular domain of APP directly interacts with flotillin-1 (134). Our unpublished findings suggest that both flotillin-1 and flotillin-2 directly interact with APP, suggesting that both flotillins could facilitate recruitment of APP into microdomains.

Flotillins and other lipid raft-associated proteins might also be involved in other human neuronal diseases. The study by Shin *et al.* (135) showed an increased level of the lipid raft associated proteins caveolin-1, -2, and -3 in the spinal cord during the early stage of experimental autoimmune encephalomyelitis (EAE). EAE is an experimental animal model, mostly used in rodents, of inflammatory demyelinating diseases of the central nervous system (CNS), including multiple sclerosis (reviewed in (136)). Similar results with the caveolin data were obtained for flotillin-1 during the peak stage of EAE. Immunohistochemical analysis showed an enhanced expression of flotillin-1 in the dorsal horn lamina and in some flotillin-1-positive macrophages and astrocytes, in which it colocalized with the lysosomal marker cathepsin D (137). Due to that, they postulated that flotillin-1 inherits an important function in immune and neuronal cells within the CNS during EAE, possibly via the activation of signal transduction and lysosomal activity.

Parkinson's disease (PD) is one of the most common, progressive neurological disorders. The pathological hallmark of PD is the extensive loss of dopamine secreting cells within the substantia nigra, particularly affecting the ventral component of the pars compacta (reviewed in (138)), which can lead to uncontrolled muscle contraction and movement, dementia, depression and anxiety. Flotillin-1 staining in rat brain sections showed a prominent labeling in the cytoplasm of catecholamine releasing cells (dopamine, norepinephrine, and epinephrine) and an upregulated gene expression of flotillin-1 in the substantia nigra of Parkinson's brain by RT-PCR (139). Although the molecular function of flotillin-1 in Parkinson's disease is still not known, this study implies that flotillin-1 may be involved in the neuronal changes occurring during Parkinson's disease.

Flotillins and pathogens

During evolution, many pathogens have developed mechanisms to use host-cell lipid rafts as signaling and entry platforms to escape the host immune system (reviewed in (140, 141)). Several studies demonstrated that lipid rafts are often used as entry sites for bacteria, e.g., *Salmonella enterica (142)* or *Listeria monocytogenes* (143). In regard to flotillins, Li *et al.* (144) showed that flotillin-1 accumulates at bacteria entry sites and around intracellular enteropathogenic *Escherichia coli* (EPEC). This bacterium causes diarrheal disease by disrupting the integrity of tight junctions, which are essential structures for physiological homeostasis and defense against pathogen invasion. Furthermore, they detected a shift of flotillin-1 and occludin, a major protein of tight junctions, from Triton X-100 insoluble fractions to Triton X-100 soluble fractions following EPEC infection. This led to the conclusion that the loss of tight junction barrier function might be accounted to the redistribution of occludin and flotillin-1 after EPEC infection.

Not only bacteria use lipid raft domains as preferred entry sites in host-cells, but also various enveloped and non-enveloped viruses are dependent on an intact lipid raft structure and the presence of cholesterol for successful virus entry (reviewed in (145)). In the case of the retrovirus human immunodeficiency virus-1 (HIV-1), flotillin-1 was suggested to play a role of in the cellular response to the viral infection since the protein level of flotillin-1 was increased in peripheral blood mononuclear cells after treatment with the HIV-1 component gp120 (146). The primary HIV-1 receptor CD4 and the co-receptor CCR5, both of which are important for HIV-1 host-cell entry, were also shown to associate with flotillin-1 containing lipid rafts in monocytes (147). Recently, flotillin-1 was also identified as an interaction partner of the overexpressed rhesus monkey TRIM5α (148). TRIM5α is a member of tripartite motif (TRIM) protein family, and plays an important role during host cell defense against retroviruses such as HIV-1 especially in old world monkeys, but not in humans (reviewed in (149)). The function of flotillin-1/TRIM5α interaction is still unknown, as flotillin-1 knockdown or overexpression did not affect HIV-1 transduction efficiency, leading to the suggestion that flotillin-1 at least plays no role in the post-entry restriction of HIV-1 in fetal rhesus monkey kidney (FRhK4) cells.

Flotillins and diabetes mellitus

Flotillins seem to be of functional relevance in insulin signaling (see above) and the metabolic disease diabetes mellitus, as first demonstrated by Baumann *et al.* (63). A year later, James *et al.* showed an increased protein level of flotillin and caveolin-1 in muscle tissue and myoblast lysates derived from stroke-prone spontaneously hypertensive (SHRSP) rats as compared to male Wistar-Kyoto control rats (150). It is important to note that SHRSP rats are a model of human insulin resistance, defined by the decreased ability of cells or tissues to respond to physiological levels of insulin especially in skeletal muscles and adipose tissue. Insulin resistance is of major importance in several human diseases, e.g. diabetes type 2 (151). The results of both the above studies lead to the assumption that flotillins might play a role in insulin signaling in the skeletal muscle and adipose tissue. Furthermore, during steady state conditions, flotillin-1 was found in perinuclear regions in differentiated skeletal muscle cells, but at the plasma membrane in adipocytes (31). This observation suggested that the role of flotillin-1 in targeting GLUT4 to the plasma membrane after insulin stimulation may be different between muscle and adipose tissue. In fact in skeletal muscle cells, the insulin-stimulated signaling cascade leading to the translocation of GLUT4 to the plasma membrane is dependent on flotillin-1 and the muscle-specific protein caveolin-3 (103).

Lipid rafts also play a role in diabetic xerostomia, or dry mouth. This disease, when associated with diabetes mellitus, is caused by degenerative changes in the salivary glands leading to increased infectious conditions in the oral cavity and in the long-range aggravates the risk of atherosclerosis and cardiovascular diseases (reviewed in (152)). Wang *et al.* (153) tried to clarify the mechanisms leading to diabetic xerostomia by testing the subcellular localization of aquaporin 5 (AQP5), a water channel protein, in parotid glands of steptozotocin-induced diabetic rats during stimulation with the muscarinic agonist cevimeline. In parotid acinar cells derived from control rats, AQP5 colocalized with flotillin-2 in the cytoplasm and at the apical plasma membrane ten minutes after cemivelime treatment. In contrast, in the parotid acinar cells derived from diabetic rats, the translocation of these proteins did not occur. In summary, the results showed that AQP5 translocation is a lipid raft-dependent process and inhibition of the muscarinic agonist-induced translocation might be the cause of diabetic xerostomia.

6. Conclusions

It has become evident that flotillins play a key role in the regulation of cellular signaling and membrane trafficking. Although flotillins are not essential for life in metazoans, including mammals, as shown by the recent studies in flotillin knockout mice, they appear to be extremely important for many processes in cultured cells. This would suggest that especially mammals are capable compensating for the loss of flotillins by upregulating the expression of other proteins and thus overcoming the defects in e.g. signaling and cell adhesion. This feature is observed in both our flotillin-2 knockout mice and cultured cells with a constitutive flotillin knockdown (our unpublished data). In the future, it will be important to study what the molecular mechanisms of the compensation of loss of flotillin function might be. It will also be of major interest to study if the original function of flotillins in neuronal regeneration can also be observed in the mammalian knockout model. Furthermore, the functional significance of flotillin modifications can now be studied in the context of mammalian organisms when knockout/knock-in mice with specific mutations become available. Thus, the recent development of flotillin-1 and flotillin-2 knockout mice has brought the studies of flotillin functions to a new exciting era, and important data on the physiological function of flotillins can be expected in the near future.

Author details

Nina Kurrle, Bincy John, Melanie Meister and Ritva Tikkanen*
Institute of Biochemistry, Medical Faculty, University of Giessen, Giessen, Germany

Acknowledgement

The research in the Tikkanen lab is supported by the German Research council DFG (Grants Ti291/6-1 and Ti291/6-2), the Von Behring-Röntgen Foundation and the state of Hessen (LOEWE program "Non-neuronal Cholinergic Systems"), whose support is gratefully acknowledged.

---

* Corresponding Author

7. References

[1] Bickel PE, Scherer PE, Schnitzer JE, Oh P, Lisanti MP, Lodish HF. Flotillin and epidermal surface antigen define a new family of caveolae-associated integral membrane proteins. J Biol Chem. 1997 May 23;272(21):13793-802.

[2] Schulte T, Paschke KA, Laessing U, Lottspeich F, Stuermer CA. Reggie-1 and reggie-2, two cell surface proteins expressed by retinal ganglion cells during axon regeneration. Development. 1997 Jan;124(2):577-87.

[3] Morrow IC, Rea S, Martin S, Prior IA, Prohaska R, Hancock JF, et al. Flotillin-1/reggie-2 traffics to surface raft domains via a novel golgi-independent pathway. Identification of a novel membrane targeting domain and a role for palmitoylation. J Biol Chem. 2002 Dec 13;277(50):48834-41.

[4] Neumann-Giesen C, Falkenbach B, Beicht P, Claasen S, Luers G, Stuermer CA, et al. Membrane and raft association of reggie-1/flotillin-2: role of myristoylation, palmitoylation and oligomerization and induction of filopodia by overexpression. Biochem J. 2004 Mar 1;378(Pt 2):509-18.

[5] Salzer U, Prohaska R. Stomatin, flotillin-1, and flotillin-2 are major integral proteins of erythrocyte lipid rafts. Blood. 2001 Feb 15;97(4):1141-3.

[6] Simons K, Ikonen E. Functional rafts in cell membranes. Nature. 1997 Jun 5;387(6633):569-72.

[7] Simons K, Gerl MJ. Revitalizing membrane rafts: new tools and insights. Nat Rev Mol Cell Biol. 2010 Oct;11(10):688-99.

[8] Melkonian KA, Ostermeyer AG, Chen JZ, Roth MG, Brown DA. Role of lipid modifications in targeting proteins to detergent-resistant membrane rafts. Many raft proteins are acylated, while few are prenylated. J Biol Chem. 1999 Feb 5;274(6):3910-7.

[9] Fernow I, Icking A, Tikkanen R. Reggie-1 and reggie-2 localize in non-caveolar rafts in epithelial cells: cellular localization is not dependent on the expression of caveolin proteins. Eur J Cell Biol. 2007 Jun;86(6):345-52.

[10] Schroeder WT, Siciliano MJ, Stewart-Galetka SL, Duvic M. The human gene for an epidermal surface antigen (M17S1) is located at 17q11-12. Genomics. 1991 Oct;11(2):481-2.

[11] Hazarika P, Dham N, Patel P, Cho M, Weidner D, Goldsmith L, et al. Flotillin 2 is distinct from epidermal surface antigen (ESA) and is associated with filopodia formation. J Cell Biochem. 1999 Oct 1;75(1):147-59.

[12] Deininger SO, Rajendran L, Lottspeich F, Przybylski M, Illges H, Stuermer CA, et al. Identification of teleost Thy-1 and association with the microdomain/lipid raft reggie proteins in regenerating CNS axons. Mol Cell Neurosci. 2003 Apr;22(4):544-54.

[13] Glebov OO, Bright NA, Nichols BJ. Flotillin-1 defines a clathrin-independent endocytic pathway in mammalian cells. Nat Cell Biol. 2006 Jan;8(1):46-54.

[14] Stuermer CA, Lang DM, Kirsch F, Wiechers M, Deininger SO, Plattner H. Glycosylphosphatidyl inositol-anchored proteins and fyn kinase assemble in noncaveolar plasma membrane microdomains defined by reggie-1 and -2. Mol Biol Cell. 2001 Oct;12(10):3031-45.

[15] Malaga-Trillo E, Solis GP, Schrock Y, Geiss C, Luncz L, Thomanetz V, et al. Regulation of embryonic cell adhesion by the prion protein. PLoS Biol. 2009 Mar 10;7(3):e55.

[16] Babuke T, Tikkanen R. Dissecting the molecular function of reggie/flotillin proteins. Eur J Cell Biol. 2007 Sep;86(9):525-32.

[17] Lopez D, Kolter R. Functional microdomains in bacterial membranes. Genes Dev. 2010 Sep 1;24(17):1893-902.

[18] Haney CH, Long SR. Plant flotillins are required for infection by nitrogen-fixing bacteria. Proc Natl Acad Sci U S A. 2010 Jan 5;107(1):478-83.

[19] Otto GP, Nichols BJ. The roles of flotillin microdomains--endocytosis and beyond. J Cell Sci. 2012 Dec 1;124(Pt 23):3933-40.

[20] Edgar AJ, Polak JM. Flotillin-1: gene structure: cDNA cloning from human lung and the identification of alternative polyadenylation signals. Int J Biochem Cell Biol. 2001 Jan;33(1):53-64.

[21] Browman DT, Hoegg MB, Robbins SM. The SPFH domain-containing proteins: more than lipid raft markers. Trends Cell Biol. 2007 Aug;17(8):394-402.

[22] Tavernarakis N, Driscoll M, Kyrpides NC. The SPFH domain: implicated in regulating targeted protein turnover in stomatins and other membrane-associated proteins. Trends Biochem Sci. 1999 Nov;24(11):425-7.

[23] Solis GP, Hoegg M, Munderloh C, Schrock Y, Malaga-Trillo E, Rivera-Milla E, et al. Reggie/flotillin proteins are organized into stable tetramers in membrane microdomains. Biochem J. 2007 Apr 15;403(2):313-22.

[24] Volonte D, Galbiati F, Li S, Nishiyama K, Okamoto T, Lisanti MP. Flotillins/cavatellins are differentially expressed in cells and tissues and form a hetero-oligomeric complex with caveolins in vivo. Characterization and epitope-mapping of a novel flotillin-1 monoclonal antibody probe. J Biol Chem. 1999 Apr 30;274(18):12702-9.

[25] Yokoyama H, Fujii S, Matsui I. Crystal structure of a core domain of stomatin from Pyrococcus horikoshii Illustrates a novel trimeric and coiled-coil fold. J Mol Biol. 2008 Feb 22;376(3):868-78.

[26] Ha H, Kwak HB, Lee SK, Na DS, Rudd CE, Lee ZH, et al. Membrane rafts play a crucial role in receptor activator of nuclear factor kappaB signaling and osteoclast function. J Biol Chem. 2003 May 16;278(20):18573-80.

[27] Amaddii M, Meister M, Banning A, Tomasovic A, Mooz J, Rajalingam K, et al. Flotillin-1/reggie-2 plays a dual role in the activation of receptor tyrosine kinase/map kinase signaling. J Biol Chem. 2012 Jan 9.

[28] Langhorst MF, Reuter A, Jaeger FA, Wippich FM, Luxenhofer G, Plattner H, et al. Trafficking of the microdomain scaffolding protein reggie-1/flotillin-2. Eur J Cell Biol. 2008 Jan 29.

[29] Langhorst MF, Reuter A, Luxenhofer G, Boneberg EM, Legler DF, Plattner H, et al. Preformed reggie/flotillin caps: stable priming platforms for macrodomain assembly in T cells. FASEB J. 2006 Apr;20(6):711-3.

[30] Neumann-Giesen C, Fernow I, Amaddii M, Tikkanen R. Role of EGF-induced tyrosine phosphorylation of reggie-1/flotillin-2 in cell spreading and signaling to the actin cytoskeleton. J Cell Sci. 2007 Feb 1;120(Pt 3):395-406.

[31] Liu J, Deyoung SM, Zhang M, Dold LH, Saltiel AR. The stomatin/ prohibitin/ flotillin/ HflK/C domain of flotillin-1 contains distinct sequences that direct plasma membrane localization and protein interactions in 3T3-L1 adipocytes. J Biol Chem. 2005 Apr 22;280(16):16125-34.
[32] Rajendran L, Beckmann J, Magenau A, Boneberg EM, Gaus K, Viola A, et al. Flotillins are involved in the polarization of primitive and mature hematopoietic cells. PLoS One. 2009;4(12):e8290.
[33] Rajendran L, Masilamani M, Solomon S, Tikkanen R, Stuermer CA, Plattner H, et al. Asymmetric localization of flotillins/reggies in preassembled platforms confers inherent polarity to hematopoietic cells. Proc Natl Acad Sci U S A. 2003 Jul 8;100(14):8241-6.
[34] Frick M, Bright NA, Riento K, Bray A, Merrified C, Nichols BJ. Coassembly of flotillins induces formation of membrane microdomains, membrane curvature, and vesicle budding. Curr Biol. 2007 Jul 3;17(13):1151-6.
[35] Hansen CG, Nichols BJ. Molecular mechanisms of clathrin-independent endocytosis. J Cell Sci. 2009 Jun 1;122(Pt 11):1713-21.
[36] Langhorst MF, Solis GP, Hannbeck S, Plattner H, Stuermer CA. Linking membrane microdomains to the cytoskeleton: regulation of the lateral mobility of reggie-1/flotillin-2 by interaction with actin. FEBS Lett. 2007 Oct 2;581(24):4697-703.
[37] Affentranger S, Martinelli S, Hahn J, Rossy J, Niggli V. Dynamic reorganization of flotillins in chemokine-stimulated human T-lymphocytes. BMC Cell Biol. 2011;12:28.
[38] de Gassart A, Geminard C, Fevrier B, Raposo G, Vidal M. Lipid raft-associated protein sorting in exosomes. Blood. 2003 Dec 15;102(13):4336-44.
[39] Staubach S, Razawi H, Hanisch FG. Proteomics of MUC1-containing lipid rafts from plasma membranes and exosomes of human breast carcinoma cells MCF-7. Proteomics. 2009 May;9(10):2820-35.
[40] Street JM, Barran PE, Mackay CL, Weidt S, Balmforth C, Walsh TS, et al. Identification and proteomic profiling of exosomes in human cerebrospinal fluid. J Transl Med. 2012;10:5.
[41] Strauss K, Goebel C, Runz H, Mobius W, Weiss S, Feussner I, et al. Exosome secretion ameliorates lysosomal storage of cholesterol in Niemann-Pick type C disease. J Biol Chem. 2010 Aug 20;285(34):26279-88.
[42] Dermine JF, Duclos S, Garin J, St-Louis F, Rea S, Parton RG, et al. Flotillin-1-enriched lipid raft domains accumulate on maturing phagosomes. J Biol Chem. 2001 May 25;276(21):18507-12.
[43] Santamaria A, Castellanos E, Gomez V, Benedit P, Renau-Piqueras J, Morote J, et al. PTOV1 enables the nuclear translocation and mitogenic activity of flotillin-1, a major protein of lipid rafts. Mol Cell Biol. 2005 Mar;25(5):1900-11.
[44] Gkantiragas I, Brugger B, Stuven E, Kaloyanova D, Li XY, Lohr K, et al. Sphingomyelin-enriched microdomains at the Golgi complex. Mol Biol Cell. 2001 Jun;12(6):1819-33.
[45] Lang DM, Lommel S, Jung M, Ankerhold R, Petrausch B, Laessing U, et al. Identification of reggie-1 and reggie-2 as plasmamembrane-associated proteins which cocluster with activated GPI-anchored cell adhesion molecules in non-caveolar micropatches in neurons. J Neurobiol. 1998 Dec;37(4):502-23.

[46] Pust S, Dyve AB, Torgersen ML, van Deurs B, Sandvig K. Interplay between toxin transport and flotillin localization. PLoS One. 2010;5(1):e8844.

[47] Kokubo H, Helms JB, Ohno-Iwashita Y, Shimada Y, Horikoshi Y, Yamaguchi H. Ultrastructural localization of flotillin-1 to cholesterol-rich membrane microdomains, rafts, in rat brain tissue. Brain Res. 2003 Mar 7;965(1-2):83-90.

[48] Carcea I, Ma'ayan A, Mesias R, Sepulveda B, Salton SR, Benson DL. Flotillin-mediated endocytic events dictate cell type-specific responses to semaphorin 3A. J Neurosci. 2010 Nov 10;30(45):15317-29.

[49] Riento K, Frick M, Schafer I, Nichols BJ. Endocytosis of flotillin-1 and flotillin-2 is regulated by Fyn kinase. J Cell Sci. 2009 Apr 1;122(Pt 7):912-8.

[50] Resh MD. Fatty acylation of proteins: new insights into membrane targeting of myristoylated and palmitoylated proteins. Biochim Biophys Acta. 1999 Aug 12;1451(1):1-16.

[51] Johnson DR, Bhatnagar RS, Knoll LJ, Gordon JI. Genetic and biochemical studies of protein N-myristoylation. Annu Rev Biochem. 1994;63:869-914.

[52] Dietrich LE, Ungermann C. On the mechanism of protein palmitoylation. EMBO Rep. 2004 Nov;5(11):1053-7.

[53] Li Y, Martin BR, Cravatt BF, Hofmann SL. DHHC5 protein palmitoylates flotillin-2 and is rapidly degraded on induction of neuronal differentiation in cultured cells. J Biol Chem. 2012 Jan 2;287(1):523-30.

[54] Koegl M, Zlatkine P, Ley SC, Courtneidge SA, Magee AI. Palmitoylation of multiple Src-family kinases at a homologous N-terminal motif. Biochem J. 1994 Nov 1;303 (Pt 3):749-53.

[55] Ali MH, Imperiali B. Protein oligomerization: how and why. Bioorg Med Chem. 2005 Sep 1;13(17):5013-20.

[56] Babuke T, Ruonala M, Meister M, Amaddii M, Genzler C, Esposito A, et al. Hetero-oligomerization of reggie-1/flotillin-2 and reggie-2/flotillin-1 is required for their endocytosis. Cell Signal. 2009 Aug;21(8):1287-97.

[57] Langhorst MF, Jaeger FA, Mueller S, Sven Hartmann L, Luxenhofer G, Stuermer CA. Reggies/flotillins regulate cytoskeletal remodeling during neuronal differentiation via CAP/ponsin and Rho GTPases. Eur J Cell Biol. 2008 Dec;87(12):921-31.

[58] Haglund K, Ivankovic-Dikic I, Shimokawa N, Kruh GD, Dikic I. Recruitment of Pyk2 and Cbl to lipid rafts mediates signals important for actin reorganization in growing neurites. J Cell Sci. 2004 May 15;117(Pt 12):2557-68.

[59] Ludwig A, Otto GP, Riento K, Hams E, Fallon PG, Nichols BJ. Flotillin microdomains interact with the cortical cytoskeleton to control uropod formation and neutrophil recruitment. J Cell Biol. 2011 Nov 15;191(4):771-81.

[60] Munderloh C, Solis GP, Bodrikov V, Jaeger FA, Wiechers M, Malaga-Trillo E, et al. Reggies/flotillins regulate retinal axon regeneration in the zebrafish optic nerve and differentiation of hippocampal and N2a neurons. J Neurosci. 2009 May 20;29(20):6607-15.

[61] von Philipsborn AC, Ferrer-Vaquer A, Rivera-Milla E, Stuermer CA, Malaga-Trillo E. Restricted expression of reggie genes and proteins during early zebrafish development. J Comp Neurol. 2005 Feb 14;482(3):257-72.

[62] Stuermer CA. Microdomain-forming proteins and the role of the reggies/flotillins during axon regeneration in zebrafish. Biochim Biophys Acta. 2011 Mar;1812(3):415-22.

[63] Baumann CA, Ribon V, Kanzaki M, Thurmond DC, Mora S, Shigematsu S, et al. CAP defines a second signalling pathway required for insulin-stimulated glucose transport. Nature. 2000 Sep 14;407(6801):202-7.

[64] Katanaev VL, Solis GP, Hausmann G, Buestorf S, Katanayeva N, Schrock Y, et al. Reggie-1/flotillin-2 promotes secretion of the long-range signalling forms of Wingless and Hedgehog in Drosophila. Embo J. 2008 Feb 6;27(3):509-21.

[65] Limpert AS, Karlo JC, Landreth GE. Nerve growth factor stimulates the concentration of TrkA within lipid rafts and extracellular signal-regulated kinase activation through c-Cbl-associated protein. Mol Cell Biol. 2007 Aug;27(16):5686-98.

[66] Lin C, Wu Z, Lin X, Yu C, Shi T, Zeng Y, et al. Knockdown of FLOT1 impairs cell proliferation and tumorigenicity in breast cancer through upregulation of FOXO3a. Clin Cancer Res. 2011 May 15;17(10):3089-99.

[67] Sugawara Y, Nishii H, Takahashi T, Yamauchi J, Mizuno N, Tago K, et al. The lipid raft proteins flotillins/reggies interact with Galphaq and are involved in Gq-mediated p38 mitogen-activated protein kinase activation through tyrosine kinase. Cell Signal. 2007 Jun;19(6):1301-8.

[68] Helms JB, Zurzolo C. Lipids as targeting signals: lipid rafts and intracellular trafficking. Traffic. 2004 Apr;5(4):247-54.

[69] McMahon HT, Boucrot E. Molecular mechanism and physiological functions of clathrin-mediated endocytosis. Nat Rev Mol Cell Biol. 2011 Aug;12(8):517-33.

[70] Staubach S, Hanisch FG. Lipid rafts: signaling and sorting platforms of cells and their roles in cancer. Expert Rev Proteomics. 2011 Apr;8(2):263-77.

[71] Otto GP, Nichols BJ. The roles of flotillin microdomains--endocytosis and beyond. J Cell Sci. 2011 Dec 1;124(Pt 23):3933-40.

[72] Ait-Slimane T, Galmes R, Trugnan G, Maurice M. Basolateral internalization of GPI-anchored proteins occurs via a clathrin-independent flotillin-dependent pathway in polarized hepatic cells. Mol Biol Cell. 2009 Sep;20(17):3792-800.

[73] Blanchet MH, Le Good JA, Mesnard D, Oorschot V, Baflast S, Minchiotti G, et al. Cripto recruits Furin and PACE4 and controls Nodal trafficking during proteolytic maturation. EMBO J. 2008 Oct 8;27(19):2580-91.

[74] Cremona ML, Matthies HJ, Pau K, Bowton E, Speed N, Lute BJ, et al. Flotillin-1 is essential for PKC-triggered endocytosis and membrane microdomain localization of DAT. Nat Neurosci. 2011 Apr;14(4):469-77.

[75] Schneider A, Rajendran L, Honsho M, Gralle M, Donnert G, Wouters F, et al. Flotillin-dependent clustering of the amyloid precursor protein regulates its endocytosis and amyloidogenic processing in neurons. J Neurosci. 2008 Mar 12;28(11):2874-82.

[76] Ge L, Qi W, Wang LJ, Miao HH, Qu YX, Li BL, et al. Flotillins play an essential role in Niemann-Pick C1-like 1-mediated cholesterol uptake. Proc Natl Acad Sci U S A. 2011 Jan 11;108(2):551-6.
[77] Orth JD, Krueger EW, Weller SG, McNiven MA. A novel endocytic mechanism of epidermal growth factor receptor sequestration and internalization. Cancer Res. 2006 Apr 1;66(7):3603-10.
[78] Sigismund S, Argenzio E, Tosoni D, Cavallaro E, Polo S, Di Fiore PP. Clathrin-mediated internalization is essential for sustained EGFR signaling but dispensable for degradation. Dev Cell. 2008 Aug;15(2):209-19.
[79] Solis GP, Schrock Y, Hulsbusch N, Wiechers M, Plattner H, Stuermer CA. Reggies/Flotillins regulate E-cadherin-mediated cell contact formation by affecting EGFR trafficking. Mol Biol Cell. 2012 Mar 21.
[80] Wiley HS, Cunningham DD. The endocytotic rate constant. A cellular parameter for quantitating receptor-mediated endocytosis. J Biol Chem. 1982 Apr 25;257(8):4222-9.
[81] Masui H, Castro L, Mendelsohn J. Consumption of EGF by A431 cells: evidence for receptor recycling. J Cell Biol. 1993 Jan;120(1):85-93.
[82] Schroeder WT, Stewart-Galetka S, Mandavilli S, Parry DA, Goldsmith L, Duvic M. Cloning and characterization of a novel epidermal cell surface antigen (ESA). J Biol Chem. 1994 Aug 5;269(31):19983-91.
[83] Hoehne M, de Couet HG, Stuermer CA, Fischbach KF. Loss- and gain-of-function analysis of the lipid raft proteins Reggie/Flotillin in Drosophila: they are posttranslationally regulated, and misexpression interferes with wing and eye development. Mol Cell Neurosci. 2005 Nov;30(3):326-38.
[84] Yap AS, Brieher WM, Gumbiner BM. Molecular and functional analysis of cadherin-based adherens junctions. Annu Rev Cell Dev Biol. 1997;13:119-46.
[85] Bodrikov V, Solis GP, Stuermer CA. Prion protein promotes growth cone development through reggie/flotillin-dependent N-cadherin trafficking. J Neurosci. 2011 Dec 7;31(49):18013-25.
[86] Pommereit D, Wouters FS. An NGF-induced Exo70-TC10 complex locally antagonises Cdc42-mediated activation of N-WASP to modulate neurite outgrowth. J Cell Sci. 2007 Aug 1;120(Pt 15):2694-705.
[87] Taulet N, Comunale F, Favard C, Charrasse S, Bodin S, Gauthier-Rouviere C. N-cadherin/p120 catenin association at cell-cell contacts occurs in cholesterol-rich membrane domains and is required for RhoA activation and myogenesis. J Biol Chem. 2009 Aug 21;284(34):23137-45.
[88] Chartier NT, Laine MG, Ducarouge B, Oddou C, Bonaz B, Albiges-Rizo C, et al. Enterocytic differentiation is modulated by lipid rafts-dependent assembly of adherens junctions. Exp Cell Res. 2011 Jun 10;317(10):1422-36.
[89] Tomasovic A, Traub S, Tikkanen R. Molecular Networks in FGF Signaling: Flotillin-1 and Cbl-Associated Protein Compete for the Binding to Fibroblast Growth Factor Receptor Substrate 2. PLoS ONE. 2012;7(1): e29739. doi:10.1371.

[90] Kato N, Nakanishi M, Hirashima N. Flotillin-1 regulates IgE receptor-mediated signaling in rat basophilic leukemia (RBL-2H3) cells. J Immunol. 2006 Jul 1;177(1):147-54.

[91] Gotoh N, Manova K, Tanaka S, Murohashi M, Hadari Y, Lee A, et al. The docking protein FRS2alpha is an essential component of multiple fibroblast growth factor responses during early mouse development. Mol Cell Biol. 2005 May;25(10):4105-16.

[92] Lax I, Wong A, Lamothe B, Lee A, Frost A, Hawes J, et al. The docking protein FRS2alpha controls a MAP kinase-mediated negative feedback mechanism for signaling by FGF receptors. Mol Cell. 2002 Oct;10(4):709-19.

[93] Wu Y, Chen Z, Ullrich A. EGFR and FGFR signaling through FRS2 is subject to negative feedback control by ERK1/2. Biol Chem. 2003 Aug;384(8):1215-26.

[94] Hofman EG, Ruonala MO, Bader AN, van den Heuvel D, Voortman J, Roovers RC, et al. EGF induces coalescence of different lipid rafts. J Cell Sci. 2008 Aug 1;121(Pt 15):2519-28.

[95] Ueda Y, Hirai S, Osada S, Suzuki A, Mizuno K, Ohno S. Protein kinase C activates the MEK-ERK pathway in a manner independent of Ras and dependent on Raf. J Biol Chem. 1996 Sep 20;271(38):23512-9.

[96] Zou Y, Komuro I, Yamazaki T, Aikawa R, Kudoh S, Shiojima I, et al. Protein kinase C, but not tyrosine kinases or Ras, plays a critical role in angiotensin II-induced activation of Raf-1 kinase and extracellular signal-regulated protein kinases in cardiac myocytes. J Biol Chem. 1996 Dec 27;271(52):33592-7.

[97] Kouhara H, Hadari YR, Spivak-Kroizman T, Schilling J, Bar-Sagi D, Lax I, et al. A lipid-anchored Grb2-binding protein that links FGF-receptor activation to the Ras/MAPK signaling pathway. Cell. 1997 May 30;89(5):693-702.

[98] Roskoski R, Jr. The ErbB/HER receptor protein-tyrosine kinases and cancer. Biochem Biophys Res Commun. 2004 Jun 18;319(1):1-11.

[99] Ribon V, Herrera R, Kay BK, Saltiel AR. A role for CAP, a novel, multifunctional Src homology 3 domain-containing protein in formation of actin stress fibers and focal adhesions. J Biol Chem. 1998 Feb 13;273(7):4073-80.

[100] Ribon V, Printen JA, Hoffman NG, Kay BK, Saltiel AR. A novel, multifuntional c-Cbl binding protein in insulin receptor signaling in 3T3-L1 adipocytes. Mol Cell Biol. 1998 Feb;18(2):872-9.

[101] Kimura A, Baumann CA, Chiang SH, Saltiel AR. The sorbin homology domain: a motif for the targeting of proteins to lipid rafts. Proc Natl Acad Sci U S A. 2001 Jul 31;98(16):9098-103.

[102] Zhang M, Kimura A, Saltiel AR. Cloning and characterization of Cbl-associated protein splicing isoforms. Mol Med. 2003 Jan-Feb;9(1-2):18-25.

[103] Fecchi K, Volonte D, Hezel MP, Schmeck K, Galbiati F. Spatial and temporal regulation of GLUT4 translocation by flotillin-1 and caveolin-3 in skeletal muscle cells. FASEB J. 2006 Apr;20(6):705-7.

[104] Huang EJ, Reichardt LF. Trk receptors: roles in neuronal signal transduction. Annu Rev Biochem. 2003;72:609-42.

[105] Kaplan DR, Miller FD. Neurotrophin signal transduction in the nervous system. Curr Opin Neurobiol. 2000 Jun;10(3):381-91.

[106] Delahaye L, Rocchi S, Van Obberghen E. Potential involvement of FRS2 in insulin signaling. Endocrinology. 2000 Feb;141(2):621-8.

[107] Meakin SO, MacDonald JI, Gryz EA, Kubu CJ, Verdi JM. The signaling adapter FRS-2 competes with Shc for binding to the nerve growth factor receptor TrkA. A model for discriminating proliferation and differentiation. J Biol Chem. 1999 Apr 2;274(14):9861-70.

[108] Ong SH, Hadari YR, Gotoh N, Guy GR, Schlessinger J, Lax I. Stimulation of phosphatidylinositol 3-kinase by fibroblast growth factor receptors is mediated by coordinated recruitment of multiple docking proteins. Proc Natl Acad Sci U S A. 2001 May 22;98(11):6074-9.

[109] Saslowsky DE, Cho JA, Chinnapen H, Massol RH, Chinnapen DJ, Wagner JS, et al. Intoxication of zebrafish and mammalian cells by cholera toxin depends on the flotillin/reggie proteins but not Derlin-1 or -2. J Clin Invest. 2010 Dec;120(12):4399-409.

[110] Ludwig A, Otto GP, Riento K, Hams E, Fallon PG, Nichols BJ. Flotillin microdomains interact with the cortical cytoskeleton to control uropod formation and neutrophil recruitment. J Cell Biol. 2010 Nov 15;191(4):771-81.

[111] Rossy J, Schlicht D, Engelhardt B, Niggli V. Flotillins interact with PSGL-1 in neutrophils and, upon stimulation, rapidly organize into membrane domains subsequently accumulating in the uropod. PLoS One. 2009;4(4):e5403.

[112] Even-Ram S, Doyle AD, Conti MA, Matsumoto K, Adelstein RS, Yamada KM. Myosin IIA regulates cell motility and actomyosin-microtubule crosstalk. Nat Cell Biol. 2007 Mar;9(3):299-309.

[113] Shih W, Yamada S. Myosin IIA dependent retrograde flow drives 3D cell migration. Biophys J. 2010 Apr 21;98(8):L29-31.

[114] Rajalingam K, Rudel T. Ras-Raf signaling needs prohibitin. Cell Cycle. 2005 Nov;4(11):1503-5.

[115] Rajalingam K, Wunder C, Brinkmann V, Churin Y, Hekman M, Sievers C, et al. Prohibitin is required for Ras-induced Raf-MEK-ERK activation and epithelial cell migration. Nat Cell Biol. 2005 Aug;7(8):837-43.

[116] Ande SR, Gu Y, Nyomba BL, Mishra S. Insulin induced phosphorylation of prohibitin at tyrosine 114 recruits Shp1. Biochim Biophys Acta. 2009 Aug;1793(8):1372-8.

[117] Han EK, McGonigal T, Butler C, Giranda VL, Luo Y. Characterization of Akt overexpression in MiaPaCa-2 cells: prohibitin is an Akt substrate both in vitro and in cells. Anticancer Res. 2008 Mar-Apr;28(2A):957-63.

[118] Chiu CF, Ho MY, Peng JM, Hung SW, Lee WH, Liang CM, et al. Raf activation by Ras and promotion of cellular metastasis require phosphorylation of prohibitin in the raft domain of the plasma membrane. Oncogene. 2012 Mar 12.

[119] Da Cruz S, Parone PA, Gonzalo P, Bienvenut WV, Tondera D, Jourdain A, et al. SLP-2 interacts with prohibitins in the mitochondrial inner membrane and contributes to their stability. Biochim Biophys Acta. 2008 May;1783(5):904-11.

[120] Hazarika P, McCarty MF, Prieto VG, George S, Babu D, Koul D, et al. Up-regulation of Flotillin-2 is associated with melanoma progression and modulates expression of the thrombin receptor protease activated receptor 1. Cancer Res. 2004 Oct 15;64(20):7361-9.
[121] Doherty SD, Prieto VG, George S, Hazarika P, Duvic M. High flotillin-2 expression is associated with lymph node metastasis and Breslow depth in melanoma. Melanoma Res. 2006 Oct;16(5):461-3.
[122] Sasaki Y, Oshima Y, Koyama R, Maruyama R, Akashi H, Mita H, et al. Identification of Flotillin-2, a Major Protein on Lipid Rafts, as a Novel Target of p53 Family Members. Mol Cancer Res. 2008 Feb 22.
[123] Haass C, Lemere CA, Capell A, Citron M, Seubert P, Schenk D, et al. The Swedish mutation causes early-onset Alzheimer's disease by beta-secretase cleavage within the secretory pathway. Nat Med. 1995 Dec;1(12):1291-6.
[124] Kao SC, Krichevsky AM, Kosik KS, Tsai LH. BACE1 suppression by RNA interference in primary cortical neurons. J Biol Chem. 2004 Jan 16;279(3):1942-9.
[125] Small SA, Gandy S. Sorting through the cell biology of Alzheimer's disease: intracellular pathways to pathogenesis. Neuron. 2006 Oct 5;52(1):15-31.
[126] Tikkanen R, Banning A, Meister M. Trafficking and endocytosis of Alzheimer amyloid precursor protein. in: Dowler BC, editor Endocytosis: Structural Components, Functions and Pathways Nova Publishers pp 1-38. 2010.
[127] Riddell DR, Christie G, Hussain I, Dingwall C. Compartmentalization of beta-secretase (Asp2) into low-buoyant density, noncaveolar lipid rafts. Curr Biol. 2001 Aug 21;11(16):1288-93.
[128] Lee SJ, Liyanage U, Bickel PE, Xia W, Lansbury PT, Jr., Kosik KS. A detergent-insoluble membrane compartment contains A beta in vivo. Nat Med. 1998 Jun;4(6):730-4.
[129] Parkin ET, Hussain I, Karran EH, Turner AJ, Hooper NM. Characterization of detergent-insoluble complexes containing the familial Alzheimer's disease-associated presenilins. J Neurochem. 1999 Apr;72(4):1534-43.
[130] Kokubo H, Lemere CA, Yamaguchi H. Localization of flotillins in human brain and their accumulation with the progression of Alzheimer's disease pathology. Neurosci Lett. 2000 Aug 25;290(2):93-6.
[131] Rajendran L, Knobloch M, Geiger KD, Dienel S, Nitsch R, Simons K, et al. Increased Abeta production leads to intracellular accumulation of Abeta in flotillin-1-positive endosomes. Neurodegener Dis. 2007;4(2-3):164-70.
[132] Kokubo H, Saido TC, Iwata N, Helms JB, Shinohara R, Yamaguchi H. Part of membrane-bound Abeta exists in rafts within senile plaques in Tg2576 mouse brain. Neurobiol Aging. 2005 Apr;26(4):409-18.
[133] Girardot N, Allinquant B, Langui D, Laquerriere A, Dubois B, Hauw JJ, et al. Accumulation of flotillin-1 in tangle-bearing neurones of Alzheimer's disease. Neuropathol Appl Neurobiol. 2003 Oct;29(5):451-61.
[134] Chen TY, Liu PH, Ruan CT, Chiu L, Kung FL. The intracellular domain of amyloid precursor protein interacts with flotillin-1, a lipid raft protein. Biochem Biophys Res Commun. 2006 Mar 31;342(1):266-72.

[135] Shin T, Kim H, Jin JK, Moon C, Ahn M, Tanuma N, et al. Expression of caveolin-1, -2, and -3 in the spinal cords of Lewis rats with experimental autoimmune encephalomyelitis. J Neuroimmunol. 2005 Aug;165(1-2):11-20.

[136] Constantinescu CS, Farooqi N, O'Brien K, Gran B. Experimental autoimmune encephalomyelitis (EAE) as a model for multiple sclerosis (MS). Br J Pharmacol. 2011 Oct;164(4):1079-106.

[137] Kim H, Ahn M, Moon C, Matsumoto Y, Sung Koh C, Shin T. Immunohistochemical study of flotillin-1 in the spinal cord of Lewis rats with experimental autoimmune encephalomyelitis. Brain Res. 2006 Oct 9;1114(1):204-11.

[138] Davie CA. A review of Parkinson's disease. Br Med Bull. 2008;86:109-27.

[139] Jacobowitz DM, Kallarakal AT. Flotillin-1 in the substantia nigra of the Parkinson brain and a predominant localization in catecholaminergic nerves in the rat brain. Neurotox Res. 2004;6(4):245-57.

[140] Manes S, del Real G, Martinez AC. Pathogens: raft hijackers. Nat Rev Immunol. 2003 Jul;3(7):557-68.

[141] Vieira FS, Correa G, Einicker-Lamas M, Coutinho-Silva R. Host-cell lipid rafts: a safe door for micro-organisms? Biol Cell. 2010 Jul;102(7):391-407.

[142] Knodler LA, Vallance BA, Hensel M, Jackel D, Finlay BB, Steele-Mortimer O. Salmonella type III effectors PipB and PipB2 are targeted to detergent-resistant microdomains on internal host cell membranes. Mol Microbiol. 2003 Aug;49(3):685-704.

[143] Seveau S, Bierne H, Giroux S, Prevost MC, Cossart P. Role of lipid rafts in E-cadherin--and HGF-R/Met--mediated entry of Listeria monocytogenes into host cells. J Cell Biol. 2004 Aug 30;166(5):743-53.

[144] Li Q, Zhang Q, Wang C, Li N, Li J. Invasion of enteropathogenic Escherichia coli into host cells through epithelial tight junctions. FEBS J. 2008 Dec;275(23):6022-32.

[145] Chazal N, Gerlier D. Virus entry, assembly, budding, and membrane rafts. Microbiol Mol Biol Rev. 2003 Jun;67(2):226-37, table of contents.

[146] Cicala C, Arthos J, Selig SM, Dennis G, Jr., Hosack DA, Van Ryk D, et al. HIV envelope induces a cascade of cell signals in non-proliferating target cells that favor virus replication. Proc Natl Acad Sci U S A. 2002 Jul 9;99(14):9380-5.

[147] Carter GC, Bernstone L, Sangani D, Bee JW, Harder T, James W. HIV entry in macrophages is dependent on intact lipid rafts. Virology. 2009 Mar 30;386(1):192-202.

[148] Ohmine S, Sakuma R, Sakuma T, Thatava T, Solis GP, Ikeda Y. Cytoplasmic body component TRIM5{alpha} requires lipid-enriched microdomains for efficient HIV-1 restriction. J Biol Chem. 2010 Nov 5;285(45):34508-17.

[149] Nakayama EE, Shioda T. Role of Human TRIM5alpha in Intrinsic Immunity. Front Microbiol. 2012;3:97.

[150] James DJ, Cairns F, Salt IP, Murphy GJ, Dominiczak AF, Connell JM, et al. Skeletal muscle of stroke-prone spontaneously hypertensive rats exhibits reduced insulin-stimulated glucose transport and elevated levels of caveolin and flotillin. Diabetes. 2001 Sep;50(9):2148-56.

[151] Collison M, Glazier AM, Graham D, Morton JJ, Dominiczak MH, Aitman TJ, et al. Cd36 and molecular mechanisms of insulin resistance in the stroke-prone spontaneously hypertensive rat. Diabetes. 2000 Dec;49(12):2222-6.

[152] Ship JA. Diabetes and oral health: an overview. J Am Dent Assoc. 2003 Oct;134 Spec No:4S-10S.

[153] Wang D, Yuan Z, Inoue N, Cho G, Shono M, Ishikawa Y. Abnormal subcellular localization of AQP5 and downregulated AQP5 protein in parotid glands of streptozotocin-induced diabetic rats. Biochim Biophys Acta. 2011 May;1810(5):543-54.

Chapter 11

Role of Tyrosine Kinase A Receptor (TrkA) on Pathogenicity of *Clostridium perfringens* Alpha-Toxin

Masataka Oda, Masahiro Nagahama, Keiko Kobayashi and Jun Sakurai

Additional information is available at the end of the chapter

http://dx.doi.org/10.5772/48515

1. Introduction

Clostridium perfringens (*C. perfringens*) is a toxin-producing anaerobic Gram-positive bacterium, which is well known for its role in human tissue infections and food poisoning. It is readily isolated from soil and a component of normal human intestinal and vaginal flora in many individuals. Apart from the classic clostridial myonecrosis of gas gangrene, *C. perfringens* can be responsible for a range of other clinical scenarios including sepsis, aspiration pneumonia, brain abscess, and enteritis necroticans. The potent exotoxins produced by various strains of *C. perfringens* are central to their effectiveness as pathogens, and include four major toxins used in strain classification: a phospholipase C (alpha-toxin, PLC), two pore-forming toxins (beta and epsilon toxins); and an ADP-ribosylation toxin (iota toxin). *C. perfringens* gas gangrene is one of the most fulminant necrotizing infections affecting humans. The infection can become well established in traumatized tissues in as little as 6-8 h and the destruction of adjacent healthy muscle can progress several inches per hour despite appropriate antibiotic coverage. Shock and organ failure occur in 50% of patients, and 40% of these individuals die. Even with modern medical advances and intensive care regimens, the centuries-old practice of radical amputation on an emergent basis remains the single best treatment. Histologically, this infection is characterized by widespread destruction of muscle and the absence of polymorphonuclear leukocytes at the site of infection. Instead, leukocytes accumulate within adjacent vessels.

C. perfringens alpha-toxin is the major virulence factor in gas gangrene with inflammatory myopathies (Williamson and Titball 1993, Awad et al. 1995). The toxin, which exhibits phospholipase C (PLC) and sphingomyelinase activities, causes hemolysis, necrosis, and death, and the activation of neutrophils and release of cytokines (Sakurai, Nagahama and Oda 2004). Bryant reported that the intramuscular injection of alpha-toxin caused a rapid and irreversible decline in skeletal muscle blood flow due to toxin-induced intravascular aggregates of plates, leukocytes and fibrin (Bryant et al. 2000a, Bryant et al. 2000b). Neutrophils in these aggregates often bordered the endothelium but all remained intravascular (Bryant et al. 2000a). These findings suggested that the large heterotypic aggregates of platelets and leukocytes generated by alpha-toxin also contributed to impairment of the tissue inflammatory response. We have reported that alpha-toxin-induced activation of endogenous PLC and sphingomyelinase via a pertussis toxin (PT)-sensitive GTP-binding protein (Gi) plays an important role in the hemolysis of rabbit and sheep erythrocytes, respectively (Ochi et al. 1996, Ochi et al. 2004, Oda et al. 2008).

Recently, we revealed that the tyrosine kinase A (TrkA) receptor plays an important role in the release of superoxides and cytokines (Oda et al. 2006, Oda et al. 2008). This review will present findings about the signal transduction via TrkA receptor induced by alpha-toxin and summarize information about its likely role in inflammatory disease, especially septic shock.

2. Role of TrkA on a inflammation induced by alpha-toxin

2.1. Signal transduction via TrkA receptor

The TrkA receptor is a 140-kDa transmembrane protein encoded by a proto-oncogene located on chromosome 1 (Martin-Zanca, Hughes and Barbacid 1986). The family of Trk receptor tyrosine kinases consists of TrkA, TrkB and TrkC. While these family members have highly conserved sequences, they are activated by different neurotrophins: TrkA by nerve growth factor (NGF), TrkB by Brain-derived neurotrophic factor (BDNF) or neurotrophin 4 (NT4), and TrkC by NT3. TrkA regulates proliferation and is important for development and maturation of the nervous system (Pierotti and Greco 2006). This receptor comprises a tyrosine-kinase domain in its intra-cytoplasmic region and five extracellular domains, including two immunoglobulin-like domains involved in NGF binding and responsible for the specific selectivity to bind NGF (Wiesmann et al. 1999). In humans, the TrkA receptor is expressed on cells throughout the nervous system (Muragaki et al. 1995) as well as on structural cells and other non-neuronal cells in the immune and neuroendocrine systems (Levi-Montalcini et al. 1995, Aloe et al. 1997, Bonini et al. 2002, Levi-Montalcini 1987). When NGF binds to the TrkA receptor, it induces receptor homodimerization, which initiates kinase activation and transphosphorylation (Kaplan et al. 1991). This kinase activation involves small G proteins (Ras, Rac, Rap-1), PLCγ, protein kinase C (PKC) and phosphatidylinositol-3 kinase (PI3K) in neural cells (Obermeier et al. 1993b, Obermeier et al. 1993a, Melamed et al. 1999, York et al. 2000, Wu, Lai and Mobley 2001). Phosphorylation at Tyr490 is required for association with Shc and activation of the Ras-MAP kinase cascade. Residues Tyr674/675 lie within the catalytic domain, and phosphorylation at this site reflects TrkA kinase activity (Segal and Greenberg 1996, Stephens et al. 1994, Obermeier et al. 1993a, Obermeier et al. 1993b, Yao and Cooper 1995). Point mutations, deletions and chromosomal rearrangements (chimeras) cause ligand-independent receptor dimerization and activation of TrkA.

The mitogen-activated protein kinase (MAPK) pathways are activated next: extracellular-regulated protein kinase (ERK) by the small G proteins; ERK, p38 and JUN-N-terminal kinase (JNK) MAPK by PKC; and p38 and JNK by PI3K (Kaplan and Miller 1997). PI3K in turn induces activation of protein kinase B (PKB or Akt) and PKCξ (York et al. 2000)(Fig. 1).

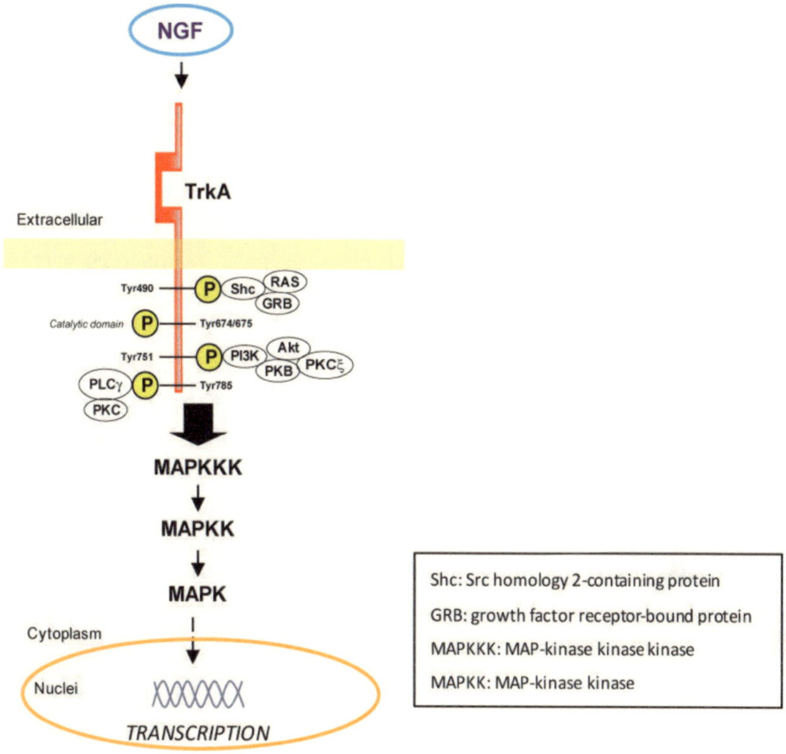

Figure 1. Signal transduction pathways of the TrkA receptor

2.2. Mechanism for the superoxide generation induced by alpha-toxin

The generation of superoxide in neutrophils has been reported to be stimulated by zymosan, 12-*O*-tetradecanoylphorbol 13-acetate (TPA), Ca^{2+} ionophores, and bacterial chemotatic peptides (Babior 1999). The signal transduction process leading to the stimulation has been studied extensively using *N*-formyl-methionyl-leucyl-phenylalanine (fMLP) (Kusunoki et al. 1992), platelet-activating factor (Yasaka, Boxer and Baehner 1982), and TPA (Nick et al. 1997, Pongracz and Lord 1998). It has been reported that these stimuli activated MAPK or PI3K in neutrophils (Shenoy, Gleich and Thomas 2003, Yamamori et al. 2004). Furthermore, these studies have demonstrated that the interaction of the ligands with receptors on neutrophils activates endogenous PLC with the formation of diacylglycerol (DG), which activates PKC, and inositol 1, 4, 5-trisphosphate (IP_3), inducing the release of Ca^{2+} from the endoreticulum, and that these products act synergistically to generate superoxide. Several studies also reported that phosphorylation of tyrosine kinases and activation of phospholipase D (PLD) were closely related to the generation of superoxide in neutrophils stimulated with agonists

(Garland 1992, Mitsuyama, Takeshige and Minakami 1993) and that activation of PLD resulted in the formation of PA, which was linked to the activation of NADPH oxidase (Bellavite et al. 1988, Olson, Tyagi and Lambeth 1990). We revealed that alpha-toxin-induced generation of superoxide is closely related to the activation of endogenous PKCθ via a combination of two events: production of DG on activation of PLC through a PT-sensitive GTP-binding protein and activation of phosphatidylinositide kinase 1 (PDK1) through the TrkA receptor (Oda et al. 2006).

There are three classes of PKC isotypes: classical PKC isotypes (PKCα, -β, and -γ) which have a C1 and C2 domain, bind DG, 1-oleoyl-2-acetyl-3-phosphoglycerol (OAG) and TPA, and are regulated by DG and Ca^{2+}; novel PKC isotypes (PKCδ, -ε, -η, and -θ), which have a C1 domain and novel C2 domain and are regulated by DG but not Ca^{2+}; and atypical isotypes (ζ/λ), which do not bind DG and are not regulated by these classical ligands (Le Good et al. 1998). Alpha-toxin induced phosphorylation of PKCθ and PKCζ/λ, and the generation of superoxide induced by the toxin was inhibited by rottlerin and calphostin C, an inhibitor of PKCθ. We reported that the formation of DG induced by alpha-toxin in rabbit neutrophils plays an important role in the generation of superoxide (Ochi et al. 2002). It therefore appears that the toxin-induced generation of superoxide is dependent on the activation of PKCθ, through binding of PKCθ phosphorylated by PDK1 to DG (Parekh, Ziegler and Parker 2000, Toker and Newton 2000). PKCθ has been reported to play an important role in activation of the protein 1 and NF-κB signaling pathway in T cells, production of interleukin-2, and apoptosis (Altman, Isakov and Baier 2000, Fan et al. 2004, Villalba et al. 1999, Villunger et al. 1999). Our data may provide clues to the role of PKCθ in neutrophils.

We reported that the alpha-toxin-stimulated generation of superoxide was related to the formation of DG through activation of endogenous PLC by a PT-sensitive GTP-binding protein in rabbit neutrophils (Ochi et al. 2002). U73122, an inhibitor of endogenous PLC, blocked the toxin-induced generation of superoxide and formation of DG in the cells, supporting that the toxin-induced increase in superoxide is dependent on the formation of DG by endogenous PLC. However, when the level of OAG incorporated into the cells was the same as the level of DG in the cells treated with 25 nM of the toxin, the level of OAG did not induce superoxide generation in the absence of the toxin but did in the presence of a near threshold dose (2.5 nM) of the toxin which did not induce production of DG. The result shows that the toxin-induced production of superoxide requires not only the formation of DG, but also the activation of other events.

It has been reported that the PI3K signaling pathway has an important role in several effector functions including the generation of superoxide (Yamamori et al. 2004). PI3K is known to generate phosphatidylinositol 3, 4, 5-trisphosphate (PIP_3), which is recognized by a pleckstrin homology domain identified as a specialized lipid-binding module (Le Good et al. 1998). Several papers have reported that PDK1 requires PIP_3 as its activator for effective catalytic activity (Le Good et al. 1998). Le Good et al. reported that there is a cascade involving PI3K, PDK1, and various members of the PKC superfamily in signal transduction (Le Good et al. 1998). Furthermore, the function of PKC family members is reported to depend on the phosphorylation of an activation loop by PDK1 (Le Good et al. 1998). LY294002 and wortmannin, both PI3K inhibitors, inhibited alpha-toxin-induced generation of superoxide and phosphorylation of PDK1 but did not affect the toxin-induced formation of DG. The result shows that the toxin-induced activation of PI3K occurs upstream of the phosphorylation of PDK1, which is an important step in the toxin-induced generation of superoxide. It is likely that the toxin-induced phosphorylation of PDK1 is a process independent of the toxin-induced formation of DG.

Tyrosine phosphorylation is thought to be crucial to the regulation of effector functions in neutrophils (Rollet et al. 1994). It is known that stimuli that induce tyrosine kinase activity in cells evoke the generation of PIP_1, PIP_2, and PIP_3. This tyrosine kinase activity is linked to the NGF receptors with intrinsic tyrosine kinase activity. Kannan et al. reported that NGF enhances the generation of superoxide induced by TPA in murine neutrophils (Kannan et al. 1991). Ehrhard et al. reported that human monocytes express the *trk* proto-oncogene, encoding the signal-transducing receptor unit for NGF, and that the interaction of NGF with monocytes triggers respiratory burst activity (Ehrhard et al. 1993). NGF, which did not induce the generation of superoxide in rabbit neutrophils, potentiated the events triggered by the toxin and caused superoxide to form in the presence of OAG, suggesting that a combination of the production of DG and stimulation of the NGF receptor induces severe activity in the generation of superoxide. The TrkA receptor was detected in rabbit neutrophils and found to be phosphorylated when the cells were treated with the toxin. Furthermore, immunoprecipitation using the anti-TrkA receptor antibody revealed direct binding of the toxin to the TrkA receptor. In addition, the antibody inhibited the toxin-induced generation of superoxide. These observations indicate that the interaction of alpha-toxin with TrkA receptors is important to the production of superoxide. In rabbit neutrophils, K252a, a TrkA inhibitor, and LY294002 inhibited the toxin-induced generation of superoxide and phosphorylation of PDK1 within specific concentration ranges, but PP2, a Src inhibitor, and AG1478, a epidermal growth factor receptor inhibitor, did not, supporting the finding that the TrkA receptor is involved in the toxin-induced increase in superoxide. The results obtained with the anti-TrkA antibody, LY294002, and K252a show that the activation of PI3K through direct binding of the toxin to the TrkA receptor results in production of PIP_3, which activates PDK1. In addition, PT inhibited the alpha-toxin-induced generation of superoxide and formation of DG, but not phosphorylation of PDK1, suggesting that a PT-sensitive GTP-binding protein plays a crucial role in the coupling to endogenous PLC, but not phosphorylation of PDK1. These observations indicate that the toxin independently induces activation of both endogenous PLC via a PT-sensitive GTP-binding protein and PDK1 via the TrkA receptor.

NGF, which binds to the TrkA receptor, is reported to be required for the differentiation and survival of sympathetic and some sensory and cholinergic neuronal populations (Howe et al. 2001). Furthermore, it has been reported that NGF is involved in inflammatory responses, an increase in mast cells in neonatal rats (Woolf et al. 1996), the degranulation of rat peritoneal mast cells (Woolf et al. 1996), and the differentiation of specific granulocytes (Kannan et al. 1991). The injection of *C. perfringens* cells or alpha-toxin into tissues is known to cause inflammation. Therefore, it is possible that the activation of the TrkA receptor by alpha-toxin is related to inflammation caused by *C. perfringens* in humans and animals.

H148G induced phosphorylation of PKCθ, but not production of DG, suggesting that the enzymatic activity of the toxin is essential for activation of endogenous PLC, but not activation of the TrkA receptor. It has been reported that binding of the C-domain, which does not contain the enzymatic site, to erythrocytes is important for the hemolysis induced by the toxin (Nagahama et al. 2002). It therefore is possible that the C-domain, the binding domain of alpha-toxin, plays a role in the binding of the toxin to the TrkA receptor and in the activation of signal transduction via the TrkA receptor.

Several studies have reported that the activation of PKC by various stimuli results in the generation of superoxide via the activation of MAPK systems (Coxon et al. 2003, Dewas et al. 2000, McLeish et al. 1998, Zu et al. 1998). K252a and U73122 inhibited the toxin-induced phosphorylation of PKCθ and ERK1/2 and generation of superoxide, suggesting that the toxin-induced production of superoxide is linked to the stimulation of the MAPK system via the activation of PKCθ. The toxin causes phosphorylation of ERK1/2, but not p38 and SAPK/JNK, implying that the process is dependent on a MAPK system containing MEK1/2 and MAPK/ERK1/2, but not systems containing p38 and SAPK/JNK.

It has been reported that PA directly or indirectly activated NADPH oxidase in a cell-free system of neutrophils (Erickson et al. 1999) and that PKCδ regulates phosphorylation of $p67^{phox}$ in human monocytes (Zhao et al. 2005). PKC also has been reported to activate directly NADPH oxidase (Johnson et al. 1998). However, PD98059 almost completely inhibited the toxin-induced production of superoxide near the inhibitory threshold dose of the inhibitor. Thus, it is unlikely that PA and PKC directly activate NADPH oxidase under the conditions used here.

We have shown that alpha-toxin induces formation of DG through the activation of endogenous PLC by a PT-sensitive GTP-binding protein and phosphorylation of PDK1 via stimulation of the TrkA receptor, so that DG and PDK1 synergistically activate PKCθ, and that the activation of PKCθ stimulates generation of superoxide through MAPK-associated signaling events in rabbit neutrophils (Fig. 2).

2.3. Mechanism for the cytokine release induced by alpha-toxin

Cytokines are immunoregulatory peptides with a potent inflammatory action, mediating the immune/metabolic response to an external noxious stimulus and fueling the transition from sepsis to septic shock, multiple organ dysfunction syndromes, and/or multiple organ failure (Tracey et al. 1987, Dinarello 2004, Riedemann, Guo and Ward 2003). It is thought that synergistic interactions between cytokines can cause or attenuate tissue injury (Calandra, Bochud and Heumann 2002). TNF-α, which is released early from neutrophils and macrophages, is one of the important cytokines involved in the pathophysiology of sepsis (Tracey et al. 1987, Lum et al. 1999). TNF-α-induced tissue injury is largely mediated through neutrophils, that respond by producing elastase, superoxide ion, hydrogen

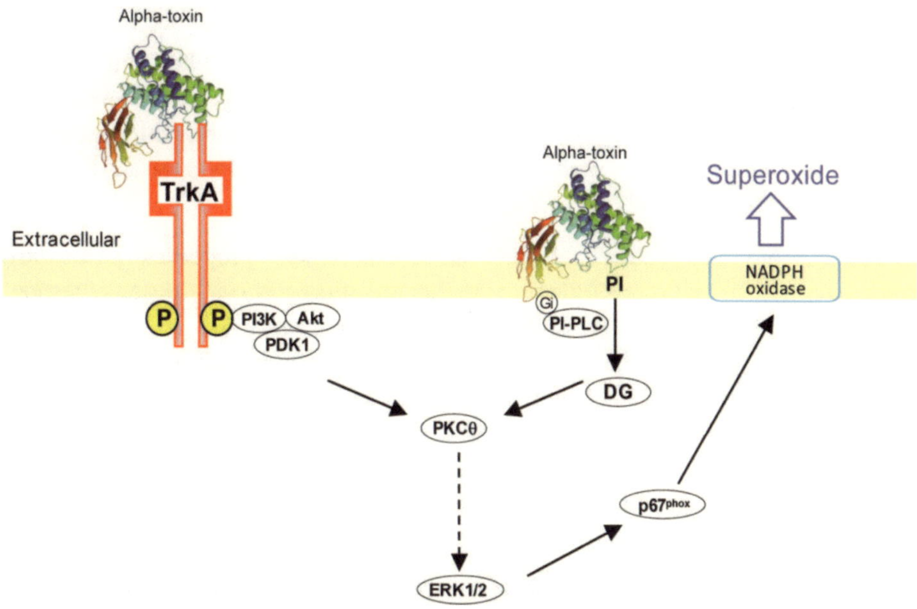

Figure 2. Signaling events involved in alpha-toxin-activated generation of superoxide

peroxide, sPLA2, PAF, leukotriene B1, and thromboxane A2 (Aldridge 2002). IL-1 stimulates the synthesis and release of prostagrandins, elastases, and collagenases and transendothelial microvascular cells, which respond by releasing the powerful neutrophil-stimulating agents, PAF and IL-8 (Leirisalo-Repo 1994). IL-1 and TNF-α are synergistic and share many biological effects in sepsis (Herbertson et al. 1995).

Anti-TNF-α antibody inhibited the death of mice induced by alpha-toxin. Furthermore, TNF-α-deficient mice were resistant to alpha-toxin. These observations suggest that the lethal effect of alpha-toxin is closely related to the release of TNF-α into the bloodstream. Stevens et al. and Bunting et al. suggested that alpha-toxin contributes indirectly to shock by stimulating production of endogenous mediators such as TNF-α and platelet-activating factor (Bunting et al. 1997, Stevens and Bryant 1997). It therefore appears that TNF-α released by alpha-toxin is important in enhancing the toxic actions of alpha-toxin in vivo. Consequently, inhibitors for release and expression of TNF-α may be worth pursuing as a novel therapeutic approach to the treatment of gas gangrene and sepsis caused by *C. perfringens*.

Cytokines such as the pro-inflammatory TNF-α, interleukin-1β (IL-1β) or transforming growth factor-β (TGF-β), increase the synthesis of NGF in airway structural cells. This stimulation has been evidenced in vitro in human pulmonary fibroblasts (Olgart and Frossard 2001, Micera et al. 2001), A549 epithelial cells (Pons et al. 2001) and bronchial smooth muscle cells (Freund et al. 2002). Studies also show that pro-inflammatory cytokines can act in concert to stimulate additional NGF secretion: TNF-α, for example, increases the secretion of NGF induced by IL-1β and interferon γ (IFN-γ) in fibroblasts (Hattori et al. 1994) and by interleukin-4 (IL-4) in astrocytes (Brodie et al. 1998). NGF synthesis in inflammatory conditions has also been demonstrated in vivo: elevated NGF concentrations are observed in cutaneous inflammation (Safieh-Garabedian et al. 1995) and in asthmatic airways (Olgart and Frossard 2001, Kassel, da Silva and Frossard 2001, Virchow et al. 1998). Taken together, these results suggest that pro-inflammatory cytokines, which are present at high levels in the airways of patients with asthma (Tillie-Leblond et al. 1999), might contribute to the elevated levels of NGF synthesis.

Corticosteroids are well known for their anti-inflammatory properties, particularly in asthmatic airways. Numerous studies report that the glucocorticoids dexamethasone and budesonide affect NGF expression. They cause a significant reduction in the increased NGF expression induced by pro-inflammatory cytokines; in one study, this action was shown to result from the repression of NGF gene transcription in endoneural fibroblasts from the rat sciatic nerve (Lindholm et al. 1990). Olgart and Frossard have reported that glucocorticoid treatment decreases the NGF secretion that the pro-inflammatory cytokines IL-1β and TNF-α stimulate in cultures of human pulmonary fibroblasts (Olgart and Frossard 2001) and in A549 epithelial cells (Pons et al. 2001).

These results suggested that the initial release of pro-inflammatory cytokines induced by alpha-toxin in vivo leads to the production of NGF, and the NGF released synergistically causes systemic inflammation such as sepsis and shock via activation of the TrkA receptor (Fig. 3).

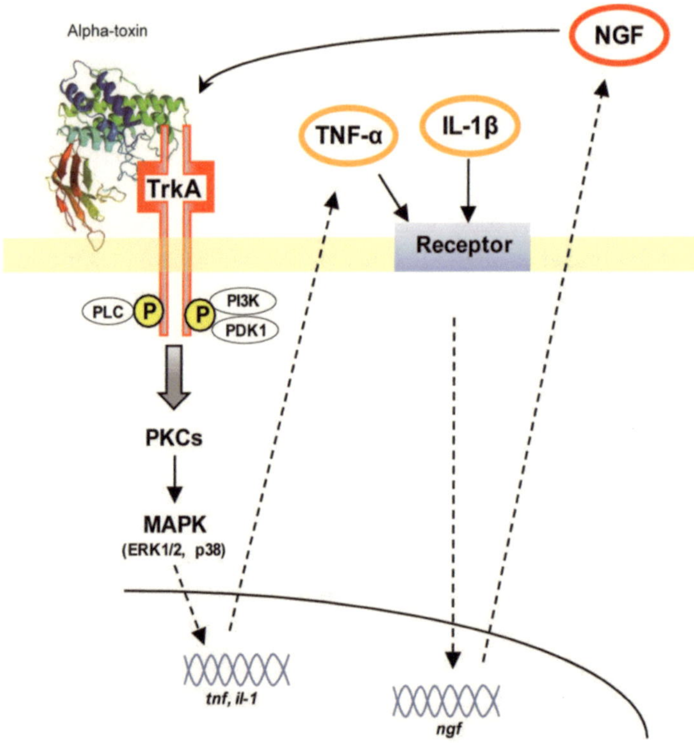

Figure 3. Alpha-toxin-induced release of pro-inflammatory cytokines and NGF

3. Conclusion

C. perfringens alpha-toxin, the main agent involved in the development of gas gangrene and septicemia, induces death, hemolysis, and the activation of macrophages and neutrophils. The toxin activated the MAPK-associated signal transduction from phospholipid metabolism and phosphorylation of TrkA. Penicillin is known to be highly effective in preventing the growth of microorganisms. In conclusion, treatment with TrkA inhibitors (tyrosine kinase inhibitors) and high doses of penicillin would be effective against diseases caused by *C. perfringens*.

Author details

Masataka Oda, Masahiro Nagahama, Keiko Kobayashi and Jun Sakurai
Faculty of Pharmaceutical Sciences, Tokushima Bunri University, Japan

4. References

Aldridge, A. J. (2002) Role of the neutrophil in septic shock and the adult respiratory distress syndrome. *Eur J Surg,* 168, 204-14.

Aloe, L., L. Bracci-Laudiero, S. Bonini & L. Manni (1997) The expanding role of nerve growth factor: from neurotrophic activity to immunologic diseases. *Allergy,* 52, 883-94.

Altman, A., N. Isakov & G. Baier (2000) Protein kinase Ctheta: a new essential superstar on the T-cell stage. *Immunol Today,* 21, 567-73.

Awad, M. M., A. E. Bryant, D. L. Stevens & J. I. Rood (1995) Virulence studies on chromosomal alpha-toxin and theta-toxin mutants constructed by allelic exchange provide genetic evidence for the essential role of alpha-toxin in *Clostridium perfringens*-mediated gas gangrene. *Mol Microbiol,* 15, 191-202.

Babior, B. M. (1999) NADPH oxidase: an update. *Blood,* 93, 1464-76.

Bellavite, P., F. Corso, S. Dusi, M. Grzeskowiak, V. Della-Bianca & F. Rossi (1988) Activation of NADPH-dependent superoxide production in plasma membrane extracts of pig neutrophils by phosphatidic acid. *J Biol Chem,* 263, 8210-4.

Bonini, S., A. Lambiase, G. Lapucci, F. Properzi, M. Bresciani, M. L. Bracci Laudiero, M. J. Mancini, A. Procoli, A. Micera, G. Sacerdoti, F. Levi-Schaffer, G. Rasi & L. Aloe (2002) Nerve growth factor and asthma. *Allergy,* 57 Suppl 72, 13-5.

Brodie, C., N. Goldreich, T. Haiman & G. Kazimirsky (1998) Functional IL-4 receptors on mouse astrocytes: IL-4 inhibits astrocyte activation and induces NGF secretion. *J Neuroimmunol,* 81, 20-30.

Bryant, A. E., R. Y. Chen, Y. Nagata, Y. Wang, C. H. Lee, S. Finegold, P. H. Guth & D. L. Stevens (2000a) Clostridial gas gangrene. I. Cellular and molecular mechanisms of microvascular dysfunction induced by exotoxins of *Clostridium perfringens*. *J Infect Dis,* 182, 799-807.

Bryant, A. E., R. Y. Chen, Y. Nagata, Y. Wang, C. H. Lee, S. Finegold, P. H. Guth & D. L. Stevens (2000b) Clostridial gas gangrene. II. Phospholipase C-induced activation of platelet gpIIbIIIa mediates vascular occlusion and myonecrosis in *Clostridium perfringens* gas gangrene. *J Infect Dis,* 182, 808-15.

Bunting, M., D. E. Lorant, A. E. Bryant, G. A. Zimmerman, T. M. McIntyre, D. L. Stevens & S. M. Prescott (1997) Alpha toxin from *Clostridium perfringens* induces proinflammatory changes in endothelial cells. *J Clin Invest,* 100, 565-74.

Calandra, T., P. Y. Bochud & D. Heumann (2002) Cytokines in septic shock. *Curr Clin Top Infect Dis,* 22, 1-23.

Coxon, P. Y., M. J. Rane, S. Uriarte, D. W. Powell, S. Singh, W. Butt, Q. Chen & K. R. McLeish (2003) MAPK-activated protein kinase-2 participates in p38 MAPK-dependent and ERK-dependent functions in human neutrophils. *Cell Signal,* 15, 993-1001.

Dewas, C., M. Fay, M. A. Gougerot-Pocidalo & J. El-Benna (2000) The mitogen-activated protein kinase extracellular signal-regulated kinase 1/2 pathway is involved in formyl-methionyl-leucyl-phenylalanine-induced p47phox phosphorylation in human neutrophils. *J Immunol,* 165, 5238-44.

Dinarello, C. A. (2004) Therapeutic strategies to reduce IL-1 activity in treating local and systemic inflammation. *Curr Opin Pharmacol,* 4, 378-85.

Ehrhard, P. B., U. Ganter, A. Stalder, J. Bauer & U. Otten (1993) Expression of functional trk protooncogene in human monocytes. *Proc Natl Acad Sci U S A,* 90, 5423-7.

Erickson, R. W., P. Langel-Peveri, A. E. Traynor-Kaplan, P. G. Heyworth & J. T. Curnutte (1999) Activation of human neutrophil NADPH oxidase by phosphatidic acid or diacylglycerol in a cell-free system. Activity of diacylglycerol is dependent on its conversion to phosphatidic acid. *J Biol Chem,* 274, 22243-50.

Fan, Y. Y., L. H. Ly, R. Barhoumi, D. N. McMurray & R. S. Chapkin (2004) Dietary docosahexaenoic acid suppresses T cell protein kinase C theta lipid raft recruitment and IL-2 production. *J Immunol,* 173, 6151-60.

Freund, V., F. Pons, V. Joly, E. Mathieu, N. Martinet & N. Frossard (2002) Upregulation of nerve growth factor expression by human airway smooth muscle cells in inflammatory conditions. *Eur Respir J,* 20, 458-63.

Garland, L. G. (1992) New pathways of phagocyte activation: the coupling of receptor-linked phospholipase D and the role of tyrosine kinase in primed neutrophils. *FEMS Microbiol Immunol,* 5, 229-37.

Hattori, A., S. Iwasaki, K. Murase, M. Tsujimoto, M. Sato, K. Hayashi & M. Kohno (1994) Tumor necrosis factor is markedly synergistic with interleukin 1 and interferon-gamma in stimulating the production of nerve growth factor in fibroblasts. *FEBS Lett,* 340, 177-80.

Herbertson, M. J., H. A. Werner, C. M. Goddard, J. A. Russell, A. Wheeler, R. Coxon & K. R. Walley (1995) Anti-tumor necrosis factor-alpha prevents decreased ventricular contractility in endotoxemic pigs. *Am J Respir Crit Care Med,* 152, 480-8.

Howe, C. L., J. S. Valletta, A. S. Rusnak & W. C. Mobley (2001) NGF signaling from clathrin-coated vesicles: evidence that signaling endosomes serve as a platform for the Ras-MAPK pathway. *Neuron,* 32, 801-14.

Johnson, J. L., J. W. Park, J. E. Benna, L. P. Faust, O. Inanami & B. M. Babior (1998) Activation of p47(PHOX), a cytosolic subunit of the leukocyte NADPH oxidase.

Phosphorylation of ser-359 or ser-370 precedes phosphorylation at other sites and is required for activity. *J Biol Chem,* 273, 35147-52.

Kannan, Y., H. Ushio, H. Koyama, M. Okada, M. Oikawa, T. Yoshihara, M. Kaneko & H. Matsuda (1991) 2.5S nerve growth factor enhances survival, phagocytosis, and superoxide production of murine neutrophils. *Blood,* 77, 1320-5.

Kaplan, D. R., B. L. Hempstead, D. Martin-Zanca, M. V. Chao & L. F. Parada (1991) The trk proto-oncogene product: a signal transducing receptor for nerve growth factor. *Science,* 252, 554-8.

Kaplan, D. R. & F. D. Miller (1997) Signal transduction by the neurotrophin receptors. *Curr Opin Cell Biol,* 9, 213-21.

Kassel, O., C. da Silva & N. Frossard (2001) The stem cell factor, its properties and potential role in the airways. *Pulm Pharmacol Ther,* 14, 277-88.

Kusunoki, T., H. Higashi, S. Hosoi, D. Hata, K. Sugie, M. Mayumi & H. Mikawa (1992) Tyrosine phosphorylation and its possible role in superoxide production by human neutrophils stimulated with FMLP and IgG. *Biochem Biophys Res Commun,* 183, 789-96.

Le Good, J. A., W. H. Ziegler, D. B. Parekh, D. R. Alessi, P. Cohen & P. J. Parker (1998) Protein kinase C isotypes controlled by phosphoinositide 3-kinase through the protein kinase PDK1. *Science,* 281, 2042-5.

Leirisalo-Repo, M. (1994) The present knowledge of the inflammatory process and the inflammatory mediators. *Pharmacol Toxicol,* 75 Suppl 2, 1-3.

Levi-Montalcini, R. (1987) The nerve growth factor 35 years later. *Science,* 237, 1154-62.

Levi-Montalcini, R., R. Dal Toso, F. della Valle, S. D. Skaper & A. Leon (1995) Update of the NGF saga. *J Neurol Sci,* 130, 119-27.

Lindholm, D., B. Hengerer, R. Heumann, P. Carroll & H. Thoenen (1990) Glucocorticoid Hormones Negatively Regulate Nerve Growth Factor Expression In Vivo and in Cultured Rat Fibroblasts. *Eur J Neurosci,* 2, 795-801.

Lum, L., B. R. Wong, R. Josien, J. D. Becherer, H. Erdjument-Bromage, J. Schlondorff, P. Tempst, Y. Choi & C. P. Blobel (1999) Evidence for a role of a tumor necrosis factor-alpha (TNF-alpha)-converting enzyme-like protease in shedding of TRANCE, a TNF family member involved in osteoclastogenesis and dendritic cell survival. *J Biol Chem,* 274, 13613-8.

Martin-Zanca, D., S. H. Hughes & M. Barbacid (1986) A human oncogene formed by the fusion of truncated tropomyosin and protein tyrosine kinase sequences. *Nature,* 319, 743-8.

McLeish, K. R., C. Knall, R. A. Ward, P. Gerwins, P. Y. Coxon, J. B. Klein & G. L. Johnson (1998) Activation of mitogen-activated protein kinase cascades during priming of human neutrophils by TNF-alpha and GM-CSF. *J Leukoc Biol,* 64, 537-45.

Melamed, I., H. Patel, C. Brodie & E. W. Gelfand (1999) Activation of Vav and Ras through the nerve growth factor and B cell receptors by different kinases. *Cell Immunol,* 191, 83-9.

Micera, A., E. Vigneti, D. Pickholtz, R. Reich, O. Pappo, S. Bonini, F. X. Maquart, L. Aloe & F. Levi-Schaffer (2001) Nerve growth factor displays stimulatory effects on human skin and lung fibroblasts, demonstrating a direct role for this factor in tissue repair. *Proc Natl Acad Sci U S A,* 98, 6162-7.

Mitsuyama, T., K. Takeshige & S. Minakami (1993) Tyrosine phosphorylation is involved in the respiratory burst of electropermeabilized human neutrophils at a step before diacylglycerol formation by phospholipase C. *FEBS Lett*, 322, 280-4.

Muragaki, Y., N. Timothy, S. Leight, B. L. Hempstead, M. V. Chao, J. Q. Trojanowski & V. M. Lee (1995) Expression of trk receptors in the developing and adult human central and peripheral nervous system. *J Comp Neurol*, 356, 387-97.

Nagahama, M., M. Mukai, S. Morimitsu, S. Ochi & J. Sakurai (2002) Role of the C-domain in the biological activities of *Clostridium perfringens* alpha-toxin. *Microbiol Immunol*, 46, 647-55.

Nick, J. A., N. J. Avdi, S. K. Young, C. Knall, P. Gerwins, G. L. Johnson & G. S. Worthen (1997) Common and distinct intracellular signaling pathways in human neutrophils utilized by platelet activating factor and FMLP. *J Clin Invest*, 99, 975-86.

Obermeier, A., H. Halfter, K. H. Wiesmuller, G. Jung, J. Schlessinger & A. Ullrich (1993a) Tyrosine 785 is a major determinant of Trk--substrate interaction. *EMBO J*, 12, 933-41.

Obermeier, A., R. Lammers, K. H. Wiesmuller, G. Jung, J. Schlessinger & A. Ullrich (1993b) Identification of Trk binding sites for SHC and phosphatidylinositol 3'-kinase and formation of a multimeric signaling complex. *J Biol Chem*, 268, 22963-6.

Ochi, S., K. Hashimoto, M. Nagahama & J. Sakurai (1996) Phospholipid metabolism induced by *Clostridium perfringens* alpha-toxin elicits a hot-cold type of hemolysis in rabbit erythrocytes. *Infect Immun*, 64, 3930-3.

Ochi, S., T. Miyawaki, H. Matsuda, M. Oda, M. Nagahama & J. Sakurai (2002) *Clostridium perfringens* alpha-toxin induces rabbit neutrophil adhesion. *Microbiology*, 148, 237-45.

Ochi, S., M. Oda, H. Matsuda, S. Ikari & J. Sakurai (2004) *Clostridium perfringens* alpha-toxin activates the sphingomyelin metabolism system in sheep erythrocytes. *J Biol Chem*, 279, 12181-9.

Oda, M., S. Ikari, T. Matsuno, Y. Morimune, M. Nagahama & J. Sakurai (2006) Signal transduction mechanism involved in *Clostridium perfringens* alpha-toxin-induced superoxide anion generation in rabbit neutrophils. *Infect Immun*, 74, 2876-86.

Oda, M., T. Matsuno, R. Shiihara, S. Ochi, R. Yamauchi, Y. Saito, H. Imagawa, M. Nagahama, M. Nishizawa & J. Sakurai (2008) The relationship between the metabolism of sphingomyelin species and the hemolysis of sheep erythrocytes induced by *Clostridium perfringens* alpha-toxin. *J Lipid Res*, 49, 1039-47.

Olgart, C. & N. Frossard (2001) Human lung fibroblasts secrete nerve growth factor: effect of inflammatory cytokines and glucocorticoids. *Eur Respir J*, 18, 115-21.

Olson, S. C., S. R. Tyagi & J. D. Lambeth (1990) Fluoride activates diradylglycerol and superoxide generation in human neutrophils via PLD/PA phosphohydrolase-dependent and -independent pathways. *FEBS Lett*, 272, 19-24.

Parekh, D. B., W. Ziegler & P. J. Parker (2000) Multiple pathways control protein kinase C phosphorylation. *EMBO J*, 19, 496-503.

Pierotti, M. A. & A. Greco (2006) Oncogenic rearrangements of the NTRK1/NGF receptor. *Cancer Lett*, 232, 90-8.

Pongracz, J. & J. M. Lord (1998) Superoxide production in human neutrophils: evidence for signal redundancy and the involvement of more than one PKC isoenzyme class. *Biochem Biophys Res Commun,* 247, 624-9.

Pons, F., V. Freund, H. Kuissu, E. Mathieu, C. Olgart & N. Frossard (2001) Nerve growth factor secretion by human lung epithelial A549 cells in pro- and anti-inflammatory conditions. *Eur J Pharmacol,* 428, 365-9.

Riedemann, N. C., R. F. Guo & P. A. Ward (2003) Novel strategies for the treatment of sepsis. *Nat Med,* 9, 517-24.

Rollet, E., A. C. Caon, C. J. Roberge, N. W. Liao, S. E. Malawista, S. R. McColl & P. H. Naccache (1994) Tyrosine phosphorylation in activated human neutrophils. Comparison of the effects of different classes of agonists and identification of the signaling pathways involved. *J Immunol,* 153, 353-63.

Safieh-Garabedian, B., S. Poole, A. Allchorne, J. Winter & C. J. Woolf (1995) Contribution of interleukin-1 beta to the inflammation-induced increase in nerve growth factor levels and inflammatory hyperalgesia. *Br J Pharmacol,* 115, 1265-75.

Sakurai, J., M. Nagahama & M. Oda (2004) *Clostridium perfringens* alpha-toxin: characterization and mode of action. *J Biochem,* 136, 569-74.

Segal, R. A. & M. E. Greenberg (1996) Intracellular signaling pathways activated by neurotrophic factors. *Annu Rev Neurosci,* 19, 463-89.

Shenoy, N. G., G. J. Gleich & L. L. Thomas (2003) Eosinophil major basic protein stimulates neutrophil superoxide production by a class IA phosphoinositide 3-kinase and protein kinase C-zeta-dependent pathway. *J Immunol,* 171, 3734-41.

Stephens, R. M., D. M. Loeb, T. D. Copeland, T. Pawson, L. A. Greene & D. R. Kaplan (1994) Trk receptors use redundant signal transduction pathways involving SHC and PLC-gamma 1 to mediate NGF responses. *Neuron,* 12, 691-705.

Stevens, D. L. & A. E. Bryant (1997) Pathogenesis of *Clostridium perfringens* infection: mechanisms and mediators of shock. *Clin Infect Dis,* 25 Suppl 2, S160-4.

Tillie-Leblond, I., J. Pugin, C. H. Marquette, C. Lamblin, F. Saulnier, A. Brichet, B. Wallaert, A. B. Tonnel & P. Gosset (1999) Balance between proinflammatory cytokines and their inhibitors in bronchial lavage from patients with status asthmaticus. *Am J Respir Crit Care Med,* 159, 487-94.

Toker, A. & A. C. Newton (2000) Cellular signaling: pivoting around PDK-1. *Cell,* 103, 185-8.

Tracey, K. J., Y. Fong, D. G. Hesse, K. R. Manogue, A. T. Lee, G. C. Kuo, S. F. Lowry & A. Cerami (1987) Anti-cachectin/TNF monoclonal antibodies prevent septic shock during lethal bacteraemia. *Nature,* 330, 662-4.

Villalba, M., S. Kasibhatla, L. Genestier, A. Mahboubi, D. R. Green & A. Altman (1999) Protein kinase ctheta cooperates with calcineurin to induce Fas ligand expression during activation-induced T cell death. *J Immunol,* 163, 5813-9.

Villunger, A., N. Ghaffari-Tabrizi, I. Tinhofer, N. Krumbock, B. Bauer, T. Schneider, S. Kasibhatla, R. Greil, G. Baier-Bitterlich, F. Uberall, D. R. Green & G. Baier (1999) Synergistic action of protein kinase C theta and calcineurin is sufficient for Fas ligand expression and induction of a crmA-sensitive apoptosis pathway in Jurkat T cells. *Eur J Immunol,* 29, 3549-61.

Virchow, J. C., P. Julius, M. Lommatzsch, W. Luttmann, H. Renz & A. Braun (1998) Neurotrophins are increased in bronchoalveolar lavage fluid after segmental allergen provocation. *Am J Respir Crit Care Med,* 158, 2002-5.

Wiesmann, C., M. H. Ultsch, S. H. Bass & A. M. de Vos (1999) Crystal structure of nerve growth factor in complex with the ligand-binding domain of the TrkA receptor. *Nature,* 401, 184-8.

Williamson, E. D. & R. W. Titball (1993) A genetically engineered vaccine against the alpha-toxin of *Clostridium perfringens* protects mice against experimental gas gangrene. *Vaccine,* 11, 1253-8.

Woolf, C. J., Q. P. Ma, A. Allchorne & S. Poole (1996) Peripheral cell types contributing to the hyperalgesic action of nerve growth factor in inflammation. *J Neurosci,* 16, 2716-23.

Wu, C., C. F. Lai & W. C. Mobley (2001) Nerve growth factor activates persistent Rap1 signaling in endosomes. *J Neurosci,* 21, 5406-16.

Yamamori, T., O. Inanami, H. Nagahata & M. Kuwabara (2004) Phosphoinositide 3-kinase regulates the phosphorylation of NADPH oxidase component p47(phox) by controlling cPKC/PKCdelta but not Akt. *Biochem Biophys Res Commun,* 316, 720-30.

Yao, R. & G. M. Cooper (1995) Requirement for phosphatidylinositol-3 kinase in the prevention of apoptosis by nerve growth factor. *Science,* 267, 2003-6.

Yasaka, T., L. A. Boxer & R. L. Baehner (1982) Monocyte aggregation and superoxide anion release in response to formyl-methionyl-leucyl-phenylalanine (FMLP) and platelet-activating factor (PAF). *J Immunol,* 128, 1939-44.

York, R. D., D. C. Molliver, S. S. Grewal, P. E. Stenberg, E. W. McCleskey & P. J. Stork (2000) Role of phosphoinositide 3-kinase and endocytosis in nerve growth factor-induced extracellular signal-regulated kinase activation via Ras and Rap1. *Mol Cell Biol,* 20, 8069-83.

Zhao, X., B. Xu, A. Bhattacharjee, C. M. Oldfield, F. B. Wientjes, G. M. Feldman & M. K. Cathcart (2005) Protein kinase Cdelta regulates p67phox phosphorylation in human monocytes. *J Leukoc Biol,* 77, 414-20.

Zu, Y. L., J. Qi, A. Gilchrist, G. A. Fernandez, D. Vazquez-Abad, D. L. Kreutzer, C. K. Huang & R. I. Sha'afi (1998) p38 mitogen-activated protein kinase activation is required for human neutrophil function triggered by TNF-alpha or FMLP stimulation. *J Immunol,* 160, 1982-9.

Chapter 12

Modulation of HER2 Tyrosine/Threonine Phosphorylation and Cell Signalling

Yamuna D. Gandaharen, Rachel S. Welt, David Kostyal and Sydney Welt

Additional information is available at the end of the chapter

http://dx.doi.org/10.5772/50472

1. Introduction

Cell-surface transmembrane tyrosine kinase signalling receptors EGFR, HER3 and HER4 are activated by specific ligand binding, reference in [1] which, induces signalling through intra-cellular domain kinase-dependant phosphorylation sites, see [2]. The intensity and specificity of the transmitted signal are modulated by homo and hetero-dimerization, allowing other family members to be recruited and thereby amplifying the signal [3]. HER2, which does not have a defined activating ligand, plays a key role in its capacity to amplify the signal [4] by being the preferred partner for hetero-dimerization. Both HER2 hetero and homo dimers maintain their intracellular kinase and phosphorylation sites in an activated state [3,5,6,]. HER2 hetero and homodimers both maintain their intracellular kinase and phosphorylation sites in an active state [5,6] Dimerization with HER2 increases receptor-ligand affinity and receptor-ligand stability, further enhancing activation [4,7]. In vivo enzymatic processing releases the HER2 extra-cellular domain (95 kD), including the dimerization site [8] from the membrane, but the role this plays in signal modulation remains undefined [9]. HER2-dependant activation signals promote a highly phosphorylated tyrosine state in the intra-cellular domain, which is then recognized by a family of specific cytoplasmic signal transducers [10]. These signal transducers regulate cell proliferation, apoptosis and cell characteristics associated with the transformed state [1,2 5,6]. Mitogen-activated protein kinases (MAPKs), and phosphatidylinositol 3-OH kinase (PI3K- AKT) pathways [11,12] have been particularly well studied as downstream signal pathways of HER2 leading to the concept of an oncogenic unit [13]. Accumulating experimental and clinical data link anti-HER2 treatment to inhibition of these downstream pathways suggesting that they are critical mediators of the activated HER2 state and cell survival [14]. However, whether the trastuzumab mediated inhibition of signalling is due to reduced HER2 phosphorylation/kinase activity, inhibition of HER2 dimerization, decreased HER2 levels, altered metabolic processing of HER2, binding dependant allosteric effects on HER2 or HER2-HER1/3/4 or a combination of these mechanisms is unknown.

In most cases, amplification of HER2 in breast cancer is associated with an amplicon comprising genes mapped to the 17q12-q21 region [15-18] that includes several genes involved with cell proliferation [16], transformation [17], adhesion [16] and chemotherapy sensitivity [18]. Clinically, the amplicon gene copy number is a parameter closely linked to trastuzumab and lapatinib efficacy [19,20].

Experimental evidence now suggests that nuclear localization of growth factors and receptors is not uncommon and also occurs with members of the EGFR family [21]. More recently, specific products derived from the HER2 receptor have been shown to have independent gene regulatory effects by virtue of a nuclear localization motif encoded in the HER2 protein [21,22] and by alternate splicing of the HER2 mRNA [21]. For example, the nuclear localization sequence preferentially targets a HER2 derived peptide to bind to sequences, one of which is in the COX-2 promoter region, leading to up-regulation of COX-2 expression [22]. Whether there are other HER2 derived peptides and the role they may play in the signalling cascade and whether any of the current anti-HER2 treatments modulate these factors remains is an area of current interest.

The original anti-HER2 mouse monoclonal antibody, 4D5, was shown to inhibit HER2 tyrosine phosphorylation [23] and breast cancer cell proliferation [23]. This antibody was humanized through genetic engineering to become trastuzumab [24,25]. A second antibody now in development (pertuzumab) binds to an extra-cellular HER2 epitope in close proximity to the dimerization site and has been shown to block dimerization [26-, 28]. A small molecule HER2/1 tyrosine kinase inhibitor, lapatinib has shown single agent activity in the clinic [20,29,30], providing further evidence that the disruption of the EGFR1/HER2 activation pathway, specifically by blocking phosphorylation [29-32], leads to cell death.

The focus of this investigation was to examine the effects of trastuzumab and lapatinib on breast cancer cell lines containing the HER2 amplicon under conditions of steady state anti-HER2 growth inhibitory effects. The quantifiable end point was the inhibition of proliferation as determined by MTT and Tritiated thymidine incorporation. These assays were used as evidence that the trastuzumab or lapatinib treatments had interrupted signalling pathways. Using immune detection of three distinct HER2 protein sites, four distinct HER2 tyrosine phosphorylation (P-Tyr) sites, a threonine phosphorylation (P-Thr) site and actin, changes in these parameters were monitored during anti-HER2 treatment. The demonstration of the restricted tyrosine kinase inhibitory activity of lapatinib further validated the specificity of the anti-HER2 phospho-tyrosine/threonine (P-Tyr/ P-Thr) antibodies selected for this investigation.

2. Materials and methods

Breast cancer cell lines were obtained from the American Type Culture Collection (ATCC, Manassas, VA) specifically for these experiments and maintained in RPMI 1640 with 50 units penicillin/streptomycin, 2 mM glutamine, 7.5 % fetal bovine serum, and incubated at 37º C in 5% CO_2. The ATCC authenticates and tests cell lines provide for research as per their protocols.

Four drug treatments and a control, done in quadruplicate, were analyzed using Western blot techniques. Cell concentrations were adjusted to 375,000 cells/ml in complete media and 1 ml was added to each well of a 12 well tissue culture plate. Cells were allowed to adhere to the plates for 24 hrs. Drugs or control solutions were added at a final concentration of 100 microgram/ml trastuzumab, (Herceptin) or control rituximab (Rituxin), (Genentech, San Francisco, Ca). Preliminary dose finding experiments were carried out at 2-250 micrograms/ml. 0.1% DMSO and 0.1%DMSO + 10 ηM Lapatinib (Tykerb) (GlaxoSmithKline Research Triangle Park, NC) was also tested following this same procedure .The cells were incubated at 37º C in 5% CO_2 for 8 or 48 hrs. The cells were lysed with either 400 μl of SDS loading buffer (58 mM Tris 6.8, 1.6 % SDS, 6% glycerol, 0.83% BME, 0.002% bromphenol blue) or NP-40 (0.5% NP-40, 50 mM Tris 7.4, 120 mM NaCl, 2.5 mM EGTA). Additional cell growth inhibitory studies were carried out for incubations up to 9 days in 6-well plates, and cells were tested serially every other day by pulse Tritiated thymidine incorporation and MTT assays

For Western blotting, samples were boiled in electrophoresis sample buffer containing 0.0625M Tris-HCl (pH6.8), 10% glycerol, 2% SDS and 5% BME, for 10 minutes then separated on 12% SDS-PAGE gels (mini-protean, Bio-Rad, Richmond, CA) at 100 V until the dye front reached the bottom then transferred overnight (47 mA) to nitrocellulose membranes (Bio-Rad). Membranes were blocked with a 5% w/v solution of non-fat dry milk in TPBS for 2 hours at room temperature (RT). The blots were then probed with primary antibodies according to the respective titers provided by their manufacturers and the membranes were rocked for 2 hours at RT. The blots were washed 1X with TPBS and a 1:10,000 dilution of secondary antibody (either goat anti-rabbit alkaline phosphatase or goat anti mouse alkaline phosphatase (Sigma, ST Louis, MO) was added, and the blots rocked at RT for 1 hour. The blots were washed 3X with TPBS and the membrane developed in the alkaline phosphate substrate NBT/BCIP (Promega Corp., Madison, WI).

Rabbit anti-P-Tyr 877, P-Tyr 1112, P-Tyr 1221/1222, P-Tyr 1248 P-Tyr 877, P-Tyr 1221/1222, and anti-amino acid peptide containing residue 1222, were purchased from Cell Signalling Technology, Inc,(Danvers, MA). Anti-P-Tyr 4G10, was purchased from Millipore, (Billerica, MA). Anti-extracellular HER2, Neu (9G6):sc-08, anti-HER2 P-Thr 686, p-Neu (7F8):sc81508, anti-HER2 P-Tyr 1112, p-Neu (19G5):sc-81528, anti-extracellular HER2, Neu(ER23):sc-74241, were purchased from Santa Cruz Biotechnology (Santa Cruz, CA). Anti-HER2 (AA 7570-987) was purchased from ProMab Biotechnologies, Inc. (Albany, CA). All antibodies were used per the manufacturer's recommendations. Membrane fractions were isolated using the Perfect-Focus Membrane Protein kit, (G Biosciences, Maryland Heights, MO), according to the manufacturer's protocol.

Human serum samples from patients and normal volunteers were collected under an Institutional Review Board approved research protocol and stored in our serum bank of de-identified serum specimens, stored at -78 degrees Celsius.

3. Results

3.1. Cell growth-inhibitory and viability assays

To define the experimental time points where anti-HER2 therapy modulation of downstream signalling could be demonstrated, breast cancer cell lines were tested for trastuzumab/lapatinib growth inhibitory effects by Tritiated thymidine incorporation and MTT assays. Three HER2 amplicon-containing cell lines were examined, BT-474, SK-BR-3, MDA-MB-453, and amplicon (-) MCF7 served as a control [29,31]. Cells were treated in log phase growth under conditions where factors such as confluence inhibition were minimized. Antibody controls included isotype matched human/mouse IgG1 chimeric (rituximab) and fully humanized IgG1 antibody (bevacizumab). In addition, IgG1 cetuximab, which blocks EGFR1 signalling, was used as an additional control; as in a separate set of experiments, we confirmed that bit did not induce a proliferation or inhibitory state in these cell lines, in agreement with reports by others, nor did we find any effect on HER2 tyrosine phosphorylation [29]. Trastuzumab was tested at a continuous cell exposure dose of 100 micrograms/ml with select experiments carried out at 2- 250 micrograms/ml. Cell cultures were assayed at various time points up to 9 days of treatment. Results of cumulative and pulsed-chased Tritiated thymidine incorporation and MTT assays were in agreement, demonstrating a reproducible inhibitory effect of trastuzumab on cell growth and division. This is best demonstrated by the cell line BT-474. Cell lines SK-Br-3 and MDA-MB-453 exhibited lesser effects and no effect was seen on HER2 amplicon negative control MCF7 cells. These results are consistent with previous reports [29,31]. The Tritiated thymidine incorporation experiments suggested that a trastuzumab-mediated continuous cell-growth inhibitory state is established throughout the incubation period by demonstrating reduced incorporation per cell at each time point tested in the trastuzumab treated cultures (Table 1). Significant cell death was not observed with trastuzumab up to the 9-day time point. Of note was that the maximum cell-growth inhibition by both MTT and Tritiated thymidine incorporation assays was observed at 5 micrograms/ml of trastuzumab, thus the assays described below were carried out at 20-50 times the active biological dose. The 100 micrograms/ml dose was selected as it most closely matches doses achieved in patients.

Effective doses for lapatinib in the cell culture assays ranged from 1 nanogram/ml to 1 microgram/ml. In contrast to results with trastuzumab, lapatinib induced significant cell death by day five (> 90%) under conditions of continued cell exposure at a constant drug dose of ≥10 nanograms. Lapatinib cell cultures beyond five days had no measurable MTT signal, lack of Tritiated thymidine incorporation (< 1% initial values) and few viable adherent cells by microscopic examination. Experiments with lapatinib included a dimethyl sulfoxide (DMSO) control, as it was the solvent used for this lipophilic drug. Control DMSO had a small effect on growth kinetics but no cell death was observed. In order to examine the comparative biologic/phosphorylation inhibition effects of these two agents, time points of 8 hours and 48 hours were selected for further analysis. The critical feature of these two time points is that cell viability appeared high in both trastuzumab and lapatinib cultures as demonstrated by the MTT assay, Tritiated thymidine incorporation, protein levels of HER2 and actin in cell cultures as assessed by Western blots, and the continued adherence of cells up to 48 hours as determined by microscopic examination. These experiments would therefore allow for the examination of molecular events prior to cell death, distinguishing between events that may be related to induction of cell death versus changes resulting from cell death.

TRASTUZUMAB	DAYS	1	3	5	7	9
% ^{3}H-thymidine incorporation	Cell lines					
	BT474	76.3	81.5	76.7	68.5	66.2
	SK-BR-3	84.4	80.2	80.4	77.6	65.1
	MDA-MB-543	81.4	84.3	78.3	73.9	67.7
	MCF-7	98.7	97.9	101.6	99.0	100.7
% MTT						
	BT474	99.3	95.4	87.6	62.1	45.4
	SK-BR-3	97.7	93.6	75.5	70.1	65.3
	MDA-MB-543	99.7	97.3	90.3	82.1	71.2
	MCF7	97.7	99.8	102.2	100.6	101.0
LAPATINIB	DAYS	1	3	5	7	9
% ^{3}H-thymidine incorporation	Cell lines					
	BT474	80.3	77.2	6.6	1.1	----
	SK-BR-3	84.7	82.1	8.8	----	----
	MDA-MB-543	88.7	82.0	8.4	----	----
	MCF-7	102.0	101.2	96.7	98.5	97.9
% MTT						
	BT474	97.6	88.4	4.7	----	----
	SK-BR-3	99.9	96.8	14.3	----	----
	MDA-MB-543	100.5	97.9	13.6	----	----
	MCF-7	104.1	97.9	97.6	101.7	100.6

Values are expressed as %-treated cells/controls for each time point. Data shown represents experiments carried out with trastuzumab 100 micrograms/ml and lapatinib 10 nanograms/ml While the MTT assay represents relative total viable cell counts of treated cells compared to controls, the ^{3}H-thymidine counts/minute (cpm) were corrected for number of viable cells using the MTT assay data (cpm treated/cpm control/MTT treated/MTT control). The paired data sets were evaluated by Student's t-test for significance and those values achieving statistical significance are **bolded.** ---- indicates no measurable signal.

Table 1. Relative growth inhibitory values

3.2. Western blot experiments

3.2.1. HER2 protein levels

Protein level changes for HER2 and actin, associated with trastuzumab or lapatinib treatment at two selected treatment time points (8 and 48 h) were analyzed by Western blot analysis. Three specific polyclonal antibody sera detecting HER2 were tested, one recognizing epitopes in the ectodomain (amino acid 182-373), and two detecting epitopes in the cytoplasmic domains (amino acids 750-987 and a determinant in proximity to the Tyr 1222 amino acid). These experiments were carried out at least four times each and representative panels of a single experiment are shown in Figure 1. The three controls shown here were cells grown in media alone, cells grown in the presence of rituximab, and cells grown in DMSO. All controls gave very similar bands for the three anti-HER2 antibody sera. Small changes are inHER2 levels are first detected at 48 hours in cell line SK-Br-3 treated with lapatinib, while actin levels remain unchanged at this time point. This finding is consistent in each of the four separate experiments and confirms the increase in cell surface HER2 levels associated with lapatinib treatment as previously reported for cell line SK-Br-3 [31]. This time point is just prior to the onset of events associated with apoptosis and may represent a consequence of cellular pathway disruption, as increased HER2 mRNA levels were not observed. In separate experiments, cells grown in the presence of cetuximab or bevacizumab (not shown) resulted in western blots identical to controls indicating a lack of modulation of HER2 protein expression by anti-EGFR or VEGF therapy in these cell lines. These results are consistent with our previously reported analysis of EGFR, HER2, HER3 and HER4 mRNA levels by gene expression mRNA array analysis of mRNA extracted from these breast cancer cell lines treated with trastuzumab compared to these controls [30]. These parallel experiments used extracts from these breast cancer cell lines treated with trastuzumab or cetuximab, or control antibodies, under these same defined conditions and time points.

No difference in actin levels was noted in each set of these experiments. As the cell count number in the first 48 hours showed <10% difference, the amount of cell extract applied to the gel while corrected for cell number at each time point had very little variance. Thus, these results are consistent with those of the Tritiated thymidine and MTT assays indicating the minor growth inhibitory effects of these agents up to 48 hours. These finding also support the contention that biologic events occurring up to 48 hours of treatment precede cell death events and are possible activators of critical pathways leading to cell death.

3.2.2. Tyrosine and threonine phosphorylation levels in the control cultures:

Four site specific anti-P-Tyr antibodies (Tyr 877, 1112, 1222 and 1248) and one anti-P-Thr (Thr 686) were tested on cell extracts collected at specific timed intervals (Figure 1). The controls showed consistent pattern of staining at the two time points examined for each cell line, but different patterns of relative intensity for each tyrosine or threonine were observed for each cell line. These results suggest that each cell line has a distinct net P-Tyr signalling oncogenic unit, rather than a HER2 specific net down-stream signalling motif.

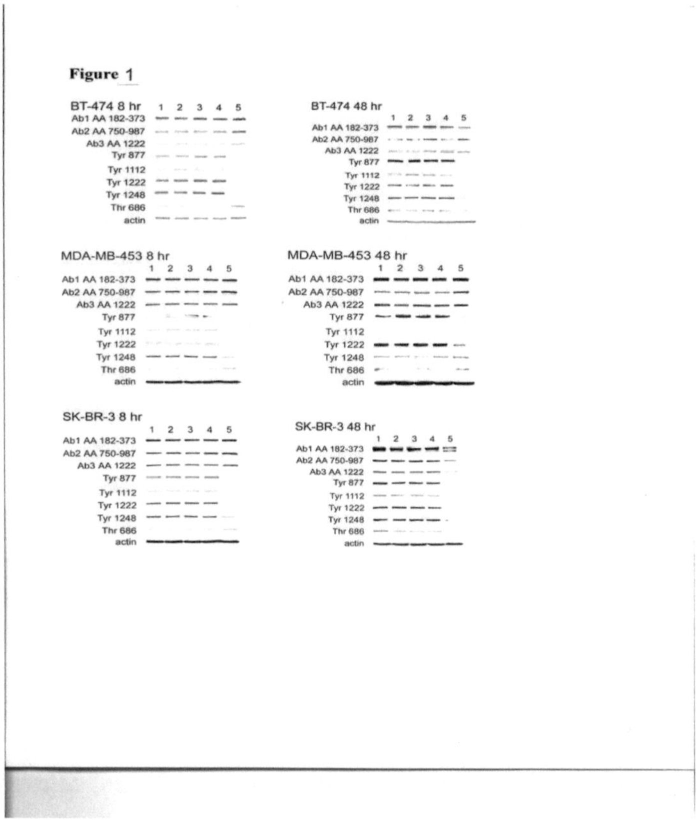

Figure 1. Shows Western blots bands of HER2, phosphorylated tyrosines/threonines, and actin from representative experiments of three cell lines growing in the presence of trastuzumab or lapatinib, or their controls, tested at 8 hours and 48 hours after drug administration. Primary antibodies were used at 1:5,000 for anti-P-Tyr/Thr and anti-HER2 antibodies and 1:10,000 for anti-actin antibodies and secondary antibodies. Labelled lanes show trastuzumab-treated cells in *lane* 2 with its controls in *lane* 1 (media alone) and 3 (control antibody). *Lane* 5 shows lapatinib-treated cells and the control grown in lapatinib solvent, (DMSO) in *lane* 4. Blots show the p185 band with secondary reagent as shown, and actin is presented as proof of viability and equivalent cell number applied to each *lane*. These gels demonstrate the contrast in phosphorylated tyrosines detected comparing lapatinib to trastuzumab and confirm the TKI activity of lapatinib. At 8 hours, lapatinib almost completely blocked tyrosine phosphorylation with virtually no discernible difference in the in the HER2 protein levels. The 48 hour time point was selected as it represented the last time point tested prior to lapatinib-induced cell death, which was almost complete by day 6.

Compared to the media controls, the DMSO controls did not differ in phosphorylation levels of these specific P-Tyr or P-Thr. While the intensity of the bands were similar for each cell line at each of the two time points, exceptions were noted for Tyr 877 and cell lines BT-474 and MDA MD 453, where phosphorylation is clearly increased from the 8 hour to the 48 hour time point. Similarly, P-Tyr 1222 also demonstrated increased intensity from 8 to 48 hours in cell line MDA-MB-453. Whether these findings suggest that the cells are not completely recruited into log phase growth at the 8-hour time point or cell-cell contact plays a role is unclear. The actin and HER2 bands strongly suggest equivalence of cell number applied to each lane at each of these time points.

3.2.3. Tyrosine and threonine phosphorylation levels in trastuzumab and lapatinib treated cells

No discernable change in phosphorylation of the P-Tyr or P-Thr was detected for trastuzumab-treated cells despite ongoing inhibition of cell growth at these time points. The unexpected lack of trastuzumab inhibition of tyrosine phosphorylation prompted experiments that replaced fetal calf serum (FCS) with human serum to determine if a component of FCS was responsible for inhibiting the full trastuzumab activity. Cells grown in media with 10% human serum from breast cancer patients or normal females, pre or postmenopausal, or male serum did not affect these findings (data not shown). Doses of trastuzumab up to 250 micrograms/ml did also did not change the patterns of phosphorylation. In contrast to the results demonstrating constant HER2 protein steady state levels, P-Tyr levels in lapatinib treated cells are markedly reduced (Tyr 1248) or absent (Tyr 687, 1116 and 1223), consistent with its role as a HER2 tyrosine kinase inhibitor (Figure 1). In addition, the P-Thr level is not affected by lapatinib exposure, demonstrating the tyrosine backbone specificity of lapatinib. As the lapatinib Western blots demonstrate, HER2 and actin protein levels are maintained through 48 hours, these results strongly suggests that changes in detected phosphorylation levels are due to kinase inhibition rather than the substantial in HER2 protein or cell death. We suggest that these early findings are related to the lapatinib mechanism of cell death that is apparent 2-3 days later.

3.3. MRNA expression patterns in trastuzumab treated breast cancer cells

3.3.1. Detection of a small molecular weight HER2-like product

Cell fractionation experiments were carried out to determine whether HER2 derived products with nuclear localization motifs could be identified by Western Blot analysis and to determine if trastuzumab or lapatinib altered their molecular processing mechanism. Differential generation of enzymatically derived nuclear localizing products could be responsible for trastuzumab mediated trans-membrane growth inhibitory effects. The results indicate that these techniques were not sensitive enough to detect, or were not of the correct immune-specificity to detect HER2 derived product in concentrates of nuclear or cytoplasmic cell fractions (data not shown).

However, using the anti-HER2 external domain antibody (AA 182-373), we detected a small molecular weight (20 kD) external domain-like HER2-derived product associated with the cell (Figure 2). This peptide segment is too far from the hydrophobic transmembrane segment to contain a transmembrane anchoring component to explain its association with the cell pellet, as it is too small (approximately 180 amino-acids in length) to extend from position 373 to the transmembrane domain. This peptide was not detected in supernatant or concentrates of supernatants. Cells exposed to acid conditions (pH 4.0, 0.5 M acetate, 0.15 N NaCl) to elute this 20 kD segment from the cell surface demonstrated that the 20 kD peptide could not be eluted under these conditions and was still found associated and concentrated in the cell pellet fraction (figure 2). Because concentrates of cytoplasmic fractions and nuclear fractions did not demonstrate the presence of this 20 kD peptide segment, a Triton X-114 fraction of the cell membrane was assayed and found to have high levels of this product (Figure 2). These results suggest that this product is derived from the extra-cellular domain of HER2 by enzymatic processing and binds avidly to a cell membrane-anchored determinant or is internalized into a sub-membrane compartment, co-purifying with the membrane fraction, or that it is a membrane protein cross reactive with antibody to extracellular domain (AA 183-373). The significance of this finding is that this peptide appears to be inhibited by lapatinib treatment while the intact HER2 levels remain constant and expression of this protein is unaffected by trastuzumab treatments (Figure 2). Thus, this small molecular weight product may be related to the unphosphorylated state of HER2.

4. Discussion

HER2 transmembrane activation signals promote a high level of selected intracellular domain P-Tyr sites, which are then recognized by specific cytoplasmic signal transducer molecules [10]. Thus, HER2 acts as an oncogenic unit transmitting cell survival, growth, and cell proliferation signals to critical intracellular pathways such as Mitogen-activated protein kinases (MAPKs), AKT and phoshatidylinositol 3-OH kinase (PI3K) pathways[11,12,29]. Here, we show that the relative level of specific P-Tyr is different for each HER2 amplicon-positive cell line examined, and thus, each oncogenic unit may be distinct in each tumour [13]r. Linkage of anti-HER2 treatment to the inhibition of these downstream pathways is well established, suggesting that these specific P-Tyr are critical mediators of the downstream signalling effects of the activated HER2 state and cell survival [7,10-12,29,30]. The molecular mechanism by which trastuzumab, a humanized IgG1, modulates the intracellular tyrosine kinase site from its extra-cellular binding site has remained unanswered. For example, cetuximab binds to, or near, the ligand binding site of EGFR thus acting as an antagonist [1,2,30-32]. Defining the molecular mechanism by which trastuzumab mediates its anti-HER2 effects could reveal a general non-ligand site-specific strategy for development of receptor inhibitory monoclonal antibodies in other receptor kinase systems.

The primary focus of this investigation was to determine the key molecular mechanism(s) governing trastuzumab's transmembrane modulation of downstream effects. Here, we show that trastuzumab binding does not appear to alter the net steady state levels of p185 HER2 protein as detected by all three of the anti-HER2 antibodies tested. Previous gene mRNA expression array findings demonstrate that no significant change in mRNA levels for HER2 or the other members of the ERBb family were induced by trastuzumab binding [33]. Taken together, these results strongly argue against an antibody-dependent alteration in natural turnover rate or internalization kinetics of HER2 [34]. We conclude that in the absence of demonstrable modulation of HER2 membrane mass on the cell surface, HER2 protein synthesis, and thus, alteration of kinetics of internalization or HER2 metabolism, net membrane HER2 levels could not be implicated as a mechanism to down-regulate HER2 signalling. Despite these observations for HER2, our gene mRNA expression array data did suggest numerous intracellular pathway modulations mediated by trastuzumab binding to the target cells examined here [33]. These findings confirm transmembrane signal transduction modulation directed and specific to trastuzumab binding [33-35]. For example, we found that, the ubiquitin pathway is up-regulated upon trastuzumab binding to HER2 [35], as has been reported by others through ligase activity at tyrosine 1112 [35,36].

Trastuzumab has not been definitively shown to retain the tyrosine kinase inhibitory activity of the parent 4D5 mouse monoclonal antibody [23]. Here we show that the level of HER2-P-Tyr/Thr corrected to cell number, actin levels, and the steady-state levels of intact extractable HER2, is not altered by exposure to trastuzumab. The finding that both P-Tyr levels and HER2 levels in each of these assays reveal no change further supports the conclusions derived from the gene mRNA expression array data [33]. Thus, examination of HER2 steady-state protein levels and key phosphorylation sites [10] did not reveal the molecular perturbation responsible for well-documented trastuzumab inhibition of cell proliferation and downstream pathways.

In contrast to trastuzumab, lapatinib treatment almost completely abrogates the HER2-P-Tyr as a signalling element while leaving HER2 protein levels unchanged. Thus, lapatinib acts through the blockage of tyrosine phosphorylation rather than the modulation of internalization or metabolism of the HER2 protein. We further show a sequential relationship between lapatinib-induced blockage of HER2-P-Tyr (8 and 48 hours) and induction of cell death at day 5-6 of drug exposure. At this late time point, MTT, Tritiated thymidine, actin levels and microscopy all support a lapatinib induction of cell lyses.

The inhibition of cell growth was used to define the conditions of ongoing drug-induced biological effects. The cell growth experiments described here are in agreement with similar reports by others [24,31]. Trastuzumab induced slower growth but did not suppress net increases in cell numbers over time. This *in vitro* effect of trastuzumab parallels the clinical observation that a prolonged stable disease is a common outcome of treatment [37].

Treatment of amplicon-positive breast cancer cells with cetuximab confirms reports by others that anti-EGFR therapy does not inhibit proliferation, induce cell death, nor inhibit HER2 phosphorylation in these cell lines [31]. Furthermore, we did not find that combinations of cetuximab and trastuzumab augment inhibition of cell growth or promote apoptotic events [31]. Cell growth inhibition and phosphorylation experiments with cetuximab have not been in agreement with results of similar investigations using small molecules with EGFR tyrosine kinase inhibitory activity (TKI) [38,39]. However, drugs such as gefitinib, which are believed to be relatively specific for EGFR, are also found to block HER2 phosphorylation at higher doses [38], complicating the interpretation of its mechanism of action [38]. Whether there is an independent anti-EGFR activity cross-inhibiting HER2 phosphorylation (cross-talk) or whether this observation is a consequence of the direct anti-HER2-phosphorylation activity of gefitinib is unclear. Results of these *in vitro* experiments may mislead investigators into attributing findings to cross-talk between receptor pathways rather than cross-reactivity of the reagent tested. We may over estimate biologic activity when reagents are used at too high of a concentration or too long of an exposure. Results of these experiments may mislead investigators into attributing findings to cross-talk between receptor pathways rather than the cross reactivity of the reagent tested. Thus, we conclude that results of experiments testing cetuximab's biologic effects more closely represent, and are more specific to, the pure anti-EGFR blockade. We clearly show here, in agreement with previous reports by others that pure anti-EGFR1 inhibition of signalling does not result in cell death or modulation of HER2 phosphorylation levels [29].

These observations suggest that the anti-EGFR1 tyrosine kinase effects of lapatinib are not contributing to its anti-HER2 effects. Thus, the results of the panel of anti-HER2-P-Tyr-antibodies demonstrating almost complete abrogation of HER2 phosphorylation by lapatinib and its associated delayed cell cytotoxicity (day 5-6) establishes a specific and unique link between HER2 tyrosine phosphorylation and cell survival. Importantly, these results also suggest that additional signalling through HER3 and HER4 may not be critical for apoptosis [40], except as it may ultimately be mediated through HER2 tyrosine kinase inhibition (reduction in hetero-dimerization) [40]. Thus, blocking dimerization by itself, which is unlikely to affect steric change in the intracellular domain, will not induce a modulation of P-Tyr levels. Taken together, these data suggest that testing the effect of a specific and robust HER2 tyrosine kinase inhibitory reagent is warranted.

In the clinic, where the anti-EGFR toxicity of lapatinib is dose limiting (diarrhea and skin rash) and prohibits dose escalation, the testing of a small molecule TKI manifesting pure HER2 kinase inhibition would be of great interest. Recently a pan ErbB TKI was tested and shown to be dose limited by the EGFR-mediated bowel toxicity, further supporting the conclusions presented here [41]. A pure anti-HER2 agent would be even more compelling if one could demonstrate upon dose escalation increased tumor cytotoxicity and a lack of other intervening non-HER2 related dose-limiting toxicities. Close examination of many of the TKIs demonstrate widespread promiscuity with many unexpected cross-reactivities [42]. In general, clinical success of a widely reactive kinase inhibitor is not informative as an identifier of the key pathway(s) responsible for mediating anti-tumor effects and often leads to "assumed" mechanisms of activity.

Using the four anti-P-Tyr sera, we could not find any diminution in the phosphorylation levels as assayed by Western blots, in cells treated up to nine days in the presence of trastuzumab. In addition, the anti-phospho-threonine reagent was used as a negative control, and was found not to be blocked by lapatinib demonstrating the specificity of the drug and the kinase activity. Thus, we propose that the kinase inhibition that was originally described by the mouse antibody 4D5 [23] has been lost in the humanization process [25]. The abundance of well-documented evidence that inhibition of specific downstream pathways is a consequence of trastuzumab-cell binding remains unexplained.

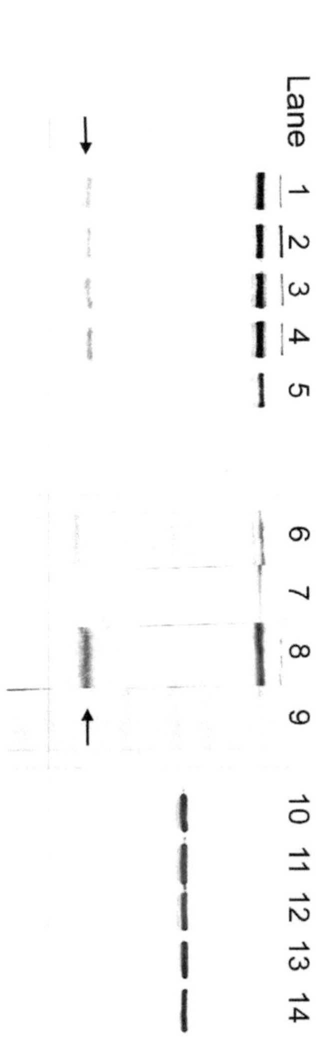

Figure 2. Demonstrates a series of experiments evaluating a 20 kD protein detected by anti-HER2 extracellular domain (AA 182-373) anti-sera at 48 hours. *Lanes 1-5* demonstrate the full Western blot gel of BT-474 (48 hours, from Figure 1) showing two bands: the p185 HER2 protein and the 20 kD protein (arrow on left) *lanes 1-4.* Note that this protein in not detected in *lane 5* which represents lapatinib-treated cells, while the p185 HER2 is mildly reduced in *lane 5. Lanes 1- 14* show the corresponding actin control confirming that equal numbers of cell were applied to *lanes 1-5.* Exposing BT-475to cells to an acid wash of pH 4.0 does not elute the protein as *lane 7* is the acid wash and the cell pellet that remains is shown in *lane 6,* has both p185 and the 20 kD protein. Using the Triton X Perfect Focus Membrane Protein kit methodology shows a clearer picture of localization of the 20 kD band with membrane HER2 protein and the 20 kD band (arrow) both in *lane 8* (membrane protein concentrate) and corresponding cell pellet, run in *lane 9,* is negative.

One hypothesis to be considered is that the trastuzumab effect is a weaker version of what is seen with lapatinib and while we cannot demonstrate a small loss of P-Tyr activity in culture, more sensitive techniques might be informative. Alternatively, trastuzumab inhibition may be allosteric or conformational in nature and at the level of the cytoplasmic signal transducers [10] ability to detect the phosphate moieties in the context of an altered peptide conformation [43]. One may further speculate that due to the unique binding epitope of trastuzumab, which is in extra-cellular proximal domain, trans-membrane tertiary structural changes may be induced. Cross-linking HER2 (dimers) at the extracellular proximal domain may disrupt the P-Tyr access to cytoplasmic signal transducers by physical constraints. This hypothesis would suggest that other membrane receptor systems could also be modulated in a similar fashion.

Our results demonstrate the presence of a small 20 kD protein concentrated in the extracted membrane fraction which is immunologically similar to an extra-cellular segment of HER2 protein. This may provide further evidence of specific enzymatic digestion of HER2 into novel biologic agents [44,45]. The low molecular weight of this identified fragment and its association with the membrane fraction raises the possibility that it may function as a ligand for another, as yet unidentified, receptor. Thus, we hypothesize that HER2 may not be a classical receptor as has been suspected by the lack of a ligand binding moiety but rather a pre-ligand entity which requires regulated and specific digestion to be activated. The differential expression of this moiety with lapatinib in contrast to trastuzumab treatment, demonstrates the complexity of this system and the difficulty in attributing a single molecular mechanism in transmembrane signal transduction.

These observations are not informative regarding the precise cytotoxic mechanism of trastuzumab activity in the clinic. Models based on preclinical animal studies favor immune mechanisms as key in mediating tumor shrinkage [46]. Studies of patients treated in the neo-adjuvant setting also support these findings [43]. However the clinical effects of trastuzumab could be divided into two distinct effects, a growth inhibitory effect as seen in vitro and which manifests clinically as long term stable disease and a cytotoxic effect as one might expect from immune mediated cell lysis which results in rapid tumor shrinkage in the clinic, especially as seen in neo-adjuvant studies [47].

In addition to these hypotheses, there is evidence that HER2 induced downstream effects actually amplify pro-inflammatory factors such as COX-2 [22] creating a micro-environment for promoting immune cell mediated tumor cell killing. These data are in agreement with modulation of a prostaglandin pathway identified by gene mRNA expression array experiments [33] in trastuzumab treated cells. Thus downstream events induced by HER2 or regulated by trastuzumab binding, may promote the immune mediated killing of tumor cells by trastuzumab. These findings provide a strong rational for combining other anti-breast cancer cell antibodies with trastuzumab therapy. Furthermore the additional anti-tumor efficacy observed with combinations of trastuzumab and chemotherapy could also be attributable to the known effects of certain chemotherapeutic agents, which render tumor cells more sensitive to immune attack [48]. If this is the case, research should be focused on mechanisms by which chemotherapy may damage tumor cells sufficiently to allow more efficient killing by immune mechanisms rather than focus on apoptotic pathways that enhance chemotherapy cytotoxic effects.

Author details

Yamuna D. Gandaharen and Sydney Welt
Welt Bio-Molecular Pharmaceutical, LLC. Molecular Research, Armonk, NY, U.S.A.

Rachel S. Welt
Department of Biological Sciences, Fordham University, NYC, NY, U.S.A.

David Kostyal
ARD Laboratories, Biologic Research, Akron, OH, U.S.A.

Acknowledgement

Funding and support-PA State Department of Health Project Cure Award SAP # 4100031280 and the Cantwell Foundation Fund of Coudersport Pennsylvania 16901.

Disclosure statement

The authors declare that there are no competing financial interests in carrying out this study.

5. References

[1] Yarden, Y Sliwowski, MX. Untangling the ErbB signalling network. *Nat Rev Mol Biol* 2:127-137, 2001.

[2] Pinkas-Kramarski, R Soussan, L Waterman, H Levkowitz, G Alroy, I *et al*. Diversification of Neu differentiation factor and epidermal growth factor signalling by combinatorial receptor interactions. *Embo J* 15: 2452-2467, 1996.

[3] Graus-Porta, D, Beerli, RR Daly, JM Hynes, NF. ErbB-2, the preferred heterodimerization partner on all Erb receptors, is mediator of lateral signalling. *Embo J* 16:1647-1655, 1997.

[4] Wang, LM Kuo, A Alimandi, M Veri, MC Lee, CC. *et al*. ErbB expression increases the spectrum and potency of ligand-mediated signal transduction through ErbB. *Proc Natl Acad Sci U S A* 95:6809-6814, 1998.

[5] Worthylake, R Opresko, LK Wiley, HS. ErbB-2 amplification inhibits down-regulation and induces constitutive activation of both ErbB and epidermal growth factor receptors. *J Biol Chem* 274:8865-8874, 1999.

[6] Desmedt, C Sperindle, J Piette, F Huang, W Jin, X. *et al*. Quantitation of HER2 expression or HER2:HER2 dimers and differential survival in a cohort of metastatic breast cancer patients carefully for trastuzumab treatment primarily by FISH. *Diagn Mol Pathol*. 18:22-29, 2009.

[7] Wolf-Yardin, A Kumer, N Zhang, Y Hautaniememi, S Zaman, M *et al*. Effects of HER2 overexpression on cell signalling networks governing proliferation and migration. *Mol Syst Biol* 2:55-60, 2006.

[8] Yuan, CX Lasut, AL Wynn, R Neff, NT Hollis, GF. Purification of Her-2 extracellular domain and identification of its cleavage site. *Protein Expr Purif*.29:217-22, 2003

[9] Molina, MA Codony-Servat, J Albanell, J Rojo, F Arribas, J. *et al*. Trastuzumab (herceptin), a humanized anti-Her2 receptor monoclonal antibody, inhibits basal and activated Her2 ectodomain cleavage in breast cancer cells. *Cancer Res*. 61: 4744-4749, 2001.

[10] Dankort D, Jeyabalan N, Jones N, Dumont DJ, Muller WJ. Multiple ErbB-2/Neu Phosphorylation Sites Mediate Transformation through Distinct Effector Proteins. J Biol Chem. Oct 19;276(42):38921-8, 2001

[11] Zhou, BP Liao, Y Xia, W Spohn, L Lee, MH. *et al*. Cytoplasmic localization of p21 Cip1/WAF1 by Akt-induced phosphorylation in HER-2/neu-over expressing cells. *Nature Cell Biol*; 3: 245-252, 2001.

[12] Fedi, P Pierce, JH di Fiore, PP. Efficient coupling with phosphotidylinositol 3-kinase, but not phospholipase C gamma or GTPase-activating protein, distinguishes ERB-3 signalling from that of other ERB/EGFR family receptors. *Mol Cell Biol* 14:492-500, 1994.

[13] Holbro T, Beerli RR, Maurer F, et al The ErbB2/ErbB3 heterodimer functions as an oncogenic unit: ErbB2 requires ErbB3 to drive breast cell proliferation. Proc Natl Acad Sci U S A 100:88933-8938 2003.

[14] Mohsin SK, Weiss HL, Gutierrez MC, Chamness GC, Schiff R, Digiovanna MP, Wang CX, Hilsenbeck SG, Osborne CK, Allred DC, Elledge R, Chang JC. Neoadjuvant trastuzumab induces apoptosis in primary breast cancer J Clin Oncolol 23: 7238-7240, 2005

[15] Kauraniemi P, Barlund M, Monni O, Kallioniemi. New amplified and Highly Expressed Genes Discovered in ERBB2 Amplicon in Breast Cancer by cDNA Microarrays Cancer Res: 61 8235-8240, 2001

[16] Mackay A, Jones C, Dexter T, LA Silva R, Bulmer K, JonesA, Simpson P, Harris RA, Jat PS, Neville AM, Ries LFL, Lakhani SR, O'Hare MJ c DNA microarray analysis of genes associated with ERBB2 (HER2/neu) overexpression in human mammary luminal epithelial cells. Oncogene 22; 2680-2688, 2003

[17] Kauraniemi P, Kallioniemi A. Activation of multiple cancer-associated genes at the ERBB2 amplicon in breast cancer.Endocr Relat Cancer. 13:39-49, 2006

[18] Arriola E, Marchio C, Tan DS, Drury SC, Lambros MB, Natrajan R, Rodriguez-Pinilla SM, Mackay A, Tamber N, Fenwick K, Jones C, Dowsett M, Ashworth A, Reis-Filho JS.

Genomic analysis of the HER2/TOP2A amplicon in breast cancer and breast cancer cell lines. Lab Invest. 88:491-503, 2008.

[19] Fornier M, Risio M, Van Poznak c, Seidman A Her2 testing and correlation with efficacy of trastuzumab therapy. Oncology 16: 1340-1348, 2002.

[20] Press MF, HER-2 gene amplification, HER-2 and epidermal growth factor mRNA and protein expression, and lapatinib efficacy in women with metastatic breast cancerClin Can Res. 14:7861-70 2008

[21] Chen QQ, Chen XY, Jiang YY, Liu J. Identification of novel nuclear localization signal within the ErbB-2 protein. Cell Res. 15:504-10, 2005.

[22] Wang C S, Lien HC, Xia W, Chen IF, Lo HW, Wang Z, Ali-Sayed M, Lee DF, Bartholomeusz G, Yang FO, Giri DK, Hung MC, Binding at transactivation of the COX-2 promoter by nuclear tyrosine kinase receptor Erb-2. Cancer Cell. 6: 251-261, 2004.

[23] Kumar R, Shepard HM, Mendelsohn J. Regulation of phosphorylation of the c-erbB-2/HER2 gene product by a monoclonal antibody and serum growth factor(s) in human mammary carcinoma cells. Mol Cell Biol. Feb;11(2):979-86, 1991.

[24] Lewis GD, Figari I, Fendly B, Wong WL, Carter P, Gorman C, Shepard HM. Differential responses of human tumor cell lines to anti-p185HER2 monoclonal antibodies. Cancer Immunol Immunother. Sep;37(4):255-63, 1993

[25] Carter P, Presta L, Gorman CM, Ridgway JB, Henner D, et al. Humanization of an ati-p185HER2 antibody for human cancer therapy. Proc Natl Acad Sci USA 89:4285-4289, 1992.

[26] Franklin, MC, Carey KD, Vajdos FF, Leahy DJ, de Vos AM, et al. Insights into ErbB signalling from the structure of the ErbB-pertuzumab complex. Cancer Cell 5:317-328, 2004.

[27] Agus DB, Gordon MS, Taylor C, et al. Phase I clinical study of pertuzumab, a novel HER dimerization inhibitor, in patients with advanced cancer. J Clin Oncol. 23:2534-2543, 2005.

[28] Freiss T, Scheuer W, Hasmann M. Superior antitumor activity after combination treatment with pertuzumab and trastuzumab against NSCLC and breast cancer xenograft tumors. Program and abstracts of the 31st European Society for Medical Oncology Congress; Istanbul, Turkey. September 29-October 3, 2006; Abstract 96PD.

[29] Chen WW, Input-output behaviour of ErbB signalling pathways as revealed by mass action model trained against dynamic data. Mol Syst Biol 5:239-58. 2006

[30] Xia W, Mullin RJ, Keith BR, Liu LH, Ma H, et al. Anti-tumor activity of GW572016: a dual tyrosine kinase inhibitor blocks EGF activation of EGFR/erbB2 and downstream Erk1/2 and AKT pathways. Oncogene. Sep 12;21(41):6255-63, 2002.

[31] Brockhoff G, Heckel B, Schmidt-Brueken E, Plander M, Hofstaedter F. Differential impact of Cetuximab, Pertuzumab and Trastuzumab on BT474 and SK-BR-3 breast cancer cell proliferation. Cell Prolif 40:488-507, 2007.

[32] Scaltriti M Lapatinib, A HER2 tyrosine kinase inhibitor, induced stabilization of HER2 and potentiates trastuzunmab-depedent cell cytotoxicity. Oncogene. 28: 803-14 2009

[33] Welle S, Welt S, Shay T, Lanning C, Horton K, et al. The use of gene array analysis to determine down-stream molecular expression patterns of trastuzumab (T) treatment. J Clin Onc, 2007 ASCO Annual Meeting Proceedings Part I, 25:14135,2007

[34] Mosesson Y, Mills GB, Yarden Y. Derailed endocytosis: an emerging feature of cancer. Nat Rev Cancer 9: 835-850, 2009.

[35] Klapper LN, Waterman H, Sela M, Yarden Y. Tumor-inhibitory antibodies to HER-2/ErbB-2 may act by recruiting c-Cbl and enhancing ubiquitination of HER-2. Cancer Res 60:3384-8, 2000.

[36] Binhua PZ, Yong L, Weiya X, Yiyu Z, Spohn B, et al. Her-2/ neu induces p53 ubiquination via Akt-mediated MDM2 phosphorylation. Nat Cell Biol. 3:973-982, 2001.

[37] Vogel CL, Cobleigh MA, Tripathy D, Gutheil JC, Harris LN, et al. First-line Herceptin monotherapy in metastatic breast cancer. Oncology. 61 Suppl 2:37-42, 2001.

[38] Moasser MM, Basso A, Averbuch SD, Rosen N. The tyrosine kinase inhibitor ZD1839 ("Iressa") inhibits HER-2 driven signaling and suppresses the growth of HER2-overexpressing tumor cells. Cancer Res. 61:7184-8, 2001.

[39] Moulder SL, Yakes FM, Muthuswamy SK, Bianco R, Simpson JF. Epidermal growth factor (HER1) tyrosine kinase inhibitor ZD1839 (Iressa) inhibits HER/neu (erbB2)-overexpressing breast cancer cells in vitro. Cancer Res. 2001. 61:8887-95.

[40] Sergina NV, Rausch M, Wang D, Blair J, Hann B, et al. Escape from Her-family tyrosine inhibitor therapy by kinase inhibitor therapy by the kinase-inactive HER3. Nature 445:437-441 2007.

[41] Wong KK, Fracasso PM, Bukowski RM, Lynch TJ, Munster PN, et al. A phase I study with neratinib (HKI-272), an irreversible pan ErbB receptor tyrosine kinase inhibitor, in patients with solid tumors. Clin Cancer Res. Apr 1;15(7):2552-8, 2009.

[42] Karaman MW, Herrgard S, Treiber DK, Gallant P, Atteridge CE, et al. A quantitative analysis of kinase inhibitor selectivity. Nat Biotechnol. Jan;26(1):127-32, 2008.

[43] Schulze WX, Deng L, Mann M. Phosohotyrosine interactome of the erbB-receptor kinase family, Mol Syst Biol. 10:1-13, 2005.

[44] Strohecker AM, Yehiely F, Chen F, Cryns VL. Caspase cleavage of HER-2 releases a Bad-like cell death effector. J Biol Chem. Jun 27;283(26):18269-82, 2008.

[45] Pedersen K A naturally occurring HER2 carboxyl-terminal fragment promotes mammary tumor growth and metastases. Mol Cell Biol 29:3319-31 2009

[46] Clynes RA, Towers TL, Presta LG, Ravetch JV. Inhibitory Fc receptors modulate in vivo cytoxicity against tumor targets. Nat Med. Apr;6(4):373-4, 2000.

[47] Gennari R, Menard S, Fagnoni F, Ponchio L, Scelsi M, et al. Pilot study of the mechanism of action of preoperative trastuzumab in patients with primary operable breast tumors overexpressing HER2. Clin Cancer Res. Sep 1;10(17):5650-5, 2004.

[48] Segerling M, Ohanian SH, Boros T. Chemotherapeutic drugs increase killing of tumor cells by antibody and complement. Science 188: 55-57, 1975.

Section 4

Protein Kinases and Phosphatases in Cell Cycle Regulation

Chapter 13

Protein Phosphorylation is an Important Tool to Change the Fate of Key Players in the Control of Cell Cycle Progression in *Saccharomyces cerevisiae*

Roberta Fraschini, Erica Raspelli and Corinne Cassani

Additional information is available at the end of the chapter

http://dx.doi.org/10.5772/47809

1. Introduction

Protein phosphorylation is a reversible posttranslational modification that can modulate protein role in several physiological processes in almost every possible way. These include modification of its intrinsic biological activity, subcellular location, half-life and binding with other proteins. Protein phosphorylation is particularly important for the regulation of key proteins involved in the control of cell cycle progression.

Protein phosphorylation is the covalent binding of a phosphate group to some critical residues of the polypeptide. The phosphorylation state of a protein is given by a balance between the activity of protein kinases and protein phosphatases. Eukaryotic protein kinases transfer phosphate groups (PO_4^{3-}) from ATP to an hydroxyl group of the lateral chain of specific serine, threonine or tyrosine residues on peptide substrates. In simple eukaryotic cells, like yeasts, Ser/Thr kinases are more common, while more complex eukaryotic cells, like human cells, have many Tyr kinases. Protein kinases recognize their substrates specifically and their active site consists of an activation loop and a catalytic loop between which substrates bind. Protein kinases differ from each other in the structure of their catalitic domain. A second class of enzymes, protein phosphatases, is responsible for the reverse reaction in which phosphate groups are removed from a protein. Phosphatases gain specificity by binding protein cofactors which facilitate binding to specific phosphoproteins. The active phosphatase often consists of a complex of the phosphatase catalytic subunit and a regulatory subunit.

The use of protein phosphorylation/dephosphorylation as a control mechanism has many advantages since it is rapid, it does not require new proteins to be made or degraded and it is easily reversible. The phosphorylation of specific residues induces structural changes that regulate protein functions by modulating protein folding, substrate affinity, stability and activity. For example, phosphorylation can cause switch-like changes in protein function, which can also lead to major modifications in the catalytic function of enzymes, including kinases and phosphatases. In addition, protein phosphorylation often leads to rearrangement in the structure of the protein that can induce changes in interacting partners or subcellular localization.

Phosphorylation acts as a molecular switch for many regulatory events in signalling pathways that drive cell division, proliferation, differentiation and apoptosis. In order to ensure an appropriate balance of protein phosphorylation, the cell can compartmentalize both protein kinases and phosphatases. Another kind of regulation can be achieved by the spatial distribution of kinases and phosphatases, that creates a gradient of phosphorylated substrates across different subcellular compartments. This spatial separation can also control the activity of other proteins or enzymes and the occurrence of other posttranslational modifications.

Even in a simple organism like budding yeast, approximately 3% of its proteins are kinases or phosphatases. Some of these enzymes are extremely specific, indeed that are able to phosphorylate or dephosphorylate only a few target proteins, while others can act broadly on many proteins. The examples of known targets of phosphorylation include most protein components of the cell like enzymes, structural proteins, cell receptors, ion channels and signaling factors. If a protein is controlled by its phosphorylation state, its activity will be directly dependent on the activity of the kinases and phosphatases that act on it. It is quite common for a phosphate group to be added or removed from a protein continually, a cycle that allows a protein to switch rapidly from one state to another.

A protein can be modified by the addition of a single phosphate group or it can undergo multisite phosphorylation, these events can be driven by a single kinase or by multiple kinases that act in concert. Multisite phosphorylation can determine the extent and duration of a cellular response and can integrate multiple signals on the same protein. For example, many protein kinases involved in the cell cycle control function by generating phosphoSer/Thr-containing sequence motifs in their substrates that are then recognized by phosphoSer/Thr binding proteins. In several cases the phosphopeptide binding domain targets the kinase to prephosphorylated (primed) sites and then mediates processive phosphorylation of the substrate. An important example of this regulation is given by some budding yeast proteins that are phosphorylated by the catalitic subunit of the Cyclin-Dependent Kinase (CDK), Cdc28, that "primes" the protein in order to bind and to be phosphorylated by the Polo-like kinase (Plk) Cdc5.

Cdks are the master regulators of the cell cycle and Cdc5 plays key roles during all stages of mitosis and in the cell cycle checkpoint response to genotoxic stress [1,2]. The protein kinase Cdc28 drives every cell cycle transition and its activity is tightly regulated by phosphorylation/dephosphorylation events and by its association with a class of proteins called cyclins. Cyclins levels fluctuate during the cell cycle and their binding to Cdc28 activates its catalitic domain and allows its binding to specific substrates. Polo-like kinases have a conserved Ser/Thr kinase domain and a noncatalytic C-terminal region composed by two homologous boxes Polo Box Domain (PBD) [3], that appear to target the kinase to mitotic substrates. In addition, it has been shown that phosphopeptide binding to the PBD stimulates kinase activity, suggesting a conformational switching mechanism for Plk regulation and a double function for the PBD.

It is the simplicity, reversibility and flexibility of phosphorylation that explains why it has been adopted as the most general control mechanism of the cell. Below we describe how phosphorylation and dephosphorylation events can finely regulate in space and time some key proteins in the control of cell cycle progression in *Saccharomyces cerevisiae* .

2. The protein kinase Swe1 is regulated at several levels

Budding yeast cyclin-dependent kinase Cdk1 is the motor that drives cell cycle progression. Cdk1 activity is regulated at multiple levels in different cell cycle phases by interactions with different proteins, called cyclins, and by phosphorylation and dephosphorylation events. In G2 phase of the cell cycle, the protein kinase Swe1 inhibits Cdk1 by phosphorylating the conserved Y19 residue of its catalytic subunit Cdc28 [4], thus blocking both switch from polar to isotropic bud growth and nuclear division, since both these events rely on G2/M Cdk activity. This inhibitory phosphorylation is reversed by the Mih1 phosphatase [5], leading to Cdk1 activation and entry into mitosis. Swe1 phosphorylates and inhibits Cdc28 during every cell cycle and in case of problems in the bud neck, bud formation, actin cytoskeleton and abnormal cell shape. Successful bud formation leads to Swe1 degradation in late G2 phase, while morphological defects block this degradation, thus delaying entry into mitosis. Swe1 has therefore a critical role in coordinating cell morphogenesis with nuclear division.

Swe1 levels are controlled by the "morphogenesis checkpoint", a pathway that is activated in response to alterations in the actin cytoskeleton or in septin organization. The activation of this checkpoint ultimately leads to Swe1 stabilization and a subsequent delay in nuclear division [6]. In an unperturbed cell cycle, Swe1 is recruited to the mother-bud neck in S phase; this change in its localization, which is promoted by the interaction with its regulators Hsl1 and Hsl7, is essential for subsequent Swe1 multiphosphorylation, an event that leads to its ubiquitylation and degradation, thus allowing entry into mitosis. The morphogenesis checkpoint causes Swe1 stabilization by interfering with its localization to the bud neck, acting directly on Swe1 or on its regulators Hsl1 and Hsl7, thus preventing modifications that lead to its degradation [7]. Accordingly, the lack of septin localization at the bud neck results in Swe1 stabilization [7-9], and even subtle perturbations in septin structure interfere with Hsl1 and Swe1 localization to the bud neck [7]. Moreover, actin depolymerization in budded cells causes both stabilization of Swe1 and its displacement from the bud neck without altering Hsl1 localization [7], indicating that morphogenesis checkpoint activation prevents Swe1 degradation by interfering with Swe1 localization to the bud neck, thus inhibiting its phosphorylation.

Swe1 is subjected to multiple regulations that change its phosphorylation state (35-40 phosphorylated sites have been identified *in vivo*), subcellular localization and protein levels (Figure 1). During S phase, Swe1 accumulates in the nucleus where it is phosphorylated by Clb-Cdc28 before being exported to the cytoplams and then to the daughter side of the bud neck. Swe1 nuclear export is essential for its degradation in G2/M in fact a Swe1 variant that cannot be exported from the nucleus is largely stabilized [10]. Clb-Cdc28 phosphorylates Swe1 at multiple sites [11] and these events can occur in the nucleus, in the cytoplasm or at the bud neck. This multiphosphorylation by Cdc28-Clb has different roles: on one hand it promotes Swe1 activity generating a feedback loop, while on the other hand it promotes Swe1 degradation [12]. At the mother-bud neck, filaments of conserved proteins called septins (Cdc3, Cdc10, Cdc11, Cdc12 and Shs1 in *S. cerevisiae*) form a dynamic ring structure [13] that is essential for the recruitment of a number of proteins involved in the control of cell cycle progression [14,15]. Among these, the septin ring acts as a platform to recruit several Swe1 regulators, such as the Hsl1 protein kinase and its adaptor Hsl7, both essential for Swe1 localization to the bud neck and for its phosphorylation [7,9]. Hsl1, whose kinase activity requires assembled septins, undergoes autophosphorylation [8,16] and phosphorylates Hsl7 [9] but does not seem to phosphorylates Swe1 [17] although its kinase activity is required for Swe1 recruitment at the bud neck [18]. The fact that Hsl1 activation requires assembled septins ensures that Swe1 degradation does not begin until a bud has formed, thus providing a link between bud formation and entry into mitosis [18]. Also the PAK (p21-activated kinase) kinase Cla4 associates with the septin ring and is involved in Swe1 phosphorylation, probably during S phase [19]. Moreover Swe1 phosphorylation by Clb-Cdc28 promotes subsequent phosphorylation by the Polo-like kinase Cdc5; in fact the synergistic phosphorylation that can be observed *in vitro* on Swe1 by Clb2-Cdc28 and Cdc5 is the result of priming Swe1 by Cdc28, in which the resulting phosphorylated Swe1 becomes a better substrate for Cdc5 [20]. An additional level of Swe1 regulation involves the Cdc55 regulatory subunit of protein phosphatase PP2A, that has been implicated in its degradation since loss of Cdc55 function causes Swe1 stabilization [21]. However, how this control happens at the molecular level is not clear. In addition, a mathematical model for the morphogenesis checkpoint activation suggested that a subset of Swe1 phosphorylations could inhibit its activity whereas other phosphorylations could target Swe1 for degradation [22]. In any case, hyperphosphorylated Swe1 species are recognized by a still unidentified ubiquitin ligase and ubiquitylated [23]. Subsequently, Swe1 is degraded via the proteasome and this event allows mitotic entry [23]. However, how bud neck-localized Swe1 is targeted to degradation after phosphorylation is still obscure. There are Swe1 variants that do not undergo degradation although they show proper bud neck localization, phosphorylation and interaction with known Swe1 regulators [23], indicating that still unknown Swe1 regulators exist.

So, Swe1 regulation is governed by complex pathways that are still partially unidentified. In particular, the involvement of the ubiquitylation pathway and the identity of the related ubiquitin ligase(s) involved in Swe1 degradation are unknown. A possible role in this control can be hypothesized for the functionally redundant budding yeast proteins Dma1 and Dma2, which belong to the same FHA-RING ubiquitin ligase family as *S. pombe* Dma1 and human Chfr and Rnf8. FHA domains are phosphothreonine-binding modules [24] frequently found in DNA repair and checkpoint proteins [25,26] and RING domains are typical of E3 ubiquitin ligases [26]. The presence of an FHA domain implies that one or more protein kinases function upstream of these proteins. An intact FHA domain is required for checkpoint function of all characterized FHA-RING ubiquitin ligases. All these proteins appear to control different aspects of the mitotic cell cycle, but several molecular details of their functions are still obscure [for review, see 27]. In particular, the *S. cerevisiae* Dma proteins are involved in mitotic checkpoints and contribute to control septin ring dynamics and cytokinesis by unknown mechanisms [28,29]. Moreover, *in vitro* ubiquitin ligase activity of Dma1 and Dma2 has been described [30], although their *in vivo* targets are still unknown.

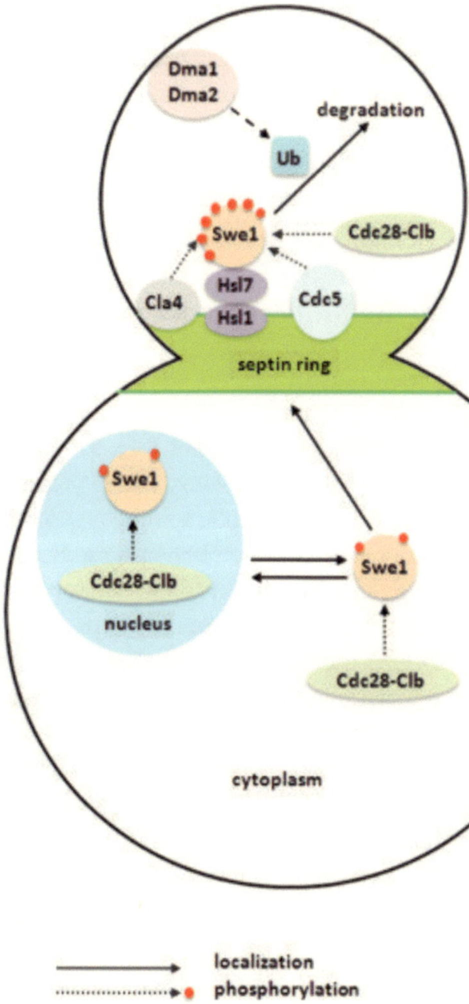

Figure 1. Model for Swe1 regulation. Swe1 shuttles from the nucleus to the cytoplasm and then it is translocated to the septin ring at the bud neck. These events are controlled through phosphorylation by Cdc28-Clb kinase. Once at the bud neck, Swe1 undergoes other phosphorylation events that drive its ubiquitylation and ultimately lead to its degradation via the proteasome. Dashed line indicates that Dma1 and Dma2 ubiquitin ligases are involved, directly or indirectly, in Swe1 ubiquitylation.

Recently, we provided genetic and biochemical evidence that Dma proteins are involved in promoting Swe1 ubiquitylation *in vivo* and contribute to the regulation of Swe1 stability by acting in a step following the recruitment of Swe1 to the bud neck and its phosphorylation [31]. Indeed, the lack of Dma proteins leads to accumulation of fully phosphorylated and bud neck localized Swe1. However, as *dma1Δ dma2Δ* cells are viable while Swe1 degradation is essential for cell viability, other yet unidentified ubiquitin ligases likely ubiquitylate Swe1 during an unperturbed cell cycle. The Dma-dependent Swe1 down-regulation, whose lack does not significantly affect unperturbed cell cycle progression when the other Swe1 regulatory pathways are proficient, appears to be crucial for proper response to DNA replication stress.

Collectively, the complex Swe1 regulation is an example of how phosphorylation events drive the fate of a protein. Indeed, Swe1 undergoes multiple phosphorylations that are crucial for its localization, its activity and its interaction with an E3 ubiquitin ligase that promote its degradation; moreover also some Swe1 regulators are regulated by phosphorylation, showing how this modification is largely involved in the control of cellular events.

3. The complex regulation of the protein kinase Kin4, a key player of the spindle position checkpoint

The spindle position checkpoint (SPOC) is the important pathway that blocks mitotic exit and cytokinesis in case of mitotic spindle misalignment [32]. This pathway is crucial for budding yeast since the division site is determined early in the yeast cell cycle, in late G1 concomitantly with bud site selection, while the mitotic spindle is assembled after this event. So, in order to allow proper chromosome distribution between mother and daugher cell, the mitotic spindle must be correctly aligned with respect to the mother bud axis before mitotic exit. The SPOC monitors this event and arrests mitotic progression in case of spindle misalignment. The target of the SPOC is the GTPase Tem1, that acts at the top of the Mitotic Exit Network (MEN). The MEN is a signaling cascade of protein kinases that controls both exit from mitosis and cytokinesis. At the top of the pathway, the GTPase Tem1 activates Cdc15 kinase that leads to Dbf2/Dbf20 and Mob1 activation. The MEN ultimately activates the protein phosphatase Cdc14 that leads to Cdk1 inactivation, a key event for both mitotic exit and cytokinesis [33]. The localization of all these proteins is important for their activity. The spindle pole body (SPB) component Nud1 is the platform for most MEN components localization to the spindle poles during mitosis [34]. During every cell cycle, Tem1 is kept inactive until the mitotic spindle is properly aligned respect to the mother-bud axis, thus coupling mitotic exit with nuclear division [35-37]. Tem1 regulation is complex: it is positively regulated by Lte1 [35] and it is kept inactive by the dimeric GTPase-activating protein (GAP) Bub2-Bfa1, which is the target of two protein kinases, Cdc5 and Kin4 [38-41]. Cdc5 is the budding yeast Polo-like kinase, it plays multiple functions in mitosis and cytokinesis through phosphorylation of different substrates. Cdc5 inhibits Bfa1 by phosphorylation at the anaphase onset [40,41], thus promoting timely Tem1 activation and mitotic exit. Kin4 is a non essential serine/threonine protein kinase that plays only a minor role in mitotic progression in normal growth conditions. But, importantly, Kin4 kinase participates in the SPOC and indeed it is essential to delay cell cycle progression of cells with a misaligned spindle. In case of spindle mispositioning, Kin4 maintains Bub2-Bfa1 GAP complex active through phosphorylation of Bfa1 on residues Ser150 and Ser180 [42], these events counteract Cdc5 action on Bfa1 and thereby inhibit mitotic exit.

As already said, the subcellular localization of MEN and SPOC components is critical for their function, indeed the asymmetric distribution of MEN activators and inhibitors is one element that couples mitotic exit with correct nuclear migration. During an unperturbed cell cycle the Bub2-Bfa1 complex and Tem1 preferentially associates with the SPB that enters the daughter cell (dSPB) [35,37]. Instead the Lte1 protein, which positively regulates Tem1, is confined in the bud from the G1/S transition to telophase, when it diffuses throughout the cytoplasm of both mother cell and bud [37]. During anaphase, the SPB-associated Bub2-Bfa1 GAP complex keeps Tem1 inactive until the SPB and spindle enter the bud, where Tem1 is activated by its encounter with Lte1, thus promoting mitotic exit. Similarly to MEN factors, Kin4 binds the SPB in a Nud1 dependent manner [34,43]. During normal cell cycle progression, Kin4 localizes to the cortex of the mother cell by interaction of its C-terminal regulatory domain and this binding is a prerequisit for its loading on mother-bound SPB (mSPB) during midanaphase [44]. When spindles is correctly oriented, Kin4 and Bub2-Bfa1 are asymmetrically localized to opposite SPBs. With anaphase onset, Bub2-Bfa1 then becomes inhibited by the Cdc5 kinase thus promoting mitotic exit. On the contrary, in case of spindle misalignment, Kin4 and Bub2-Bfa1 are brought together at both SPBs [45-48]; in these conditions Kin4 prevents Bfa1 phosphorylation by Cdc5, thereby inhibiting mitotic exit and this regulation is essential for survival of cells with a misaligned spindle.

So, Kin4 subcellular localization and activity are finely regulated during an unperturbed cell cycle and in response to spindle misalignment and these events involve its phosphorylation state (Figure 2). Kin4 phosphorylation state changes during the cell cycle: it is hyperphosphorylated during late stages of mitosis but is hypophosphorylated during S-phase and early mitosis [49]. At present, the relationship between Kin4 function, phosphorylation and localization is not fully understood, but at least three regulators of Kin4 have been identified: Lte1, the protein phosphatase PP2A-Rts1 and the bud neck kinase Elm1.

Recent data indicate that Lte1 can regulate Kin4 by controlling its phosphorylation status [50]: Lte1 binds Kin4 and promotes its hyperphosphorylation and this event restricts Kin4 binding to the mSPB and prevents Kin4 that escapes the mother cell from associating with the dSPB. Importantly, this Lte1-mediated exclusion of Kin4 from the dSPB is essential for proper mitotic exit of cells with a correctly aligned spindle. Therefore, Lte1 promotes mitotic exit by inhibiting Kin4 activity at the dSPB. However, how this regulation happens remains to be determined. Indeed, Lte1 might regulate Kin4 activity itself, the Kin4 phosphatase PP2A-Rts1, the Kin4 kinase Elm1, other Kin4 kinases or the availability of Kin4 itself to be phosphorylated. So the SPOC function could be linked to the spatial restriction of the MEN regulators Kin4 and Lte1 and inhibition of Kin4 by Lte1 [50].

On the basis of the correlation between phosphorylation status and time of Kin4 activation during the cell cycle, it was hypothesized that dephosphorylated Kin4 might be its active form and that phosphatases that promote accumulation of this form would be required for Kin4 function. Recently, the protein phosphatase PP2A and its regulatory subunit Rts1 have been identified as Kin4 regulators. In particular, the phosphatase PP2A-Rts1 is required for Kin4 dephosphorylation during cell cycle entry and to maintain Kin4 in the dephosphorylated state during S phase and mitosis [49]. In addition, PP2A-Rts1 is crucial for proper localization of Kin4 to the mother cortex and SPBs both during the cell cycle and in response to spindle position defects [49]. The phosphatase does not appear to affect Kin4 kinase activity but instead it promotes its association with SPBs, which is essential for SPOC activity. So, PP2A-Rts1 functions upstream of Kin4, regulating its phosphorylation and localization during an unperturbed cell cycle and during SPOC activation, thus defining the phosphatase as a key regulator of SPOC function [49]. However, it is still unclear how Rts1 mobilizes Kin4 at the cortex and enables its association with SPBs, indeed it might dephosphorylate Kin4 or a Kin4 interactor at SPBs.

Another key player of Kin4 regulation is the bud neck-localized Elm1 kinase [51,52]. Elm1 has been previously implicated in septin organization, bud morphogenesis, bud neck integrity and cell cycle progression [53-55]. Recently it has been shown that Elm1 contributes to the SPOC by promoting Kin4 kinase activity. Indeed, Elm1 activates Kin4 by direct phosphorylation on Thr209, a residue in the activation loop, and on additional sites at the C terminus of Kin4 [51,52]. Kin4 phosphorylation by Elm1 is critical for its kinase activity and subsequent hyperphosphorylation [49,51,52]. At present, the molecular mechanism by which phosphorylation of Thr209 influences Kin4 catalytic function is unclear. Structural studies of kinases regulated by activation loop phosphorylation indicate that the loop might function as a "sensitive switch" that controls substrate binding triggered by phosphorylation-dependent conformational changes [56]. However, the lack of Kin4 kinase activity and hyperphosphorylation observed in *elm1Δ* cells lead to reduced Kin4 binding to the mother cell cortex and SPOC deficiency. So, Elm1 function in the SPOC upstream of Kin4 by controlling its activity and localization.

Interestingly, we have recently described a new level of complexity in SPOC regulation. Indeed, we have implicated the E3 ubiquitin ligases Dma1 and Dma2 in the control of Elm1 bud neck localization [29]. Elm1 mislocalization in *dma1Δ dma2Δ* cells results in reduced levels of Kin4 kinase activity and asymmetry of Bub2-Bfa1 at the spindle poles of mispositioned spindles. So, Dma1, Dma2, Elm1 and Kin4 are part of the same SPOC regulatory module, with Dma proteins controlling Elm1 localization, that is in turn required for full Kin4 activation. Importantly, it is worth noting that Dma1, Dma2, Elm1 and Kin4 all are required to prevent mitotic exit in response to spindle mispositioning but not to spindle depolymerization, differently from Bub2 and Bfa1 [28,39,52].

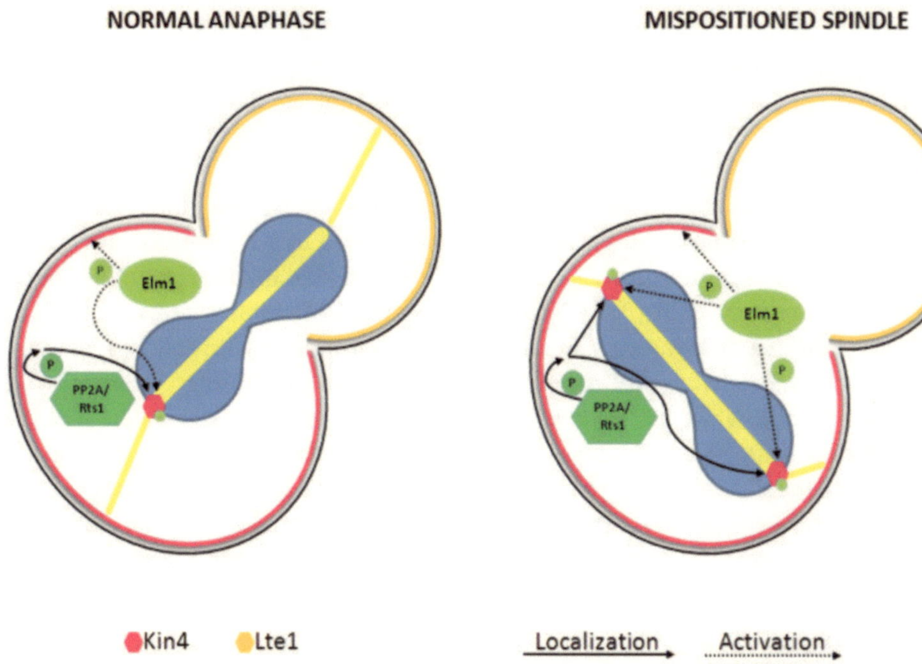

Figure 2. Model for Kin4 regulation. Kin4 is localized to the mother cell cortex and to the mother bound spindle pole body (SPB) when the mitotic spindle is correctly oriented. On the contrary, in case of spindle misalignment, Kin4 is present at both SPBs. The protein phosphatase PP2A-Rts1 is crucial for the proper localization of Kin4 to the mother cortex and SPBs both during the cell cycle and in response to spindle position defects. The protein kinase Elm1 activates Kin4 by direct phosphorylation and controls its localization.

4. Budding yeast cytokinesis is controlled by several phosphoproteins

Cytokinesis is the spatially and temporally regulated process by which, after chromosome segregation, eukaryotic cells divide their cytoplasm and membranes in order to produce two daughter cells. In budding yeast, the activity of the components of the citokinetic machinery is tightly controlled and their recruitment to the mother-bud neck follows a hieralchical order of assembly during the cell cycle. Most of these regulations are driven by phosphorylation and dephosphorylation events.

Cytokinesis completion is driven by complex and partially redundant pathways that regulate the assembly and contraction of an actomyosin ring (AMR) and the deposition of a trilaminary septum between mother and bud. In particular, the AMR is involved in constricting the plasma membrane at the division site to complete closure [57,58] and AMR contraction is coupled to the centripetal growth of the primary septum (PS).

The first step towards cytokinesis is the assembly of a septin ring, which forms at the bud neck concomitantly with bud emergence as soon as cells enter S phase, and marks the position where constriction between mother and daughter cell will take place at the end of mitosis. During S phase, the septin ring becomes an hourglass shaped structure that serves as a scaffold for recruiting other proteins to the bud neck, among which the type II myosin heavy chain Myo1 that forms a ring at the presumptive bud site during early S phase [57]. This Myo1 ring persists at the mother-bud neck until the end of anaphase, when a coincident ring of F-actin assembles and the resulting AMR eventually contracts, accomplishing septum formation. In late anaphase Hof1, Cyk3 and Inn1 are recruited sequentially to the bud neck. All these proteins are required to activate the chitin synthase Chs2 [59-61], which is in turn recruited to the division site after mitotic exit and is required to build the primary septum (PS) which is mostly made of chitin. Once the cytokinetic apparatus is fully assembled, AMR contraction, membrane invagination and PS synthesis all begin almost immediately. After completion of the PS, at either side of this structure, secondary septa (SS), which are made of the same components as the cell wall, i. e. glucans and mannan, are synthetized [62]. At this point, mother and daughter cells are connected by a trilaminar septum. Afterwards, cell separation is driven by the action of endochitinase, Cts1, and glucanases, Dse2 Dse4 Egt2, that degrade the PS from the daughter side [63,64]. Then mother and daughter cells separate permanently from each other leaving a disk of chitin, called "bud scar", on the mother cell surface.

The events leading to cytokinesis must be tightly controlled and coordinated with chromosome segregation and mitotic exit in order to ensure the genetic stability during cell growth and thereby the fate of daughter cells. Several pathways are able to regulate the last event of the cell cycle including the Mitotic Exit Network (MEN). The MEN seems to control not only the exit from mitosis but also the timing of cytokinesis. In fact, several MEN components localize to the division site after mitotic exit and they likely play a direct role in the regulation of cytokinesis. Indeed, as mitotic Cdk1 activity decrease, MEN kinases Cdc15, Dbf2/Dbf20, Mob1, Cdc5 and the protein phosphatase Cdc14 associate with the bud neck [65-69], in addition some MEN mutants fail to undergo cytokinesis [70,71]. Here we describe examples of regulation by phosphorylation and/or dephosphorylation during cytokinesis catalyzed by Cdc28-Clb2 and/or Dbf2-Mob1 kinases and also by Cdc14 phosphatase, and how these post-translational modifications can regulate the function of three important cytokinetic proteins, Cyk3, Hof1 and Chs2, in space and time.

Cyk3 is an SH3-domain protein and was isolated as high-copy suppressor of lethality in an *iqg1Δ* strain [72] and in a *myo1Δ* strain [73]. Cyk3 interacts with Hof1 and both cooperate to recruit Inn1 [61,74], that is essential for activation of chitin synthase and therefore for primary septum formation [60,61]. Overexpression of *CYK3* leads to an actomyosin independent recruitment of Inn1 to the bud neck [74], indicating that Cyk3 plays a central role in a rescue mechanism for cytokinesis in the absence of a functional AMR. Cyk3 activity and localization are positively regulated by phosphorylation events (Figure 3). Cyk3 total levels are constant throughout the cell cycle, but interestingly Cyk3 phosphorylated species begin to accumulate after mitotic exit and this leads to its recruitment to the bud neck. This phosphorylation event requires the MEN activity [75]. In particular, it has been proposed that Cyk3 is phosphorylated by Dbf2-Mob1 kinase but if it is its direct substrate has not been determined.

It has instead been demonstrated that the Dbf2-Mob1 kinase, that appears at the division site just before AMR contraction [76,77], directly phosphorylates Hof1, a member of the F-BAR (Fes/CIP4 homology Bin/Amphiphysin/Rvsp) protein family conserved from yeast to mammals [78]. Hof1 protein levels, activity and localization are regulated by many phosphorylation events. Hof1 protein levels are regulated during the cell cycle, in particular Hof1 accumulates from G1/S phase, it disappears after mitotic exit, concomitantly with AMR contraction, and it remains unstable during the G1 phase of the following cell cycle. Hof1 colocalizes with the septin ring from S phase to late anaphase, then it interacts with the AMR before its contraction [79]. Efficient AMR contraction and cell separation are allowed by subsequent degradation of Hof1 by the action of the E3 ubiquitin ligase complex SCF (Skp, Cullin, F-box containing complex)/Grr1 [80] that can recognize its PEST (Proline, glutamin acid (E), Serine and Threonine) domain. Hof1 is directly phosphorylated by three kinases that act in concert to regulate its activity: Clb2-Cdc28, Cdc5 and Dbf2-Mob1 [81]. During mitosis, Hof1 undergoes Clb2-Cdc28 phosphorylation that does not seem to control its localization, but it primes Hof1 for subsequent phosphorylation by Cdc5 at Ser517. This event facilitates Hof1 binding to Mob1. The Dbf2-Mob1 kinase then phosphorylates several residues at both N- and C- terminal of Hof1 [81]. These modifications do not influence the physical interaction between Hof1 and Cyk3 or Inn1, instead they promote Hof1 release from the septin ring and localization to the AMR (Figure 3). There, phosphorylated Hof1 promotes AMR contraction by an unknown mechanism.

The third example is the regulation of the chitin synthase that builds the PS. Chs2 is an integral membrane protein that polymerizes chitin from its precursor UDP-N-acetyl-glucosamine. The chitin synthase 2 is synthetized in G2/M and accumulates in the endoplasmic reticulum (ER). The N-terminal and the central catalytic domain are located in the cytoplasm while the hydrophobic C-terminal domain is integrated into the ER membrane. During the metaphase to anaphase transition, Chs2 is phosphorylated in several Ser-Pro sites at its N-terminus exposed into the cytoplasm by Cdc28-Clb2 [82,83]. These phosphorylations events are important for Chs2 retention into the ER and therefore for its inibition. At the end of mitosis, MEN activation leads to the decrease of Cdc28-Clb2 activity and Chs2 can be exported from the ER and targeted to the division site [75,84-86]. The molecular mechanism of this release was unclear, but recent data indicate that Chs2 N-terminus is directly dephosphorylated by the protein phosphatase Cdc14 [86]. Then dephosphorylated Chs2 is traslocated to Golgi and, through secretory vescicoles, is delivered to the plasma membrane at the bud neck (Figure 3) [85,87]. There, Chs2 is active and promotes centripetally deposition of PS that occurs concomitantly with AMR contraction and membrane ingression. After PS completion Chs2 is removed from the bud neck by endocytosis and transferred to the vacuole where it is degraded by the action of the protease Pep4 [87]. The signal that leads to Chs2 endocytosis is currently unknown.

In summary, Cyk3, Hof1 and Chs2 regulations are good examples of how phosphorylation events can change the fate of a protein and underline the relevance of this posttranslational modification in the control of a very important cell cycle process, the cytokinesis.

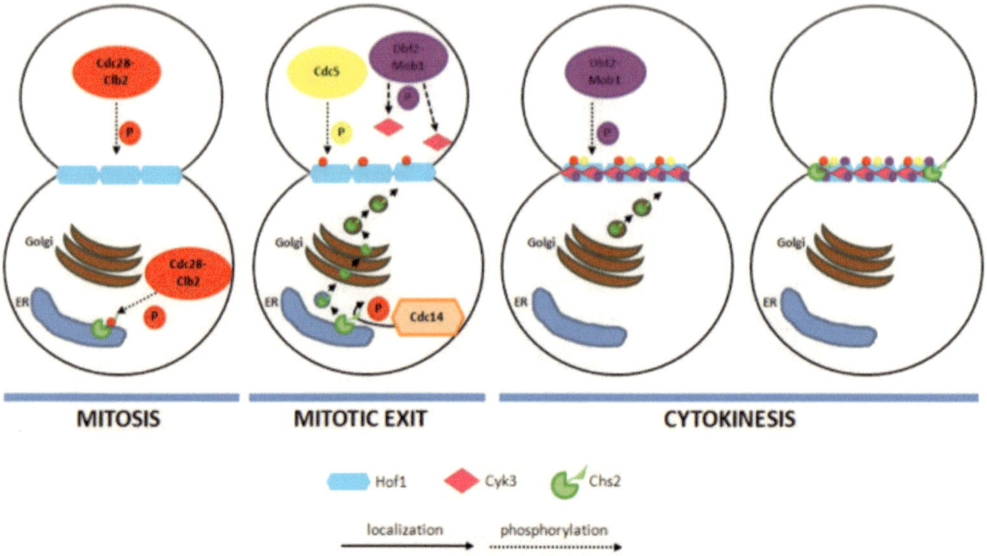

Figure 3. Model for Cyk3, Hof1 and Chs2 regulation. Cyk3 is likely phosphorylated by Dbf2-Mob1 kinase (dashed line) and recruited to the bud neck. Septin bound Hof1 is "primed" by Cdc28-Clb2 phosphorylation and then it is phosphorylated by polo-like kinase Cdc5 and by Dbf2-Mob1 kinase. These modifications promote Hof1 release from the septin ring and localization to the actomyosin ring. Chs2 accumulates in the endoplasmic reticulum (ER) with its N-terminus exposed into the cytoplasm, this tail is phosphorylated by Cdc28-Clb2. These phosphorylations events are important for Chs2 retention into the ER. At the end of mitosis, Chs2 N-terminus is directly dephosphorylated by the protein phosphatase Cdc14, then dephosphorylated Chs2 is traslocated to Golgi and, through secretory vescicoles, is delivered to the plasma membrane at the bud neck.

5. Conclusion

The phosphorylation of a protein is a simple mechanism that alters its conformation, and so its ability to function, in a reversibile way. As we can learn from the examples of protein regulation that we have focused on, phosphorylation is a flexible mechanism that regulates the target protein in several ways. Indeed, phosphorylation is not simply used to switch the activity of a protein on or off, but can have many additional roles. It can influence its ability to form complexes with other proteins, it can affect the rate at which a protein is degraded or its ability to localize to a particular subcellular location. For example, phosphorylation events on the protein kinases Swe1 and Kin4, and on the cytokinetic proteins Cyk3, Hof1 and Chs2 lead to change in their localization.

The action of kinases is counteracted by phosphatases and both controls are essential to determine the phosphorylation state of the target proteins. The balance of phosphorylation and dephosphorylation can also be critical in determining the strength and duration of the response. Therefore, kinases and phosphatases must be regulated spatiotemporally in order to obtain the proper cellular response.

In addition, a protein can be modified by the addition of a single phosphate group or by multiple phosphates, by a single protein kinase or by multiple kinases. Multisite phosphorylation is a strategy that enables two or more effects to operate in the same protein. Indeed, some phosphorylation events "prime" the protein in order to be phosphorylated by another kinase that acts subsequently in the same cellular compartment or in another location. The protein kinase Swe1 is a very good example of this kind of regulation, in fact several kinases act sequentially leading to the accumulation of hyperphosphorylated bud neck localized Swe1. Also the cytokinetic proteins Hof1 and Chs2 are the target of at least two different protein kinases that change Hof1 and Chs2 activity and localization. Alternatively, a phosphorylation event can inhibit the phosphorylation of other residues on the same protein. For example, Bfa1 phosphorylation by Kin4 inhibits phosphate group addition by the polo-like kinase Cdc5 and so keeps Bfa1 active.

Another important issue is the crosstalk between phosphorylation and other posttranslational modifications. Crosstalks can be positive or negative, thus promoting or inhibiting the subsequent modification. About phosphorylation and ubiquitylation, an increasing number of phosphoproteins are then ubiquitylated. Both Hof1 and Swe1 are hyperphosphorylated and afterwards ubiquitylated, subsequently they are targeted to degradation via the proteasome. A very interesting issue is how the specificity is determined. Indeed, phosphorylated residues of serine, threonine and tyrosine recognition by phosphobinding domains depends on the sequence of amino acids immediately around the phosphorylated residue, whereas recognition of monoUb by ubiquitin binding domains does not seem to be influenced by the primary sequence bearing the ubiquitinated lysine.

Even if there are several open questions regarding the molecular mechanisms that control the phosphoproteins that we have described, they are good examples of how the phosphorylation event can change the fate of a protein.

Author details

Roberta Fraschini*, Erica Raspelli† and Corinne Cassani
Università degli Studi di Milano-Bicocca, Dipartimento di Biotecnologie e Bioscienze, Milano, Italy

Acknowledgement

Roberta Fraschini's research is supported by grants from PRIN (Progetti di Ricerca di Interesse Nazionale) 2008. C. C. is supported by a fellowship from Fondazione Confalonieri.

6. References

[1] Morgan DO (2007) The Cell Cycle: Principles of Control. Oxford University Press.

* Corresponding Author
† Equally Contributing Authors

[2] Nigg EA (1998) Polo-like kinases: positive regulators of cell division from start to finish. Curr Opin Cell Biol. 10:776-83.

[3] Sonnhammer EL, Eddy SR, Birney E, Bateman A, Durbin R (1998) Pfam: multiple sequence alignments and HMM-profiles of protein domains. Nucleic Acids Res. 26: 320–322.

[4] Booher RN, Deshaies RJ, Kirschner MW (1993) Properties of *Saccharomyces cerevisiae* wee1 and its differential regulation of p34CDC28 in response to G1 and G2 cyclins. EMBO J. 12: 3417-26.

[5] Russell P, Moreno S, Reed SI (1989) Conservation of mitotic controls in fission and budding yeasts. Cell. 57: 295-303.

[6] Lew DJ (2003) The morphogenesis checkpoint: how yeast cells watch their figures. Curr Opin Cell Biol 15: 648-53.

[7] Longtine MS, Theesfeld CL, McMillan JN, Weaver E, Pringle JR, Lew DJ (2000) Septin-dependent assembly of a cell cycle-regulatory module in *Saccharomyces cerevisiae*. Mol Cell Biol. 20: 4049-61.

[8] Barral Y, Parra M, Bidlingmaier S, Snyder M (1999) Nim1-related kinases coordinate cell cycle progression with the organization of the peripheral cytoskeleton in yeast. Genes Dev 13: 176-87.

[9] Shulewitz MJ, Inouye CJ, Thorner J (1999) Hsl7 localizes to a septin ring and serves as an adapter in a regulatory pathway that relieves tyrosine phosphorylation of Cdc28 protein kinase in *Saccharomyces cerevisiae*. Mol Cell Biol.19: 7123-37.

[10] Keaton MA, Szkotnicki L, Marquitz AR, Harrison J, Zyla TR, Lew DJ (2008) Nucleocytoplasmic trafficking of G2/M regulators in yeast. Mol Biol Cell. 19: 4006-18.

[11] Harvey SL, Charlet A, Haas W, Gygi SP, Kellogg DR (2005) Cdk1-dependent regulation of the mitotic inhibitor Wee1. Cell. 122: 407-20.

[12] Keaton MA, Lew DJ (2006) Eavesdropping on the cytoskeleton: progress and controversy in the yeast morphogenesis checkpoint. Curr Opin Microbiol. 9: 540-6.

[13] Versele M, Thorner J (2005) Some assembly required: yeast septins provide the instruction manual. Trends Cell Biol. 15: 414-24.

[14] Longtine MS, Bi E (2003) Regulation of septin organization and function in yeast. Trends Cell Biol. 13: 403-9.

[15] Gladfelter AS, Kozubowski L, Zyla TR, Lew DJ (2005) Interplay between septin organization, cell cycle and cell shape in yeast. J Cell Sci. 118: 1617-28.

[16] McMillan JN, Longtine MS, Sia RA, Theesfeld CL, Bardes ES, Pringle JR, Lew DJ (1999) The morphogenesis checkpoint in *Saccharomyces cerevisiae*: cell cycle control of Swe1p degradation by Hsl1p and Hsl7p. Mol Cell Biol. 19: 6929-39.

[17] Cid VJ, Shulewitz MJ, McDonald KL, Thorner J (2001) Dynamic localization of the Swe1 regulator Hsl7 during the *Saccharomyces cerevisiae* cell cycle. Mol Biol Cell.12: 1645-69.

[18] Theesfeld CL, Zyla TR, Bardes EG, Lew DJ (2003) A monitor for bud emergence in the yeast morphogenesis checkpoint. Mol Biol Cell. 14: 3280-91.

[19] Sakchaisri K, Asano S, Yu LR, Shulewitz MJ, Park CJ, Park JE, Cho YW, Veenstra TD, Thorner J, Lee KS (2004) Coupling morphogenesis to mitotic entry. Proc Natl Acad Sci U S A. 101: 4124-9.

[20] Asano S, Park JE, Sakchaisri K, Yu LR, Song S, Supavilai P, Veenstra TD Lee KS (2005). Concerted mechanism of Swe1/Wee1 regulation by multiple kinases in budding yeast. EMBO J. 24: 2194–2204.

[21] Yang H, Jiang W, Gentry M, Hallberg RL (2000) Loss of a protein phosphatase 2A regulatory subunit (Cdc55p) elicits improper regulation of Swe1p degradation. Mol Cell Biol. 20: 8143-56.

[22] Ciliberto A, Novak B, Tyson JJ (2003) Mathematical model of the morphogenesis checkpoint in budding yeast. J Cell Biol.163: 1243-54.

[23] McMillan JN, Theesfeld CL, Harrison JC, Bardes ES, Lew DJ (2002). Determinants of Swe1p degradation in *Saccharomyces cerevisiae*. Mol Biol Cell.13: 3560-75.

[24] Hofmann K, Bucher P (2005) The FHA domain: a putative nuclear signalling domain found in protein kinases and transcription factors. Trends Biochem Sci. 20:347-9.

[25] Durocher D, Jackson SP (2002) The FHA domain. FEBS Lett 513: 58–66.

[26] Lorick KL, Jensen JP, Fang S, Ong AM, Hatekeyama S, Wissman AM (1999) RING fingers mediate ubiquitin-conjugating enzyme (E2)-dependent ubiquitination. PNAS 28: 11364-9.

[27] Brooks L 3rd, Heimsath EG Jr, Loring GL, Brenner C (2008) FHA-RING ubiquitin ligases in cell division cycle control. Cell Mol Life Sci. 65: 3458-66.

[28] Fraschini R, Bilotta D, Lucchini G, Piatti S (2004) Functional characterization of Dma1 and Dma2, the budding yeast homologues of *Schizosaccharomyces pombe* Dma1 and human Chfr. Mol Biol Cell 15: 3796-810.

[29] Merlini L, Fraschini R, Boettcher B, Barral Y, Lucchini G, Piatti S (2012) Budding yeast Dma proteins control septin dynamics and the spindle position checkpoint by promoting the recruitment of the Elm1 kinase to the bud neck. Plos Genetics, in press.

[30] Loring GL, Christensen KC, Gerber SA, Brenner C (2008) Yeast Chfr homologs retard cell cycle at G1 and G2/M via Ubc4 and Ubc13/Mms2-dependent ubiquitination. Cell Cycle 7: 96-105.

[31] Raspelli E, Cassani C, Lucchini G, Fraschini R (2011) Budding yeast Dma1 and Dma2 participate in regulation of Swe1 levels and localization. Mol. Biol. Cell. 22: 2185-2197.

[32] Fraschini R, Venturetti M, Chiroli E, Piatti S (2008) The spindle position checkpoint: how to deal with spindle misalignment during asymmetric cell division in budding yeast. Biochemical Society Transactions Volume 36, part 3, 416-420.

[33] Stegmeier F, Amon A (2004) Closing mitosis: the functions of the Cdc14 phosphatase and its regulation. Annu Rev Genet. 38: 203-32.

[34] Gruneberg U, Campbell K, Simpson C, Grindlay J, Schiebel E (2000) Nud1p links astral microtubule organization and the control of exit from mitosis. EMBO J. 19: 6475-88.

[35] Bardin AJ, Visintin R, Amon A (2000) A mechanism for coupling exit from mitosis to partitioning of the nucleus. Cell 102: 21-31.

[36] Bloecher A, Venturi GM, Tatchell K (2000) Anaphase spindle position is monitored by the BUB2 checkpoint. Nat Cell Biol 2: 556-558.

[37] Pereira G, Hofken T, Grindlay J, Manson C, Schiebel E (2000) The Bub2p spindle checkpoint links nuclear migration with mitotic exit. Mol Cell 6: 1-10.

[38] Pereira G, Schiebel E (2005) Kin4 kinase delays mitotic exit in response to spindle alignment defects. Mol Cell 19: 209-221.

[39] D'Aquino KE, Monje-Casas F, Paulson J, Reiser V, Charles GM, et al (2005) The protein kinase Kin4 inhibits exit from mitosis in response to spindle position defects. Mol Cell 19: 223-234.

[40] Geymonat M, Spanos A, Walzer PA, Johnston LH, Sedgwick SG (2003) In vitro regulation of budding yeast Bfa1/Bub2 GAP activity by Cdc5. J Biol Chem. 278: 14591-4.

[41] Hu F, Wang Y, Liu D, Li Y, Qin J, Elledge SJ (2001) Regulation of the Bub2/Bfa1 GAP complex by Cdc5 and cell cycle checkpoints. Cell. 107: 655-65.

[42] Maekawa H, Priest C, Lechner J, Pereira G, Schiebel E (2007) The yeast centrosome translates the positional information of the anaphase spindle into a cell cycle signal. J Cell Biol 179: 423-436.

[43] Stegmeier F, Amon A (2004) Closing Mitosis: The Functions of the Cdc14 Phosphatase and Its Regulation. Annu Rev Genet 38: 203-232.

[44] Chan LY, Amon A (2010) Spindle position is coordinated with cell-cycle progression through establishment of mitotic exit-activating and -inhibitory zones. Mol Cell. 39: 444-54.

[45] Caydasi AK, Pereira G (2009) Spindle alignment regulates the dynamic association of checkpoint proteins with yeast spindle pole bodies. Dev Cell 16: 146-156.

[46] Molk JN, Schuyler SC, Liu JY, Evans JG, Salmon ED, et al (2004) The differential roles of budding yeast Tem1p, Cdc15p, and Bub2p protein dynamics in mitotic exit. Mol Biol Cell 15: 1519-1532.

[47] Monje-Casas F, Amon A (2009) Cell polarity determinants establish asymmetry in MEN signaling. Dev Cell 16: 132-145.

[48] Pereira G, Tanaka TU, Nasmyth K, Schiebel E (2001) Modes of spindle pole body inheritance and segregation of the Bfa1p- Bub2p checkpoint protein complex. Embo J. 20: 6359-6370.

[49] Chan LY, Amon A (2009) The protein phosphatase 2A functions in the spindle position checkpoint by regulating the checkpoint kinase Kin4. Genes Dev 23: 1639–1649.

[50] Jill E, Falk L, Chan Y, Amon A (2011) Lte1 promotes mitotic exit by controlling the localization of the spindle position checkpoint kinase Kin4 PNAS 108: 12584-590.

[51] Caydasi AK, Kurtulmus B, Orrico MI, Hofmann A, Ibrahim B, et al (2010) Elm1 kinase activates the spindle position checkpoint kinase Kin4. J Cell Biol 190: 975-989.

[52] Moore JK, Chudalayandi P, Heil-Chapdelaine RA, Cooper JA (2010) The spindle position checkpoint is coordinated by the Elm1 kinase. J Cell Biol 191: 493-503.

[53] Edgington NP, Blacketer MJ, Bierwagen TA, Myers AM. (1999) Control of *Saccharomyces cerevisiae* filamentous growth by cyclin-dependent kinase Cdc28. Mol Cell Biol. 19:1369-80.

[54] Sreenivasan A, Kellogg D. (1999) The elm1 kinase functions in a mitotic signaling network in budding yeast. Mol Cell Biol. 19: 7983-94.

[55] Bouquin N, Barral Y, Courbeyrette R, Blondel M, Snyder M, Mann C. (2000) Regulation of cytokinesis by the Elm1 protein kinase in Saccharomyces cerevisiae. J Cell Sci. 113: 1435-45.

[56] Adams JA (2003) Activation loop phosphorylation and catalysis in protein kinases: is there functional evidence for the autoinhibitor model? Biochemistry. 42: 601-7.

[57] Bi E, Maddox P, Lew DJ, Salmon ED, McMillan JN, Yeh E, Pringle JR (1998) Involvement of an actomyosin contractile ring in *Saccharomyces cerevisiae* cytokinesis. J. Cell Biol. 142: 1301-12.

[58] Lippincott J, Li R (1998) Sequential assembly of myosin II, an IQGAP-like protein, and filamentous actin to a ring structure involved in budding yeast cytokinesis. J. Cell Biol. 140: 355-66.

[59] Yeong FM (2005) Severing all ties between mother and daughter: cell separation in budding yeast. Mol Microbiol. 55: 1325-31.

[60] Sanchez-Diaz A, Marchesi V, Murray S, Jones R, Pereira G, Edmondson R, Allen T, Labib K (2008) Inn1 couples contraction of the actomyosin ring to membrane ingression during cytokinesis in budding yeast. Nat Cell Biol. 4: 395-406.

[61] Nishihama R, Schreiter JH, Onishi M, Vallen EA, Hanna J, Moravcevic K, Lippincott MF, Han H, Lemmon MA, Pringle JR, Bi E (2009) Role of Inn1 and its interactions with Hof1 and Cyk3 in promoting cleavage furrow and septum formation in *S. cerevisiae.* J Cell Biol. 185: 995-1012.

[62] Lesage G, Bussey H (2006) Cell wall assembly in *Saccharomyces cerevisiae.* Microbiol Mol Biol Rev. 70: 317-43.

[63] Kuranda MJ, Robbins PW (1991) Chitinase is required for cell separation during growth of *Saccharomyces cerevisiae*. J Biol Chem. 266: 19758-67.

[64] Colman-Lerner A, Chin TE, Brent R (2001) Yeast Cbk1 and Mob2 activate daughter-specific genetic programs to induce asymmetric cell fates Cell. 107: 739-50.

[65] Bembenek J, Kang J, Kurischko C, Li B, Raab JR, Belanger KD, Luca FC, Yu H (2005) Crm1-mediated nuclear export of Cdc14 is required for the completion of cytokinesis in budding yeast. Cell Cycle. 4: 961-71.

[66] Frenz LM, Lee SE, Fesquet D, Johnston LH (2000) The budding yeast Dbf2 protein kinase localises to the centrosome and moves to the bud neck in late mitosis. J Cell Sci. 19: 3399-408.

[67] Luca FC, Mody M, Kurischko C, Roof DM, Giddings TH, Winey M (2001) *Saccharomyces cerevisiae* Mob1p is required for cytokinesis and mitotic exit. Mol Cell Biol. 21: 6972-83.

[68] Song S, Grenfell TZ, Garfield S, Erikson RL, Lee KS (2000) Essential function of the polo box of Cdc5 in subcellular localization and induction of cytokinetic structures. Mol Cell Biol. 20: 286-98.

[69] Xu S, Huang HK, Kaiser P, Latterich M, Hunter T (2000) Phosphorylation and spindle pole body localization of the Cdc15p mitotic regulatory protein kinase in budding yeast. Curr Biol. 10: 329-32.

[70] Lippincott J, Shannon KB, Shou W, Deshaies RJ, Li R (2001) The Tem1 small GTPase controls actomyosin and septin dynamics during cytokinesis. J Cell Sci. 114: 1379-86.

[71] Hwa Lim H, Yeong FM, Surana U (2003) Inactivation of mitotic kinase triggers translocation of MEN components to mother-daughter neck in yeast. Mol Biol Cell. 14: 4734-43.

[72] Korinek WS, Bi E, Epp JA, Wang L, Ho J, Chant J (2000) Cyk3, a novel SH3-domain protein, affects cytokinesis in yeast. Curr Biol. 10: 947-50.

[73] Ko N, Nishihama R, Tully GH, Ostapenko D, Solomon MJ, Morgan DO, Pringle JR (2007) Identification of yeast IQGAP (Iqg1p) as an anaphase-promoting-complex substrate and its role in actomyocin-ring-independent cytokinesis. Mol Biol Cell. 18: 5139-53.

[74] Jendretzki A, Ciklic I, Rodicio R, Schmitz HP, Heinisch JJ (2009) Cyk3 acts in actomyosin ring independent cytokinesis by recruiting Inn1 to the yeast bud neck. Mol Genet Genomics. 282: 437-51.

[75] Meitinger F, Petrova B, Lombardi IM, Bertazzi DT, Hub B, Zentgraf H, Pereira G (2010) Targeted localization of Inn1, Cyk3 and Chs2 by the mitotic-exit network regulates cytokinesis in budding yeast. J Cell Sci. 123: 1851-61.

[76] Frenz LM, Lee SE, Fesquet D, Johnston LH (2000) The budding yeast Dbf2 protein kinase localises to the centrosome and moves to the bud neck in late mitosis. J Cell Sci. 19: 3399-408.

[77] Yoshida S, Toh-e A (2001) Regulation of the localization of Dbf2 and Mob1 during cell division of *Saccharomyces cerevisiae*. Genes Genet. Syst. 76:141–47.

[78] Aspenström P (2009) Roles of F-BAR/PCH proteins in the regulation of membrane dynamics and actin reorganization. Int Rev Cell Mol Biol. 272: 1-31.

[79] Vallen EA, Caviston J, Bi E (2000) Roles of Hof1p, Bni1p, Bnr1p, and Myo1 in cytokinesis in *Saccharomyces cerevisiae*. Mol Biol Cell. 11: 593-611.

[80] Blondel M, Bach S, Bamps S, Dobbelaere J, Wiget P, Longaretti C, Barral Y, Meijer L, Peter M (2005) Degradation of Hof1 by SCF(Grr1) is important for actomyosin contraction during cytokinesis in yeast. EMBO J. 24: 1440-52.

[81] Meitinger F, Boehm ME, Hofmann A, Hub B, Zentgraf H, Lehmann WD, Pereira G (2011) Phosphorylation-dependent regulation of the F-BAR protein Hof1 during cytokinesis. Genes Dev. 25: 875-88.

[82] Martínez-Rucobo FW, Eckhardt-Strelau L, Terwisscha van Scheltinga AC (2009) Yeast chitin synthase 2 activity is modulated by proteolysis and phosphorylation. Biochem J. 417: 547-54.

[83] Teh EM, Chai CC, Yeong FM (2009) Retention of Chs2p in the ER requires N-terminal CDK1-phosphorylation sites. Cell Cycle 8: 2964–2974.

[84] VerPlank L, Li R (2005) Cell cycle-regulated trafficking of Chs2 controls actomyosin ring stability during cytokinesis. Mol Biol Cell. 16: 2529-43.

[85] Zhang G, Kashimshetty R, Ng KE, Tan HB, Yeong FM (2006) Exit from mitosis triggers Chs2p transport from the endoplasmic reticulum to mother-daughter neck via the secretory pathway in budding yeast. J Cell Biol. 174: 207–220.

[86] Chin CF, Bennett AM, Ma WK, Hall MC, Yeong FM (2012) Dependence of Chs2 ER export on dephosphorylation by cytoplasmic Cdc14 ensures that septum formation follows mitosis. Mol Biol Cell. 23: 45-58.

[87] Chuang JS, Schekman RW (1996) Differential trafficking and timed localization of two chitin synthase proteins, Chs2p and Chs3p. J Cell Biol.135: 597-610.

Chapter 14

Phosphorylation Mediated Regulation of Cdc25 Activity, Localization and Stability

C. Frazer and P.G. Young

Additional information is available at the end of the chapter

http://dx.doi.org/10.5772/ 48315

1. Introduction

Dual specificity phosphatases of the Cdc25 family are critically important regulators of the cell cycle. They activate cyclin-dependent kinases (CDKs) at key cell cycle transitions such as the initiation of DNA synthesis and mitosis. They also represent key points of regulation for pathways monitoring DNA integrity, DNA replication, growth factor signaling and extracellular stress. Since their mis-regulation allows cells to function in a genetically unstable state, it is not surprising that these phosphatases are involved in transformation to a cancerous state. Cdc25 phosphatases are heavily regulated by phosphorylation. Many regulatory phosphorylation sites on Cdc25 influence catalytic activity, substrate specificity, subcellular localization and stability. This chapter summarizes the current literature on the phospho-regulation of these proteins.

2. Yeast genetics and Xenopus oocyte maturation – Setting the stage

The study of cell division in eukaryotes was dramatically changed with the isolation of temperature sensitive "cell division cycle" (*cdc*⁻) mutants of the yeasts *Schizosaccharomyces pombe* and *Saccharomyces cerevisiae*. These mutants arrested uniformly at a particular cell cycle stage and uncoupled cell growth from cell cycle progression.[1-3] *S. pombe* cells are cylindrical cells growing from the tips while keeping a constant diameter.[3] At the restrictive temperature, fission yeast *cdc*⁻ mutants arrest at their restriction point and become abnormally elongated. Within the fission yeast *cdc*⁻ collection was the *cdc25-22* mutation which arrests at mitotic entry when incubated at its restrictive temperature.[3] The collection also included *cdc9-50* which divided at approximately half the length of a wildtype cell; it was later renamed *wee1-50* in reference to its small size.[4] The *wee1-50* mutation suppresses the cell cycle phenotype of *cdc25-22* demonstrating that these two proteins act in opposition during the G2/M transition.[5] Analysis of these mutations showed that Cdc2 is rate limiting for mitotic entry and is inhibited by Wee1 and activated by Cdc25.[6,7] Regulation of Cdc2 by Wee1 and Cdc25 in fission yeast was one of the first connected pathways in cell cycle research in any organism. The gene names Cdc25 and Wee1 are used in almost all organisms today.

Concurrently, Maturation Promoting Factor (MPF) was discovered through a series of elegant cytoplasmic transfer experiments conducted on frog, starfish and sea urchin oocytes [8-10]. Immature *Xenopus* oocytes arrest at prophase I. Progesterone induced MPF activation induces maturation whereby oocytes complete meiosis I and arrest at meiotic metaphase II.[9,11] Microinjection of cytoplasm from a mature oocyte into an immature oocyte also induces maturation.[8,9] This bioassay for maturation promoting factor (MPF) activity allowed it to be tracked through the meiotic and later mitotic cycles. Activity falls after anaphase I, rising again as cells enter prophase II. Although MPF activity is high, mature oocytes arrest due to the presence of a second soluble factor called Cyto-Static Factor (CSF).[9] Subsequent entry of the sperm nucleus causes an influx of extracellular calcium, ultimately removing CSF inhibition and serving as the trigger for completion of meiosis and the start of mitotic divisions. Extracts from prophase II arrested mature oocytes can be induced to undergo alternating DNA synthesis and mitotic phases by the addition of calcium, providing an excellent cell free system for studying MPF regulation.[12] A peak of MPF activity accompanies each round of mitosis, reaching maximal activity during meiotic prophase, followed by a catastrophic drop as chromosomes segregate at anaphase. Fertilization is followed by a rapid succession of 12 rounds of DNA synthesis and cell division with no intervening gap phases, driven solely by maternally derived mRNA.[13] Gap phases are re-established at the mid-blastula transition followed by typical somatic cell cycles.[14] MPF consists of three proteins: Cdk1 kinase, cyclin B (Cdc2 [19-21] and Cdc13 [22,23] respectively in fission yeast) and the small regulatory protein Suc1.[15-19] The activator of both MPF in *Xenopus* and the Cdc2-Cdc13 complex in *S. pombe* is Cdc25 phosphatase.[24,25]

The cytoplasmic transfer experiments showed that MPF activity correlates with increased protein phosphorylation in donor oocytes [26], targeting a large number of nuclear proteins.[27,28] MPF is a histone H1 kinase, an activity which is still used today to measure CDK function.[29] MPF induces many of the cytological changes associated with mitosis such as nuclear envelope breakdown, chromosome condensation and mitotic spindle formation.[30-32] Mass spectrometry has shown that the single Cdk1 homologue in budding yeast (CDC28) phosphorylates 547 sites on 308 proteins *in vivo.*[33] The regulation of only about 75 of these CDC28 substrates has been examined in any detail.[34] Undoubtedly, the network of CDK mediated phosphorylation events in vertebrate cells will turn out to be far more complex.

3. Taxonomic distribution, duplication and divergence of Cdc25 homologues

Cdc25 is present in all eukaryotic cells. The yeasts, *S. cerevisiae* and *S. pombe,* possess a single Cdc25 protein (referred to as MIH1 in the former).[35] Duplication and divergence led to three Cdc25 paralogues in vertebrates, Cdc25A, Cdc25B, and Cdc25C.[36,36-40] Cdc25A acts early in the cell cycle, regulating the G1/S transition, whereas Cdc25B and Cdc25C act at G2/M. Human Cdc25A, Cdc25B and Cdc25C have several isoforms through alternative splicing.[41-44] Cdc25C was discovered based on sequence similarity to fission yeast Cdc25 by using degenerate PCR primers to conserved residues in the catalytic region.[38] Human Cdc25A and Cdc25B were cloned by complementation of the temperature sensitive *cdc25-22*^{ts} allele of *S. pombe,* demonstrating the strong conservation of function in this protein family.[37] *Xenopus* Cdc25A and Cdc25C were initially discovered based on sequence similarity to human Cdc25C.[40,45] Injection of recombinant *Xenopus* Cdc25A or Cdc25C into oocytes induces their maturation, the first direct indication that this protein was a positive regulator of MPF.[40,45,46] *Xenopus* Cdc25C also complements the *cdc25-22*^{ts} mutation in fission yeast.[45] Four Cdc25 homologues are present in *Caenorhabditis* [47], whereas *Drosophila* contains two, *string* and *twine.*[48,49] The conserved C-terminal domain of *string* contains the intrinsic phosphatase activity against a Cdk1-derived peptide containing phosphorylated Y15 and against the synthetic substrate *p*-nitrophenyl phosphate.[50] Few plant Cdc25 homologues can be found by sequence comparison in the NCBI database and those only in unicellular algae, eg *Ostreococcus tauri*.[51] In *Arabidopsis thaliana* [52] the full length protein is only 146 residues long representing only the phosphatase domain and it shows marginal similarity to vertebrate and fission yeast Cdc25. Overexpression of *A. thaliana* Cdc25 causes premature mitotic entry in fission yeast.[53]

4. Regulation of cell cycle transitions by Cdc25

4.1. The fission yeast G2/M transition – The prototype Cdc25/cyclin-CDK circuit

Regulation of the transition from G2 to mitosis in *S. pombe* is typical of the positive feedback loops seen between Cdc25 and CDKs in all systems. Cdc2 (Cdk1) drives all cell cycle transitions in fission yeast.[20] During G2 and early mitosis Cdc2 complexes with the B-type cyclin Cdc13 [54,55], the only essential cyclin in fission yeast.[56] Whereas Cdc2 is constitutively expressed throughout the cell cycle [57], Cdc25 and Cdc13 begin to accumulate in G2 and are degraded during mitotic entry.[58-60] Prior to M-phase, the Cdc2-Cdc13 complex is kept inactive by phosphorylation of threonine 14 (T14) and tyrosine 15 (Y15).[61,62] Y15 is phosphorylated by the S-phase specific kinase Mik1 [63,64] and T14 and Y15 are modified by Wee1.[63,65-67] In G2 Cdc25 translocates to the nucleus via the importin-β homologue Sal3.[68] After cells grow to a critical size for mitotic entry, Cdc25 becomes active and dephosphorylates Cdc2 Y15.[69] Cdc25 is activated and hyperphosphorylated by Cdc2 as the cell enters mitosis.[58, 70] CDKs phosphorylate a serine or threonine residue in the context of a consensus site (S/T)PX(K/R).[71,72] The positions of the Cdc2 phosphorylation sites on Cdc25 have not been determined, but mutagenesis of 15 potential CDK consensus sites abrogates phosphorylation by Cdc2-Cdc13.[73] In *S. pombe*, the feedback loop between Cdc25 and Cdc2-Cdc13 is strengthened by the involvement of the *S. pombe* Polo kinase homologue Plo1 which phosphorylates Cdc25 downstream of Cdc2 activation.[74] After the metaphase-anaphase transition, Polo kinase activation encourages cyclin degradation through activation of the anaphase promoting complex (APC).[75] Thus, this kinase simultaneously ensures that Cdc2 activation will be robust, and brief, as its cyclin partner Cdc13 is degraded by the APC immediately following anaphase initiation.

4.2 Vertebrate cell cycle

While fission yeast Cdc25 is solely involved in the G2/M transition, Cdc25 orthologues in vertebrates also play a role in G1 and S-phase progression. Vertebrates have several CDK-cyclin complexes which participate in these transitions through positive feedback loops with Cdc25. In addition to associating with cyclin B, Cdk1 associates with cyclin A during late S-phase and G2.[76] A second CDK, Cdk2, was discovered as a cDNA which could complement the loss of the budding yeast Cdk1 homologue, CDC28.[77] Cdk2 functions early in the cell cycle and is likewise negatively regulated by phosphorylation of Y15.[78,79] It forms a complex with Cyclin A and Cyclin E.[80,81] Cdk4 and Cdk6 operate early in G1 in association with D-type cyclins.[82] In many cases a particular cyclin class (ie. A, B, D, E) has multiple members. For the sake of clarity, cyclins will be referred to by their subtype only. Furthermore, only the CDKs and cyclins directly responsible for cell cycle transitions in concert with Cdc25 orthologues will be discussed. For instance, Cdk1/cyclin B is activated by a CDK-Activating Kinase (CAK), a complex of Cdk7 and cyclin H [83], but as CAKs are not activated by Cdc25 they are outside the scope of this review.

4.2.1. Cell cycle re-entry from G_0

Most somatic cells spend their time in G_0. Cells in G_0 may commit to entry into the cell cycle when they receive stimuli in the form of growth factors The cells then deactivate the cell cycle repressors which have kept them in G_0 and transcribe the positive regulators of the next cell cycle transition, G1/S.

In non-dividing cells, the Retinoblastoma protein (Rb) binds to E2F thus preventing transcription of genes required for cell cycle progression including cyclin D, cyclin A and Cdc25A.[84-87] (Figure 1) After exposure to growth factors, cells in G_0 re-enter the cell cycle through activation of the Ras pathway via the Raf/MAP (Mitogen Activated Protein) kinase pathway.[88] This leads to the degradation of the Cdk4 inhibitors $p15^{INK4B}$ and $p16^{INK4A}$ and the Cdk2 inhibitors $p27^{KIP}$, $p21^{CIP}$ and induction of cyclin D. Cdk4 and Cdk6 bound to cyclin D inhibit the Rb protein [89] allowing transcription of cyclin E and cyclin A.[89,90] Cdc25A activates Cdk4-cyclin D but not Cdk6-cyclin D *in vitro*.[91] Cyclin E associates with Cdk2 in late G1 and helps complete the inhibition of Rb.[89,92]

4.2.2. The G1/S transition

Cdc25A is transcribed following relief of Rb-mediated transcriptional repression, reaching its maximal level at the end of G1 and dephosphorylating Y15 on Cdk2.[87,91] Cdk2 is phosphorylated on Y15 by Wee1.[93] Dephosphorylation of Cdk2 takes place via both

Cdc25A and Cdc25B.[94-97] Cdk2 immunoprecipitated from cell lysates where Cdc25A has been overexpressed has high histone H1 kinase activity and low levels of Y15 phosphorylation.[91] Such overexpression accelerates entry into S-phase through activation of Cdk2-cyclin E.[91,98] DNA-synthesis can be blocked in these cells by injecting them with anti-Cdc25A antibodies.[99] Cdk2-cyclin E and Cdc25A are mutually activated by a positive feedback loop allowing passage of the G1/S boundary.[95] Depletion of Cdk2 or cyclin E prevents phosphorylation of Cdc25A and recombinant Cdc25A can be activated by Cdk2-cyclin E *in vitro*.[95] In addition phosphorylation of Cdc25A by Cdk2 destabilizes the phosphatase. Conversely, exposure of cells to CDK inhibitors roscovitine and olomoucine causes stabilization of Cdc25A.[99]

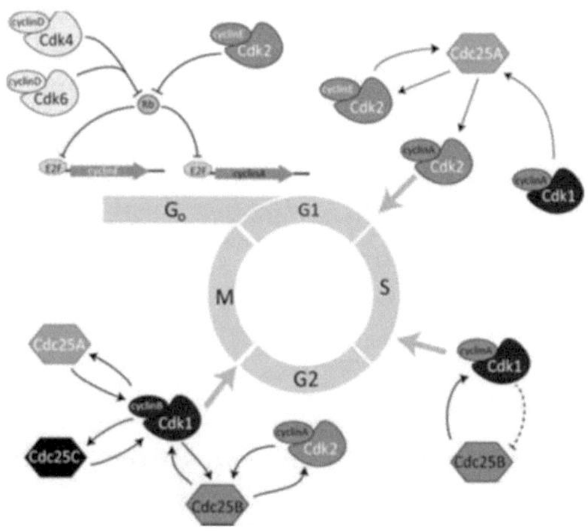

Figure 1. Positive feedback loops between Cdk-cyclin complexes and Cdc25 family members drive cell cycle transitions.

S-phase initiation requires activation of DNA replication proteins by Cdk2-cyclin A. Injecting G1 cells with anti-cyclin A antibodies stops entry into S-phase.[100] Phosphorylation of the essential DNA replication initiator Cdc6 by Cdk2-cyclin A leads to its nuclear import.[101,102] Cdk2 is recruited to chromatin by the replication initiation factor Cdc45 where it phosphorylates histone H1 and induces chromosome de-condensation.[103] As S-phase progresses high Cdk2-cyclin A activity induces degradation of Cdc6, preventing re-initiation of DNA synthesis at origins which have already fired.[102]

Cdc25B has a role late in S-phase as Cdc25B immunoprecipitated from late S-phase HeLa cell extracts is phosphorylated, activated, and able to dephosphorylate Cdk2-cyclin A.[97] The murine homologue of Cdc25B purified from S-phase extracts promotes cyclin A and cyclin E associated histone H1 kinase activity *in vitro*.[94] In addition, siRNA knockdown of human Cdc25B causes a delay in initiation of DNA synthesis.[104] The Cdk1-cyclin A complex regulates late origin firing in S-phase. A constitutively activated Cdk1 allele increases firing of late S-phase origins, whereas a loss of function temperature sensitive allele of Cdk1 has a defect in late origin firing at the restrictive temperature.[76]

4.2.3. The G2/M transition

Unlike the simple circuit of Cdc25-Cdc2 activation in fission yeast, the vertebrate G2/M transition involves a series of interconnected loops with positive and negative inputs from a variety of pathways. This led to what could be considered the "traditional model" of G2/M transition in vertebrates with respect to Cdc25 regulation by CDK-cyclin complexes. In reality things may be more complex. Cdc25C is not explicitly required for mitotic entry; siRNA knockdown of Cdc25C does not prevent the G2/M transition.[105] In addition, mouse lines which lack Cdc25B and/or Cdc25C are viable with the only obvious phenotype being a defect in oocyte maturation observed in *cdc25B*$^{-/-}$ mice.[106-108] In addition, the creation of CDK and cyclin knockout mice has revealed a network of compensatory mechanisms which cloud the traditional model. Cdk2$^{-/-}$, Cdk4$^{-/-}$, or Cdk6$^{-/-}$ mice show some abnormalities as adults, but are not embryonic lethal indicating that these Cdks are not individually essential for cell division.[92] There is considerable redundancy. Mitotic entry is best viewed as a three step process. First, Cdc25B and CDK-cyclin A are activated followed by basal activation of Cdk1-cyclin B at the centrosome.[109] Second, Cdk1-cyclinB, Cdc25B and Cdc25C localize to the nucleus. Third, Cdk1-cyclin B and Cdc25C mutually activate. Cdk1-cyclin B then induces overt mitotic events such as breakdown of the nuclear envelope and spindle formation. [81,110,111]

4.2.4. Activation of Cdc25B and Cdk1/2-cyclinA

Phosphorylation of human Cdc25B by Cdk1-cyclin A during G2 causes Cdc25B activation but also destabilizes the protein.[112,113] Cdc25B activates Cdk2-cyclinA in a positive feedback loop.[114] Cdk2-cyclin A mediated destabilization of Cdc25B has not been reported, although the Cdk1 and Cdk2 kinase complexes modify Cdc25B to approximately the same degree and have a similar set of substrates.[113,115] However, Cdk2 is the preferred binding partner of cyclin A and is more active than Cdk1-cyclin A during G2.[80,100] Cdk2 cyclin A has two peaks of activation, one during S-phase and one prior to G2/M. [80,116] Inhibition of Cdk2-cyclin A delays mitotic entry.[109] Depletion of Cdk1-cyclin A, activation of the CDK inhibitor p21^{cip} , or addition of an inhibitory ATP analogue destabilizes Cdc25B in *Sf9* cell extracts.[112] Similarly, in cycloheximide treated cells Cdc25B, but not Cdc25A or Cdc25C, is unstable and uniquely labile during the cell cycle.[117]

Cyclin B accumulates throughout G2 but Cdc25A and Cdc25B are required to induce formation of the Cdk1-cyclin B complex at G2/M.[118] Cdk1-cyclin B interaction occurs earlier in G2 when Cdc25A or Cdc25B are overexpressed. Cdk1 and cyclin B are almost exclusively cytoplasmic during interphase with a small portion of the complex associating with the centrosome at G2/M.[119-121] A population of Cdk2-cyclinA is likewise localized to the centrosomes prior to prophase.[116] In *Xenopus*, centrosomal localization of Cdk1-cyclin B requires Aurora kinase.[122] Aurora is involved in a diverse set of mitotic events such as spindle assembly, centrosome maturation, and cytokinesis.[123] Aurora can also phosphorylate Cdc25B at S353 *in vivo*, activating the phosphatase.[124] (Table 1) Although some Cdk1-cyclin B is activated by Cdc25B [120,125], this does not represent a full mitotic activation and is only sufficient for progression as far as prophase. Injection of a dominant-negative mutant of Cdc25B into HeLa cells causes arrest in prophase with condensed chromosomes and disassembled nucleoli, but without nuclear envelope breakdown [109]. Microinjection of Cdk1-cyclin B lets cells pass this block and complete mitosis.

Species	Member	Kinase	Site(s)	References
S. pombe	Cdc25	Cds1/Chk1/Srk1	S99, S148, S178, S192, S204, S206, T226, S234, S359, T561, S567, T569	[60, 156, 157, 162]
Human	Cdc25A	Cdk1-cyclin B	S18, S40, S88, S116, S261, S283, S321	[149, 151, 167]
		Chk1	S76, S124, S178, T507	[168-173, 200]
		Chk2	S124, S278	[173, 175]
		Casein Kinase 1ε	S82	[199]
		Casein Kinase 1α	S79, S82	[198]
		p38	S76, S124	[168, 175]
		GSK-3β	S76	[193, 194]
		NEK11	S82, S88	[187]
		Plk3	S80	[193, 194]
	Cdc25B*	Cdk1-cyclinB	S50, S160, S321	[135, 136, 246]
		Chk1	S151, S230, S323, S563	[236, 238, 239]
		Aurora	S353	[124]
		Casein Kinase 2	S186, S187	[235]
		JNK	S101, S103	[280]
		MEK/ERK	S249	[259]
		p38	S323	[208]
		MK2	S323	[210]
		Plk1	T167, S209, T404, S465	[136]
	Cdc25C	Cdk1/cyclin B	T48, T67, S122, T130, S168, S214	[42, 143, 145, 246]
		Chk1	S216, S247, S263	[219-221, 225, 226]
		Chk2	S216	[209, 242]
		Casein Kinase 2	T236	[234]
		MK2	S216	[210]
		C-TAK1	S216	[276]
		JNK	S168	[281, 282]
		MEK/ERK	S216	[278]
		Plk1	S198	[140]
		Plk3	S191, S198	[141]
Xenopus	Cdc25A	Chk1	S73, T504	[201, 207]
	Cdc25C	Cdk1/cylinB Cdk1-cyclinA	T48, T67, T138, S205, S285;	[193, 247, 249]
		Chk1	S287, T533	[207, 229-231, 241]
		p42	S48, T138, S205	[272]
		$p90^{rsk}$	S287	[269, 270]
		Rsk2	S317, S318, S319	[271]

Table 1. Summary of known phosphorylation sites on Cdc25 family members and the kinases responsible

4.2.5. Everybody into the nucleus

Cyclin B has a cytoplasmic retention sequence which is sufficient to induce cytoplasmic localization of the normally nuclear protein and contains a nuclear export signal (NES).[126]

Nuclear export is blocked by phosphorylation of S126 at the end of prophase.[127-129] Cyclin B is phosphorylated by Cdk1-Cyclin B as starfish oocytes pass the prophase II to metaphase II arrest.[130] Human cyclin B S126 is followed by a proline residue suggesting Cdk1-cyclin B autophosphorylation. Cyclin B is phosphorylated by the *Xenopus* Polo kinase homologue Plx1 on S133 and S147 (homologous to human cyclin B S177 and S181) enhancing its nuclear import.[125,131] Initial Cdc25B mediated activation of Cdk1-cyclin B may result in a priming autophosphorylation of S126 followed by docking of Polo kinase and inhibition of nuclear export. Such a Cdk1 mediated priming phosphorylation has been shown to induce Plx1 phosphorylation of Cdc25B (see below). Human Polo kinase Plk1 also deactivates Cdk1-cyclin B inhibitory kinases. Plk1 inhibits the cytoplasmic Cdk1 inhibitory kinase Myt1.[132,133] Wee1 is phosphorylated on S53 and S123 by Plk1 and Cdk1-cyclin B, respectively, resulting in its degradation by β-TrCP.[134]

The activated cytoplasmic pool of Cdk1-cyclin B phosphorylates Cdc25B on S160 inducing its nuclear import. [135] (All phosphorylated residues on human Cdc25B are numbered according to the sequence of the longest splice variant Cdc25B3). Overexpression of human Cdc25B causes an increase in cells with condensed chromatin, whereas overexpression of Cdc25B-S160G does not induce mitotic entry. S160 phosphorylation does not affect the *in vitro* activity of human Cdc25B against a fluorescein diphosphate substrate, but instead positively regulates its nuclear import. *In vitro* phosphorylation assays show Cdk1-cyclin B can phosphorylate residues on Cdc25B which are not targeted by Cdk1-cyclin A or Cdk2-cyclin A.[113] Interestingly, Cdk1-cyclin A cannot phosphorylate Cdc25B that has previously been phosphorylated by Cdk1-cyclin B.[112]

Plk1 is involved in human Cdc25B nuclear import following the initial activation of Cdk1-cyclin B. After addition of the Plk1 inhibitor thiophene benzimidazole, nuclear accumulation of GFP-Cdc25B is reduced. Conversely, expression of a constitutively active Plk1 mutant enhances Cdc25 nuclear localization.[136] Co-overexpression of Plk1 and Cdc25B in U2OS osteosarcoma cells induces chromosome condensation to a greater degree compared to cells expressing Plk1 or Cdc25B alone. This is partially dependent on the presence of a functional nuclear localization signal (NLS) in Cdc25B. Plk1 docking to Cdc25B requires prior phosphorylation of S50 by Cdk1/cyclin B.[137] Mass spectrometry identified thirteen phosphorylated Plk1 sites on Cdc25B *in vitro* and showed that T167, S209, T404, S465 and S513 appear to be particularly strong targets.[137] Plk1 is required for Cdk1-cyclin B activation, at least in part by negatively regulating Cdc25C nuclear export. Depletion of Plx1 from oocyte extracts prevents the activation of Cdc25C and Cdk1-cyclin B.[138] Unlike Cdc25B, phosphorylation of Cdc25C by Cdk1 is not a prerequisite for Plk1 targeting the phosphatase; Plk1 affects Cdc25C phosphatase activity and its localization. *In vitro* phosphorylation of Cdc25C enhances its ability to dephosphorylate kinase dead Cdc2 on Y15.[139] Plk1 phosphorylates human Cdc25C on S198 which resides within the nuclear export signal (NES) of the phosphatase, promoting its nuclear localization.[140] Polo kinase family member Plk3 also interacts with human Cdc25C and phosphorylates it on S191, and S198 to a lesser degree.[141] Substitutions S191D, S198D or Plk3 overexpression result in constitutive nuclear localization, while siRNA knockdown of Plk3 or substitutions S191A and S198A leads to nuclear exclusion.[141] Another polo family member, Plk4, phosphorylates human Cdc25C on undetermined sites.[142]

4.2.6. *Full activation of Cdk1-CyclinB and Cdc25C*

Activated Cdk1-cyclin B phosphorylates human Cdc25C on T48, T67, S122, T130, S168 and S214 *in vitro* and *in vivo*, driving a positive feedback loop which culminates in the phosphorylation of mitotic Cdk1 substrates.[42,143] Cdk1 phosphorylated Cdc25C has an increased Cdk1 Y15 phosphatase activity.[143] Recombinant Cdc25C can activate Cdk1 thereby increasing its histone H1 kinase activity.[144] Use of phospho-specific antibodies recently showed that phosphorylation of T48, T67 and T130 occur on spatially separate pools of human Cdc25C.[145] T67-phosphorylated Cdc25C is chromatin associated from prophase until telophase while T130-phosphorylated Cdc25C localizes to the centrosomes. T130 phosphorylation creates a Plk1 binding site on Cdc25C. Three distinct pools of T48, T67 and T130 mono-phosphorylated Cdc25C protein can be detected by immunoprecipitation with each individual phospho-specific antibody; Cdc25C pulled down with one antibody is not bound by the other two. In *Xenopus* oocyte extracts Cdc25C is heavily phosphorylated while cells undergo germinal vesicle breakdown (meiosis I).[45] *Xenopus* Cdc25C residues T48, T67, T138, S205 and S285 are phosphorylated by Cdk1-cyclin A and Cdk1-cyclin B *in vitro.*[146] Mutation of the major targets, T48, T67 and T138, to alanine prevents *Xenopus* Cdc25C activation *in vitro.*[147] Although G2/M is not normally associated with Cdc25A function, it also contributes to Cdk1-cyclin B activation. Depleting cells of Cdc25A reduces Cdk1-cyclin B activation by approximately fifty percent.[148] In cells arrested in mitosis by addition of nocodazole, a microtubule polymerization inhibitor and spindle poison, Cdc25A is phosphorylated by Cdk1-cyclin B on S18 and S116. Substitution of these residues with alanine leads to Cdc25A instability. Cdc25A S40, S88, S261 and S283 are also Cdk1-cyclin B phosphorylated *in vitro.*[149]

4.2.7. *Mitotic exit*

Following chromosome alignment on the metaphase plate a cascade of APC mediated degradation events occurs to reset conditions for the start of the next cell cycle.[150] The APC regulates two important processes required for completion of mitosis. First, it targets Securin, the inhibitory subunit of Separase, which is responsible for Cohesin cleavage and chromosome separation. Second, it targets cyclin A and cyclin B for destruction, inactivating Cdk1. Cyclin B is degraded after the metaphase-anaphase transition while cyclin A is degraded during metaphase. [121] Cdk1 mediated phosphorylation of Cdc25 paralogues is reversed by Cdc14 family phosphatases. Cdk1-cyclin B phosphorylates human Cdc25A S18, S40, S88, S116, S261 and S283 *in vitro.*[149] Of these sites, human Cdc14A dephosphorylates S116, Cdc14B targets S88 and S261, while both phosphatases can dephosphorylate S40. Cdc14A was independently identified as also dephosphorylating Cdc25A S321.[151] siRNA knockdown of Cdc14B leads to accumulation of phosphorylated Cdc25B and Cdc25C.[149] In *S. pombe* Cdc14 homologue Clp1 dephosphorylates Cdc25 and this is required for its ubiquitination and APC mediated proteolysis at the end of mitosis.[73] Similarly, in vertebrates Cdc25A and Cdc25B are targeted by the APC at mitotic exit.[152,153]

5. Cdc25 phosphorylation by the DNA damage and replication checkpoint

DNA damage causes activation of checkpoints which delay cell cycle transitions to allow sufficient time for repair. Stalling of replication forks causes a similar cell cycle arrest, with additional need for stabilizing replication forks and/or modulating replication origin firing until the cause of the stalling is eliminated. Checkpoint effector kinases impinge on the central cell cycle machinery by phosphorylating Cdc25. This modification variously inhibits Cdc25 phosphatase activity, induces degradation or creates binding sites for 14-3-3 proteins which modify localization of the protein.

5.1. Fission yeast

Cell cycle arrest following DNA damage requires that Cdc2 is kept in a Y15-phosphorylated, inhibited state.[154] Cdc25 is inhibited through phosphorylation by Chk1 and Cds1 kinases in response to DNA damage and replication fork arrest, respectively.[155-157] Cells over-expressing Cdc25 or expressing a Y15F phospho-mimetic mutation of Cdc2 fail to arrest cell cycle progression after exposure to ionizing radiation.[154] In the absence of Cds1, Chk1 can cause cell cycle arrest following stalling of replication forks by hydroxyurea (HU) exposure. Cells lacking both kinases are unable to arrest.[155] Cds1 also phosphorylates multiple substrates to stabilize stalled replication forks and prevent the occurrence of inappropriate recombination events.[158] Upstream regulation of the DNA damage and replication checkpoint pathway occurs through activation of the ATM (Ataxia-telangiectasia mutated) homologue Rad3 through a well conserved signaling cascade.[159]

Phosphorylation of Cdc25 by Chk1 and Cds1 creates binding sites for the 14-3-3 homologues Rad24 and Rad25.[160,161] Phosphorylation and 14-3-3 binding stabilizes Cdc25, a phenomena referred to as "stockpiling", thought to allow the cell to rapidly re-enter the cell cycle once replication or DNA damage arrest has been lifted.[70] The first Chk1/Cds1 phosphorylated Cdc25 residue identified, S99, partially impairs the replication and DNA damage checkpoint when mutated to alanine.[157] S99 modified Cdc25 is also phosphorylated on S192 and S359 by Cds1 and Chk1 *in vivo* and *in vitro*.[156] By phosphorylating Cdc25 *in vitro* with Cds1, nine additional sites were identified by mass spectrometry (S148, S178, S204, S206, T226, S234, T561, S567, T569) as well as the three sites previously known.[162] Nine sites between S99 and S359 are distributed through the poorly conserved N-terminal two thirds of the protein, while three sites reside in the extreme C-terminus. Alanine substitutions of all nine sites in the amino two thirds of Cdc25, *cdc25(9A)*, overrides the DNA replication checkpoint when expressed under control of a relatively weak heterologous promoter.[162] However, when *cdc25(9A)* is expressed from the native *cdc25*$^{+}$ locus under the control of its own promoter it does not cause a cell cycle phenotype, and the cell is checkpoint competent.[60] In addition, Cdc25(9A) is unstable following replication arrest suggesting redundancy in checkpoint control, such that Cdc25 which cannot be inhibited by Cds1 is eliminated from the cell. The S-phase specific Cdc2-Y15 kinase Mik1 is sufficient to prevent mitotic entry in these cells. Alanine substitutions of only the three C-terminal Cdc25 sites (T561, S567, T569) have a clear replication checkpoint defect in a *mik1*⁻ background and appear to be involved in maintenance, but not establishment, of the DNA damage checkpoint. [305]

5.2. Vertebrate Cdc25 regulation by DNA damage and replication checkpoints

In vertebrate cells detection of DNA damage is relayed through ATM and ATR (ATM-Related) to two checkpoint effectors, Chk1 and Chk2. While the *S. pombe* ATM homologue Rad3 is involved in activation of both Chk1 and Cds1; DNA damage signaling in vertebrates shows separation of ATR-Chk1 and ATM-Chk2 axes.[163,164] The target of these effector proteins is determined by the cell cycle stage at which the damage occurs and the nature of the damage itself. ATM-Chk2 signaling is initiated by double strand breaks, while ATR-Chk1 is activated by stalled replication forks and single stranded breaks. The p38 MAP kinase pathway is critical for cell cycle arrest following UV induced DNA damage. (Figure 2)

5.2.1. G1/S and Intra-S checkpoints

The G1/S checkpoint prevents the start of DNA synthesis in the presence of DNA damage while the Intra-S checkpoint protects replication forks, prevents activation of late replication origins, and keeps the cell from entering mitosis until S-phase is completed. G1-S checkpoint arrest is manifested through inhibition of Cdc25A, thus preventing activation of Cdk4-cyclin D and Cdk2-cyclin E. The checkpoint also activates p53 resulting in the induction of the Cdk2 inhibitor $p21^{CIP}$ and the targeting of Cyclin E to the SCF complex to reinforce Cdk2 inhibition.[165] In rat fibroblasts UV induced DNA damage during G1 results in cell cycle arrest at the G1/S transition requiring inhibition of Cdc25A and phosphorylation of Cdk4-Y14.[166] In U2OS osteosarcoma cells Cdk2-cyclin E kinase activity decreases and Y15 phosphorylation increases coincident with Cdc25A degradation following UV exposure.[167] Conversely, Cdc25A overexpression in UV exposed U2OS osteosarcoma cells results in bypass of the checkpoint and dephosphorylation of Cdk2-cyclin E. Cdc25A inhibition involves a combination of destabilization and inhibition of phosphatase activity by Chk1.[167] Treatment with caffeine (an ATM/ATR inhibitor) or the Chk1 inhibitor UNC-01, or depletion of Chk1, stabilizes the phosphatase.[167,168] In humans, Chk1 phosphorylates Cdc25A S76, S124 , S178, and T507.[168-170] Cdc25A catalytic activity is reduced three-fold when it is phosphorylated by hChk1 *in vitro*.[169] S76 and S124 are phosphorylated following ionizing radiation resulting in Cdc25A instability.[168,169,171-173] Mutation of S76 to alanine stabilizes human Cdc25A [171,172]; however, neither S76A nor S124A overrides checkpoint arrest following ionizing radiation or UV.[168] Mouse cells homozygous for the Cdc25A S124A mutation display Cdc25A stabilization following ionizing radiation;[174] however, there are no changes in proportion of cells in S-phase, or radiation resistant DNA synthesis indicating their S-phase checkpoint is intact.

Human Cdc25A S76, S124 and/or S178 are identified in several publications as "S75, S123 and S177," respectively.[168,169,174-176] In the original cloning of human Cdc25A.[37], there are several substitutions in the N-terminus (Accession: AAA58415.1) and a one residue gap corresponding to residue R12 in all other full length human Cdc25A sequences in the NCBI database (Accession: P30304). Residues have been re-numbered as per "P30304" for the sake of consistency.

Cdc25A S76, S124, S178 and T507 match the consensus site for 14-3-3 binding, RXX_pS/T [177] However, only the Chk1 dependent phosphorylation of S178 and T507 results in association with 14-3-3.[170] Substitution of these residues to alanine results in a complete loss of 14-3-3 interaction *in vivo*. Phosphorylation of T507 in particular, and subsequent 14-3-3 binding, interferes with Cdk1-cyclin B association by blocking a cyclin B docking site. A recent study suggests that a ternary complex between Cdc25A, 14-3-3γ and Chk1 is formed following ionizing radiation.[178] The Chk1/14-3-3γ interaction requires auto-phosphorylation of Chk1 S296. Substituting Chk1 S296 for alanine precludes 14-3-3 binding and Cdc25A S76 phosphorylation and deactivates the DNA damage checkpoint.[178] 14-3-3 proteins preferably exist as thermostable homo- and heterodimers. Each isoform in a heterodimer binding a different protein provides a common mechanism for bringing enzymes and their substrate proteins into close proximity.[179,180]

Defects in the Intra-S checkpoint allow replication of damaged DNA.[173,176,181] In mammalian cells, DNA damage results in destabilization of Cdc25A and inhibition of Cdk2.[173] Cdk2 is involved in loading the Cdc45 origin binding factor. Inhibition of Cdc25A stops further origin firing once DNA damage is detected.[182] Cdc25A is also unstable after HU induced replication fork stalling, which unlike in fission yeast, is controlled by activation of Chk1 in mammalian cells.[183]

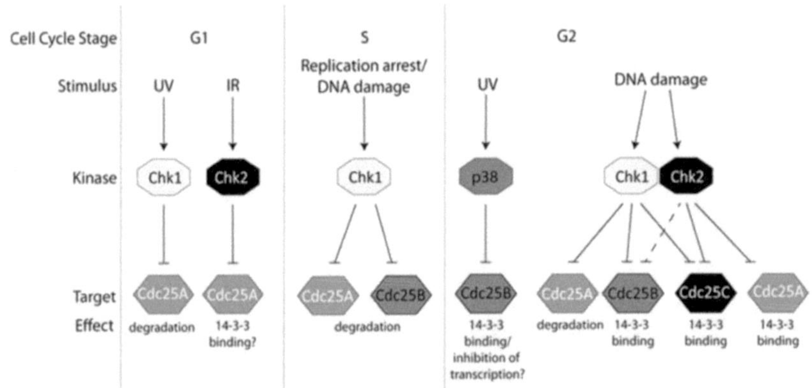

Figure 2. Inhibitory phosphorylation of Cdc25 family members following DNA damage and replication arrest

5.2.1.1. Phosphorylation mediated degradation of Cdc25A by the SCF- βTrCP complex

The mechanism by which Cdc25A is destabilized following DNA structure checkpoint activation is well understood (Figure 3). Human Cdc25A phosphorylation by Chk1 following S-phase DNA damage causes degradation by F-box protein β-TrCP associated with the Skp1-cullin-Fbox (SCF) complex.[171,184] Mutating the destruction box or KEN box (APC interaction motifs) of Cdc25A does not stabilize the protein following exposure to ionizing radiation.[152] This indicates that SCF-mediated degradation of Cdc25A after DNA damage is independent of the cell cycle regulated APC-mediated degradation which occurs at mitotic exit. β-TrCP recognizes a degron motif of DSG(X)$_4$S where both serine residues are phosphorylated.[185] siRNA knockdown of β-TrCP causes stabilization of Cdc25A, and radiation-resistant DNA synthesis in cells exposed to ionizing radiation.[171,184] Human Cdc25A contains such a motif: DS$_{82}$GFCLDS$_{88}$. The S88A substitution does not stabilize the phosphatase, suggesting that S88 phosphorylation is not explicitly required for β-TrCP binding to Cdc25A.[171] Following ionizing radiation, Chk1 primes Cdc25A for destruction through phosphorylation of S76.[171,186] The NimA-related NEK11 kinase targets Cdc25A S82 and S88, within the DSG degron sequence.[187] Depletion of NEK11 causes a marked decrease in S82 and S88 phosphorylation *in vivo*, and prevents Cdc25A degradation following IR. NEK11, itself thought to be a Chk1 substrate, can directly phosphorylate S82 and S88 *in vitro*.

Following ATM activation, Chk2 phosphorylates and activates the oncogene p53, and inhibits its negative regulator MDM2 after ionizing radiation.[188-191] p53 then induces the Cdk2-cyclin E inhibitor p21^{WAF}.[192] p53 also activates Glycogen Synthase Kinase (GSK-3β), which phosphorylates human Cdc25A S76 following a priming phosphorylation of S80 which can be targeted *in vitro* by Plk3.[193,194] Plk3 is unique among Polo kinase family members in causing Cdc25A stabilization when knocked down with siRNA.[194] In Plk3 null mice Cdc25A is stabilized following DNA damage.[195] Plk3 also phosphorylates and activates p53 following DNA damage and contributes to Chk2 activation.[196,197] In HeLa cells, Casein Kinase 1α (CK1α) sequentially phosphorylates both S79 and S82 following priming phosphorylation of S76 by Chk1 or GSK-3β.[198] The CK1ε isoform negatively regulates Cdc25A by S82 phosphorylation in HEK293 cells.[199] S82 phosphorylation *in vitro* and *in vivo* takes place in response to DNA damage, dependent on CK1α first phosphorylating S79.[198] S79A substitution prevents S82 phosphorylation. S76 phosphorylation appears to be the first target in the cascade, since it does not require prior phosphorylation of S79, T80, S82 or S88. Only alanine substitutions of S76, S79 and S82 impair β-TrCP interaction with Cdc25A and stabilize the phosphatase suggesting that T80 and S88 are not critical for Cdc25A degradation. Additional sites (S107, S156, S192, S279 S293) are phosphorylated by Chk1 or Cds1 *in vitro* but mutating any of these sites does not eliminate β-TrCP binding.[200] Although an interaction between phosphorylated *Xenopus* Cdc25A and β-TrCP has not been demonstrated, Chk1 is required for Cdc25A degradation at the mid-blastula transition through phosphorylation of S73.[201] Interestingly, *Xenopus* Cdc25A lacks the first serine in the DSG(X)$_4$S degron motif found in human Cdc25A, instead possessing DDG. *Xenopus* Cdc25A S73 lies just upstream of the mutated degron and is analogous to S76 in human Cdc25A. The DAG motif of *Xenopus* Cdc25A lies within a larger PEST motif which regulates stability of the phosphatase through β-TrCP binding, independent of Chk1.[202] In mouse embryonic stem cells, which lack a G1/S DNA damage response, Cdk2 kinase activity is not affected by Cdc25A degradation following exposure to ionizing radiation.[203] Cdc25A degradation is independent of Chk1 and Chk2 but instead dependent on GSK-3β. Like Cdc25A, mammalian Cdc25B is unstable following HU induced arrest.[117] Cdc25B binds β-TrCP strongly and contains the residues DAG rather than the DSG degron motif.[202,204] In contrast, Cdc25B accumulates following G2 DNA damage checkpoint arrest induced by a variety of agents.[205] This is reminiscent of the "stockpiling" phenomena noted earlier in *S. pombe*.[70] β-TrCP interaction with Cdc25B may also be required for mitotic exit.[204] A Cdc25B-DDA degron mutant which cannot bind β-TrCP accelerates mitotic entry slightly, but has a significant delay completing mitosis and progressing to G1. This mitotic delay is due to an extended metaphase in which Cdc25B-DDA shows a high proportion of lagging, misaligned and bridged chromosomes as well as mis-oriented spindles.[204]

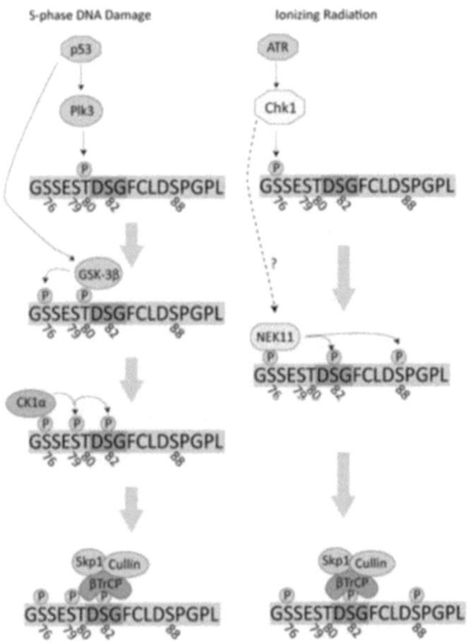

Figure 3. Multi-step phosphorylation cascades involved in targeting human Cdc25A for degradation by the β-TrCP SCF complex following DNA damage in S-phase and G2.

5.2.1.2. Cdc25A inhibition by 14-3-3 binding

Cdc25A S76, S124, S178 and T507 match the consensus site for 14-3-3 binding RXX_pS/T [177] However, only the Chk1 dependent phosphorylation of S178 and T507 results in association with 14-3-3.[170] Substitution of these residues to alanine results in a complete loss of 14-3-3 interaction *in vivo*. Phosphorylation of T507 in particular, and subsequent 14-3-3 binding, interferes with Cdk1-cyclin B association by blocking a cyclin B docking site. A recent study suggests that a ternary complex between Cdc25A, 14-3-3γ and Chk1 is formed following ionizing radiation.[178] The Chk1/14-3-3γ interaction requires auto-phosphorylation of Chk1 S296. Substituting Chk1 S296 to alanine precludes 14-3-3 binding and Cdc25A S76 phosphorylation and deactivates the DNA damage checkpoint.[178] 14-3-3 proteins preferably exist as thermostable homo- and heterodimers. Each isoform in a heterodimer binding a different protein provides a common mechanism for bringing enzymes and their substrate proteins into close proximity.[179,180]

Following exposure to ionizing radiation during G1 phosphorylation of Cdc25A on S124 by Chk2 prevents entry to S-phase .[173] Chk2 cannot efficiently phosphorylate Cdc25A on S76 and so cannot induce Cdc25A degradation by the β-TrCP route.[206] The mechanism by which S124 phosphorylation induces Cdc25A degradation is not clear because it is not required for degradation via β-TrCP.[173] S124 conforms to a 14-3-3 phospho-serine binding site, but doesn't bind 14-3-3.[170]In contrast to the effects of Cdc25A phosphorylation sites discussed thus far, modification of *Xenopus* Cdc25A T504 by Chk1 negatively regulates interaction with Cdk1-cyclin A, Cdk1-cyclin B and Cdk2-cyclin E but in a 14-3-3 independent manner.[207]

5.2.2. G2/M DNA damage checkpoint

The response to damage in G2 is dependent on the nature of the damage signal. Exposure to UV activates p38 MAP kinase and checkpoint arrest is independent of ATM and ATR since the arrest is not caffeine sensitive.[208] The primary target following UV irradiation is Cdc25B and although p38 can phosphorylate Cdc25C *in vitro,* UV exposure does not affect the Cdc25C/14-3-3 interaction.[208] Ionizing radiation activates ATM and ATR and results in Cdc25C phosphorylation by Chk1 and Chk2.[209]

5.2.2.1. Cdc25B inhibition following UV induced DNA damage

A number of conflicting reports have appeared relating to Cdc25B regulation following UV exposure. Some groups have reported that UV has no effect on Cdc25B protein levels [208,210], but others have shown that UV causes either MAP kinase mediated Cdc25B degradation or Cdc25B accumulation.[205,208,211] Cell line specific effects have no doubt contributed to these inconsistencies as human molecular biology relies heavily on transformed cell lines and mis-regulation of Cdc25B is a common phenomenon in tumors.[212] Cdc25B isolated from UV irradiated A2058 melanoma cells still retains a substantial portion of its Y15 phosphatase activity and is localized to the nucleus.[213] In HeLa cells Cdc25B is localized almost exclusively to the cytoplasm as detected by cell fractionation and immunofluorescence.[120] Variation in the apparatus used for UV irradiation could also have contributed to contradictory accounts of Cdc25B regulation. A recent re-examination of the effect of UV on Cdc25B showed that after 10 J/m^2 exposure, Cdc25B levels did not decrease, although following 60 J/m^2 Cdc25B was clearly downregulated.[214] Exposure of U2OS osteosarcoma cells to 10 J/m^2 UV leads to Cdc25B nuclear export. Based on chemical inhibitor experiments Cdc25B downregulation is not mediated by ATM/ATR, p38 MAPK or JNK, but rather following 60 J/m^2, by inhibiting Cdc25 translation. The eukaryotic initiation factor regulating Cdc25B expression, eIF2α, is phosphorylated and inhibited following UV exposure.[215] UV mediated DNA damage during G2 involves human Cdc25B S323 phosphorylation through the p38 kinase during interphase.[208] ATM/ATR inhibitor caffeine and the Chk1 inhibitor UNC-01 have no effect on UV mediated checkpoint arrest. Isoforms 14-3-3β and 14-3-3ε bind preferentially to Cdc25B phosphorylated S323, allowing its nuclear export.[216] Nuclear export of Cdc25B is abolished in cells expressing the Cdc25B S323A substitution, regardless of which 14-3-3 isoform is co-expressed.[216] Two amino-truncated Cdc25B isoforms localize to the nucleus *in vivo* and regulate recovery from G2/M checkpoint arrest but neither is required for mitotic entry.[44] Although one of these isoforms contains the DDG degron described above, both are more stable than the full length Cdc25B.

5.2.2.2. Inhibition of Cdc25C following DNA damage

Cdk1 activation is prevented by UV induced checkpoint activity coincident with the appearance of a phosphorylated form of Cdc25C.[213] In contrast with fission yeast Cdc25, which gradually accumulates in the nucleus during G2, human Cdc25C is primarily localized to the cytoplasm during interphase and only enters the nucleus at mitotic entry.[217] Thus, nuclear export of Cdc25C is not a requirement for G2 DNA damage response, since the phosphatase is already cytoplasmic at this time. However, exposure to ionizing radiation decreases the enzymatic activity of human Cdc25C.[218] Several research groups showed relatively early in the Cdc25 phosphorylation story that residue S216 is phosphorylated by Chk1 [219-221] and Chk2 *in vitro*.[209,222] Phosphorylation of S216 results in 14-3-3 binding and nuclear export.[219] Residues surrounding S216, RSPS$_{216}$MP, correspond to the canonical 14-3-3 consensus binding site RSX$_p$SXP.[177] Cdc25C S216A mutants are unable to bind 14-3-3.[219] This is likely due to close proximity of S216 to the NLS, leading to the obstruction of the import signal and trapping of the phosphatase in the cytoplasm.[221,223] A higher proportion of cells expressing Cdc25 S216A have nuclear abnormalities indicative of progression to mitosis prior to completion of DNA synthesis; this effect is exacerbated by addition of HU.[217,219] Such cells also have reduced ability to delay entry to mitosis following ionizing radiation exposure.[224]

Although Cdc25C S216A is a relatively poor substrate for Chk1 compared to the wildtype protein, Chk1 can still execute some degree of phosphorylation on the mutant phosphatase.[220] This observation suggests the possibility that additional Cdc25C phosphorylation negatively regulates its enzymatic activity. Recent bioinformatics approaches to generate profiles from peptide binding arrays based on three diverse 14-3-3 binding sites have generated an improved 14-3-3 binding motif consensus.[225] This helped to identify two additional phosphorylated Cdc25C residues, Ser247 and Ser263, which interact with 14-3-3. Mutation of either residue to alanine reduces 14-3-3 binding, but neither of these mutant peptides was affected by Cdc25 S216 phosphorylation when expressed in cells. S263 was previously identified in an isolated report which showed phosphorylation of this residue induces Cdc25B nuclear export.[226] Cdc25C purified from cells treated with the topoisomerase II inhibitor etoposide is phosphorylated on S263, but S263A substitution results in enhanced nuclear localization. The kinase targeting this residue has yet to be determined experimentally. However, the residues surrounding S263 (KKTV$_p$SLCD) conform to a Chk1 consensus site as Chk1 can tolerate a lysine (K) at the -3 position relative to the phosphorylated serine or threonine *in vitro*.[227]

Regulation of *Xenopus* Cdc25C localization is similar to its human counterpart. In cultured *Xenopus* tissue Cdc25C is primarily in the cytoplasm while the Cdc25C S287A mutant, corresponding to S216 in human Cdc25C, is almost exclusively nuclear.[228] Cdc25C is phosphorylated on multiple sites by Chk1 but only S287 phosphorylation is required for 14-3-3 binding.[229-231] Although *Xenopus* Cdc25C can be made exclusively cytoplasmic by co-expression with 14-3-3ε, Cdc25C S287A is not affected. Nuclear export depends on the intrinsic 14-3-3ε nuclear export signal and re-import is prevented by blocking Cdc25C association with importin-α.[228] In egg extracts depleted of endogenous Cdc25C, expressing Cdc25C S287A accelerates mitotic entry relative to overexpression of the wildtype protein.[229] However, Cdc25C S287A has a less than two fold increase of *in vitro* Cdk1 Y15 dephosphorylation activity over wildtype Cdc25C when pre-incubated with 14-3-3ε. Thus, it seems likely that *Xenopus* Cdc25C phosphorylation and 14-3-3 binding regulates the phosphatase at the level of cellular localization, rather than inhibiting its activity *per se*.

Cdc25A is considered to regulate the G1/S transition in the "Traditional Model" of the human cell cycle but it also has a significant role in mitotic entry. As such, Cdc25A is an important target of the DNA damage checkpoint. In fact, mice lacking Cdc25B and Cdc25C do not have a G2/M checkpoint defect.[106,107] Phosphorylation by Chk1 causes degradation of Cdc25A following DNA damage during G2 ionizing radiation and exposure to the DNA intercalating agent adriamycin.[172,181]

5.3. Chk1 regulation of Cdc25 orthologues in unperturbed cell cycles

Cdc25A, B and C are all phosphorylated by Chk1 in the absence of externally induced DNA damage. As Cdc25 phosphatases are such potent positive regulators of cell cycle transitions it is perhaps not surprising that the cell maintains their activity at a low level until their precise point of activation. Chk1 regulates human Cdc25A stability during unperturbed cell cycles. Phosphorylation of S82 and S88 can be detected using phospho-specific antibodies in unperturbed cells.[184] Depletion of the S82/S88 kinase NEK1 and S76 kinase CK1ε by siRNA, results in Cdc25A stabilization in the absence of DNA damage.[187,199] Cdc25A S124 phosphorylation by Chk1 also occurs in the absence of damage and destabilizes the phosphatase.[168,169,200] Inhibiting ATM/ATR, or a variety of upstream checkpoint components, also stabilizes in the absence of externally induced DNA damage which may indicate there is some basal level of spontaneous damage checkpoint signaling.[232] Cdc25A is also phosphorylated by Casein kinase 2β (CK2β) in a damage independent manner.[233] CK2 phosphorylates human Cdc25C T236 adjacent to the NLS *in vitro*.[234] A T236D mutation reduces β-importin binding, thus excluding Cdc25 from the nucleus.[234] CK2 phosphorylates Cdc25B on residues S186 and S187, just downstream from the KEN box, modestly increases its phosphatase activity, and potentially blocking APC mediated degradation.[235]

Human Cdc25B is phosphorylated *in vitro* by Chk1 at S230 and S563 in the absence of DNA damage.[236] S230 phosphospecific antibodies show that Cdc25B modified on this residue is centrosome associated from S-phase until mitosis.[236] A population of Chk1 is localized to the centrosome during G2 and can prevent promiscuous Cdk1-cyclin B activation by Cdc25B.[237] S323 was previously identified as the major 14-3-3 binding site.[238] S151 and S230 account for the remainder of the interaction, but both need to be dephosphorylated before interaction with 14-3-3 is lost.[239] Human Cdc25B S563 resides in the extreme C-terminus of Cdc25B and is analogous to Cdc25A S504 and *S. pombe* Cdc25 T569. Cdc25B lacking the S323 phosphorylation site is almost exclusively nuclear. It is interesting that this residue is targeted by Chk1, but does not appear to bind 14-3-3 when phosphorylated. If the function of this phosphorylation is conserved between Cdc25A S504 and Cdc25B S563, phosphorylation may affect interaction with Cdk1-cyclin B.[240]

Chk1 phosphorylation of human Cdc25C and nuclear export by 14-3-3 binding keeps the phosphatase cytoplasmic during unperturbed cell cycles.[217] Nuclear localization of Cdc25C(S216A) is enhanced, suggesting that part of the function of 14-3-3 binding is to obscure the NLS located adjacent to this residue.[224] Overexpression of Cdc25C(S216A) induces a higher degree of premature mitotic entry.[217] *Xenopus* Cdc25C is likewise phosphorylated on S287 by Chk1 during interphase.[228,241] Phospho-S287 is bound by 14-3-3ε and 14-3-3ζ obscuring the NLS and preventing nuclear import.[228] *Xenopus* Cdc25C is phosphorylated on T533 by Chk1, but not Chk2.[207] Injecting Cdc25C T533A mRNA into *Xenopus* oocytes results in more rapid dephosphorylation of Cdk1 Y15.[207] Again, this suggests that regulation of CDK-cyclin interaction with Cdc25 orthologues by C-terminal phosphorylation is a common mechanism for inhibiting cell cycle progression.

Although Cdc25A and Cdc25B are dispensable for embryonic development, Chk1 and ATR kinases are essential.[242,243] The Cdc25B/14-3-3 interaction is important for maintaining G2 arrest, and inhibiting germinal vesicle breakdown in *Xenopus* oocytes prior to progesterone exposure.[244]

In *S. pombe*, Chk1 does not appear to negatively regulate Cdc25 in the absence of DNA damage. Loss of a negative regulator of Cdc25 is expected to cause the cell to divide at a reduced length. However, deletion of Chk1 does not cause a cell cycle phenotype.[245] In addition, expressing Cdc25 where all twelve putative Cds1/Chk1 phosphorylation sites are mutated to alanine does not cause acceleration of the cell cycle.[60]

5.4. Cdk1 phosphorylation of Cdc25 precludes checkpoint mediated inhibition during mitosis

If Cdc25C is phosphorylated and inactivated during interphase via 14-3-3 binding, how is it then activated at mitotic entry? Cdk1-cyclin B phosphorylation of Cdc25C causes 14-3-3 dissociation and allows removal of interphase phosphorylations. Re-phosphorylation of these residues is simultaneously blocked. Cdk1-cyclin B thus potentiates Cdc25C for its pro-mitotic function and ensures that it remains active. The region surrounding S216 in human Cdc25C and S287 in *Xenopus* Cdc25C is a well conserved stretch in the N-terminal region of the two proteins; LYRSPS$_{216}$MPE is identical between Human and *Xenopus* and contains S216 and S287, respectively.(Figure 4) In both organisms, the two serine residues upstream of the major phosphorylated 14-3-3 binding residue, S214 in human and S285 in *Xenopus*, is targeted by Cdk1-cyclin B.[42,246-248] In human cells phosphorylation of S214 precludes phosphorylation of S216 by Chk1 and 14-3-3 binding.[42,246] Substituting S214D prevents phosphorylation of S216.[246] S216 is not phosphorylated during M-phase *in vivo*, and ionizing radiation in M-phase cells cannot induce its phosphorylation.[246] 14-3-3 is unable to bind Cdc25C immunoprecipitated from cells arrested in mitosis with nocodazole.[219] In *Xenopus*, Cdc25C S285 phosphorylation prevents the phosphorylation of S287.[247,249] S285 can be phosphorylated by both Cdk1-cyclin B and Cdk1-cyclin A *in vitro*.[146] Until the mid-blastula transition, *Xenopus* Cdc25C is phosphorylated on S285 which precludes Chk1 mediated phosphorylation of S287 and subsequent 14-3-3 binding.[247] Human Cdc25C S214 is also phosphorylated in maturing human oocytes.[250] Removal of phospho-S287 bound 14-3-3 and phosphorylation of *Xenopus* Cdc25C S285 requires prior phosphorylation of Cdc25C T138.[249] T138 is a substrate of Cdk1-cyclin B.[146] However, selective depletion of Cdk2 from *Xenopus* egg extracts using the N-terminus of the Cdk2 inhibitor p21, completely prevents removal of 14-3-3 from Cdc25C.[251] In *Xenopus* egg extracts Cdk2 is required for mitotic entry.[81] Other CDK phosphorylation sites on *Xenopus* Cdc25C such as T48 and T67 negatively regulate its activity in an S287 independent manner.[249] Phosphorylation of T138 is not sufficient to cause 14-3-3 dissociation.[248] How is 14-3-3 physically removed from phospho-S287? The pelleted fraction from ultracentrifuged interphase egg extracts contains a 14-3-3 dissociating activity, which was determined to be the intermediate filament component Keratin 8/18[248]. Keratin is phosphorylated during mitosis, binds 14-3-3, and has a role in mitotic progression in hepatocytes.[252] Keratin may act as a "14-3-3 sink" during mitosis, stripping 14-3-3 from S287.[248] *Xenopus* Cdc25C T138 corresponds with T130 in human Cdc25C. A phospho-T130 specific antibody shows that Cdc25C phosphorylated on this site localizes to the centrosome.[145] A localization for the de-inhibition of Cdc25C fits well with the putative centrosomal localization of Cdc25C activation.

PP1 phosphatase removes S287 phosphorylation once 14-3-3 has dissociated.[251] Binding of PP1 to *Xenopus* Cdc25C requires a docking motif "VXF", amino acids 105-107, the loss of which prevents S287 dephosphorylation.[251] Phosphorylation of *Xenopus* Cdc25C S285 by Cdk1-cyclin B enhances recruitment of phosphatase PP1 to Cdc25C, inducing the dephosphorylation of S287.[249] PP2A/B56δ dephosphorylates *Xenopus* Cdc25C T138 during interphase, mitotic exit and following replication arrest.[248] This maintains the phosphatase in a state where it can be inhibited by S287 phosphorylation. Inhibition of PP2A by okadaic acid prematurely induces mitotic entry in *Xenopus* egg extracts.[253] T138 is also dephosphorylated during replication arrest where B56δ is itself phosphorylated by Chk1, enhancing complex formation with PP2A.[248] PP2A mediated dephosphorylation of Cdc25 is assisted by the action of the Pin1 prolyl isomerase. Pin1 isomerizes the peptide bond between phospho-serine/threonine and proline placing their R-groups in a *trans* orientation.[254] This isomerization makes the phosphorylated residue a better substrate for the PP2A phosphatase.[255] *In vitro*, Pin1 decreases the catalytic activity of Cdc25C that has previously been phosphorylated by Cdk1.[256] Pin1 is also involved in maintenance of replication checkpoint arrest in *Xenopus* encouraging the reversal of Cdk1 mediated Cdc25C phosphorylation.[257] In Humans, Cdc25C is deactivated in a similar manner. T130 on Cdc25C is dephosphorylated by PP2A.[258] Mitotic exit is delayed when PP2A is knocked down, suggesting that dephosphorylation of Cdc25C T130 in human cells is also important for the transition from M to G1 of the next cycle. A similar situation may exist where human Cdc25B1

S321 phosphorylation blocks phosphorylation of the major 14-3-3 binding residue S323 by p38.[246] Expression of the phosphorylation-mimicking Cdc25B1 S321D prevents p38 mediated phosphorylation of S323 and abolishes binding by 14-3-3β and 14-3-3ε.[246,259] 14-3-3σ binding is unaffected by S321 phosphorylation.[259] 14-3-3σ preferentially interacts with Cdc25B3 S230 [216] and is induced by p53 following activation by ATM/Chk2.[260]

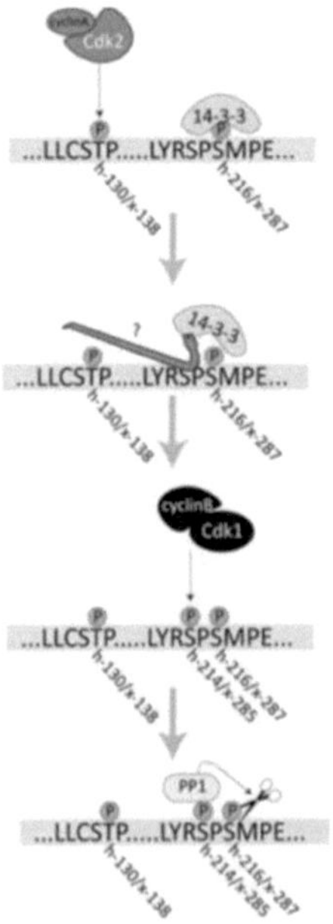

Figure 4. Cdk-cyclin mediated removal of inhibitory S216/S287 phosphorylation and 14-3-3 binding in human and *Xenopus* Cdc25C, respectively.

There are no Cdc2 phosphorylation motifs (S/TP) directly upstream of any of the twelve Cds1 *in vitro* phosphorylation sites in *S. pombe*. Large scale phosphoproteome analysis has detected S99, S178 and S359 phosphorylation of fission yeast Cdc25 in M-phase arrested cells.[261] Thus it appears that the vertebrate mechanism for reversing and preventing Chk1 phosphorylation of Cdc25C evolved relatively recently. However, parallels exist between some aspects of Cdc25 dephosphorylation between fission yeast and vertebrates. Treatment with okadaic acid or deletion of PP2A homologue Ppa2 causes premature mitotic entry in fission yeast.[262,263] Loss of *ppa2* suppresses the *cdc25-22*^{ts} mutation, a genetic interaction indicative of a negative regulator.[263] Loss of PP1 homologue Dis2 results in cell elongation, suggesting its role as a positive regulator of Cdc25 is conserved in *S. pombe*.[264] Temperature sensitive *dis2* mutants have a defect in exit from mitosis, similar to the effect of siRNA inhibition of human PP2A.[258,264]

6. Cdc25 phosphorylation by MAP kinase cascades

In addition to regulation by DNA damage and DNA replication checkpoints, Cdc25 is the target of several MAPK cascades responding to stress and mitogenic signals. A detailed description of the variety of MAPK pathways is outside of the scope of this manuscript, but excellent reviews are available.[265]. In general, MAP kinase cascades involve the sequential activation of three kinases; a MAP kinase kinase kinase (MAPKKK) phosphorylates a MAP kinase kinase (MAPKK), which phosphorylates a MAP kinase (MAPK). There are three such cascades which are salient to our discussion of Cdc25 regulation.

6.1. Raf/MEK/ERK

The ERK1/ERK2 MAPKs are activated by Raf MAPKKKs working on MEK1/MEK2 MAPKKs. This cascade is primarily activated by extracellular signaling through receptor tyrosine kinases in response to mitogenic signals.[266] During Cyto-Static Factor arrest in mature *Xenopus* oocytes metaphase II arrest is enforced by the combined activity of the MEK/ERK pathway upregulating ribosomal subunit S6 kinase/CamKII homologue $p90^{rsk}$, and APC inhibition by the Emi2 kinase.[267] Calcium influx as a result of fertilization activates $p90^{rsk}$ (a Ca^{2+}/calmodulin dependent kinase II homologue) which phosphorylates Emi2.[268] This allows APC activation, cyclin B degradation, and progression through meiosis II. Cdc25C is phosphorylated on S287 by $p90^{Rsk}$ *in vitro* resulting in its inhibition via 14-3-3 binding.[269,270] Conversely, *Xenopus* Cdc25C S317, T318 and S319 are phosphorylated by $p90^{rsk}$ orthologue Rsk2 which serves to activate the phosphatase in mature oocyte extracts.[271] The *Xenopus* ERK homologue, p42, phosphorylates Cdc25C T48, T138 and S205 *in vitro.*[272] T138 and S205 are also Cdk1-cyclinB targets [146], but T48 is uniquely phosphorylated by p42. In HeLa cells after activation of MEK/ERK signaling by addition of 12-O-tetradecanoylphorbol-13- acetate (TPA), G2/M transition is inhibited by degradation of Cdc25B.[273] This is mediated through MEK dependent phosphorylation of Cdc25B S249 by CamKII, an activator of human Cdc25C.[274] Inhibition of CamKII results in a G2 arrest. Overexpression of CamKII can also arrest cells in G2, but with a high level of Cdk1/Cyclin B activity.[275] Another member of the CamKII family, C-TAK1, phosphorylates human Cdc25C on S216 resulting in inhibition via 14-3-3 binding and nuclear export.[276] *Xenopus* Cdc25C can be phosphorylated by CamKII *in vitro.*[277] Lastly, $p14^{arf}$ upregulation in response to anti-proliferative signals results in human Cdc25C downregulation through MEK/ERK MAPK signaling.[278] Human Cdc25C becomes phosphorylated on S216 and is subsequently ubiquitinated and degraded.[278]

6.2. p38 and JNK MAPKs

The p38 and JNK kinases activate in response to extracellular stimuli such as heatshock, oxidative stress, ionizing radiation, UV and growth factor deprivation. Both are activated by MAPKKs of the MKK family which are themselves activated by a large variety of MAPKKKs. We have already discussed the function of p38 in response to UV irradiation. p38 also phosphorylates human Cdc25A on S124 and S76 in response to osmotic stress, destabilizing the protein [168] and a 42 C heatshock causes p38 and Chk2 to phosphorylate S76 and S178 of human Cdc25A, respectively.[175] MAPKAP kinase 2 (MK2) functions downstream of p38 and regulates G1 and S-phase cell cycle progression in response to UV.[210] Downstream of p38, it phosphorylates RxxS/T motifs and activation of MK2 correlates with increased binding of 14-3-3 to Cdc25B. p38 and MK2 kinase form a tight complex and are imported into the nucleus together, so previous work showing that p38 directly phosphorylates S216 on Cdc25C and S323 on Cdc25B may in fact have been inadvertently monitoring MK2 activity.[279] Cdc25A may also be an MK2 substrate as MK2 knockdowns ablate the G1 and S-phase checkpoints. JNK activity targets two serines within the region DAGLCMDS_{101}PS_{103}P of the DSG degron on human Cdc25B.[280] Simultaneous S101A and S103A substitution prevents β-TrCP binding and Cdc25B ubiquitination. JNK also phosphorylates Cdc25C on S168 inhibiting its phosphatase activity.[281,282] This residue is transiently phosphorylated *in vivo* on nuclear Cdc25C prior to and after mitotic entry.[281] S168 is phosphorylated following UV irradiation and osmotic shock.[281,282]

6.3. The *S. pombe* stress activated MAP kinase pathway

In fission yeast, Cdc25 is phosphorylated by the CamKII homologue Srk1 in response to extracellular stress.[283] Srk1 is activated downstream of the Spc1 MAPK, Wis1 MAPKK, and Win1 or Wak1MAPKKKs.[284] This phosphorylation occurs on residues also targeted by Cds1 as Cdc25(9A) is not sensitive to Srk1 mediated inhibition.[283] Srk1 phosphorylation of Cdc25 results in its nuclear export, similar to the response to DNA damage and replication arrest.

7. Other kinases which phosphorylate Cdc25s

PKA prevents oocyte maturation by inhibition of Polo kinase mediated Cdc25 activation, and deactivating the Mos/MEK/ERK MAP kinase cascade which inhibits Myt1.[285] Progesterone exposure in *Xenopus* oocytes down regulates adenylate cyclase, lowering cyclicAMP levels and consequently deactivating PKA. Prior to maturation, *Xenopus* Cdc25C is also inhibited by PKA phosphorylation of S287 and T318 *in vitro*.[286] Murine PKA phosphorylates Cdc25B S321, negatively regulating the phosphatase; S321A mutants cause enhanced germinal vesicle breakdown when injected into mouse oocytes.[287]

Pim1 is a serine/threonine kinase induced by the SAT3 and SAT5 transcription factors following cytokine exposure thus linking pro-proliferative signals to the cell cycle control machinery.[288] Pim1 phosphorylates and activates Cdc25A and represses the Cdk4/6 inhibitor $p21^{CIP}$ to encourage the G1/S transition.[289,290] Pim1 is also able to phosphorylate and inhibit the CamKII homologue c-TAK and accelerate Cdc25C mediated mitotic entry.[291]PAR-1/MARK (partitioning-defective 1/Microtubule affinity-Regulating Kinase) protein homologue pEG3 phosphorylates human Cdc25A S263, Cdc25B S169 and Cdc25C S216.[292,293] Overexpressing pEg3 results in G2 arrest which can be reversed by co-expressing Cdc25B.[292] Anti-phospho PAR1 S169 antibodies stain spindle pole and centrosome in immunofluorescence experiments.[293] In *C. elegans* the first cell division is unequal which produces a larger anterior cell and a smaller posterior one. The next cell division is asynchronous with the anterior cell dividing prior to the posterior one.[294] Rapid anterior cell cycle timing is due to enrichment of Polo kinase and Cdc25.1 in the anterior cell. This is dependent on a network of polarity proteins, including Par1.[295]

8. Cdc25 and disease

Cdc25 orthologues are the subject of much attention as they are commonly upregulated in human tumors.[296] This is perhaps not surprising considering the role of Cdc25 inhibition in maintaining genomic stability and the regulation of these phosphatases by Rb, p53 and a number of other oncogenes. Cdc25A and Cdc25B themselves are oncogenes in humans.[212] Cdc25B is overexpressed in 32% of breast cancer tissue samples, and high Cdc25B levels correlate with high incidences of recurrence and decreased 10 year survival.[212] Overexpression of Cdc25A is similarly linked to poor clinical outcome.[296,297] Cells bearing oncogenic mutations of myc have elevated Cdc25A and Cdc25B levels.[298] Anti-Cdc25B autoantibody has been shown to be a predictor of poor prognosis in esophageal cancer patients.[299] Overexpression of Cdc25B has recently been shown to cause a variety of S-phase effects including increased Cdc45 recruitment to chromatin, impairment of replication fork progression DNA damage and chromosome instability.[300]

An interesting link between Cdc25 and disease comes from the finding that the HIV-1 protein vpr causes G2/M arrest.[301] When expressed in *S. pombe*, vpr activates Srk1 kinase, resulting in Cdc25 phosphorylation and 14-3-3 mediated nuclear export.[302,303] The vpr protein also acts through upregulation of PP2A phosphatase acting on both Wee1 kinase and Cdc25, reversing activating Cdc2 phosphorylation.[304]

9. Conclusion

It has been more than thirty five years since Cdc25 was first isolated as an elongated temperature-sensitive fission yeast mutant and twenty one years since its biochemical function was determined. The field of cell cycle research and the study of Cdc25 in particular are extremely active with numerous new manuscripts appearing each year. This research has revealed that Cdc25 is one of the most intricately regulated proteins in the cell. Cdc25 accepts input from numerous pathways and checkpoints monitoring whether conditions inside and outside the cell are permissive for cell cycle progression. When conditions warrant caution, Cdc25 is inhibited by phosphorylation leading to alterations in its catalytic activity, cellular localization, substrate recognition and stability. When the green light is given Cdc25 participates in an intricate series of interconnected positive feedback loops with the beating heart of cell cycle regulation, the Cyclin-CDK complex. When the cell loses control of Cdc25 regulation, the results are deadly.

Author details

C. Frazer
Department of Biomedical and Molecular Science, Queen's University, Kingston, Ontario, K7L 3N6, Canada

P.G. Young*
Department of Biology, Queen's University, Kingston, Ontario, Canada

* Corresponding Author

Acknowledgement

Thank you to Silja Freitag for her critical reading of this manuscript. This work was supported by a grant from the Natural Sciences and Engineering Research Council of Canada to PGY.

10. References

[1] Hartwell LH, Culotti J, Reid B. (1970) Genetic control of the cell-division cycle in yeast. I. Detection of mutants. Proc Natl Acad Sci U S A 66(2):352-359.

[2] Hartwell LH, Mortimer RK, Culotti J, Culotti M. (1973) Genetic control of the cell division cycle in yeast: V. Genetic analysis of *cdc* mutants. Genetics 74(2):267-286.

[3] Nurse P, Thuriaux P, Nasmyth K. (1976) Genetic control of the cell division cycle in the fission yeast *Schizosaccharomyces pombe* . Mol Gen Genet 146(2):167-178.

[4] Nurse P. (1975) Genetic control of cell size at cell division in yeast. Nature 256(5518):547-551.

[5] Fantes P. (1979) Epistatic gene interactions in the control of division in fission yeast. Nature 279(5712):428-430.

[6] Fantes PA. (1981) Isolation of cell size mutants of a fission yeast by a new selective method: characterization of mutants and implications for division control mechanisms. J Bacteriol 146(2):746-754.

[7] Thuriaux P, Nurse P, Carter B. (1978) Mutants altered in the control co-ordinating cell division with cell growth in the fission yeast *Schizosaccharomyces pombe*. Mol Gen Genet 161(2):215-220.

[8] Kishimoto T, Kanatani H. (1976) Cytoplasmic factor responsible for germinal vesicle breakdown and meiotic maturation in starfish oocyte. Nature 260(5549):321-322.

[9] Masui Y, Markert CL. (1971) Cytoplasmic control of nuclear behavior during meiotic maturation of frog oocytes. J Exp Zool 177(2):129-145.

[10] Maller JL. (1990) Xenopus oocytes and the biochemistry of cell division. Biochemistry 29(13):3157-3166.

[11] Smith LD, Ecker RE. (1971) The interaction of steroids with Rana pipiens Oocytes in the induction of maturation. Dev Biol 25(2):232-247.

[12] Murray AW, Solomon MJ, Kirschner MW. (1989) The role of cyclin synthesis and degradation in the control of maturation promoting factor activity. Nature 339(6222):280-286.

[13] Newport J, Kirschner M. (1982) A major developmental transition in early Xenopus embryos: II. Control of the onset of transcription. Cell 30(3):687-696.

[14] Newport J, Kirschner M. (1982) A major developmental transition in early Xenopus embryos: I. characterization and timing of cellular changes at the midblastula stage. Cell 30(3):675-686.

[15] Dunphy WG, Brizuela L, Beach D, Newport J. (1988) The *Xenopus* cdc2 protein is a component of MPF, a cytoplasmic regulator of mitosis. Cell 54(3):423-431.

[16] Evans T, Rosenthal ET, Youngblom J, Distel D, Hunt T. (1983) Cyclin: a protein specified by maternal mRNA in sea urchin eggs that is destroyed at each cleavage division. Cell 33(2):389-396.

[17] Gautier J, Minshull J, Lohka M, Glotzer M, Hunt T, Maller JL. (1990) Cyclin is a component of maturation-promoting factor from Xenopus. Cell 60(3):487-494.

[18] Patra D, Dunphy WG. (1996) Xe-p9, a Xenopus Suc1/Cks homolog, has multiple essential roles in cell cycle control. Genes Dev 10(12):1503-1515.

[19] Gautier J, Norbury C, Lohka M, Nurse P, Maller J. (1988) Purified maturation-promoting factor contains the product of a Xenopus homolog of the fission yeast cell cycle control gene cdc2+. Cell 54(3):433-439.

[20] Nurse P, Bissett Y. (1981) Gene required in G1 for commitment to cell cycle and in G2 for control of mitosis in fission yeast. Nature 292(5823):558-560.

[21] Beach D, Durkacz B, Nurse P. (1982) Functionally homologous cell cycle control genes in budding and fission yeast. Nature 300(5894):706-709.

[22] Hagan I, Hayles J, Nurse P. (1988) Cloning and sequencing of the cyclin-related cdc13+ gene and a cytological study of its role in fission yeast mitosis. J Cell Sci 91 (Pt 4)(Pt 4):587-595.

[23] Booher R, Beach D. (1988) Involvement of cdc13+ in mitotic control in *Schizosaccharomyces pombe*: possible interaction of the gene product with microtubules. EMBO J 7(8):2321-2327.

[24] Gautier J, Solomon MJ, Booher RN, Bazan JF, Kirschner MW. (1991) Cdc25 is a Specific Tyrosine Phosphatase that Directly Activates P34cdc2. Cell 67(1):197-211.

[25] Millar JB, McGowan CH, Lenaers G, Jones R, Russell P. (1991) $p80^{cdc25}$ mitotic inducer is the tyrosine phosphatase that activates $p34^{cdc2}$ kinase in fission yeast. EMBO J 10(13):4301-4309.

[26] Doree M, Peaucellier G, Picard A. (1983) Activity of the maturation-promoting factor and the extent of protein phosphorylation oscillate simultaneously during meiotic maturation of starfish oocytes. Dev Biol 99(2):489-501.

[27] Maller J, Wu M, Gerhart JC. (1977) Changes in protein phosphorylation accompanying maturation of Xenopus laevis oocytes. Dev Biol 58(2):295-312.

[28] Mazzei G, Guerrier P. (1982) Changes in the pattern of protein phosphorylation during meiosis reinitiation in starfish oocytes. Dev Biol 91(2):246-256.

[29] Wiblet M. (1974) Protein kinase activities during maturation in Xenopus laevis oocytes. Biochem Biophys Res Commun 60(3):991-998.

[30] Margalit A, Vlcek S, Gruenbaum Y, Foisner R. (2005) Breaking and making of the nuclear envelope. J Cell Biochem 95(3):454-465.

[31] Abe S, Nagasaka K, Hirayama Y, Kozuka-Hata H, Oyama M, Aoyagi Y, et al. (2011) The initial phase of chromosome condensation requires Cdk1-mediated phosphorylation of the CAP-D3 subunit of condensin II. Genes Dev 25(8):863-874.

[32] Glotzer M. (2009) The 3Ms of central spindle assembly: microtubules, motors and MAPs. Nat Rev Mol Cell Biol 10(1):9-20.

[33] Holt LJ, Tuch BB, Villen J, Johnson AD, Gygi SP, Morgan DO. (2009) Global analysis of Cdk1 substrate phosphorylation sites provides insights into evolution. Science 325(5948):1682-1686.

[34] Enserink JM, Kolodner RD. (2010) An overview of Cdk1-controlled targets and processes. Cell Div 5:11.
[35] Russell P, Moreno S, Reed SI. (1989) Conservation of mitotic controls in fission and budding yeasts. Cell 57(2):295-303.
[36] Nagata A, Igarashi M, Jinno S, Suto K, Okayama H. (1991) An additional homolog of the fission yeast cdc25+ gene occurs in humans and is highly expressed in some cancer cells. New Biol 3(10):959-968.
[37] Galaktionov K, Beach D. (1991) Specific activation of cdc25 tyrosine phosphatases by B-type cyclins: evidence for multiple roles of mitotic cyclins. Cell 67(6):1181-1194.
[38] Sadhu K, Reed SI, Richardson H, Russell P. (1990) Human homolog of fission yeast cdc25 mitotic inducer is predominantly expressed in G2. Proc Natl Acad Sci U S A 87(13):5139-5143.
[39] Wickramasinghe D, Becker S, Ernst MK, Resnick JL, Centanni JM, Tessarollo L, et al. (1995) Two CDC25 homologues are differentially expressed during mouse development. Development 121(7):2047-2056.
[40] Okazaki K, Hayashida K, Iwashita J, Harano M, Furuno N, Sagata N. (1996) Isolation of a cDNA encoding the X enopus homologue of mammalian Cdc25A that can induce meiotic maturation of oocytes. Gene 178(1-2):111-114.
[41] Forrest AR, McCormack AK, DeSouza CP, Sinnamon JM, Tonks ID, Hayward NK, et al. (1999) Multiple splicing variants of cdc25B regulate G2/M progression. Biochem Biophys Res Commun 260(2):510-515.
[42] Bonnet J, Mayonove P, Morris MC. (2008) Differential phosphorylation of Cdc25C phosphatase in mitosis. Biochem Biophys Res Commun 370(3):483-488.
[43] Wegener S, Hampe W, Herrmann D, Schaller HC. (2000) Alternative splicing in the regulatory region of the human phosphatases CDC25A and CDC25C. Eur J Cell Biol 79(11):810-815.
[44] Jullien D, Bugler B, Dozier C, Cazales M, Ducommun B. (2011) Identification of N-terminally truncated stable nuclear isoforms of CDC25B that are specifically involved in G2/M checkpoint recovery. Cancer Res 71(5):1968-1977.
[45] Kumagai A, Dunphy WG. (1992) Regulation of the cdc25 protein during the cell cycle in Xenopus extracts. Cell 70:139-151.
[46] Rime H, Huchon D, De Smedt V, Thibier C, Galaktionov K, Jessus C, et al. (1994) Microinjection of Cdc25 protein phosphatase into Xenopus prophase oocyte activates MPF and arrests meiosis at metaphase I. Biol Cell 82(1):11-22.
[47] Ashcroft NR, Kosinski ME, Wickramasinghe D, Donovan PJ, Golden A. (1998) The four cdc25 genes from the nematode *Caenorhabditis elegans*. Gene 214(1-2):59-66.
[48] Alphey L, Jimenez J, White-Cooper H, Dawson I, Nurse P, Glover DM. (1992) twine, a cdc25 homolog that functions in the male and female germline of Drosophila. Cell 69(6):977-988.
[49] Edgar BA, O'Farrell PH. (1989) Genetic control of cell division patterns in the Drosophila embryo. Cell 57(1):177-187.
[50] Kumagai A, Dunphy WG. (1991) The cdc25 protein controls tyrosine dephosphorylation of the cdc2 protein in a cell-free system. Cell 64(5):903-914.

[51] Khadaroo B, Robbens S, Ferraz C, Derelle E, Eychenie S, Cooke R, et al. (2004) The first green lineage cdc25 dual-specificity phosphatase. Cell Cycle 3(4):513-518.

[52] Landrieu I, da Costa M, De Veylder L, Dewitte F, Vandepoele K, Hassan S, et al. (2004) A small CDC25 dual-specificity tyrosine-phosphatase isoform in *Arabidopsis thaliana*. Proc Natl Acad Sci U S A 101(36):13380-13385.

[53] Sorrell DA, Chrimes D, Dickinson JR, Rogers HJ, Francis D. (2005) The Arabidopsis CDC25 induces a short cell length when overexpressed in fission yeast: evidence for cell cycle function. New Phytol 165(2):425-428.

[54] Booher RN, Alfa CE, Hyams JS, Beach DH. (1989) The fission yeast cdc2/cdc13/suc1 protein kinase: regulation of catalytic activity and nuclear localization. Cell 58(3):485-497.

[55] Booher R, Beach D. (1987) Interaction between cdc13+ and cdc2+ in the control of mitosis in fission yeast; dissociation of the G1 and G2 roles of the cdc2+ protein kinase. EMBO J 6(11):3441-3447.

[56] Martin-Castellanos C, Blanco MA, de Prada JM, Moreno S. (2000) The puc1 cyclin regulates the G1 phase of the fission yeast cell cycle in response to cell size. Mol Biol Cell 11(2):543-554.

[57] Durkacz B, Carr A, Nurse P. (1986) Transcription of the cdc2 cell cycle control gene of the fission yeast *Schizosaccharomyces pombe*. EMBO J 5(2):369-373.

[58] Creanor J, Mitchison JM. (1996) The kinetics of the B cyclin p56cdc13 and the phosphatase p80cdc25 during the cell cycle of the fission yeast *Schizosaccharomyces pombe* . J Cell Sci 109 (Pt 6)(Pt 6):1647-1653.

[59] Ducommun B, Draetta G, Young P, Beach D. (1990) Fission yeast cdc25 is a cell-cycle regulated protein. Biochem Biophys Res Commun 167(1):301-309.

[60] Frazer C, Young PG. (2011) Redundant mechanisms prevent mitotic entry following replication arrest in the absence of Cdc25 hyper-phosphorylation in fission yeast. PLoS One 6(6):e21348.

[61] Den Haese GJ, Walworth N, Carr AM, Gould KL. (1995) The Wee1 protein kinase regulates T14 phosphorylation of fission yeast Cdc2. Mol Biol Cell 6(4):371-385.

[62] Gould KL, Nurse P. (1989) Tyrosine phosphorylation of the fission yeast cdc2+ protein kinase regulates entry into mitosis. Nature 342(6245):39-45.

[63] Lundgren K, Walworth N, Booher R, Dembski M, Kirschner M, Beach D. (1991) Mik1 and Wee1 Cooperate in the Inhibitory Tyrosine Phosphorylation of Cdc2. Cell 64(6):1111-1122.

[64] Lee MS, Enoch T, Piwnica-Worms H. (1994) Mik1+ Encodes a Tyrosine Kinase that Phosphorylates P34cdc2 on Tyrosine 15. J Biol Chem 269(48):30530-30537.

[65] Russell P, Nurse P. (1987) Negative regulation of mitosis by wee1+, a gene encoding a protein kinase homolog. Cell 49(4):559-567.

[66] Parker LL, Atherton-Fessler S, Piwnica-Worms H. (1992) P107wee1 is a Dual-Specificity Kinase that Phosphorylates P34cdc2 on Tyrosine 15. Proc Natl Acad Sci U S A 89(7):2917-2921.

[67] Featherstone C, Russell P. (1991) Fission yeast p107wee1 mitotic inhibitor is a tyrosine/serine kinase. Nature 349:808-811.

[68] Chua G, Lingner C, Frazer C, Young PG. (2002) The sal3(+) gene encodes an importin-beta implicated in the nuclear import of Cdc25 in *Schizosaccharomyces pombe*. Genetics 162(2):689-703.

[69] Rupes I, Webb BA, Mak A, Young PG. (2001) G2/M arrest caused by actin disruption is a manifestation of the cell size checkpoint in fission yeast. Mol Biol Cell 12(12):3892-3903.

[70] Kovelman R, Russell P. (1996) Stockpiling of Cdc25 during a DNA replication checkpoint arrest in *Schizosaccharomyces pombe*. Mol Cell Biol 16(1):86-93.

[71] Moreno S, Nurse P. (1990) Substrates for p34cdc2: in vivo veritas? Cell 61(4):549-551.

[72] Shenoy S, Choi JK, Bagrodia S, Copeland TD, Maller JL, Shalloway D. (1989) Purified maturation promoting factor phosphorylates pp60c-src at the sites phosphorylated during fibroblast mitosis. Cell 57(5):763-774.

[73] Wolfe BA, Gould KL. (2004) Fission yeast Clp1p phosphatase affects G2/M transition and mitotic exit through Cdc25p inactivation. EMBO J 23(4):919-929.

[74] Mulvihill DP, Petersen J, Ohkura H, Glover DM, Hagan IM. (1999) Plo1 kinase recruitment to the spindle pole body and its role in cell division in *Schizosaccharomyces pombe*. Mol Biol Cell 10(8):2771-2785.

[75] Charles JF, Jaspersen SL, Tinker-Kulberg RL, Hwang L, Szidon A, Morgan DO. (1998) The Polo-related kinase Cdc5 activates and is destroyed by the mitotic cyclin destruction machinery in S. cerevisiae. Curr Biol 8(9):497-507.

[76] Katsuno Y, Suzuki A, Sugimura K, Okumura K, Zineldeen DH, Shimada M, et al. (2009) Cyclin A-Cdk1 regulates the origin firing program in mammalian cells. Proc Natl Acad Sci U S A 106(9):3184-3189.

[77] Elledge SJ, Spottswood MR. (1991) A new human p34 protein kinase, CDK2, identified by complementation of a cdc28 mutation in *Saccharomyces cerevisiae*, is a homolog of Xenopus Eg1. EMBO J 10(9):2653-2659.

[78] Gu Y, Rosenblatt J, Morgan DO. (1992) Cell cycle regulation of CDK2 activity by phosphorylation of Thr160 and Tyr15. EMBO J 11(11):3995-4005.

[79] Elledge SJ, Richman R, Hall FL, Williams RT, Lodgson N, Harper JW. (1992) CDK2 encodes a 33-kDa cyclin A-associated protein kinase and is expressed before CDC2 in the cell cycle. Proc Natl Acad Sci U S A 89(7):2907-2911.

[80] Rosenblatt J, Gu Y, Morgan DO. (1992) Human cyclin-dependent kinase 2 is activated during the S and G2 phases of the cell cycle and associates with cyclin A. Proc Natl Acad Sci U S A 89(7):2824-2828.

[81] Guadagno TM, Newport JW. (1996) Cdk2 kinase is required for entry into mitosis as a positive regulator of Cdc2-cyclin B kinase activity. Cell 84(1):73-82.

[82] Bates S, Bonetta L, MacAllan D, Parry D, Holder A, Dickson C, et al. (1994) CDK6 (PLSTIRE) and CDK4 (PSK-J3) are a distinct subset of the cyclin-dependent kinases that associate with cyclin D1. Oncogene 9(1):71-79.

[83] Fisher RP, Morgan DO. (1994) A novel cyclin associates with MO15/CDK7 to form the CDK-activating kinase. Cell 78(4):713-724.

[84] Weinberg RA. (1995) The retinoblastoma protein and cell cycle control. Cell 81(3):323-330.

[85] Dyson N. (1998) The regulation of E2F by pRB-family proteins. Genes Dev 12(15):2245-2262.

[86] Vidal A, Koff A. (2000) Cell-cycle inhibitors: three families united by a common cause. Gene 247(1-2):1-15.

[87] Chen X, Prywes R. (1999) Serum-induced expression of the cdc25A gene by relief of E2F-mediated repression. Mol Cell Biol 19(7):4695-4702.

[88] Malumbres M, Pellicer A. (1998) RAS pathways to cell cycle control and cell transformation. Front Biosci 3:d887-912.

[89] Sherr CJ, Roberts JM. (1999) CDK inhibitors: positive and negative regulators of G1-phase progression. Genes Dev 13(12):1501-1512.

[90] Lundberg AS, Weinberg RA. (1998) Functional inactivation of the retinoblastoma protein requires sequential modification by at least two distinct cyclin-cdk complexes. Mol Cell Biol 18(2):753-761.

[91] Blomberg I, Hoffmann I. (1999) Ectopic expression of Cdc25A accelerates the G(1)/S transition and leads to premature activation of cyclin E- and cyclin A-dependent kinases. Mol Cell Biol 19(9):6183-6194.

[92] Sherr CJ, Roberts JM. (2004) Living with or without cyclins and cyclin-dependent kinases. Genes Dev 18(22):2699-2711.

[93] Booher RN, Holman PS, Fattaey A. (1997) Human Myt1 is a cell cycle-regulated kinase that inhibits Cdc2 but not Cdk2 activity. J Biol Chem 272(35):22300-22306.

[94] Sebastian B, Kakizuka A, Hunter T. (1993) Cdc25M2 activation of cyclin-dependent kinases by dephosphorylation of threonine-14 and tyrosine-15. Proc Natl Acad Sci U S A 90(8):3521-3524.

[95] Hoffmann I, Draetta G, Karsenti E. (1994) Activation of the phosphatase activity of human cdc25A by a cdk2-cyclin E dependent phosphorylation at the G1/S transition. EMBO J 13(18):4302-4310.

[96] Gabrielli BG, Clark JM, McCormack AK, Ellem KA. (1997) Hyperphosphorylation of the N-terminal domain of Cdc25 regulates activity toward cyclin B1/Cdc2 but not cyclin A/Cdk2. J Biol Chem 272(45):28607-28614.

[97] Lammer C, Wagerer S, Saffrich R, Mertens D, Ansorge W, Hoffmann I. (1998) The cdc25B phosphatase is essential for the G2/M phase transition in human cells. J Cell Sci 111 (Pt 16)(Pt 16):2445-2453.

[98] Sexl V, Diehl JA, Sherr CJ, Ashmun R, Beach D, Roussel MF. (1999) A rate limiting function of cdc25A for S phase entry inversely correlates with tyrosine dephosphorylation of Cdk2. Oncogene 18(3):573-582.

[99] Ducruet AP, Lazo JS. (2003) Regulation of Cdc25A half-life in interphase by cyclin-dependent kinase 2 activity. J Biol Chem 278(34):31838-31842.

[100] Pagano M, Pepperkok R, Verde F, Ansorge W, Draetta G. (1992) Cyclin A is required at two points in the human cell cycle. EMBO J 11(3):961-971.

[101] Petersen BO, Lukas J, Sorensen CS, Bartek J, Helin K. (1999) Phosphorylation of mammalian CDC6 by cyclin A/CDK2 regulates its subcellular localization. EMBO J 18(2):396-410.

[102] Coverley D, Pelizon C, Trewick S, Laskey RA. (2000) Chromatin-bound Cdc6 persists in S and G2 phases in human cells, while soluble Cdc6 is destroyed in a cyclin A-cdk2 dependent process. J Cell Sci 113 (Pt 11)(Pt 11):1929-1938.

[103] Alexandrow MG, Hamlin JL. (2005) Chromatin decondensation in S-phase involves recruitment of Cdk2 by Cdc45 and histone H1 phosphorylation. J Cell Biol 168(6):875-886.

[104] Garner-Hamrick PA, Fisher C. (1998) Antisense phosphorothioate oligonucleotides specifically down-regulate cdc25B causing S-phase delay and persistent antiproliferative effects. Int J Cancer 76(5):720-728.

[105] Lindqvist A, Kallstrom H, Lundgren A, Barsoum E, Rosenthal CK. (2005) Cdc25B cooperates with Cdc25A to induce mitosis but has a unique role in activating cyclin B1-Cdk1 at the centrosome. J Cell Biol 171(1):35-45.

[106] Chen MS, Hurov J, White LS, Woodford-Thomas T, Piwnica-Worms H. (2001) Absence of apparent phenotype in mice lacking Cdc25C protein phosphatase. Mol Cell Biol 21(12):3853-3861.

[107] Lincoln AJ, Wickramasinghe D, Stein P, Schultz RM, Palko ME, De Miguel MP, et al. (2002) Cdc25b phosphatase is required for resumption of meiosis during oocyte maturation. Nat Genet 30(4):446-449.

[108] Ferguson AM, White LS, Donovan PJ, Piwnica-Worms H. (2005) Normal cell cycle and checkpoint responses in mice and cells lacking Cdc25B and Cdc25C protein phosphatases. Mol Cell Biol 25(7):2853-2860.

[109] Furuno N, den Elzen N, Pines J. (1999) Human cyclin A is required for mitosis until mid prophase. J Cell Biol 147:295-306.

[110] Mitra J, Enders GH. (2004) Cyclin A/Cdk2 complexes regulate activation of Cdk1 and Cdc25 phosphatases in human cells. Oncogene 23(19):3361-3367.

[111] Minshull J, Golsteyn R, Hill CS, Hunt T. (1990) The A- and B-type cyclin associated cdc2 kinases in Xenopus turn on and off at different times in the cell cycle. EMBO J 9(9):2865-2875.

[112] Cans C, Ducommun B, Baldin V. (1999) Proteasome-dependent degradation of human CDC25B phosphatase. Mol Biol Rep 26(1-2):53-57.

[113] Baldin V, Cans C, Knibiehler M, Ducommun B. (1997) Phosphorylation of human CDC25B phosphatase by CDK1-cyclin A triggers its proteasome-dependent degradation. J Biol Chem 272(52):32731-32734.

[114] Gabrielli BG, Lee MS, Walker DH, Piwnica-Worms H, Maller JL. (1992) Cdc25 regulates the phosphorylation and activity of the Xenopus cdk2 protein kinase complex. J Biol Chem 267(25):18040-18046.

[115] Malumbres M, Barbacid M. (2005) Mammalian cyclin-dependent kinases. Trends Biochem Sci 30(11):630-641.

[116] De Boer L, Oakes V, Beamish H, Giles N, Stevens F, Somodevilla-Torres M, et al. (2008) Cyclin A/cdk2 coordinates centrosomal and nuclear mitotic events. Oncogene 27(31):4261-4268.

[117] Nishijima H, Nishitani H, Seki T, Nishimoto T. (1997) A dual-specificity phosphatase Cdc25B is an unstable protein and triggers p34(cdc2)/cyclin B activation in hamster BHK21 cells arrested with hydroxyurea. J Cell Biol 138(5):1105-1116.

[118] Timofeev O, Cizmecioglu O, Settele F, Kempf T, Hoffmann I. (2010) Cdc25 phosphatases are required for timely assembly of CDK1-cyclin B at the G2/M transition. J Biol Chem 285(22):16978-16990.

[119] Bailly E, Doree M, Nurse P, Bornens M. (1989) p34cdc2 is located in both nucleus and cytoplasm; part is centrosomally associated at G2/M and enters vesicles at anaphase. EMBO J 8(13):3985-3995.

[120] Gabrielli BG, De Souza CP, Tonks ID, Clark JM, Hayward NK, Ellem KA. (1996) Cytoplasmic accumulation of cdc25B phosphatase in mitosis triggers centrosomal microtubule nucleation in HeLa cells. J Cell Sci 109 (Pt 5)(Pt 5):1081-1093.

[121] Pines J, Hunter T. (1991) Human cyclins A and B1 are differentially located in the cell and undergo cell cycle-dependent nuclear transport. J Cell Biol 115(1):1-17.

[122] Hirota T, Kunitoku N, Sasayama T, Marumoto T, Zhang D, Nitta M, et al. (2003) Aurora-A and an interacting activator, the LIM protein Ajuba, are required for mitotic commitment in human cells. Cell 114(5):585-598.

[123] Barr AR, Gergely F. (2007) Aurora-A: the maker and breaker of spindle poles. J Cell Sci 120(Pt 17):2987-2996.

[124] Dutertre S, Cazales M, Quaranta M, Froment C, Trabut V, Dozier C, et al. (2004) Phosphorylation of CDC25B by Aurora-A at the centrosome contributes to the G2-M transition. J Cell Sci 117(Pt 12):2523-2531.

[125] Jackman M, Lindon C, Nigg EA, Pines J. (2003) Active cyclin B1-Cdk1 first appears on centrosomes in prophase. Nat Cell Biol 5(2):143-148.

[126] Pines J, Hunter T. (1994) The differential localization of human cyclins A and B is due to a cytoplasmic retention signal in cyclin B. EMBO J 13(16):3772-3781.

[127] Hagting A, Karlsson C, Clute P, Jackman M, Pines J. (1998) MPF localization is controlled by nuclear export. EMBO J 17(14):4127-4138.

[128] Toyoshima F, Moriguchi T, Wada A, Fukuda M, Nishida E. (1998) Nuclear export of cyclin B1 and its possible role in the DNA damage-induced G2 checkpoint. EMBO J 17(10):2728-2735.

[129] Yang J, Bardes ES, Moore JD, Brennan J, Powers MA, Kornbluth S. (1998) Control of cyclin B1 localization through regulated binding of the nuclear export factor CRM1. Genes Dev 12(14):2131-2143.

[130] Borgne A, Ostvold AC, Flament S, Meijer L. (1999) Intra-M phase-promoting factor phosphorylation of cyclin B at the prophase/metaphase transition. J Biol Chem 274(17):11977-11986.

[131] Toyoshima-Morimoto F, Taniguchi E, Shinya N, Iwamatsu A, Nishida E. (2001) Polo-like kinase 1 phosphorylates cyclin B1 and targets it to the nucleus during prophase. Nature 410(6825):215-220.

[132] Okano-Uchida T, Okumura E, Iwashita M, Yoshida H, Tachibana K, Kishimoto T. (2003) Distinct regulators for Plk1 activation in starfish meiotic and early embryonic cycles. EMBO J 22(20):5633-5642.

[133] Nakajima H, Toyoshima-Morimoto F, Taniguchi E, Nishida E. (2003) Identification of a consensus motif for Plk (Polo-like kinase) phosphorylation reveals Myt1 as a Plk1 substrate. J Biol Chem 278(28):25277-25280.

[134] Watanabe N, Arai H, Nishihara Y, Taniguchi M, Watanabe N, Hunter T, et al. (2004) M-phase kinases induce phospho-dependent ubiquitination of somatic Wee1 by SCFbeta-TrCP. Proc Natl Acad Sci U S A 101(13):4419-4424.

[135] Baldin V, Pelpel K, Cazales M, Cans C, Ducommun B. (2002) Nuclear localization of CDC25B1 and serine 146 integrity are required for induction of mitosis. J Biol Chem 277(38):35176-35182.

[136] Lobjois V, Jullien D, Bouche JP, Ducommun B. (2009) The polo-like kinase 1 regulates CDC25B-dependent mitosis entry. Biochim Biophys Acta 1793(3):462-468.

[137] Lobjois V, Froment C, Braud E, Grimal F, Burlet-Schiltz O, Ducommun B, et al. (2011) Study of the docking-dependent PLK1 phosphorylation of the CDC25B phosphatase. Biochem Biophys Res Commun 410(1):87-90.

[138] Qian YW, Erikson E, Taieb FE, Maller JL. (2001) The polo-like kinase Plx1 is required for activation of the phosphatase Cdc25C and cyclin B-Cdc2 in Xenopus oocytes. Mol Biol Cell 12(6):1791-1799.

[139] Roshak AK, Capper EA, Imburgia C, Fornwald J, Scott G, Marshall LA. (2000) The human polo-like kinase, PLK, regulates cdc2/cyclin B through phosphorylation and activation of the cdc25C phosphatase. Cell Signal 12(6):405-411.

[140] Toyoshima-Morimoto F, Taniguchi E, Nishida E. (2002) Plk1 promotes nuclear translocation of human Cdc25C during prophase. EMBO Rep 3(4):341-348.

[141] Bahassi el M, Hennigan RF, Myer DL, Stambrook PJ. (2004) Cdc25C phosphorylation on serine 191 by Plk3 promotes its nuclear translocation. Oncogene 23(15):2658-2663.

[142] Bonni S, Ganuelas ML, Petrinac S, Hudson JW. (2008) Human Plk4 phosphorylates Cdc25C. Cell Cycle 7(4):545-547.

[143] Strausfeld U, Fernandez A, Capony JP, Girard F, Lautredou N, Derancourt J, et al. (1994) Activation of p34cdc2 protein kinase by microinjection of human cdc25C into mammalian cells. Requirement for prior phosphorylation of cdc25C by p34cdc2 on sites phosphorylated at mitosis. J Biol Chem 269(8):5989-6000.

[144] Honda R, Ohba Y, Nagata A, Okayama H, Yasuda H. (1993) Dephosphorylation of human p34cdc2 kinase on both Thr-14 and Tyr-15 by human cdc25B phosphatase. FEBS Lett 318(3):331-334.

[145] Franckhauser C, Mamaeva D, Heron-Milhavet L, Fernandez A, Lamb NJ. (2010) Distinct pools of cdc25C are phosphorylated on specific TP sites and differentially localized in human mitotic cells. PLoS One 5(7):e11798.

[146] Izumi T, Maller JL. (1993) Elimination of cdc2 phosphorylation sites in the cdc25 phosphatase blocks initiation of M-phase. Mol Biol Cell 4(12):1337-1350.

[147] Pines J, Hunter T. Cyclins A and B1 in the Human Cell Cycle. In: Marsh J, editor. Regulation of the Eukaryotic Cell New York: Wiley; 1992. p. 187-208.

[148] Mailand N, Podtelejnikov AV, Groth A, Mann M, Bartek J, Lukas J. (2002) Regulation of G(2)/M events by Cdc25A through phosphorylation-dependent modulation of its stability. EMBO J 21(21):5911-5920.

[149] Tumurbaatar I, Cizmecioglu O, Hoffmann I, Grummt I, Voit R. (2011) Human Cdc14B promotes progression through mitosis by dephosphorylating Cdc25 and regulating Cdk1/cyclin B activity. PLoS One 6(2):e14711.

[150] Barford D. (2011) Structural insights into anaphase-promoting complex function and mechanism. Philos Trans R Soc Lond B Biol Sci 366(1584):3605-3624.
[151] Esteban V, Vazquez-Novelle MD, Calvo E, Bueno A, Sacristan MP. (2006) Human Cdc14A reverses CDK1 phosphorylation of Cdc25A on serines 115 and 320. Cell Cycle 5(24):2894-2898.
[152] Donzelli M, Squatrito M, Ganoth D, Hershko A, Pagano M, Draetta GF. (2002) Dual mode of degradation of Cdc25 A phosphatase. EMBO J 21(18):4875-4884.
[153] Kieffer I, Lorenzo C, Dozier C, Schmitt E, Ducommun B. (2007) Differential mitotic degradation of the CDC25B phosphatase variants. Oncogene 26(57):7847-7858.
[154] Rhind N, Furnari B, Russell P. (1997) Cdc2 tyrosine phosphorylation is required for the DNA damage checkpoint in fission yeast. Genes Dev 11(4):504-511.
[155] Boddy MN, Furnari B, Mondesert O, Russell P. (1998) Replication checkpoint enforced by kinases Cds1 and Chk1. Science 280(5365):909-912.
[156] Zeng Y, Forbes KC, Wu Z, Moreno S, Piwnica-Worms H, Enoch T. (1998) Replication checkpoint requires phosphorylation of the phosphatase Cdc25 by Cds1 or Chk1. Nature 395(6701):507-510.
[157] Furnari B, Blasina A, Boddy MN, McGowan CH, Russell P. (1999) Cdc25 inhibited in vivo and in vitro by checkpoint kinases Cds1 and Chk1. Mol Biol Cell 10(4):833-845.
[158] Branzei D, Foiani M. (2010) Maintaining genome stability at the replication fork. Nat Rev Mol Cell Biol 11(3):208-219.
[159] Melo J, Toczyski D. (2002) A unified view of the DNA-damage checkpoint. Curr Opin Cell Biol 14(2):237-245.
[160] Lopez-Girona A, Furnari B, Mondesert O, Russell P. (1999) Nuclear localization of Cdc25 is regulated by DNA damage and a 14-3-3 protein. Nature 397(6715):172-175.
[161] Ford JC, al-Khodairy F, Fotou E, Sheldrick KS, Griffiths DJ, Carr AM. (1994) 14-3-3 protein homologs required for the DNA damage checkpoint in fission yeast. Science 265(5171):533-535.
[162] Zeng Y, Piwnica-Worms H. (1999) DNA damage and replication checkpoints in fission yeast require nuclear exclusion of the Cdc25 phosphatase via 14-3-3 binding. Mol Cell Biol 19(11):7410-7419.
[163] Dai Y, Grant S. (2010) New insights into checkpoint kinase 1 in the DNA damage response signaling network. Clin Cancer Res 16(2):376-383.
[164] Niida H, Nakanishi M. (2006) DNA damage checkpoints in mammals. Mutagenesis 21(1):3-9.
[165] Minella AC, Grim JE, Welcker M, Clurman BE. (2007) p53 and SCFFbw7 cooperatively restrain cyclin E-associated genome instability. Oncogene 26(48):6948-6953.
[166] Terada Y, Tatsuka M, Jinno S, Okayama H. (1995) Requirement for tyrosine phosphorylation of Cdk4 in G1 arrest induced by ultraviolet irradiation. Nature 376(6538):358-362.
[167] Mailand N, Falck J, Lukas C, Syljuasen RG, Welcker M, Bartek J, et al. (2000) Rapid destruction of human Cdc25A in response to DNA damage. Science 288(5470):1425-1429.

[168] Goloudina A, Yamaguchi H, Chervyakova DB, Appella E, Fornace AJ,Jr, Bulavin DV. (2003) Regulation of human Cdc25A stability by Serine 75 phosphorylation is not sufficient to activate a S phase checkpoint. Cell Cycle 2(5):473-478.

[169] Hassepass I, Voit R, Hoffmann I. (2003) Phosphorylation at serine 75 is required for UV-mediated degradation of human Cdc25A phosphatase at the S-phase checkpoint. J Biol Chem 278(32):29824-29829.

[170] Chen MS, Ryan CE, Piwnica-Worms H. (2003) Chk1 kinase negatively regulates mitotic function of Cdc25A phosphatase through 14-3-3 binding. Mol Cell Biol 23(21):7488-7497.

[171] Jin J, Shirogane T, Xu L, Nalepa G, Qin J, Elledge SJ, et al. (2003) SCFbeta-TRCP links Chk1 signaling to degradation of the Cdc25A protein phosphatase. Genes Dev 17(24):3062-3074.

[172] Zhao H, Watkins JL, Piwnica-Worms H. (2002) Disruption of the checkpoint kinase 1/cell division cycle 25A pathway abrogates ionizing radiation-induced S and G2 checkpoints. Proc Natl Acad Sci U S A 99(23):14795-14800.

[173] Falck J, Mailand N, Syljuasen RG, Bartek J, Lukas J. (2001) The ATM-Chk2-Cdc25A checkpoint pathway guards against radioresistant DNA synthesis. Nature 410(6830):842-847.

[174] Shreeram S, Hee WK, Bulavin DV. (2008) Cdc25A serine 123 phosphorylation couples centrosome duplication with DNA replication and regulates tumorigenesis. Mol Cell Biol 28(24):7442-7450.

[175] Madlener S, Rosner M, Krieger S, Giessrigl B, Gridling M, Vo TP, et al. (2009) Short 42 degrees C heat shock induces phosphorylation and degradation of Cdc25A which depends on p38MAPK, Chk2 and 14.3.3. Hum Mol Genet 18(11):1990-2000.

[176] Falck J, Petrini JH, Williams BR, Lukas J, Bartek J. (2002) The DNA damage-dependent intra-S phase checkpoint is regulated by parallel pathways. Nat Genet 30(3):290-294.

[177] Yaffe MB, Rittinger K, Volinia S, Caron PR, Aitken A, Leffers H, et al. (1997) The structural basis for 14-3-3:phosphopeptide binding specificity. Cell 91(7):961-971.

[178] Kasahara K, Goto H, Enomoto M, Tomono Y, Kiyono T, Inagaki M. (2010) 14-3-3gamma mediates Cdc25A proteolysis to block premature mitotic entry after DNA damage. EMBO J 29(16):2802-2812.

[179] Aitken A. (2002) Functional specificity in 14-3-3 isoform interactions through dimer formation and phosphorylation. Chromosome location of mammalian isoforms and variants. Plant Mol Biol 50(6):993-1010.

[180] Aitken A, Baxter H, Dubois T, Clokie S, Mackie S, Mitchell K, et al. (2002) Specificity of 14-3-3 isoform dimer interactions and phosphorylation. Biochem Soc Trans 30:351-360.

[181] Xiao Z, Chen Z, Gunasekera AH, Sowin TJ, Rosenberg SH, Fesik S, et al. (2003) Chk1 mediates S and G2 arrests through Cdc25A degradation in response to DNA-damaging agents. J Biol Chem 278(24):21767-21773.

[182] Costanzo V, Robertson K, Ying CY, Kim E, Avvedimento E, Gottesman M, et al. (2000) Reconstitution of an ATM-dependent checkpoint that inhibits chromosomal DNA replication following DNA damage. Mol Cell 6(3):649-659.

[183] Molinari M, Mercurio C, Dominguez J, Goubin F, Draetta GF. (2000) Human Cdc25 A inactivation in response to S phase inhibition and its role in preventing premature mitosis. EMBO Rep 1(1):71-79.

[184] Busino L, Donzelli M, Chiesa M, Guardavaccaro D, Ganoth D, Dorrello NV, et al. (2003) Degradation of Cdc25A by beta-TrCP during S phase and in response to DNA damage. Nature 426(6962):87-91.

[185] Winston JT, Strack P, Beer-Romero P, Chu CY, Elledge SJ, Harper JW. (1999) The SCFbeta-TRCP-ubiquitin ligase complex associates specifically with phosphorylated destruction motifs in IkappaBalpha and beta-catenin and stimulates IkappaBalpha ubiquitination in vitro. Genes Dev 13(3):270-283.

[186] Donzelli M, Busino L, Chiesa M, Ganoth D, Hershko A, Draetta GF. (2004) Hierarchical order of phosphorylation events commits Cdc25A to betaTrCP-dependent degradation. Cell Cycle 3(4):469-471.

[187] Melixetian M, Klein DK, Sorensen CS, Helin K. (2009) NEK11 regulates CDC25A degradation and the IR-induced G2/M checkpoint. Nat Cell Biol 11(10):1247-1253.

[188] Shieh SY, Ahn J, Tamai K, Taya Y, Prives C. (2000) The human homologs of checkpoint kinases Chk1 and Cds1 (Chk2) phosphorylate p53 at multiple DNA damage-inducible sites. Genes Dev 14(3):289-300.

[189] Khosravi R, Maya R, Gottlieb T, Oren M, Shiloh Y, Shkedy D. (1999) Rapid ATM-dependent phosphorylation of MDM2 precedes p53 accumulation in response to DNA damage. Proc Natl Acad Sci U S A 96(26):14973-14977.

[190] Maya R, Balass M, Kim ST, Shkedy D, Leal JF, Shifman O, et al. (2001) ATM-dependent phosphorylation of Mdm2 on serine 395: role in p53 activation by DNA damage. Genes Dev 15(9):1067-1077.

[191] Tritarelli A, Oricchio E, Ciciarello M, Mangiacasale R, Palena A, Lavia P, et al. (2004) p53 localization at centrosomes during mitosis and postmitotic checkpoint are ATM-dependent and require serine 15 phosphorylation. Mol Biol Cell 15:3751.

[192] el-Deiry WS, Harper JW, O'Connor PM, Velculescu VE, Canman CE, Jackman J, et al. (1994) WAF1/CIP1 is induced in p53-mediated G1 arrest and apoptosis. Cancer Res 54(5):1169-1174.

[193] Watcharasit P, Bijur GN, Zmijewski JW, Song L, Zmijewska A, Chen X, et al. (2002) Direct, activating interaction between glycogen synthase kinase-3beta and p53 after DNA damage. Proc Natl Acad Sci U S A 99(12):7951-7955.

[194] Kang T, Wei Y, Honaker Y, Yamaguchi H, Appella E, Hung MC, et al. (2008) GSK-3 beta targets Cdc25A for ubiquitin-mediated proteolysis, and GSK-3 beta inactivation correlates with Cdc25A overproduction in human cancers. Cancer Cell 13(1):36-47.

[195] Myer DL, Robbins SB, Yin M, Boivin GP, Liu Y, Greis KD, et al. (2011) Absence of polo-like kinase 3 in mice stabilizes Cdc25A after DNA damage but is not sufficient to produce tumors. Mutat Res 714(1-2):1-10.

[196] Xie S, Wu H, Wang Q, Cogswell JP, Husain I, Conn C, et al. (2001) Plk3 functionally links DNA damage to cell cycle arrest and apoptosis at least in part via the p53 pathway. J Biol Chem 276(46):43305-43312.

[197] Bahassi el M, Myer DL, McKenney RJ, Hennigan RF, Stambrook PJ. (2006) Priming phosphorylation of Chk2 by polo-like kinase 3 (Plk3) mediates its full activation by

ATM and a downstream checkpoint in response to DNA damage. Mutat Res 596(1-2):166-176.

[198] Honaker Y, Piwnica-Worms H. (2010) Casein kinase 1 functions as both penultimate and ultimate kinase in regulating Cdc25A destruction. Oncogene 29(23):3324-3334.

[199] Piao S, Lee SJ, Xu Y, Gwak J, Oh S, Park BJ, et al. (2011) CK1epsilon targets Cdc25A for ubiquitin-mediated proteolysis under normal conditions and in response to checkpoint activation. Cell Cycle 10(3):531-537.

[200] Sorensen CS, Syljuasen RG, Falck J, Schroeder T, Ronnstrand L, Khanna KK, et al. (2003) Chk1 regulates the S phase checkpoint by coupling the physiological turnover and ionizing radiation-induced accelerated proteolysis of Cdc25A. Cancer Cell 3(3):247-258.

[201] Shimuta K, Nakajo N, Uto K, Hayano Y, Okazaki K, Sagata N. (2002) Chk1 is activated transiently and targets Cdc25A for degradation at the Xenopus midblastula transition. EMBO J 21(14):3694-3703.

[202] Kanemori Y, Uto K, Sagata N. (2005) Beta-TrCP recognizes a previously undescribed nonphosphorylated destruction motif in Cdc25A and Cdc25B phosphatases. Proc Natl Acad Sci U S A 102(18):6279-6284.

[203] Koledova Z, Kafkova LR, Kramer A, Divoky V. (2010) DNA damage-induced degradation of Cdc25A does not lead to inhibition of Cdk2 activity in mouse embryonic stem cells. Stem Cells 28(3):450-461.

[204] Thomas Y, Coux O, Baldin V. (2010) betaTrCP-dependent degradation of CDC25B phosphatase at the metaphase-anaphase transition is a pre-requisite for correct mitotic exit. Cell Cycle 9(21):4338-4350.

[205] Bansal P, Lazo JS. (2007) Induction of Cdc25B regulates cell cycle resumption after genotoxic stress. Cancer Res 67(7):3356-3363.

[206] Jin J, Ang XL, Ye X, Livingstone M, Harper JW. (2008) Differential roles for checkpoint kinases in DNA damage-dependent degradation of the Cdc25A protein phosphatase. J Biol Chem 283(28):19322-19328.

[207] Uto K, Inoue D, Shimuta K, Nakajo N, Sagata N. (2004) Chk1, but not Chk2, inhibits Cdc25 phosphatases by a novel common mechanism. EMBO J 23(16):3386-3396.

[208] Bulavin DV, Higashimoto Y, Popoff IJ, Gaarde WA, Basrur V, Potapova O, et al. (2001) Initiation of a G2/M checkpoint after ultraviolet radiation requires p38 kinase. Nature 411(6833):102-107.

[209] Matsuoka S, Huang M, Elledge SJ. (1998) Linkage of ATM to cell cycle regulation by the Chk2 protein kinase. Science 282(5395):1893-1897.

[210] Manke IA, Nguyen A, Lim D, Stewart MQ, Elia AE, Yaffe MB. (2005) MAPKAP kinase-2 is a cell cycle checkpoint kinase that regulates the G2/M transition and S phase progression in response to UV irradiation. Mol Cell 17(1):37-48.

[211] Uchida S, Yoshioka K, Kizu R, Nakagama H, Matsunaga T, Ishizaka Y, et al. (2009) Stress-activated mitogen-activated protein kinases c-Jun NH2-terminal kinase and p38 target Cdc25B for degradation. Cancer Res 69(16):6438-6444.

[212] Galaktionov K, Lee AK, Eckstein J, Draetta G, Meckler J, Loda M, et al. (1995) CDC25 phosphatases as potential human oncogenes. Science 269(5230):1575-1577.

[213] Gabrielli BG, Clark JM, McCormack AK, Ellem KA. (1997) Ultraviolet light-induced G2 phase cell cycle checkpoint blocks cdc25-dependent progression into mitosis. Oncogene 15(7):749-758.

[214] Lemaire M, Ducommun B, Nebreda AR. (2010) UV-induced downregulation of the CDC25B protein in human cells. FEBS Lett 584(6):1199-1204.

[215] Deng J, Harding HP, Raught B, Gingras AC, Berlanga JJ, Scheuner D, et al. (2002) Activation of GCN2 in UV-irradiated cells inhibits translation. Curr Biol 12(15):1279-1286.

[216] Uchida S, Kuma A, Ohtsubo M, Shimura M, Hirata M, Nakagama H, et al. (2004) Binding of 14-3-3beta but not 14-3-3sigma controls the cytoplasmic localization of CDC25B: binding site preferences of 14-3-3 subtypes and the subcellular localization of CDC25B. J Cell Sci 117(Pt 14):3011-3020.

[217] Dalal SN, Schweitzer CM, Gan J, DeCaprio JA. (1999) Cytoplasmic localization of human cdc25C during interphase requires an intact 14-3-3 binding site. Mol Cell Biol 19(6):4465-4479.

[218] Barth H, Hoffmann I, Kinzel V. (1996) Radiation with 1 Gy prevents the activation of the mitotic inducers mitosis-promoting factor (MPF) and cdc25-C in HeLa cells. Cancer Res 56(10):2268-2272.

[219] Peng CY, Graves PR, Thoma RS, Wu Z, Shaw AS, Piwnica-Worms H. (1997) Mitotic and G2 checkpoint control: regulation of 14-3-3 protein binding by phosphorylation of Cdc25C on serine-216. Science 277(5331):1501-1505.

[220] Sanchez Y, Wong C, Thoma RS, Richman R, Wu Z, Piwnica-Worms H, et al. (1997) Conservation of the Chk1 checkpoint pathway in mammals: linkage of DNA damage to Cdk regulation through Cdc25. Science 277(5331):1497-1501.

[221] Ogg S, Gabrielli B, Piwnica-Worms H. (1994) Purification of a serine kinase that associates with and phosphorylates human Cdc25C on serine 216. J Biol Chem 269(48):30461-30469.

[222] Brown AL, Lee CH, Schwarz JK, Mitiku N, Piwnica-Worms H, Chung JH. (1999) A human Cds1-related kinase that functions downstream of ATM protein in the cellular response to DNA damage. Proc Natl Acad Sci U S A 96(7):3745-3750.

[223] Morris MC, Heitz A, Mery J, Heitz F, Divita G. (2000) An essential phosphorylation-site domain of human cdc25C interacts with both 14-3-3 and cyclins. J Biol Chem 275(37):28849-28857.

[224] Graves PR, Lovly CM, Uy GL, Piwnica-Worms H. (2001) Localization of human Cdc25C is regulated both by nuclear export and 14-3-3 protein binding. Oncogene 20(15):1839-1851.

[225] Chan PM, Ng YW, Manser E. (2011) A robust protocol to map binding sites of the 14-3-3 interactome: Cdc25C requires phosphorylation of both S216 and S263 to bind 14-3-3. Mol Cell Proteomics 10(3):M110.005157.

[226] Esmenjaud-Mailhat C, Lobjois V, Froment C, Golsteyn RM, Monsarrat B, Ducommun B. (2007) Phosphorylation of CDC25C at S263 controls its intracellular localisation. FEBS Lett 581(21):3979-3985.

[227] O'Neill T, Giarratani L, Chen P, Iyer L, Lee CH, Bobiak M, et al. (2002) Determination of substrate motifs for human Chk1 and hCds1/Chk2 by the oriented peptide library approach. J Biol Chem 277(18):16102-16115.

[228] Kumagai A, Dunphy WG. (1999) Binding of 14-3-3 proteins and nuclear export control the intracellular localization of the mitotic inducer Cdc25. Genes Dev 13(9):1067-1072.

[229] Kumagai A, Yakowec PS, Dunphy WG. (1998) 14-3-3 proteins act as negative regulators of the mitotic inducer Cdc25 in Xenopus egg extracts. Mol Biol Cell 9(2):345-354.

[230] Kumagai A, Guo Z, Emami KH, Wang SX, Dunphy WG. (1998) The Xenopus Chk1 protein kinase mediates a caffeine-sensitive pathway of checkpoint control in cell-free extracts. J Cell Biol 142(6):1559-1569.

[231] Hutchins JR, Dikovskaya D, Clarke PR. (2002) Dephosphorylation of the inhibitory phosphorylation site S287 in Xenopus Cdc25C by protein phosphatase-2A is inhibited by 14-3-3 binding. FEBS Lett 528(1-3):267-271.

[232] Sorensen CS, Syljuasen RG, Lukas J, Bartek J. (2004) ATR, Claspin and the Rad9-Rad1-Hus1 complex regulate Chk1 and Cdc25A in the absence of DNA damage. Cell Cycle 3(7):941-945.

[233] Kreutzer J, Guerra B. (2007) The regulatory beta-subunit of protein kinase CK2 accelerates the degradation of CDC25A phosphatase through the checkpoint kinase Chk1. Int J Oncol 31(5):1251-1259.

[234] Schwindling SL, Noll A, Montenarh M, Gotz C. (2004) Mutation of a CK2 phosphorylation site in cdc25C impairs importin alpha/beta binding and results in cytoplasmic retention. Oncogene 23(23):4155-4165.

[235] Theis-Febvre N, Filhol O, Froment C, Cazales M, Cochet C, Monsarrat B, et al. (2003) Protein kinase CK2 regulates CDC25B phosphatase activity. Oncogene 22(2):220-232.

[236] Schmitt E, Boutros R, Froment C, Monsarrat B, Ducommun B, Dozier C. (2006) CHK1 phosphorylates CDC25B during the cell cycle in the absence of DNA damage. J Cell Sci 119(Pt 20):4269-4275.

[237] Kramer A, Mailand N, Lukas C, Syljuasen RG, Wilkinson CJ, Nigg EA, et al. (2004) Centrosome-associated Chk1 prevents premature activation of cyclin-B-Cdk1 kinase. Nat Cell Biol 6(9):884-891.

[238] Forrest A, Gabrielli B. (2001) Cdc25B activity is regulated by 14-3-3. Oncogene 20(32):4393-4401.

[239] Giles N, Forrest A, Gabrielli B. (2003) 14-3-3 acts as an intramolecular bridge to regulate cdc25B localization and activity. J Biol Chem 278(31):28580-28587.

[240] Davezac N, Baldin V, Gabrielli B, Forrest A, Theis-Febvre N, Yashida M, et al. (2000) Regulation of CDC25B phosphatases subcellular localization. Oncogene 19(18):2179-2185.

[241] Stanford JS, Ruderman JV. (2005) Changes in regulatory phosphorylation of Cdc25C Ser287 and Wee1 Ser549 during normal cell cycle progression and checkpoint arrests. Mol Biol Cell 16(12):5749-5760.

[242] Brown EJ, Baltimore D. (2003) Essential and dispensable roles of ATR in cell cycle arrest and genome maintenance. Genes Dev 17(5):615-628.

[243] Liu Q, Guntuku S, Cui XS, Matsuoka S, Cortez D, Tamai K, et al. (2000) Chk1 is an essential kinase that is regulated by Atr and required for the G(2)/M DNA damage checkpoint. Genes Dev 14(12):1448-1459.

[244] Yang J, Winkler K, Yoshida M, Kornbluth S. (1999) Maintenance of G_2 arrest in the Xenopus oocyte: a role for 14-3-3-mediated inhibition of Cdc25 nuclear import. EMBO J 18(8):2174-2183.

[245] Brondello JM, Boddy MN, Furnari B, Russell P. (1999) Basis for the checkpoint signal specificity that regulates Chk1 and Cds1 protein kinases. Mol Cell Biol 19(6):4262-4269.

[246] Bulavin DV, Higashimoto Y, Demidenko ZN, Meek S, Graves P, Phillips C, et al. (2003) Dual phosphorylation controls Cdc25 phosphatases and mitotic entry. Nat Cell Biol 5(6):545-551.

[247] Bulavin DV, Demidenko ZN, Phillips C, Moody SA, Fornace AJ,Jr. (2003) Phosphorylation of Xenopus Cdc25C at Ser285 interferes with ability to activate a DNA damage replication checkpoint in pre-midblastula embryos. Cell Cycle 2(3):263-266.

[248] Margolis SS, Perry JA, Forester CM, Nutt LK, Guo Y, Jardim MJ, et al. (2006) Role for the PP2A/B56delta phosphatase in regulating 14-3-3 release from Cdc25 to control mitosis. Cell 127(4):759-773.

[249] Margolis SS, Perry JA, Weitzel DH, Freel CD, Yoshida M, Haystead TA, et al. (2006) A role for PP1 in the Cdc2/Cyclin B-mediated positive feedback activation of Cdc25. Mol Biol Cell 17(4):1779-1789.

[250] Cunat S, Anahory T, Berthenet C, Hedon B, Franckhauser C, Fernandez A, et al. (2008) The cell cycle control protein cdc25C is present, and phosphorylated on serine 214 in the transition from germinal vesicle to metaphase II in human oocyte meiosis. Mol Reprod Dev 75(7):1176-1184.

[251] Margolis SS, Walsh S, Weiser DC, Yoshida M, Shenolikar S, Kornbluth S. (2003) PP1 control of M phase entry exerted through 14-3-3-regulated Cdc25 dephosphorylation. EMBO J 22(21):5734-5745.

[252] Ku NO, Michie S, Resurreccion EZ, Broome RL, Omary MB. (2002) Keratin binding to 14-3-3 proteins modulates keratin filaments and hepatocyte mitotic progression. Proc Natl Acad Sci U S A 99(7):4373-4378.

[253] Clarke PR, Hoffmann I, Draetta G, Karsenti E. (1993) Dephosphorylation of cdc25-C by a type-2A protein phosphatase: specific regulation during the cell cycle in Xenopus egg extracts. Mol Biol Cell 4(4):397-411.

[254] Crenshaw DG, Yang J, Means AR, Kornbluth S. (1998) The mitotic peptidyl-prolyl isomerase, Pin1, interacts with Cdc25 and Plx1. EMBO J 17(5):1315-1327.

[255] Zhou XZ, Kops O, Werner A, Lu PJ, Shen M, Stoller G, et al. (2000) Pin1-dependent prolyl isomerization regulates dephosphorylation of Cdc25C and tau proteins. Mol Cell 6(4):873-883.

[256] Stukenberg PT, Kirschner MW. (2001) Pin1 acts catalytically to promote a conformational change in Cdc25. Mol Cell 7(5):1071-1083.

[257] Winkler KE, Swenson KI, Kornbluth S, Means AR. (2000) Requirement of the prolyl isomerase Pin1 for the replication checkpoint. Science 287(5458):1644-1647.

[258] Forester CM, Maddox J, Louis JV, Goris J, Virshup DM. (2007) Control of mitotic exit by PP2A regulation of Cdc25C and Cdk1. Proc Natl Acad Sci U S A 104(50):19867-19872.

[259] Astuti P, Boutros R, Ducommun B, Gabrielli B. (2010) Mitotic phosphorylation of Cdc25B Ser321 disrupts 14-3-3 binding to the high affinity Ser323 site. J Biol Chem 285(45):34364-34370.

[260] Hermeking H, Lengauer C, Polyak K, He TC, Zhang L, Thiagalingam S, et al. (1997) 14-3-3 sigma is a p53-regulated inhibitor of G2/M progression. Mol Cell 1(1):3-11.

[261] Wilson-Grady JT, Villén J, Gygi SP. (2008) Phosphoproteome analysis of fission yeast. Journal of Proteome Research 7(3):1088-1097.

[262] Kinoshita N, Ohkura H, Yanagida M. (1990) Distinct, essential roles of type 1 and 2A protein phosphatases in the control of the fission yeast cell division cycle. Cell 63(2):405-415.

[263] Kinoshita N, Yamano H, Niwa H, Yoshida T, Yanagida M. (1993) Negative regulation of mitosis by the fission yeast protein phosphatase ppa2. Genes Dev 7(6):1059-1071.

[264] Ohkura H, Adachi Y, Kinoshita N, Niwa O, Toda T, Yanagida M. (1988) Cold-sensitive and caffeine-supersensitive mutants of the *Schizosaccharomyces pombe* dis genes implicated in sister chromatid separation during mitosis. EMBO J 7(5):1465-1473.

[265] Cargnello M, Roux PP. (2011) Activation and function of the MAPKs and their substrates, the MAPK-activated protein kinases. Microbiol Mol Biol Rev 75(1):50-83.

[266] Shaul YD, Seger R. (2007) The MEK/ERK cascade: from signaling specificity to diverse functions. Biochim Biophys Acta 1773(8):1213-1226.

[267] Liu J, Grimison B, Maller JL. (2007) New insight into metaphase arrest by cytostatic factor: from establishment to release. Oncogene 26(9):1286-1289.

[268] Rauh NR, Schmidt A, Bormann J, Nigg EA, Mayer TU. (2005) Calcium triggers exit from meiosis II by targeting the APC/C inhibitor XErp1 for degradation. Nature 437(7061):1048-1052.

[269] Chun J, Chau AS, Maingat FG, Edmonds SD, Ostergaard HL, Shibuya EK. (2005) Phosphorylation of Cdc25C by pp90Rsk contributes to a G2 cell cycle arrest in Xenopus cycling egg extracts. Cell Cycle 4(1):148-154.

[270] Hutchins JR, Dikovskaya D, Clarke PR. (2003) Regulation of Cdc2/cyclin B activation in Xenopus egg extracts via inhibitory phosphorylation of Cdc25C phosphatase by Ca(2+)/calmodulin-dependent protein [corrected] kinase II. Mol Biol Cell 14(10):4003-4014.

[271] Wang R, Jung SY, Wu CF, Qin J, Kobayashi R, Gallick GE, et al. (2010) Direct roles of the signaling kinase RSK2 in Cdc25C activation during Xenopus oocyte maturation. Proc Natl Acad Sci U S A 107(46):19885-19890.

[272] Wang R, He G, Nelman-Gonzalez M, Ashorn CL, Gallick GE, Stukenberg PT, et al. (2007) Regulation of Cdc25C by ERK-MAP kinases during the G2/M transition. Cell 128(6):1119-1132.

[273] Astuti P, Pike T, Widberg C, Payne E, Harding A, Hancock J, et al. (2009) MAPK pathway activation delays G2/M progression by destabilizing Cdc25B. J Biol Chem 284(49):33781-33788.

[274] Patel R, Holt M, Philipova R, Moss S, Schulman H, Hidaka H, et al. (1999) Calcium/calmodulin-dependent phosphorylation and activation of human Cdc25-C at the G2/M phase transition in HeLa cells. J Biol Chem 274(12):7958-7968.

[275] Planas-Silva MD, Means AR. (1992) Expression of a constitutive form of calcium/calmodulin dependent protein kinase II leads to arrest of the cell cycle in G2. EMBO J 11(2):507-517.

[276] Peng CY, Graves PR, Ogg S, Thoma RS, Byrnes MJ,3rd, Wu Z, et al. (1998) C-TAK1 protein kinase phosphorylates human Cdc25C on serine 216 and promotes 14-3-3 protein binding. Cell Growth Differ 9(3):197-208.

[277] Izumi T, Maller JL. (1995) Phosphorylation and activation of the Xenopus Cdc25 phosphatase in the absence of Cdc2 and Cdk2 kinase activity. Mol Biol Cell 6(2):215-226.

[278] Eymin B, Claverie P, Salon C, Brambilla C, Brambilla E, Gazzeri S. (2006) p14ARF triggers G2 arrest through ERK-mediated Cdc25C phosphorylation, ubiquitination and proteasomal degradation. Cell Cycle 5(7):759-765.

[279] Kotlyarov A, Yannoni Y, Fritz S, Laass K, Telliez JB, Pitman D, et al. (2002) Distinct cellular functions of MK2. Mol Cell Biol 22(13):4827-4835.

[280] Uchida S, Watanabe N, Kudo Y, Yoshioka K, Matsunaga T, Ishizaka Y, et al. (2011) SCFbeta(TrCP) mediates stress-activated MAPK-induced Cdc25B degradation. J Cell Sci 124(Pt 16):2816-2825.

[281] Gutierrez GJ, Tsuji T, Cross JV, Davis RJ, Templeton DJ, Jiang W, et al. (2010) JNK-mediated phosphorylation of Cdc25C regulates cell cycle entry and G(2)/M DNA damage checkpoint. J Biol Chem 285(19):14217-14228.

[282] Goss VL, Cross JV, Ma K, Qian Y, Mola PW, Templeton DJ. (2003) SAPK/JNK regulates cdc2/cyclin B kinase through phosphorylation and inhibition of cdc25c. Cell Signal 15(7):709-718.

[283] Lopez-Aviles S, Grande M, Gonzalez M, Helgesen AL, Alemany V, Sanchez-Piris M, et al. (2005) Inactivation of the Cdc25 phosphatase by the stress-activated Srk1 kinase in fission yeast. Mol Cell 17(1):49-59.

[284] Smith DA, Morgan BA, Quinn J. (2010) Stress signalling to fungal stress-activated protein kinase pathways. FEMS Microbiol Lett 306(1):1-8.

[285] Stanford JS, Lieberman SL, Wong VL, Ruderman JV. (2003) Regulation of the G2/M transition in oocytes of xenopus tropicalis. Dev Biol 260(2):438-448.

[286] Duckworth BC, Weaver JS, Ruderman JV. (2002) G2 arrest in Xenopus oocytes depends on phosphorylation of cdc25 by protein kinase A. Proc Natl Acad Sci U S A 99(26):16794-16799.

[287] Pirino G, Wescott MP, Donovan PJ. (2009) Protein kinase A regulates resumption of meiosis by phosphorylation of Cdc25B in mammalian oocytes. Cell Cycle 8(4):665-670.

[288] Bachmann M, Moroy T. (2005) The serine/threonine kinase Pim-1. Int J Biochem Cell Biol 37(4):726-730.

[289] Mochizuki T, Kitanaka C, Noguchi K, Muramatsu T, Asai A, Kuchino Y. (1999) Physical and functional interactions between Pim-1 kinase and Cdc25A phosphatase. Implications for the Pim-1-mediated activation of the c-Myc signaling pathway. J Biol Chem 274(26):18659-18666.

[290] Wang Z, Bhattacharya N, Mixter PF, Wei W, Sedivy J, Magnuson NS. (2002) Phosphorylation of the cell cycle inhibitor p21Cip1/WAF1 by Pim-1 kinase. Biochim Biophys Acta 1593(1):45-55.

[291] Bachmann M, Hennemann H, Xing PX, Hoffmann I, Moroy T. (2004) The oncogenic serine/threonine kinase Pim-1 phosphorylates and inhibits the activity of Cdc25C-associated kinase 1 (C-TAK1): a novel role for Pim-1 at the G2/M cell cycle checkpoint. J Biol Chem 279(46):48319-48328.

[292] Davezac N, Baldin V, Blot J, Ducommun B, Tassan JP. (2002) Human pEg3 kinase associates with and phosphorylates CDC25B phosphatase: a potential role for pEg3 in cell cycle regulation. Oncogene 21(50):7630-7641.

[293] Mirey G, Chartrain I, Froment C, Quaranta M, Bouche JP, Monsarrat B, et al. (2005) CDC25B phosphorylated by pEg3 localizes to the centrosome and the spindle poles at mitosis. Cell Cycle 4(6):806-811.

[294] Nance J. (2005) PAR proteins and the establishment of cell polarity during *C. elegans* development.Bioessays 27:126-135.

[295] Rivers DM, Moreno S, Abraham M, Ahringer J. (2008) PAR proteins direct asymmetry of the cell cycle regulators Polo-like kinase and Cdc25. J Cell Biol 180(5):877-885.

[296] Kristjansdottir K, Rudolph J. (2004) Cdc25 phosphatases and cancer. Chem Biol 11(8):1043-1051.

[297] Loffler H, Syljuasen RG, Bartkova J, Worm J, Lukas J, Bartek J. (2003) Distinct modes of deregulation of the proto-oncogenic Cdc25A phosphatase in human breast cancer cell lines. Oncogene 22(50):8063-8071.

[298] Galaktionov K, Chen X, Beach D. (1996) Cdc25 cell-cycle phosphatase as a target of c-myc. Nature 382(6591):511-517.

[299] Dong J, Zeng BH, Xu LH, Wang JY, Li MZ, Zeng MS, et al. (2010) Anti-CDC25B autoantibody predicts poor prognosis in patients with advanced esophageal squamous cell carcinoma. J Transl Med 8:81.

[300] Bugler B, Schmitt E, Aressy B, Ducommun B. (2010) Unscheduled expression of CDC25B in S-phase leads to replicative stress and DNA damage. Mol Cancer 9:29.

[301] Planelles V, Benichou S. (2009) Vpr and its interactions with cellular proteins. Curr Top Microbiol Immunol 339:177-200.

[302] Huard S, Elder RT, Liang D, Li G, Zhao RY. (2008) Human immunodeficiency virus type 1 Vpr induces cell cycle G2 arrest through Srk1/MK2-mediated phosphorylation of Cdc25. J Virol 82(6):2904-2917.

[303] Matsuda N, Tanaka H, Yamazaki S, Suzuki J, Tanaka K, Yamada T, et al. (2006) HIV-1 Vpr induces G2 cell cycle arrest in fission yeast associated with Rad24/14-3-3-dependent, Chk1/Cds1-independent Wee1 upregulation. Microbes Infect 8(12-13):2736-2744.

[304] Elder RT, Yu M, Chen M, Zhu X, Yanagida M, Zhao Y. (2001) HIV-1 Vpr induces cell cycle G2 arrest in fission yeast (*Schizosaccharomyces pombe*) through a pathway involving regulatory and catalytic subunits of PP2A and acting on both Wee1 and Cdc25. Virology 287(2):359-370.

[305] Frazer C, Young, PG (2012) Carboxy-terminal phosphorylation sites in Cdc25 contribute to enforcement of the DNA damage and replication checkpoints in fission yeast. Curr Genetics , DOI 10.1007/s00294-012-0379-1

Section 5

Histidine Kinases in Two-Component Systems

Chapter 15

Bacterial Two-Component Systems: Structures and Signaling Mechanisms

Shuishu Wang

Additional information is available at the end of the chapter

http://dx.doi.org/10.5772/48277

1. Introduction

Two-component systems (TCS) are ubiquitous among bacteria. They play essential roles in signaling events in bacteria, such as cell-cell communication, adaptation to environments, and pathogenesis in the case of pathogens. Due to their absence in humans and other mammals, TCS proteins are considered potential targets for developing new antibiotics. Most bacterial TCSs consist of two proteins, a sensor histidine kinase (HK) and a response regulator (RR). The HK senses specific signals, and that leads to activation of the kinase activity and autophosphorylation of a conserved histidine residue. The phosphoryl group is subsequently transferred to a cognate response regulator to activate its activities. Most RRs are transcription regulators and turn on or off gene transcriptions in response to the signals received by sensor HKs. Recent years have seen a rapid expansion of structural data of bacterial TCS proteins. In this chapter, I will review structures of HKs and RRs and discuss their structure-function relationship and their signaling mechanisms. The chapter contains three main sections: structures of histidine kinases, structures of response regulators, and structures of complexes between a histidine kinase and a response regulator. I will conclude the chapter with the implications of these structural and functional data on developments of new therapeutics against bacterial pathogens. Analysis of structures and reaction mechanisms will focus on the extracytosolic sensor HKs and OmpR/PhoB subfamily transcription regulator RRs.

2. Structures of histidine kinases

The prototypical histidine kinase is a homodimeric integral membrane protein (Figure 1). Each protomer has two transmembrane (TM) helices with the N-terminus in the cytosol. An extracytosolic sensor domain lies between the two TM helices. After the second TM helix is a HAMP domain, which is commonly found in Histidine kinases, Adenylyl cyclases, Methyl-accepting chemotaxis proteins, and Phosphatases [1], hence the name. The HAMP domain connects TM2 to the dimerization and histidine phosphorylation domain (often abbreviated as DHp). A catalytic and ATP-binding (CA) domain lies at the carboxyl terminus. The combination of DHp and CA is sometimes referred to as the kinase domain. The TM helices, HAMP domains, and DHp domains are all involved in homodimerization. The sensor domain is likely to dimerize in the context of the entire protein. Sensor domains share little sequence identity, as is expected from their diverse functions of sensing various signals. However, available structures of sensor domains fall into a few common structural folds, suggesting conserved signal sensing mechanisms. The HAMP, DHp, and CA domains are common modules of HKs and have well conserved structures and sequences, especially DHp and CA, whose sequences contain several conserved motifs. There is an absolutely conserved histidine residue that is phosphorylated, and the phosphoryl group is then donated to an RR, in response to signals sensed by the sensor domain. How the sensor domain regulates the kinase activities is still unknown, due to the lack of full-length structures of the transmembrane sensor HKs. However, a large accumulation of structures of isolated domains in recent years has started to shed light on possible molecular mechanisms of the signal transduction. In this section, I will summarize these structures and discuss their conformational changes that transmit signals from the sensor domain to the kinase domain.

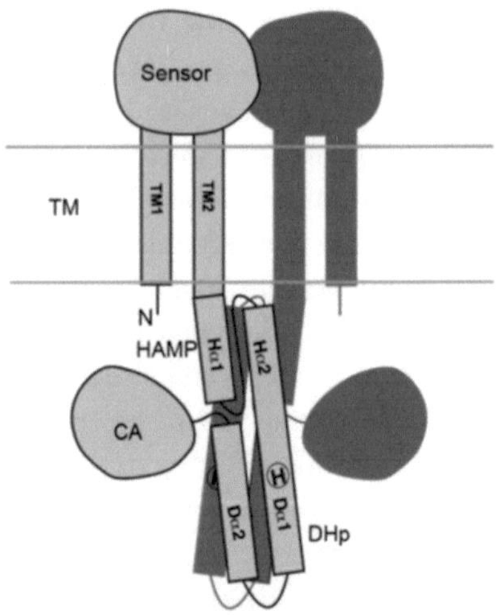

Figure 1. Schematic diagram of the modular structure of the prototypical sensor histidine kinase. At the N-terminus, a sensor domain lies between the two transmembrane (TM) helices. A HAMP domain follows TM2 with its second helix (Hα2) connected to helix Dα1 of the DHp domain. The catalytic and ATP-binding (CA) domain is at the C-terminus. The position of the phosphorylation site histidine is marked with an "H". The HAMP and DHp domains form homodimers.

2.1. Structures of sensor domains

Sensor domains of histidine kinases are located in cytosol, in membrane, or outside of cell membrane (extracytosolic). Currently, there is little structural information of the membrane-embedded sensor domains. The prototypical HK has an extracytosolic sensor domain that senses extracellular signals or conditions in the cell envelope. These sensor domains have highly diverse sequences. However, most of the known structures of extracytosolic sensor domains fall into three distinct structural folds, mixed αβ, all-helical, and β-sandwich. Unlike extracytosolic sensor domains, many cytosolic sensor domains can be annotated on the sequence level as PAS or GAF domains, which have related structural folds and are named from their occurrence in Period circadian, Aryl hydrocarbon receptor nuclear translocator, and Single-minded proteins (PAS) [2], or in cGMP-regulated cyclic nucleotide phosphodiesterases, Adenylate cyclases, and the bacterial transcriptional regulator FhlA (GAF) [3].

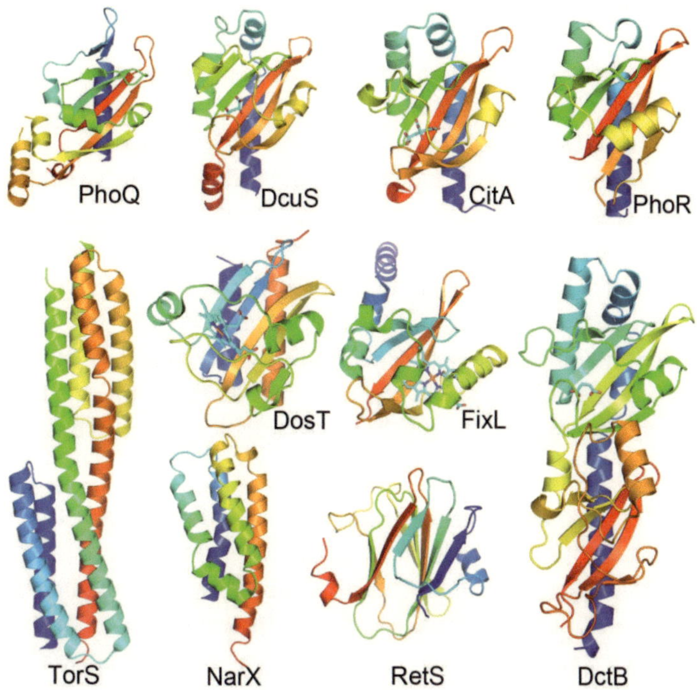

Figure 2. Structures of sensor domains. The structures are each colored in a rainbow spectrum from blue to red from the N- to C-terminus, respectively. The DosT (PDB code 2VZW, *M. tuberdulosis*) and FixL (1EW0, *R. meliloti*) sensor domains are located in the cell cytosol and belong to GAF and PAS domains, respectively; the remainders are extracytosolic domains. The PhoQ (3BQ8, *Escherichia coli*) and DcuS (3BY8, *E. coli*), and PhoR (3CWF, *Bacillus subtilis*), and CitA (2J80, *Klebsiella pneumoniae*) sensor domains have a PDC fold. DctB (3BY9, *Vibrio cholerae*) has two tandem PDC domains. The structures are shown in similar orientations with the N- and C-termini facing down for easy comparison, except DosT and FixL, which are shown with their central β-sheet having the same orientation as the PDC domains but their N- and C-termini facing other directions. The ligands and heme groups of DcuS, CitA, DctB, DosT, and FixL are shown as sticks. All of them are bound at the central β-sheet. NarX (3EZH, *E. coli*) has an all-helical sensor domain, while TorS (3I9Y, *Vibrio parahaemolyticus*) has double helical domains. The RetS (3JYB, *Pseudomonas aeruginosa*) sensor domain is currently the sole structural representative of β-sandwich fold extracytosolic sensors. The ribbon diagrams were prepared with PyMOL (Schrodinger, LLC).

DosS and DosT from *Mycobacterium tuberculosis* are soluble sensor HKs that have dual GAF domains located in the cytosol. The first GAF domain binds a heme group for sensing redox and hypoxia conditions of the cell cytoplasm to regulate the dormancy regulon *Dos*, which is believed by some researchers to allow *M. tuberculosis* to survive in a latent state for decades [4]. The structures of the N-terminal GAF domains of DosS [5] and DosT [6] reveal highly similar structures with a central five-stranded antiparallel β-sheet flanked on one side by the first and last helices and on the other side by some loops and short helices (Figure 2, DosT). The heme group is bound in the center of the β-sheet with the plane of the heme perpendicular to the β-sheet. The PAS domain of FixL from *Rhizobium meliloti* has the same topology of the central β-sheet, but has different α-helices (Figure 2) [7]. The heme binds at a different location of the sheet in a parallel manner.

The most common structural fold of the extracytosolic sensor domains is the mixed αβ fold, which has an identical topology to that of PAS domains [8]. The structures consist of a central 5-stranded antiparallel β-sheet, flanked by α-helices on both sides (Figure 2, top row). These extracytosolic sensor domains are slightly different in structure from the PAS and GAF domains. Their structures fall into a group by themselves and are named as PDC domains, referring to first three structures of this group, i.e. sensor domains of PhoQ, DcuS, and CitA [9]. Among the PDC domains, the structures are similar to each other, especially the N-terminal helix and the position of the C-terminus. The PDC domains have a long N-terminal helix, possibly continuous from the TM1 helix. The N- and C-termini of the domain are next to each other, and both are facing the same direction toward the membrane for connecting to the transmembrane helices. In some structures, there is a short helix at the C-terminus, possibly continuous to the TM2 helix.

Some HK sensor domains are all-helical, represented by those of NarX [10] and TorS [11] (Figure 2). The NarX sensor domain is an antiparallel four-helix bundle. Most of the helices have kinks or bends, suggesting mobility. TorS has two antiparallel four-helix bundles stacked along their bundle axes, with the second one inserted between the last two helices of the first bundle. Their mechanisms for signal sensing are different. NarX binds directly to nitrite and nitrate; while TorS interacts with a periplasmic binding protein TorT to detect trimethylamine-N-oxide.

The crystal structure of the sensor domain of RetS from *P. aeruginosa* reveals a β-sandwich fold (Figure 2) [12]. RetS works with two other HKs, LadS and GacS, to regulate genes for type III secretion system controlling acute infection and those for drug-resistant biofilm formation controlling chronic infection. The RetS sensor domain has two antiparallel β-sheets, with topologies β1-β3-β8-β5-β6 and β2-β9-β4-β7, stacking back-to-back. The β-sandwich fold structure resembles carbohydrate-binding modules.

2.2. Structure and function of HAMP domains

HAMP domains are widely occurring domains of prokaryotic transmembrane receptors. They follow the last TM helix and thus connect the extracytosolic sensory domain to the cytosolic signaling domains. The sequences of HAMP domains have heptad repeats, in which hydrophobic residues occupy positions a and d (Figure 3). The structures of HAMP domains are dimers with each protomer of ~50 residues forming two helices (referred to as Hα1 and Hα2) connected by a linker of ~14 residue. The four helices from two protomers associate to form a parallel four-helix bundle. The linker residues have an extended structure that spans the length of the four-helix bundle [13, 14]. Other than the hydrophobic side chains of the heptad repeats and a conserved glycine residue at the beginning of the linker, HAMP domains do not have strong sequence conservation. Nevertheless, the domains can be exchanged, yielding hybrid proteins that are still functional [15, 16], which suggests that HAMP domains share a conserved mechanism for propagating signals.

The HAMP domain of Af1503, a hypothetical receptor from the archaeon *Archaeoglobus fulgidus* [14] is the first HAMP structure determined (Figure 3). The packing of the 4 helices is different from the expected conventional knobs-into-holes geometry, in which a residue from one helix (knob) packs into a space surrounded by four side chains of the facing helix (hole). Instead, the helical packing of the Af1503 HAMP domain is described as complementary x-da, in which the x- and da-layers alternate along the helices to form mixed x-da layers. In the x-layer, side chains point straight at the central supercoil axis; and in the da-layer, side chains point side ways to form an interacting ring of residues enclosing a central cavity. This non-canonical packing geometry is stabilized by the small side chain of alanine at residue 291 [17]. Mutations of A291 with amino acids of larger side chain convert the helical packing to the knobs-into-holes conformation through a concerted axial rotation of all four helices of ~26° (Figure 3). It was hence proposed that signals propagate through the TM helices and HAMP by helix rotation around an axis perpendicular to the membrane, a so-called gearbox model [18].

The crystal structure of a tri-HAMP unit from the *P. aeruginosa* soluble receptor Aer2 shows that the three HAMP domains each form a parallel four-helix bundle similar to HAMP of Af1503 (Figure 3) [13]. This confirms that the parallel four-helix bundle is likely universal among HAMP domains. The top HAMP domain (HAMP1) is separated from HAMP2 by a helical insert that connects Hα2 of HAMP1 to Hα1 of HAMP2 by a slightly kinked helical insert. HAMP2 and HAMP3 are contiguous and form a concatenated di-HAMP structure. There are two distinct packing configurations among the three HAMP domains. HAMP1 and HAMP3 are similar to each other and resemble that of Af1503. The middle HAMP2 domain, however, has a unique helical packing, in which there is an offset of the helical register between α1 and α2 of half a helical turn (~2-3 Å). This results in side chain staggering of the buried hydrophobic core between the two helices of the same polypeptide chain. The two α1 helices coil around each other, so do the two α2 helices; but the two coiled-coils have limited interactions with each other. The unique packing of HAMP2 leads to a slightly different possible mechanism of signaling propagation by the HAMP domain: a combination of vertical movement and helical rotation, also known as screw-like motion.

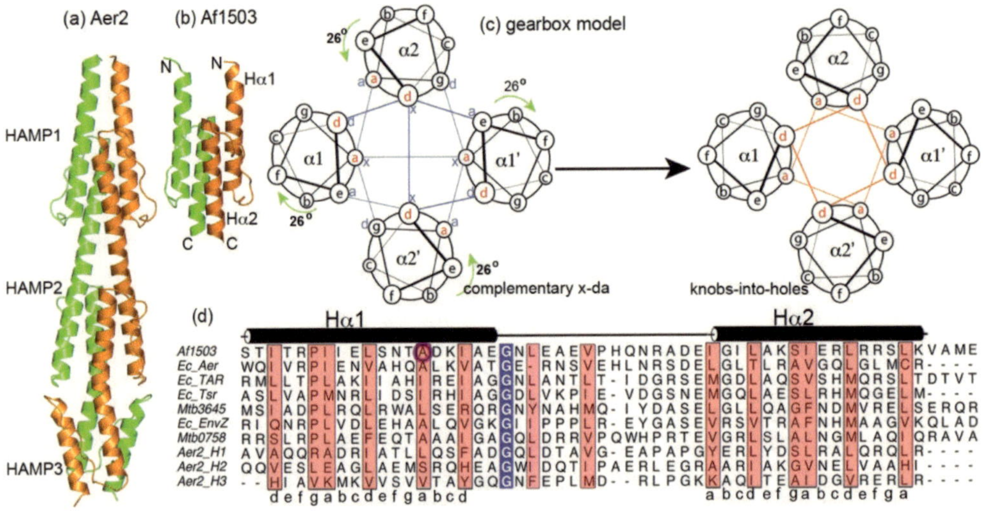

Figure 3. HAMP domain structures, a gearbox model for signal propagation, and sequences. The crystal structure of a tri-HAMP domain from Aer2 (Pdb code 3LNR) shows that all three HAMP domains have a four-helix bundle structure (a), which is similar to that of the HAMP domain of Af1503 (2L7H) (b). Each four-helix bundle is a homodimer of a parallel two-helix coiled-coil of helix Hα1 and Hα2. Af1503 has a helical packing of complementary x-da, which can be converted to the canonical knobs-into-holes supercoil by a 26 º rotation of each helix (c). (d) Sequence alignment of HK HAMP domains shows heptad repeats with hydrophobic side chains at positions a and d. Conserved hydrophobic residues are highlighted in red. There is a highly conserved Gly at the beginning of the linker, highlighted in blue. Residue A291 in Af1503 is circled. Aer2_H1, Aer2_H2, and Aer2_H3 in (d) are sequences for Aer2 HAMP1, HAMP2, and HAMP3, respectively.

2.3. The dimerization and phosphorylation domain

The dimerization and phosphorylation domain is a conserved domain of histidine kinases. This domain is often abbreviated as DHp for dimerization and histidine phosphotransfer. It is also referred to as dimerization domain or histidine kinase domain A. The sequence of DHp contains the H box that is part of the signature motifs defining histidine kinases (Figure 4). The histidine residue in the H box motif is absolutely conserved and is the site for autophosphorylation and subsequent transfer of the phosphoryl group to downstream proteins. This domain participates in dimerization of the histidine kinase. DHp is located in the cytosol and directly follows the HAMP domain, and it is immediately followed by the CA domain in the prototypical histidine kinases (Figure 1).

The structure of the DHp domain consists of two α-helices (referred to as Dα1 and Dα2), that form an antiparallel coiled-coil (also referred to as helical hairpin), and two protomers associate to form a four-helix bundle (Figure 5). The conserved histidine residue is on helix Dα1. Similar to HAMP domains, sequences of the DHp domains have heptad repeats. Several structures of DHp have been determined. The NMR structure of the *E. coli* EnvZ DHp shows a four-helix bundle that is relatively straight [19]. The phosphorylation site H243 is solvent exposed and located in the middle of helix Dα1, which is more mobile than

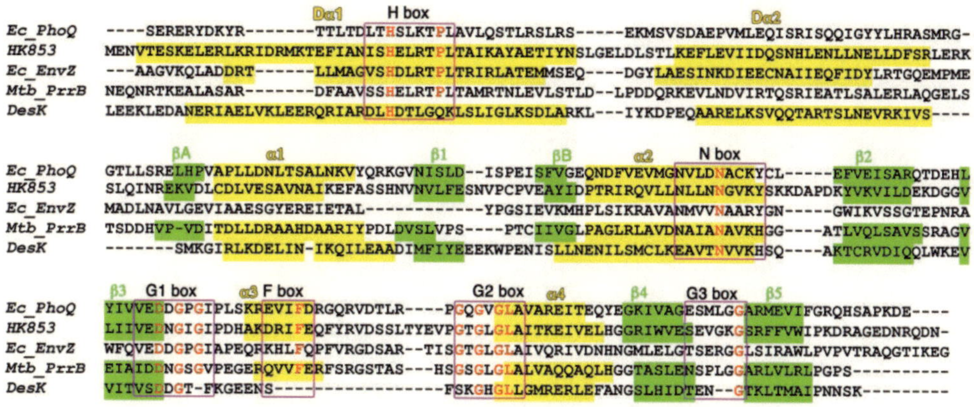

Figure 4. Sequences of the DHp and CA domains of HKs. Conserved sequence motifs H, N, G1, F, G2, and G3 boxes are in magenta boxes. Helices are highlighted in yellow, and β-strands in green.

helix Dα2, especially around the conserved H-box residues. The intra-subunit interface is mostly hydrophobic; the dimer interface, however, contains two acidic clusters. A related phosphotransferase Spo0B from *B. subtilis* has a similar dimerization domain of four-helix bundle [20]. The active site residue H30 is in the middle of helix Dα1, with its side chain protruding to the surface, similar to that of the EnvZ DHp domain.

The structure of the entire cytoplasmic portion of HK853, a putative sensor HK from *Thermotoga maritima*, shows that the DHp domain forms a four-helix bundle slightly different from that of EnvZ [21]. The HK853 four-helix bundle has a larger twist angle of ~25°, compared to that of EnvZ, which is unusually straight and parallel. The connections between hairpin helices have different topologies between the two structures. EnvZ is unique in this respect as all other known DHp structures have the same topology as HK853 (Figure 5). HK853 does not have a HAMP domain but has a linker of 22 residues between TM2 and DHp. This linker region forms a helix, possibly continuous from TM2 to Dα1. The two helices of the dimer associate to form a left-handed coiled-coil on top of the four-helix bundle. There is a kink in Dα1 induced by P265, which is near the phosphorylation site H260 and is well conserved among HKs. This kink is common among all DHp structures, even those without a proline, such as Spo0B and DesK (Figure 5).

2.4. ATP-binding domain

In prototypical sensor histidine kinases, the ATP-binding domain is located at the carboxyl terminus of the polypeptide (Figure 1). The ATP-binding domain is often abbreviated as CA for catalytic and ATP-binding. This domain binds ATP, which then donates its γ-phosphate group to the conserved histidine residue on the DHp domain. Sequences of the CA domains have well conserved N, G1, F, G2, and G3 box sequence motifs (Figure 4). Together with the H box at the DHp domain, they are the markers to annotate histidine kinases from DNA sequences.

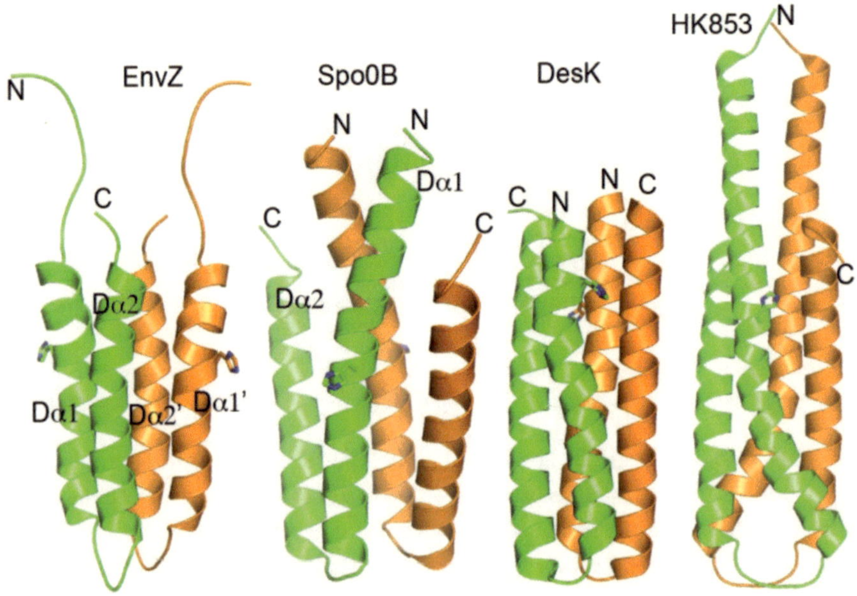

Figure 5. Structures of the DHp domains. All structures show an antiparallel helical bundle. The phosphorylation site histidine is shown as sticks. This histidine residue is located in the middle of Dα1. There is a kink of the helix right below the histidine residue, produced by a strongly conserved proline residue in EnvZ (PDB ID 1JOY) and HK853 (2C2A). DesK (3EHF) and Spo0B (1IXM) do not have this proline residue but still have a kink right below the histidine residue. Structures of DHp from Spo0B, DesK, and HK853 are a part of larger structures containing a C-terminal domain.

The structures of the CA domains are well conserved, as expected from their highly conserved sequences. The structures have an αβ sandwich fold containing two layers, a layer of mixed 5-stranded β-sheet and a layer of three α-helices (Figure 6). The CA domain of DesK from *B. subtilis* has the shortest sequence and represents the minimal core structure for this domain [22]. Most of other structures have additional α-helices, β-strands, and a longer ATP-lid (the loop covering the ATP-binding site). The ATP-binding site in DesK is much shallower due to the lack of additional structural elements and a shorter ATP-lid. Interestingly, an intact ATP molecule binds in the ATP-binding site with full occupancy, even though the phosphate groups are partially exposed to the protein surface. It is likely that in the crystal, the protein is in a conformation that shields any nucleophilic water from getting access to the phosphates, thereby protecting the ATP from hydrolysis during crystal growth. In this case, phosphotransfer will occur only in the presence of the DHp domain with the conserved histidine functioning as a nucleophile to transfer the γ-phosphate to the histidine.

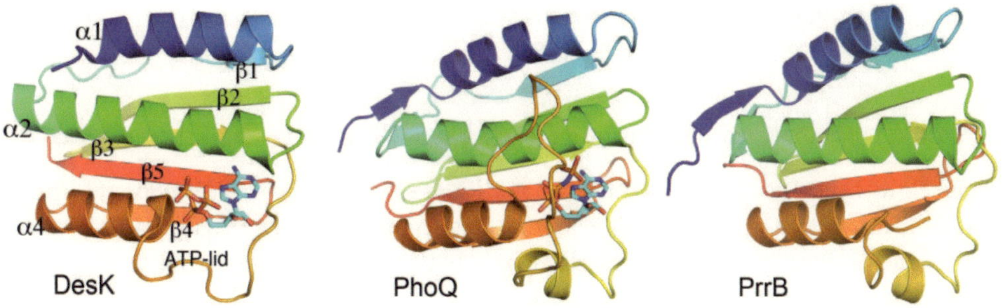

Figure 6. Ribbon diagrams of the ATP-binding domains. Each domain is colored in a rainbow spectrum with blue for the N-terminus and red for the C-terminus. Bound ATP in DesK (PDB code 3EHG) and AMPPNP in PhoQ (1ID0) are shown as sticks. The structure of PrrB (1YS3) from *M. tuberculosis* does not have a ligand bound, and part of the ATP-lid is disordered. Helices and β-strands are labeled on the structure of DesK CA. The short helix α3 in the ATP-lid is missing in DesK.

The ATP-binding site is at one end of the domain (Figure 6) and involves both absolutely conserved and partially conserved residues from the N, G1, F, G2, and G3 boxes (Figure 4). Residues from the G1 and G3 boxes are involved in binding the adenosine moiety; those from the N and G2 boxes contact both the adenosine moiety and the triphosphates-Mg^{2+} moiety. The structure of *E. coli* PhoQ in complex with AMPPNP reveals detailed binding interactions of the conserved boxes with ATP [23]. In the G1 box, the conserved Asp has a direct H-bond to the amino group and a water-mediated H-bond to N1 of adenine. In the N box, the side chains of conserved N389 and partially conserved N385 interact with the α-phosphate; the side chain oxygen of conserved N389 has a water-mediated H-bond to N1 of adenine; the partially conserved K392 and Y393 interact with the γ-phosphate through their side chains. The side chain of Y393 stacks with the adenine ring, while that of I420 from G1 box flanks the other face of the adenine ring. The side chains of partially conserved N385 (N box) and Q442 (G2 box) coordinate the divalent cation, which binds to the triphosphate group. DesK has similar binding interactions with the adenosine moiety, but slightly different binding interactions with the phosphate groups, although both proteins involve residues of the N and G2 boxes for binding the phosphate groups.

A long loop covering the ATP-binding site is called ATP-lid, which spans from the F box to the beginning of helix α4 and plays an important role in binding ATP. The ATP-lid is highly mobile; it has several glycine residues, including the conserved G2 box that contains three glycine residues (Figure 4). The bound ATP has extensive contacts with the ATP-lid residues, and thus ATP binding induces the closure of the ATP-lid. In the absence of ATP, this loop is partially disordered in crystal structures. Even in the presence of ATP, the ATP-lid shows high flexibility, indicated by high B-factors or in some cases is partially disordered in crystal structures [21-24]. The flexibility of the ATP-lid is important not only for binding ATP, but also for interacting with the DHp domain for the phosphotransfer reactions. The ATP-binding domain must adopt several positions relative to the DHp domain because the HK functions as an autokinase, phosphotransferase, or phosphatase in response to the environmental stimulates received. The flexibility of the ATP-lid allows the CA domain to bind to different regions of DHp depending on the conformation of the DHp domain and the status of the ATP-binding site of the CA domain.

2.5. Signal transduction mechanism from sensor domain to the kinase domain

Signals flow from the sensor domain to the kinase domain by conformational changes throughout the entire protein. Environmental cues received by the sensor domain cause a conformational change in the sensor domain. That conformational change is transmitted through the transmembrane helices and the HAMP domain to the kinase domain. Most of isolated sensor domains are monomers in solution. However, they are expected to form dimers in the context of the whole protein because the DHp and HAMP domains are homodimers. Therefore, ligand-induced dimerization cannot be a mechanism of signal transduction through the cell membrane. Instead, there are structural changes of the sensor domains upon ligand binding that could trigger rotation or piston-like translation movements of the TM helices [9, 25].

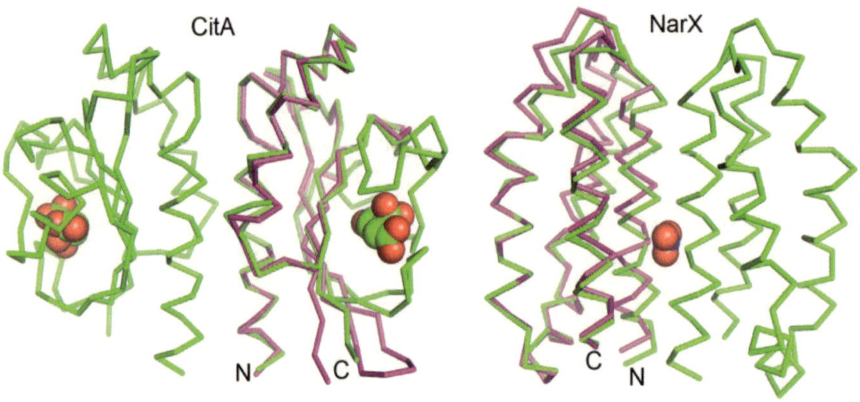

Figure 7. Piston model of ligand-induced conformational changes in the sensor domain. In both CitA (left panel, Pdb codes 2J80 and 2V9A) and NarX (right panel, 3EZH and 3EZI), ligand-bound structures are dimers in the crystal (green molecules), while ligand free forms are monomers (magenta color). Ligands are represented as space-filling models.

Comparison of structures of the sensor domain of CitA with and without citrate bound suggests a piston-type transmembrane signaling [8]. The sensor domain of CitA has a central 5-stranded anti-parallel β-sheet flanked by α-helices on both sides (Figure 2). The β-sheet curls up to one side where citrate binds. There are two loops, referred to as major loop and minor loop, which cover the citrate-binding site. The major loop is disordered in the citrate-free structure and becomes ordered in the presence of citrate in the binding site. Binding of citrate also induces more bent of the central β-sheet. This results in lifting of the C-terminus of the domain relative to the N-terminal helix (Figure 7). The C-terminus of the domain connects to the second transmembrane helix (TM2). Therefore, binding of citrate induces a piston-type movement of TM2 relative to TM1. Similar piston-type movement has been proposed for NarX from *E. coli*, whose sensor domain is a four-helix bundle that forms a dimer when binding nitrate (Figure 7) [10]. Binding of nitrate induces the movement of the N-terminal helix toward the cell membrane, relative to the C-terminal helix. Since the N- and C-terminal helices are expected to connect to TM1 and TM2, respectively, the relative movement of the two helices would push down TM1 or lift up TM2. This movement of helices could also translate into rotations of the TM helices, if winding or unwinding of helical turns occurs.

A rotation or screw-like motion of TM2 has been proposed as the signal transduction mechanism from the sensory rhodopsin into the cytosol for HtrII [26]. Based on the structure of HtrII, the transmembrane helices of prototypical HKs are expected to form a four-helix bundle [27]. A rotation or screw-like motion of the TM helices for propagating signal through membrane is compatible with that proposed for the HAMP domain, which is often found between TM2 and the DHp domain. Structural and biochemical studies suggest that HAMP domains are not rigid structures. They can alternate between different structures through helical rotation [14] or a shift in register of coiled-coils and rotation [13]. Mutation of an alanine residue of the HAMP domain of Af1503 into larger side chain residues changes the helical packing gradually from complementary x-da to the canonical knobs-into-holes mode [17]. Through these conformational changes, the HAMP domain passes the signals from the sensor domain to the downstream kinase domain.

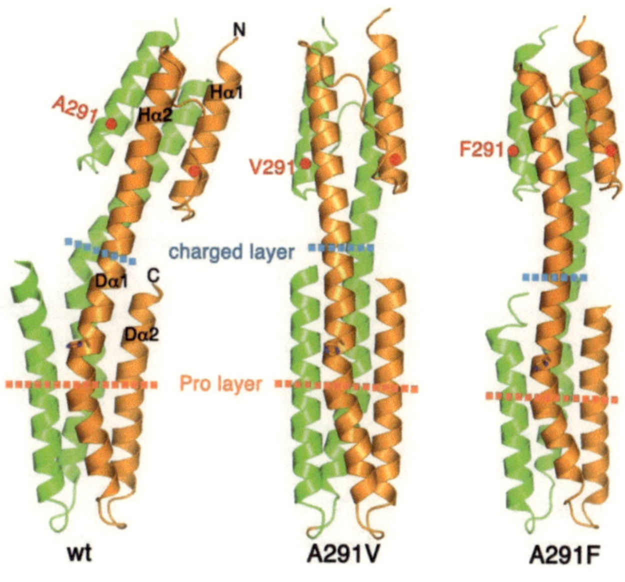

Figure 8. Crystal structures of chimeras of Af1503 HAMP fused to DHp of EnvZ. Mutations at A291 of HAMP cause conformational changes in the HAMP helical packing, which propagate to the DHp domain. The mutation sites are labeled with a red dot. Approximate positions of the charged layer and proline layer are marked. PDB codes for the structural models are 3ZRX (wt), 3ZRW (A291V), and 3ZRV (A291F).

Structures of chimeras of the Af1503 HAMP fused with the DHp domain of EnvZ show that conformational changes in the HAMP domain can trigger changes in the structure of the downstream DHp domain [18]. Figure 8 shows three crystal structures of the chimeras. The HAMP domains preserve the same conformations as their corresponding isolated domains. Mutations of A291 into amino acids with larger hydrophobic side chains change the helical packing conformation. These conformational changes in the HAMP domain propagate to the DHp domain through the connecting helices. The helices linking the HAMP domain to the DHp domain do not have a strong hydrophobic core as in the four-helix bundles but are relatively flexible, showing variations among the structures with different mutations. Conformational variation is the most pronounced at the junction between the DHp four-helix bundle and the two-helix coiled-coil where there are charged residues (charged layer, Figure 8). The induced rotational movements in helix Dα1 gradually diminish at the conserved proline, which produces a kink in the helix. Helix Dα2 also changes conformation responding to changes of Dα1, and as a result the bundle radius differs above the proline layer among variant structures.

The structural changes in DHp induced by the HAMP domain are likely to alter the activities by regulating interactions between the DHp and CA domains. Despite the structural changes triggered by varying conformations in HAMP, the phosphorylation site histidine remains little perturbed, and thus altering accessibility of the conserved histidine is unlikely to be the mechanism of signal transmission. The lower half of the DHp helical bundle (below the proline layer) remains invariant among the structures. This region contains many residues important for binding the cognate RR and contributes the majority of the interface for RR binding in the HK-RR complex structures [19, 28]. Therefore, blocking direct binding of RR is unlikely to be a mechanism for signaling either. However, the region of DHp most variable among the structures (charged layer) plays an important role in interacting with the CA domain. In the structure of HK853-RR468 complex, residues F428 and L444 of the ATP-lid interact with an exposed hydrophobic core of DHp near the charged layer, and this interaction locks the ATP-binding domain in a kinase-inactive state [28]. It is likely that conformational changes triggered by signals transmitted from the HAMP domain either promote this DHp-CA interaction (phosphatase state) or release the CA domain for it to phosphorylate the conserved histidine (kinase state).

Several structures of the entire kinase domain (DHp + CA) are available and give insights into the interactions between the two sub-domains. The crystal structure of the entire cytoplasmic portion of HK853 from *T. maritima* shows a conformational state that is ready for the phosphotransfer reaction [21]. The HK853 cytoplasmic domain forms a dimer through the DHp domain (Figure 9a). The CA domain is connected to the DHp domain through a short linker. The crystal structure contains an ADPβN, from hydrolyzed AMPPNP, in the CA domain. The ATP-lid is flexible and partially disordered, despite the presence of the ADP analog in the ATP-binding site. The H260 side chain is fully exposed to the surface of the protein. There is a sulfate ion in the crystal structure bound next to the Nε atom of H260, mimicking the phosphorylated histidine. Contacts between DHp and CA are exclusively within one polypeptide chain and involve mostly conserved hydrophobic residues. The importance of the interface residues in the HK function is confirmed by site-directed mutagenesis studies [21]. In the DHp domain, the interface involves both α helices

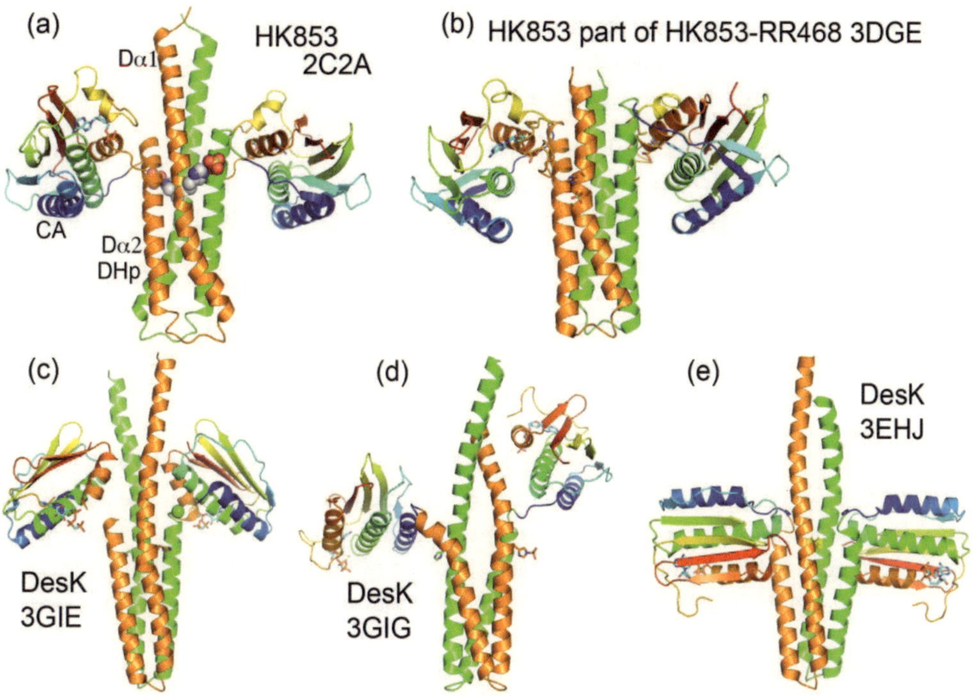

Figure 9. Structures of the entire kinase domain containing the DHp and CA subdomains. DHp domains are colored in orange for one subunit and green for the other. CA domains are colored in a rainbow spectrum. ATP analogs and the essential histidine side chains are shown as sticks except in (a) where the H260 side chains and a sulfate are shown as space-filling models. The hinge pivot residue G243 is shown as a green sphere in (c).

near the charged layer (Figures 8 and 9), and in the CA domain it involves the ATP-lid, helix α4, and residues at N-terminus of α2. The interactions are relatively weak, and thus the domain interface is dynamic, allowing the CA domain to move to other locations on DHp. The signals from the sensor domain control the interfacial stability through conformational changes of the helical bundle. The DHp-CA interface is destabilized for the kinase activity and stabilized for the phosphatase activity.

The crystal structure of HK853 complexed with RR468 reveals another binding interface between DHp and CA that is created by conformational changes in the helical packing [28]. In this structure, the CA domain moves closer to H260 of the same subunit (Figure 9b). This suggests that the autophosphorylation occurs in *cis*, although in the crystal structure, the ATP-lid interacts with the bound RR and blocks the access of the phosphorylation site histidine to ATP. The structure has a sulfate near each phosphoacceptor aspartate of RR, mimicking the phosphorylated RR. Therefore, the structure represents a conformational state poised for dephosphorylation of the RR. This phosphatase-competent state has a stronger domain interface between DHp and CA. A rotation of the helix Dα1 N-terminal coiled-coil region and a concerted inverse twist of Dα2, as in the proposed gearbox model for transmitting signals through HAMP domains (Figure 3), expose parts of the hydrophobic core of DHp near the charged layer. This allows residues F428 and L444 of ATP-lid to interact with the exposed hydrophobic pocket of DHp of the same subunit, and thus allows the CA domain to move to a new binding site.

Structural plasticity of the HK proteins is essential to allow conformational changes in order to transmit signals received at the sensor domain to the kinase domain and switch its enzymatic activities. This structural plasticity is well demonstrated by the structures of the cytoplasmic domain of the *B. substilis* DesK, a thermo-sensing histidine kinase [24]. The DHp domain is highly mobile, adopting different conformations to allow the CA domain to bind at different positions in different functional states. The structures reveal three distinct conformational states with different helical packing of the DHp domain and the relative position of the CA domain. One conformational state represents the autokinase-competent state. This conformational state is characterized by the lack of specific interactions between the DHp and CA domains, allowing the CA domain to move to a position suitable for autophosphorylation. A single rigid-body rotation of the CA domain along the interdomain hinge residue G243 can bring the ATP γ-phosphate close to the side chain of the phosphorylation site histidine of the other protomer (Figure 9c). In addition, the contact surfaces are complementary to each other in both contour and charges. The structures are consistent with a *trans* phosphorylation mechanism. That the autokinase-competent state lacks specific interdomain interactions is consistent with observations that isolated DHp domains can be phosphorylated in the presence of isolated CA domains. A second conformational state is poised for the phosphotransfer reaction, represented by structures of a phosphorylated DesK and a phosphomimetic H188E mutant. Both structures show a similar asymmetric homodimer. One of the CA domains interacts with both Dα1 helices at the coiled-coil region. This interaction precludes the binding of the other CA domain, which makes no contacts with the DHp domain in the phosphorylated DesK structure (Figure 9d), but is completely disordered in the H188E-ADP structure. The helical bending at the phosphorylation site histidine is more pronounced partially due to the negatively charged phosphohistidine associating with conserved basic residues of the opposite protomer. The third conformational state is a phosphatase-competent state, inferred from the structures of the H188V mutant. This mutation abolishes the kinase activity but retains the wild-type level phosphatase activity. The V188 side chain is buried in the hydrophobic core of the four-helix bundle (Figure 9e). This removes the kink in Dα1 and allows a tight packing rigid helical bundle. The changes in the structure of DHp also expose a patch of hydrophobic surface on Dα1 near the charged layer for a tight association with the CA domain. The CA domain interacts with the same surface of DHp as seen in the structures of HK853 [21] and KinB [29].

3. Structures of response regulators

Response regulators are simpler in structure than histidine kinases. The prototypical RR has two domains: a receiver domain that accepts a phosphoryl group from a cognate HK and an effector domain that generates the outputs of the signaling events. The structure and sequence of receiver domains are well conserved. In contrast, effector domains are variable, especially at the sequence level, reflecting their diverse output functions. The majority of RRs are transcription regulators with their effector domains as DNA-binding domains. A significant fraction of RRs have effector domains as enzymes. Many others have effector domains for binding RNA, ligands, or proteins to regulate bacterial cellular process at post-transcriptional and post-translational levels. There are also single domain RRs that have only the receiver domains such as CheY and Spo0F. RRs have been studied extensively for decades, and an extensive amount of structural data is available, as well as many well-written reviews [30]. I will focus my efforts on transcription regulator RRs and will give a summary on how phosphorylation of the receiver domain controls the activities of the effector domain with respect to their structure-function relationship.

3.1. Receiver domain structures

Receiver domains have well-conserved sequences and structures, suggesting a common signaling mechanism by two component systems to pass signals from HKs to their cognate RRs. The receiver domain is also known as the phosphorylation domain or regulatory domain. There is an invariable aspartate residue in the receiver domain that accepts a phosphoryl group from a cognate HK. Phosphorylation results in conformational changes in the domain, which is transmitted to the effector domain to regulate its activities. Receiver domains have a conserved $(\beta\alpha)_5$ fold (Figures 10 and 11), in which alternating β-strands and α-helices in the sequence fold into a central five-stranded parallel β-sheet surrounded by helices α1 and α5 on one side and helices α2, α3, and α4 on the other side. The β-sheet consists of mainly hydrophobic side chains that form a hydrophobic core. The α-helices are amphipathic and pack against the central β-sheet with their hydrophobic face. Most of the conserved residues are at the C-terminal ends of strands β1, β3, and β4. Helix α1 is involved in binding to the DHp domain of HK [28]. Although the structure and position of this helix is well conserved among RR structures, the amino acid sequence conservation is limited to the hydrophobic residues involved in packing against the hydrophobic core of the β-sheet (Figure 10). This helix is likely to play an important role in the specificity of HK-RR pairs.

The phosphorylation site is located at an acidic pocket near the C-termini of strands β1 and β3, where the conserved acidic side chains are clustered together. These acidic side chains are involved in binding a divalent cation, Mg^{2+} or Mn^{2+}, that is essential for the phosphorylation reaction [31]. An absolutely conserved aspartate at the end of the strand β3 is the phosphoacceptor. The loop β3-α3 forms a conserved structure that is held together by conserved residues: a Pro at 4 residues after the phosphorylation site aspartate and a Gly, which is at 4 residues after the Pro in sequence and the first residue of helix α3 (Figure 10).

The α4-β5-α5 face of the receiver domain has been proposed to be important for the function of RRs [32, 33]. Many RRs in the OmpR/PhoB subfamily are thought to be dimers in their active form. Structures of several RR receiver domains are found to form dimers through the α4-β5-α5 face when activated. Exposed side chains on this surface are primarily hydrophilic, suggesting that any interactions through this α4-β5-α5 face are likely to be dynamic. Comparison among receiver domain structures reveals that this face is considerably

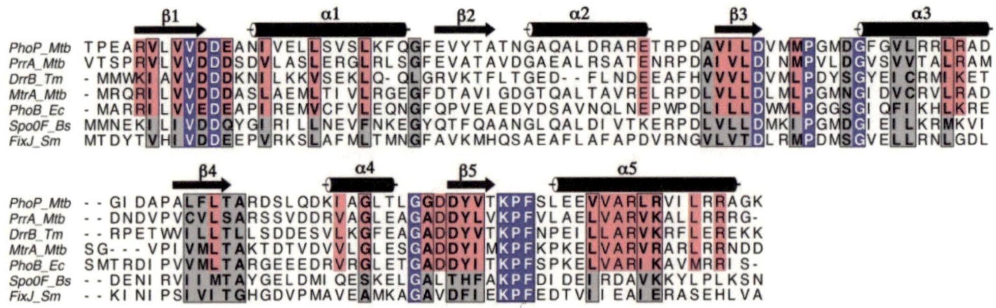

Figure 10. Sequence alignment of the response regulator receiver domains. The top five sequences, PhoP, PrrA and MtrA from *M. tuberculosis*, DrrB from *T. maritima*, and PhoB from *E. coli*, belong to the OmpR/PhoB subfamily. Spo0F from *B. subtilis* is a single domain RR. FixJ of *S. Meliloti* is in the NarL/FixJ subfamily. Identical residues for all sequences are shaded in blue. Highly conserved residues in the OmpR/PhoB subfamily are shaded in red. Moderately conserved residues across all sequences are shaded in gray.

variable. The sequence of helix α5 is well conserved among OmpR/PhoB subfamily RRs (Figure 10). Yet the length of this helix varies among known structures [34]. In the structure of PrrA from *M. tuberculosis* this helix has different lengths between two molecules in the crystal asymmetric unit [35]. Helix α4 and its flanking loops also have variable structures among RRs. Flexibility of the α4-β5-α5 elements is likely to be important for phosphorylation regulation of RR activities.

Activation of RRs by phosphorylation induces structural changes in the α4-β5-α5 face. This is accomplished by movements of two key residues, a conserved Thr/Ser at the C-terminus of β4 and a moderately conserved Tyr/Phe in the middle of β5 (Figure 11). These residues are referred to as switch residues. In the unphosphorylated RR, the side chain of Thr/Ser is oriented away from the phosphoacceptor, and that of Tyr/Phe extends outward toward the surface of the α4-β5-α5 face. Structures of activated receiver domains reveal that these side chains move in response to phosphorylation [36, 37]. All activated receiver domains of the OmpR/PhoB subfamily form a symmetric dimer through the same interface involving α4-β5-α5. Phosphorylation of the phosphoacceptor aspartate residue allows the side chain of the Thr/Ser residue to move closer to the phosphate group to make a favorable hydrogen bond. Repositioning the Thr/Ser side chain shifts the β4-α4 loop and helix α4, and makes the inward conformation of the Tyr/Phe residue more energetically favorable. Another conserved residue, a Lys in the β5-α5 loop, forms a salt bridge to the phosphoryl group and brings some modest shift in the β5-α5 loop [31]. This Lys side chain has a salt bridge to the side chain of phosphoacceptor aspartate in the unphosphorylated structure PhoP from *M. tuberculosis* [34]. It plays an important role in stabilizing the active site structure, but probably has only minor effects on structural switch between activated and non-activated RRs. Phosphorylation of NarL/FixJ subfamily RRs produces similar conformational changes in switch residues and results in dimerization through the α4-β5-α5 face, although the dimer interface are not identical to that of OmpR/PhoB RRs (Figure 11d). The difference in dimer interface might be due to lack of divalent cation in the crystal structure of FixJ [38].

Activation by BeF_3 and Mg^{2+} did not induce symmetric dimer formation of single domain response regulator RR468 [28]. However, the switch residues are in the active conformation as observed for all other RRs, suggesting that conformational changes of switch residues is the common mechanism for all RRs.

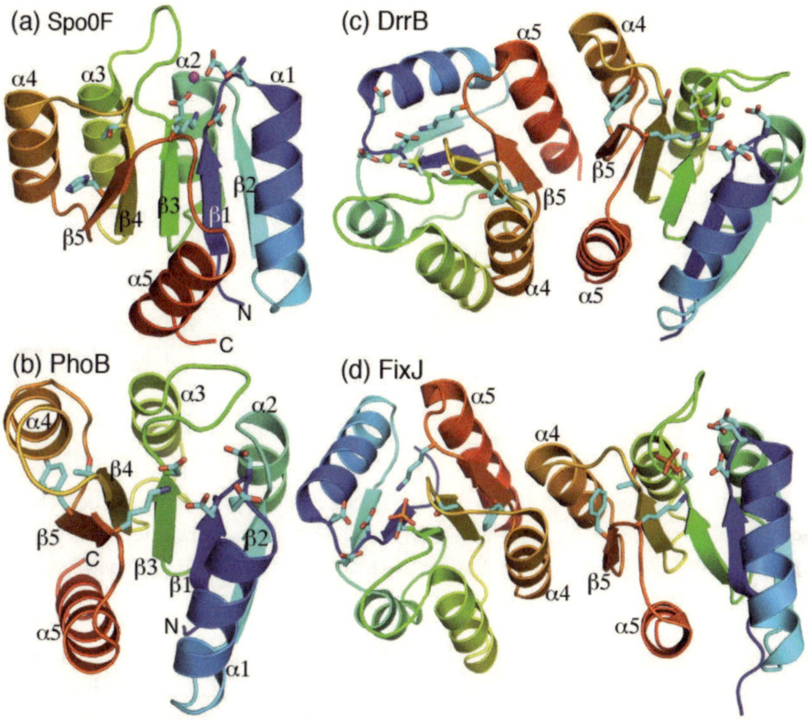

Figure 11. Structures of the receiver domains of response regulators. Each individual domain is colored from N- to C- terminus in a rainbow spectrum. Phosphorylation site residues and switch residues are shown as sticks. Spo0F (PDB code 1PEY) from *B. subtilis* binds a Mn^{2+} ion, shown in magenta. Both PhoB (1B00) from *E. coli* and Spo0B are non-activated. DrrB (3NNS) from *T. maritima* is activated with binding of BeF_3 and Mg^{2+}, shown as sticks and a green sphere, respectively. FixJ (1D5W) from *S. Meliloti* is activated by phosphorylation, but without divalent cations.

3.2. Structures of the effector domains

Unlike the receiver domains, the effector domains are very diverse, reflecting the diversity of cellular processes that are controlled by two-component systems. Effector domains are also referred to as output domains. They can be DNA-binding, RNA-binding, ligand-binding, or transporter output domains, or enzymes [30]. Except in archaea, which has almost 50% of RRs containing only the receiver domain, a great majority of bacterial RRs are transcription regulators that contain a C-terminal effector domain as a DNA-binding domain.

DNA-binding effector domains are grouped into several subfamilies based on predicted domain structures from amino acid sequences [30]. The largest subfamily is the OmpR/PhoB group, whose structure has a winged helix-turn-helix (wHTH) motif. The second largest subfamily is the NarL/FixJ group, which has a helix-turn-helix (HTH) DNA-binding motif. Another subfamily LytR/AgrA is also fairly common. A structure of a member of this subfamily, LytTR from *S. aureus*, shows that the DNA-binding domain consists mostly of β-strands [39]. The loops between the β-strands interact with DNA bases with side chains inserting into both major and minor grooves of DNA. Other subfamilies of DNA-binding response regulators are less common and are present only in certain types of bacterial species.

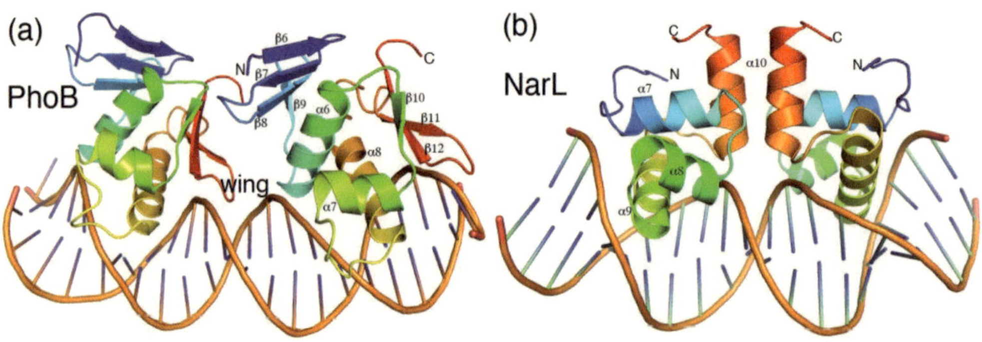

Figure 12. Structures of response regulator effector domains binding to DNA. (a) PhoB (1GXP) of *E. coli* binds to direct repeat Pho Box DNA as a tandem dimer. The PhoB effector domain has a winged HTH fold. (b) NarL (1JE8) of *E. coli* recognizes palindromic DNA sequences and forms a symmetric dimer through association of helix α10 on binding DNA.

The DNA-binding domain of the OmpR/PhoB subfamily has a conserved winged helix-turn-helix fold (Figure 12a). The structure starts with an N-terminal four-stranded anti-parallel β-sheet (β6 to β9), followed by three α-helices (α6 to α8) in the middle, and a β-hairpin (β11 and β12) at the C-terminus. A short strand (β10) between α6 and α7 assembles with the C-terminal β-hairpin to form a three-stranded anti-parallel β-sheet. The two β-sheets sandwich the three α-helices in the middle. The β-hairpin is called the wing, and α7, α8 and loop α7-α8 together constitute the helix-turn-helix motif. Helix α8 is the sequence recognition helix, which inserts into the major groove of DNA [40]. The β-hairpin (wing) binds in the minor groove of DNA. Loop α7-α8 is termed transaction loop because it is essential for transcription activation.

The C-terminal DNA-binding domain of the NarL/FixJ subfamily is a compact bundle of 4 α-helices (Figure 12). The second and third helices (α8 and α9) form a helix-turn-helix motif that interacts with the major groove of DNA [41, 42]. Helix α9 is the recognition helix that inserts into major groove of DNA with side chains interacting with DNA bases. The proteins bind DNA as a symmetric dimer to recognize palindromic DNA repeats. Helix α10 and the loop α7-α8 form the protein dimer interface in the protein-DNA complex. Isolated DNA-binding domains, however, are found to be monomeric in solution when not binding to DNA [42].

3.3. Structures of full-length response regulators and regulation mechanism

Full-length structures are available for the OmpR/PhoB and NarL/FixJ subfamilies of response regulators. Even though most RRs have only two domains, full-length structures prove to be difficult to obtain, especially for the OmpR/PhoB subfamily. This is most likely due to the dynamic nature of interactions between the receiver and effector domains. The domains are individually folded, and their associations are transient if they do associate with each other. The dynamic and transient nature of domain interactions is important for the regulation of DNA-binding activities. Signals transmitted from the HK through phosphorylation of the receiver domains must be able to relay to the DNA-binding domain by conformational changes of the receiver domain. Phosphorylation promotes dimerization of the receiver domain and in some cases releases the blockage of the DNA-binding element of the receiver domain. So far, all available structures of full-length RRs are non-activated and without DNA bound.

The full-length NarL structure in its unphosphorylated form reveals that the receiver domain is associated with the DNA-binding domain through an interface involving the DNA-binding elements [43]. The linker between the two domains forms a helix ($\alpha6$) followed by a flexible loop that is disordered in the crystal structure (Figure 13). Helix $\alpha6$ packs against $\alpha4$ of the receiver domain and $\alpha10$ of the effector domain. The domain interface also involves helices $\alpha8$ and $\alpha9$, locking the DNA-sequence-recognition helix $\alpha9$ in a manner incapable of inserting into the DNA major groove. Phosphorylation is expected to dissociate the effector domain from the receiver domain, thus allowing it to bind DNA. Unphosphorylated NarL does not bind DNA in solution. NarL binds to inverted-repeat DNA sequences as a symmetric dimer, whose interface involves helix $\alpha10$ and loop $\alpha7$-$\alpha8$ (Figure 12). Phosphorylation may also promote dimerization of the receiver domain and thus strengthens the NarL dimer.

Full-length structures of unphosphorylated StyR and DosR, which are members of the NarL/FixJ subfamily RRs, are also known (Figure 13). The receiver domain of StyR from *Pseudomonas fluorescens* has a conserved $(\beta\alpha)_5$ fold [44]. Its DNA-binding domain has the same fold as that of NarL. However, the interdomain linker forms a long helix continuous from $\alpha5$ of the receiver domain that separates the N- and C-terminal domains by more than 16 Å, exposing the helix-turn-helix motif for binding DNA in the unphosphorylated state. Phosphorylation increases DNA-binding affinity by ~10-fold, presumably through dimerization of the receiver domain that brings two effector domains next to each other for binding to DNA inverted repeats. DosR from *M. tuberculosis* forms a dimer with a unique structure [45]. Its receiver domain has a $(\beta\alpha)_4$ fold instead of the $(\beta\alpha)_5$ fold observed for all other RRs (Figure 13b), even though the conserved residues in the $\beta5$ to $\alpha5$ region are present in the DosR sequence. The sequence for the canonical $\beta5$ to $\alpha5$ region forms a long helix, pairing with a helix of linker residues to form an antiparallel coiled-coil (Figure 13b). These two helices form an antiparallel four-helix bundle with the same helices from another subunit, accounting for a major part of the dimer interface. Helices $\alpha9$ and $\alpha10$ have extensive interactions with the receiver domain, locking the structure in an inactive conformation. Activation by phosphorylation presumably causes significant structural

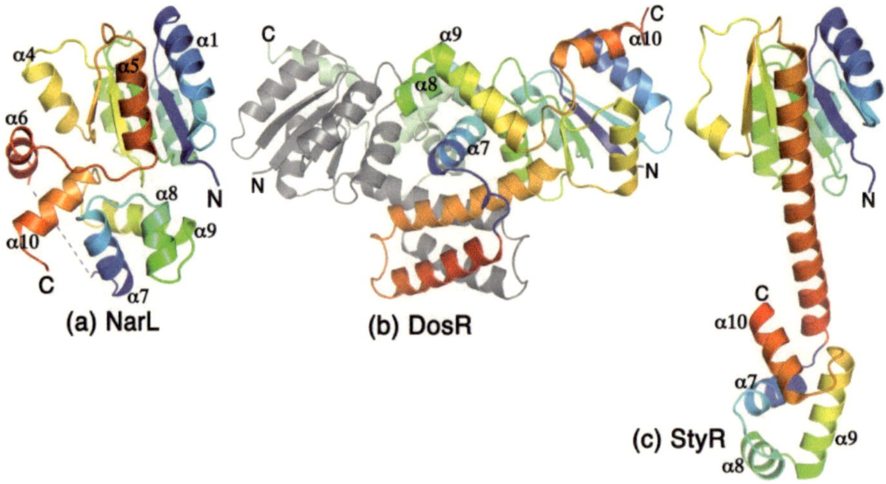

Figure 13. Full-length structures of the NarL/FixJ subfamily RRs. The receiver domains are colored in a rainbow spectrum from N-terminus in blue to the linker in red; the effector domains are separately colored in another rainbow spectrum from blue (α7) to red (α10). (a) NarL (PDB code 1RNL) has a tight packing between domains that blocks sequence recognition helix α9. Part of the linker that is disordered is depicted as a dashed line. (b) DosR (3C3W) forms a dimer, and one of the subunit is colored in gray for the receiver domain and the linker, and in pale green for the effector domain. (c) StyR (1ZN2) has a long helix α5 continuous into the linker that separates the two domains apart.

rearrangements that allows the receiver domain to form a dimer of $(\beta\alpha)_5$ fold and release the effector domain to bind DNA inverted repeats [46].

OmpR/PhoB subfamily RRs have been extensively studied in recent years. In addition to many isolated receiver and effector domain structures, there are six full-length RR structures available, DrrB [47] and DrrD [48] from *T. maritima*, and RegX3 [49], PrrA [35], MtrA [50], and PhoP [34] from *M. tuberculosis*. All structures are in the unphosphorylated forms. The interdomain interfaces are different among these structures. RegX3 forms a domain-swapped dimer in the crystal structure, exchanging the α4-β5-α5 unit between subunits. It is not clear if this domain-swapped dimer is physiologically relevant. However, consistent with the structures of the isolated receiver domains, the α4-β5-α5 unit has high mobility among the structures of full-length RRs, indicating the importance of the α4-β5-α5 face in regulating RR activities. All structures with interactions between the receiver domain and effector domain involve the α4-β5-α5 face in the interdomain interface (Figure 14).

The structures of DrrD and DrrB both reveal monomers in crystal and have interactions between domains that do not preclude DNA binding (Figure 14). The interdomain interactions are relatively weak, suggesting that in solution the domains could be free and thus phosphorylation activation mechanism is likely through dimerization of the N-terminal receiver domain. The structures of PrrA and MtrA show more extensive interdomain interactions that involve the α4-β5-α5 face and block the recognition helix. However, the interfaces are polar in nature, and the open conformation is likely to exist in solution for both proteins. All these structural data suggest that phosphorylation is likely to shift the equilibrium toward dimerization as a mechanism to activate the effector domain.

The structure of PhoP from *M. tuberculosis* supports this mechanism of activation through phosphorylation-induced dimerization of the receiver domain [34]. PhoP forms a dimer through the α4-β5-α5 face of the receiver domain (Figure 14). The effector domain is merely tethered to the receiver domain through a flexible linker, which is disordered in the crystal structure. This open conformation of unphosphorylated PhoP structure is consistent with observations that unphosphorylated PhoP binds DNA [51]. Because there is no direct interaction between the receiver domain and the effector domain, it is likely that phosphorylation regulates the DNA-binding activity by shifting the equilibrium toward dimer formation of the receiver domain [33, 44]. Although the PhoP dimer interface involves the α4-β5-α5 face, the dimer packing is less compact than the activated receiver dimers. This is because the switch residues are in the non-activated conformation, and hence the loops at the dimer interface are different in conformation from the activated structures [34]. By shifting the equilibrium toward dimer formation of the receiver domains, phosphorylation brings two DNA-binding domains in close proximity; the flexible domain linker allows the DNA-binding domains to bind two direct repeats of DNA sequence while the receiver domains adopt a symmetric dimer. The OmpR/PhoB subfamily RRs recognize DNA direct-repeat sequences as revealed in the PhoB effector domain structure in complex with DNA (Figure 12a). However, the isolated DNA-binding domain of PhoP is a monomer in solution and does not form any dimers in the crystal structure [52]. Recognition of DNA direct repeats can only be realized through dimerization of the receiver domain. Bringing two DNA-binding domains in close proximity by dimerization of the receiver domains can also increase DNA-binding affinity.

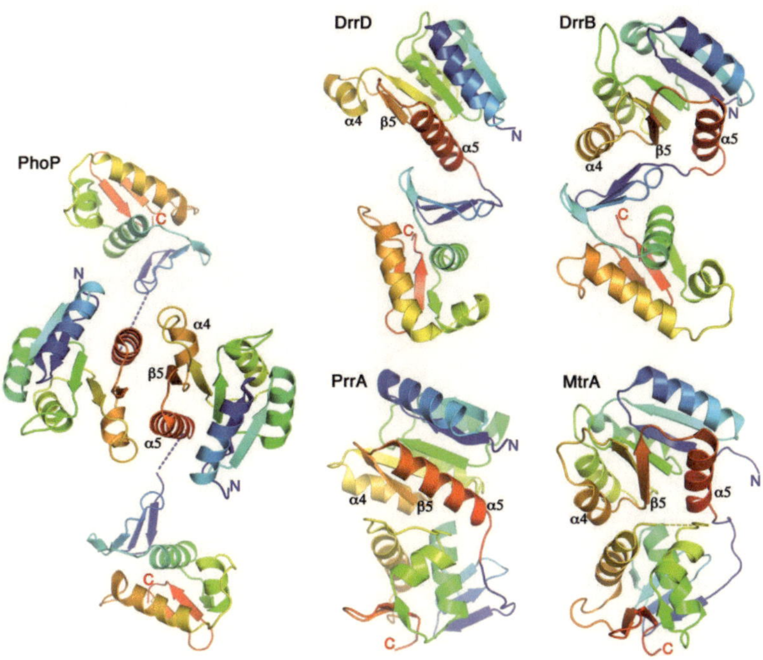

Figure 14. Full-length structures of the OmpR/PhoB subfamily RRs. Each domain is individually colored from N- to C-terminus in a rainbow spectrum. PhoP, PrrA, and MtrA are from *M. tuberculosis*; DrrD and DrrB are from *T. maritima*. The PDB codes are: PhoP, 3R0J; DrrD, 1KGS; DrrB, 1P2F; PrrA, 1YS6; MtrA, 2GWR.

4. Interactions between histidine kinases and response regulators

To complete the signaling events of two-component systems, histidine kinases, when activated, must associate with their cognate response regulators and transfer the phosphoryl group from the phosphorylated histidine to a conserved aspartate residue of RRs. Evidence suggests that HKs are also involved in dephosphorylation of RRs to turn off the signal cascade. The interactions between HK and RR must be specific because there is little cross-talk among TCS proteins. Yet, these interactions must be dynamic, as both proteins must adopt various conformations throughout the steps of the signaling event.

Several crystal structures of HK in complex with RR have been reported that offer insights into how HK and RR interact. A structure of the complex between HK853 and RR468 from *T. maritima* shows the two proteins engaged in a conformation for the phosphatase reaction [28]. The structure contains a dimer of the HK853 entire cytoplasmic portion and two RR468 molecules (Figure 15).

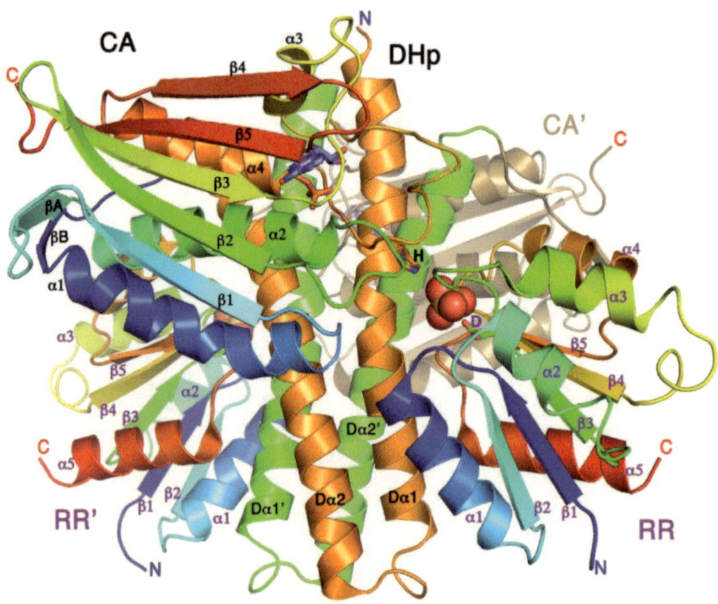

Figure 15. Structure of the HK853-RR468 complex (PDB code 3DGE). The DHp domain is colored in orange for one subunit and in green for the other. One CA domain (front) is colored in a rainbow spectrum; the other CA (back) is in sand color. Two RR molecules each individually colored in a rainbow spectrum. Secondary structural elements of HK are labeled in black, and those of RR are in purple. A sulfate between the essential histidine of HK and aspartate of RR is shown in a space-filling model.

The RR binds to the DHp domain on the helical hairpin below the phosphorylation site histidine. Helix α1 of RR interacts with both helices of the helical hairpin through hydrophobic side chains to form a six-helix bundle. Each α1 interacts only with helices of the same subunit of DHp. Loop β5-α5 also makes contacts with the DHp domain. In the crystal structure, there is a sulfate ion bound between the phosphoacceptor aspartate of RR and the phosphorylation site histidine of DHp. Binding of the sulfate mimics phosphorylation and allows the switch residues of RR to adopt the active conformation. Consequently, both loops β3-α3 and β4-α4 are also in the active conformation. These two loops interact with the ATP-lid and loop α2-β2 of the CA domain. The interactions between HK853 and RR468 would preclude dimer formation of RR through the α4-β5-α5 face, despite that the RR is in an active conformation. RR468 is a single domain protein. The structure of activated RR468 with BeF_3^- shows changes in conformation of switch residues and loops β3-α3 and β4-α4, but it is a monomer [28]. This is different from OmpR/PhoB subfamily RRs, whose activated form promotes dimerization, or NarL/FixJ family RRs, whose activated form releases the effector domain for binding DNA and might also promote dimerization. Despite these differences, binding interactions of α1 of RR with the helical hairpin of DHp is likely conserved among TCS proteins. The structure of HK853-RR468 complex is in a phosphatase-competent state because the RR is phosphorylated and the ATP-lid blocks access of the γ-phosphate of ATP by the histidine side chain. The structure indicates that the phosphorylation site histidine could play a role in the phosphatase activity by orienting a water molecule as a nucleophile.

A complex structure of ThkA/TrrA, also from *T. maritima*, has a similar binding site on HK for RR [53], and the structure also represents a phosphatase-competent state because the CA domain is locked in a position away from the phosphorylation site histidine. Similar to RR468, TrrA is also a single domain RR. The resolution of the complex structure is relatively low at 3.8 Å, and high-resolution structures of individual domains were fit into the low-resolution electron density map of the ThkA-TrrA complex. TrrA has weak electron density, indicating its high mobility in the structure. The complex puts the phosphoacceptor aspartate of TrrA facing the phosphorylation site histidine of ThkA. However, TrrA has weaker interactions with DHp. Most of interactions involve the loops around the phosphoacceptor and the N-terminal end of α1 of TrrA with Dα1 of ThkA. Unlike that of RR468, helix α1 of TrrA does not have exposed hydrophobic side chains to have coiled-coil interactions with the four-helix bundle of ThkA. The binding position of RR on DHp is similar to that of the HK853-RR468 complex, suggesting that they share a common mechanism for the phosphotransfer reaction.

A structure of the Spo0F-Spo0B complex is related to HK-RR complexes in binding interactions and the mechanism of the catalyzed reactions. Spo0B is a phosphotransferase having a DHp domain similar to that of HKs, while Spo0F is a single domain RR [54, 55]. Spo0F is phosphorylated on its phosphoacceptor aspartate by sensor HK KinA. The phosphoryl group is then transferred to the phosphorylation site histidine on spo0B, which then transfers the phosphoryl group to the response regulator Spo0A. In the structure of the Spo0F-Spo0B complex, Spo0F binds to the four-helix bundle of Spo0B in a similar manner as the HK853-RR468 complex. Helix α1 of Spo0F packs against the helical hairpin region and makes up majority of the interface with DHp, confirming that helix α1 and the lower end of the DHp four-helix bundle as the binding interface between HK and RR.

5. Therapeutic potential against bacterial pathogens

Antibiotics resistance has been a major medical problem of modern medicine. Bacterial pathogens evolve mechanisms to become resistant to antibiotics, and strains resistant to multiple drugs or the last line of antibiotics, such as methicillin-resistant *S. aureus* and vancomycin-resistant *Enterococcus* have evolved and become a major challenge for modern medicine. Emergence of multi-drug resistant (MDR) and extremely drug resistant (XDR) tuberculosis (TB) has prompted the World Health Organization to declare TB as a global emergency.

Two component systems are major signaling proteins in bacteria. They are involved in every aspect of bacterial adaptation to their environments, including sensing the existence of antibiotics and regulating cellular responses to become drug resistant. Therefore, TCSs are potential drug targets for developing new antibiotics [56]. Unlike conventional antibiotics that directly target the proteins involved in essential cellular activities, drugs inhibiting TCSs target the upstream functions that regulate these essential proteins. Thus anti-TCS drugs work in a manner different from conventional drugs and are likely to be effective against drug-resistant bacterial pathogens. Because TCS proteins are absent in animals, drugs targeting TCSs can potentially have less toxicity.

Recent advancements in structural and functional characterization of TCSs have identified several potential targets for developing new antibiotics [56]. A PhoP-PhoQ system from *S. typhimurium* is a major virulence factor that is essential for this intracellular pathogen to establish infection. Inhibitors to the kinase activity of PhoQ were studied for their interactions with the protein and the inhibition mechanism by NMR and crystallography methods [57]. The structures can serve as a platform for rational design to improve the efficacy of the lead compounds. A PhoP-PhoR system in *M. tuberculosis* was found to be an important virulence factor [58]. PhoP has a point mutation in the avirulent H37Ra strain, and this mutation plays an important role in the loss of virulence of the avirulent strain [59]. Inhibitors targeting PhoP are likely to reduce the virulence of *M. tuberculosis*. With the availability of the PhoP structure [34], it is possible to do virtual screening or rational inhibitor design to search for compounds that will disrupt phosphorylation activation by interacting with the loops near the phosphoacceptor or with helix $\alpha 1$, or binding to the $\alpha 4$-$\beta 5$-$\alpha 5$ face to prevent dimerization. Compounds inhibiting the effector domain binding DNA will also be efficient inhibitors. To develop inhibitors against PhoP-PhoR TCS, targeting the sensor domain of PhoR will be more specific and has the advantage that the compounds do not have to cross the cell membrane [58]. However, structural information of the PhoR protein is currently lacking.

Author details

Shuishu Wang
Department of Biochemistry and Molecular Biology, Uniformed Services University of the Health Sciences, Bethesda, Maryland, USA

Acknowledgement

The author thanks Dr. Chou-Zen Giam, Dr. Linda Miallau, and Dr. Issar Smith for helpful comments and revisions of the manuscript. This work was supported by a grant GM079185 from the National Institute of Health of the United States.

6. References

[1] Aravind L, Ponting CP. The cytoplasmic helical linker domain of receptor histidine kinase and methyl-accepting proteins is common to many prokaryotic signalling proteins. FEMS Microbiol Lett. 1999;176(1):111-6.

[2] Hefti MH, Francoijs KJ, de Vries SC, Dixon R, Vervoort J. The PAS fold. A redefinition of the PAS domain based upon structural prediction. Eur J Biochem. 2004;271(6):1198-208.

[3] Martinez SE, Beavo JA, Hol WG. GAF domains: two-billion-year-old molecular switches that bind cyclic nucleotides. Mol Interv. 2002;2(5):317-23.

[4] Wayne LG, Sohaskey CD. Nonreplicating persistence of mycobacterium tuberculosis. Annu Rev Microbiol. 2001;55:139-63.

[5] Cho HY, Cho HJ, Kim YM, Oh JI, Kang BS. Structural insight into the heme-based redox sensing by DosS from Mycobacterium tuberculosis. J Biol Chem. 2009;284(19):13057-67.

[6] Podust LM, Ioanoviciu A, Ortiz de Montellano PR. 2.3 A X-ray structure of the heme-bound GAF domain of sensory histidine kinase DosT of Mycobacterium tuberculosis. Biochemistry. 2008;47(47):12523-31.

[7] Miyatake H, Mukai M, Park SY, Adachi S, Tamura K, Nakamura H, et al. Sensory mechanism of oxygen sensor FixL from Rhizobium meliloti: crystallographic, mutagenesis and resonance Raman spectroscopic studies. J Mol Biol. 2000;301(2):415-31.

[8] Sevvana M, Vijayan V, Zweckstetter M, Reinelt S, Madden DR, Herbst-Irmer R, et al. A ligand-induced switch in the periplasmic domain of sensor histidine kinase CitA. J Mol Biol. 2008;377(2):512-23.

[9] Cheung J, Hendrickson WA. Sensor domains of two-component regulatory systems. Curr Opin Microbiol. 2010;13(2):116-23.

[10] Cheung J, Hendrickson WA. Structural analysis of ligand stimulation of the histidine kinase NarX. Structure. 2009;17(2):190-201.

[11] Moore JO, Hendrickson WA. Structural analysis of sensor domains from the TMAO-responsive histidine kinase receptor TorS. Structure. 2009;17(9):1195-204.

[12] Jing X, Jaw J, Robinson HH, Schubot FD. Crystal structure and oligomeric state of the RetS signaling kinase sensory domain. Proteins. 2010;78(7):1631-40.

[13] Airola MV, Watts KJ, Bilwes AM, Crane BR. Structure of concatenated HAMP domains provides a mechanism for signal transduction. Structure. 2010;18(4):436-48.

[14] Hulko M, Berndt F, Gruber M, Linder JU, Truffault V, Schultz A, et al. The HAMP domain structure implies helix rotation in transmembrane signaling. Cell. 2006;126(5):929-40.

[15] Appleman JA, Chen LL, Stewart V. Probing conservation of HAMP linker structure and signal transduction mechanism through analysis of hybrid sensor kinases. J Bacteriol. 2003;185(16):4872-82.

[16] Zhu Y, Inouye M. Analysis of the role of the EnvZ linker region in signal transduction using a chimeric Tar/EnvZ receptor protein, Tez1. J Biol Chem. 2003;278(25):22812-9.

[17] Ferris HU, Dunin-Horkawicz S, Mondejar LG, Hulko M, Hantke K, Martin J, et al. The mechanisms of HAMP-mediated signaling in transmembrane receptors. Structure. 2011;19(3):378-85.

[18] Ferris HU, Dunin-Horkawicz S, Hornig N, Hulko M, Martin J, Schultz JE, et al. Mechanism of regulation of receptor histidine kinases. Structure. 2012;20(1):56-66.

[19] Tomomori C, Tanaka T, Dutta R, Park H, Saha SK, Zhu Y, et al. Solution structure of the homodimeric core domain of Escherichia coli histidine kinase EnvZ. Nat Struct Biol. 1999;6(8):729-34.

[20] Varughese KI, Madhusudan, Zhou XZ, Whiteley JM, Hoch JA. Formation of a novel four-helix bundle and molecular recognition sites by dimerization of a response regulator phosphotransferase. Mol Cell. 1998;2(4):485-93.

[21] Marina A, Waldburger CD, Hendrickson WA. Structure of the entire cytoplasmic portion of a sensor histidine-kinase protein. Embo J. 2005;24(24):4247-59.

[22] Trajtenberg F, Grana M, Ruetalo N, Botti H, Buschiazzo A. Structural and enzymatic insights into the ATP binding and autophosphorylation mechanism of a sensor histidine kinase. J Biol Chem. 2010;285(32):24892-903.

[23] Marina A, Mott C, Auyzenberg A, Hendrickson WA, Waldburger CD. Structural and mutational analysis of the PhoQ histidine kinase catalytic domain. Insight into the reaction mechanism. J Biol Chem. 2001;276(44):41182-90.

[24] Albanesi D, Martin M, Trajtenberg F, Mansilla MC, Haouz A, Alzari PM, et al. Structural plasticity and catalysis regulation of a thermosensor histidine kinase. Proc Natl Acad Sci U S A. 2009;106(38):16185-90.

[25] Zhang Z, Hendrickson WA. Structural characterization of the predominant family of histidine kinase sensor domains. J Mol Biol. 2010;400(3):335-53.

[26] Gordeliy VI, Labahn J, Moukhametzianov R, Efremov R, Granzin J, Schlesinger R, et al. Molecular basis of transmembrane signalling by sensory rhodopsin II-transducer complex. Nature. 2002;419(6906):484-7.

[27] Goldberg SD, Clinthorne GD, Goulian M, DeGrado WF. Transmembrane polar interactions are required for signaling in the Escherichia coli sensor kinase PhoQ. Proc Natl Acad Sci U S A. 2010;107(18):8141-6.

[28] Casino P, Rubio V, Marina A. Structural insight into partner specificity and phosphoryl transfer in two-component signal transduction. Cell. 2009;139(2):325-36.

[29] Bick MJ, Lamour V, Rajashankar KR, Gordiyenko Y, Robinson CV, Darst SA. How to switch off a histidine kinase: crystal structure of Geobacillus stearothermophilus KinB with the inhibitor Sda. J Mol Biol. 2009;386(1):163-77.

[30] Galperin MY. Diversity of structure and function of response regulator output domains. Curr Opin Microbiol. 2010;13(2):150-9.

[31] Bourret RB. Receiver domain structure and function in response regulator proteins. Curr Opin Microbiol. 2010;13(2):142-9.

[32] Gao R, Stock AM. Molecular strategies for phosphorylation-mediated regulation of response regulator activity. Curr Opin Microbiol. 2010;13(2):160-7.

[33] Barbieri CM, Mack TR, Robinson VL, Miller MT, Stock AM. Regulation of response regulator autophosphorylation through interdomain contacts. J Biol Chem. 2010;285(42):32325-35.

[34] Menon S, Wang S. Structure of the response regulator PhoP from Mycobacterium tuberculosis reveals a dimer through the receiver domain. Biochemistry. 2011;50(26):5948-57.

[35] Nowak E, Panjikar S, Konarev P, Svergun DI, Tucker PA. The structural basis of signal transduction for the response regulator PrrA from Mycobacterium tuberculosis. J Biol Chem. 2006;281(14):9659-66.

[36] Bachhawat P, Stock AM. Crystal structures of the receiver domain of the response regulator PhoP from Escherichia coli in the absence and presence of the phosphoryl analog beryllofluoride. J Bacteriol. 2007;189(16):5987-95.

[37] Toro-Roman A, Wu T, Stock AM. A common dimerization interface in bacterial response regulators KdpE and TorR. Protein Sci. 2005;14(12):3077-88.

[38] Birck C, Mourey L, Gouet P, Fabry B, Schumacher J, Rousseau P, et al. Conformational changes induced by phosphorylation of the FixJ receiver domain. Structure. 1999;7(12):1505-15.

[39] Sidote DJ, Barbieri CM, Wu T, Stock AM. Structure of the Staphylococcus aureus AgrA LytTR domain bound to DNA reveals a beta fold with an unusual mode of binding. Structure. 2008;16(5):727-35.

[40] Blanco AG, Sola M, Gomis-Ruth FX, Coll M. Tandem DNA recognition by PhoB, a two-component signal transduction transcriptional activator. Structure. 2002;10(5):701-13.

[41] Maris AE, Kaczor-Grzeskowiak M, Ma Z, Kopka ML, Gunsalus RP, Dickerson RE. Primary and secondary modes of DNA recognition by the NarL two-component response regulator. Biochemistry. 2005;44(44):14538-52.

[42] Maris AE, Sawaya MR, Kaczor-Grzeskowiak M, Jarvis MR, Bearson SM, Kopka ML, et al. Dimerization allows DNA target site recognition by the NarL response regulator. Nat Struct Biol. 2002;9(10):771-8.

[43] Baikalov I, Schroder I, Kaczor-Grzeskowiak M, Grzeskowiak K, Gunsalus RP, Dickerson RE. Structure of the Escherichia coli response regulator NarL. Biochemistry. 1996;35(34):11053-61.

[44] Milani M, Leoni L, Rampioni G, Zennaro E, Ascenzi P, Bolognesi M. An active-like structure in the unphosphorylated StyR response regulator suggests a phosphorylation-dependent allosteric activation mechanism. Structure. 2005;13(9):1289-97.

[45] Wisedchaisri G, Wu M, Sherman DR, Hol WG. Crystal structures of the response regulator DosR from Mycobacterium tuberculosis suggest a helix rearrangement mechanism for phosphorylation activation. J Mol Biol. 2008;378(1):227-42.

[46] Wisedchaisri G, Wu M, Rice AE, Roberts DM, Sherman DR, Hol WG. Structures of Mycobacterium tuberculosis DosR and DosR-DNA complex involved in gene activation during adaptation to hypoxic latency. J Mol Biol. 2005;354(3):630-41.

[47] Robinson VL, Wu T, Stock AM. Structural analysis of the domain interface in DrrB, a response regulator of the OmpR/PhoB subfamily. J Bacteriol. 2003;185(14):4186-94.

[48] Buckler DR, Zhou Y, Stock AM. Evidence of intradomain and interdomain flexibility in an OmpR/PhoB homolog from Thermotoga maritima. Structure (Camb). 2002;10(2):153-64.

[49] King-Scott J, Nowak E, Mylonas E, Panjikar S, Roessle M, Svergun DI, et al. The structure of a full-length response regulator from Mycobacterium tuberculosis in a stabilized three-dimensional domain-swapped, activated state. J Biol Chem. 2007;282(52):37717-29.

[50] Friedland N, Mack TR, Yu M, Hung LW, Terwilliger TC, Waldo GS, et al. Domain orientation in the inactive response regulator Mycobacterium tuberculosis MtrA provides a barrier to activation. Biochemistry. 2007;46(23):6733-43.

[51] Gupta S, Sinha A, Sarkar D. Transcriptional autoregulation by Mycobacterium tuberculosis PhoP involves recognition of novel direct repeat sequences in the regulatory region of the promoter. FEBS Lett. 2006;580(22):5328-38.

[52] Wang S, Engohang-Ndong J, Smith I. Structure of the DNA-binding domain of the response regulator PhoP from Mycobacterium tuberculosis. Biochemistry. 2007;46(51):14751-61.

[53] Yamada S, Sugimoto H, Kobayashi M, Ohno A, Nakamura H, Shiro Y. Structure of PAS-linked histidine kinase and the response regulator complex. Structure. 2009;17(10):1333-44.

[54] Zapf J, Sen U, Madhusudan, Hoch JA, Varughese KI. A transient interaction between two phosphorelay proteins trapped in a crystal lattice reveals the mechanism of molecular recognition and phosphotransfer in signal transduction. Structure. 2000;8(8):851-62.

[55] Varughese KI, Tsigelny I, Zhao H. The crystal structure of beryllofluoride Spo0F in complex with the phosphotransferase Spo0B represents a phosphotransfer pretransition state. J Bacteriol. 2006;188(13):4970-7.

[56] Gotoh Y, Eguchi Y, Watanabe T, Okamoto S, Doi A, Utsumi R. Two-component signal transduction as potential drug targets in pathogenic bacteria. Curr Opin Microbiol. 2010;13(2):232-9.

[57] Guarnieri MT, Zhang L, Shen J, Zhao R. The Hsp90 inhibitor radicicol interacts with the ATP-binding pocket of bacterial sensor kinase PhoQ. J Mol Biol. 2008;379(1):82-93.

[58] Ryndak M, Wang S, Smith I. PhoP, a key player in Mycobacterium tuberculosis virulence. Trends Microbiol. 2008;16(11):528-34.

[59] Frigui W, Bottai D, Majlessi L, Monot M, Josselin E, Brodin P, et al. Control of M. tuberculosis ESAT-6 secretion and specific T cell recognition by PhoP. PLoS pathogens. 2008;4(2):e33.